Cranial Nerves

Guest Editor

JAN CASSELMAN, MD, PhD

CLINICS IN NEUROIMAGING

www.neuroimaging.theclinics.com

Consulting Editor
SURESH K. MUKHERJI, MD

May 2008 • Volume 18 • Number 2

Cover images courtesy of Laurie A. Loevner, MD, Professor of Radiology, University of Pennsylvania School of Medicine and Health System, Department of Radiology, Neuroradiology Division.

SAUNDERS an imprint of ELSEVIER, Inc.

W.B. SAUNDERS COMPANY
A Division of Elsevier Inc.

1600 John F. Kennedy Boulevard • Suite 1800 • Philadelphia, Pennsylvania 19103-2899

http://www.theclinics.com

NEUROIMAGING CLINICS Volume 18, Number 2
May 2008 ISSN 1052-5149, ISBN-13: 978-1-4160-5850-2, ISBN-10: 1-4160-5850-8

Editor: Lisa Richman

Neuroimaging Clinics (ISSN 1052-5149) is published quarterly by Elsevier Inc., 360 Park Avenue South, New York, NY 10010-1710. Months of issue are February, May, August, and November. Business and editorial offices: 1600 John F. Kennedy Blvd., Suite 1800, Philadelphia, PA 19103-2899. Business and editorial offices: 6277 Sea Harbor Drive, Orlando, FL 32887-4800. Periodicals postage paid at New York, NY, and additional mailing offices. Subscription prices are USD 240 per year for US individuals, USD 370 per year for US institutions, USD 123 per year for US students and residents, USD 277 per year for Canadian individuals, USD 454 per year for Canadian institutions, USD 332 per year for international individuals, USD 454 per year for international institutions and USD 166 per year for Canadian and foreign students and residents. To receive student/resident rate, orders must be accompanied by name of affiliated institution, date of term, and the *signature* of program/residency coordinator on institution letterhead. Orders will be billed at individual rate until proof of status is received. Foreign air speed delivery is included in all *Clinics* subscription prices. All prices are subject to change without notice. POSTMASTER: Send address changes to *Neuroimaging Clinics*, Elsevier Periodicals Customer Service, 6277 Sea Harbor Drive, Orlando, FL 32887-4800. **Customer Service: 1-800-654-2452 (US). From outside the United States, call 1-407-563-6020. Fax: 1-407-363-9661. E-mail: JournalsCustomerService-usa@elsevier.com.**

Reprints. For copies of 100 or more, of articles in this publication, please contact the Commercial Reprints Department, Elsevier Inc., 360 Park Avenue South, New York, New York 10010-1710. Tel.: (+1) 212-633-3813; Fax: (+1) 212-462-1935; E-mail: reprints@elsevier.com.

Neuroimaging Clinics is covered by *Excerpta Medica/EMBASE*, the RSNA Index of Imaging Literature, Index Medicus, MEDLINE/MEDLARS, SciSearch, Research Alert, and Neuroscience Citation Index.

Printed in the United States of America.

GOAL STATEMENT

The goal of *Neuroimaging Clinics of North America* is to keep practicing radiologists and radiology residents up to date with current clinical practice in radiology by providing timely articles reviewing the state of the art in patient care.

ACCREDITATION

The *Neuroimaging Clinics of North America* is planned and implemented in accordance with the Essential Areas and Policies of the Accreditation Council for Continuing Medical Education (ACCME) through the joint sponsorship of the University of Virginia School of Medicine and Elsevier. The University of Virginia School of Medicine is accredited by the ACCME to provide continuing medical education for physicians.

The University of Virginia School of Medicine designates this educational activity for a maximum of 60 *AMA PRA Category 1 Credits*™. Physicians should only claim credit commensurate with the extent of their participation in the activity.

The American Medical Association has determined that physicians not licensed in the US who participate in this CME activity are eligible for *AMA PRA Category 1 Credits*™.

Credit can be earned by reading the text material, taking the CME examination online at: http://www.theclinics.com/home/cme, and completing the evaluation. After taking the test, you will be required to review any and all incorrect answers. Following completion of the test and evaluation, your credit will be awarded and you may print your certificate.

FACULTY DISCLOSURE/CONFLICT OF INTEREST

The University of Virginia School of Medicine, as an ACCME accredited provider, endorses and strives to comply with the Accreditation Council for Continuing Medical Education (ACCME) Standards of Commercial Support, Commonwealth of Virginia statutes, University of Virginia policies and procedures, and associated federal and private regulations and guidelines on the need for disclosure and monitoring of proprietary and financial interests that may affect the scientific integrity and balance of content delivered in continuing medical education activities under our auspices.

The University of Virginia School of Medicine requires that all CME activities accredited through this institution be developed independently and be scientifically rigorous, balanced and objective in the presentation/discussion of its content, theories and practices.

All authors/editors participating in an accredited CME activity are expected to disclose to the readers relevant financial relationships with commercial entities occurring within the past 12 months (such as grants or research support, employee, consultant, stock holder, member of speakers bureau, etc.). The University of Virginia School of Medicine will employ appropriate mechanisms to resolve potential conflicts of interest to maintain the standards of fair and balanced education to the reader. Questions about specific strategies can be directed to the Office of Continuing Medical Education, University of Virginia School of Medicine, Charlottesville, Virginia.

The authors/editors listed below have identified no professional/financial affiliations for themselves or their spouse/partner:

Maher Abu Eid, MD; Matthew E. Adams, MD; Minerva Becker, MD; Andrea Borghesi, MD; Jan Casselman, MD, PhD (Guest Editor); Anne Charpiot, MD; Kenneth Coenegrachts, MD; C. Debry, MD; Joost Delanote, MD; Jacqueline Delavelle, MD; Davide Farina, MD; Ernst Garcon, MD; Enza Gatti, MD; Johan Ghekiere, MD; Volker Gudziol, MD; Thomas Hummel, MD; Hans Rolf Jäger, MD, FRCR; Romain Kohler, MD; Timo Krings, MD, PhD; Pierre Lasjaunias, MD, PhD; Jennifer Linn, MD; Anna Marconi, MD; Roberto Maroldi, MD; Koen Mermuys, MD; Katherine Anne Miszkiel, BM(Hons), MRCP, FRCR; Vitor Pereira, MD; Bruno A. Policeni, MD; Deborah L. Reede, MD; Lisa Richman (Acquiring Editor); S. Riehm, MD; Philippe Schultz, MD; Wendy R.K. Smoker, MS, MD, FACR; Joel D. Swartz, MD; Luciana Ramos Taboada, MD; Frederique Toulgoat, MD; Maria Isabel Vargas, MD; Magalie Viallon, PhD; Francis Veillon, MD; and Indra Yousry, MD, PhD.

The authors listed below have identified the following professional/financial affiliations for themselves or their spouse/partner:

Nasreddin Abolmaali, MD is an independent contractor for Medtron AG.
Randy Kardon, MD, PhD is a consultant for Ovation Pharmaceutical and Boehringer- Egleheim Pharmaceutical.
Suresh K. Mukherji, MD (Consulting Editor) is a consultant for Bracco, Bayer, Philips, and Xoran Technologies.
Augustin Ozanne, MD is employed by Bicetre Hospital.

Disclosure of Discussion of non-FDA approved uses for pharmaceutical products and/or medical devices:
The University of Virginia School of Medicine, as an ACCME provider, requires that all authors/editors identify and disclose any "off label" uses for pharmaceutical products and/or for medical devices. The University of Virginia School of Medicine recommends that each reader fully review all the available data on new products or procedures prior to instituting them with patients.

TO ENROLL

To enroll in the Neuroimaging Clinics of North America Continuing Medical Education program, call customer service at 1-800-654-2452 or sign up online at: *http://www.theclinics.com/home/cme*. The CME program is available to subscribers for an additional annual fee of USD 175.

Clinics in Neuroimaging

FORTHCOMING ISSUES

August 2008

Thyroid and Parathyroid Glands
Laurie Loevner, MD, *Guest Editor*

November 2008

Multiple Sclerosis, Volume I
Massimo Filippi, MD, *Guest Editor*

RECENT ISSUES

February 2008

Viruses and Prion in the CNS
E. Turgut Tali, MD, *Guest Editor*

November 2007

Imaging of the Mind
Carolyn Cidis Meltzer, MD, FACR, *Guest Editor*

August 2007

Angioplasty and Stenting for Atherosclerotic Cerebrovascular Disease
Colin P. Derdeyn, MD, *Guest Editor*

Contributors

CONSULTING EDITOR

SURESH K. MUKHERJI, MD
Professor; Chief, Neuroradiology and Head and Neck Radiology; Professor, Radiology, Otolaryngology Head Neck Surgery; Radiation Oncology, University of Michigan Health System, Ann Arbor, Michigan

GUEST EDITOR

JAN CASSELMAN, MD, PhD
Chairman, Department of Radiology, AZ St-Jan Brugge AV, Brugge; Consultant Radiologist, AZ St-Augustinus, Antwerp; Academic Consultant, University Ghent, Ghent, Belguim

AUTHORS

NASREDDIN ABOLMAALI, MD
OncoRay—Radiation Research in Oncology, Technical University of Dresden Medical School, Dresden, Germany

M. ABU EID, MD
Service de Radiologie I, Hôpital de Hautepierre, Strasbourg, France

MATTHEW E. ADAMS, MD
Lysholm Department of Neuroradiology, The National Hospital for Neurology and Neurosurgery, London, United Kingdom

MINERVA BECKER, MD
Chief, Section of Head and Neck and Maxillofacial Radiology, Department of Radiology; Consulting Radiologist Otorhinolaryngology, Head and Neck Surgery Clinic, Department of Neurosciences, Geneva University Hospital; Privat-Docent, Faculty of Medicine, University of Geneva, Geneva, Switzerland

ANDREA BORGHESI, MD
Department of Radiology, University of Brescia, Brescia, Italy

JAN CASSELMAN, MD, PhD
Chairman, Department of Radiology, AZ St-Jan Brugge AV, Brugge; Consultant Radiologist, AZ St-Augustinus, Antwerp; Academic Consultant, University Ghent, Ghent, Belguim

A. CHARPIOT, MD
Service d'O.R.L., Hôpital de Hautepierre, Strasbourg, France

KENNETH COENEGRACHTS, MD
Department of Radiology, AZ St-Jan Brugge AV, Brugge, Belgium

C. DEBRY, MD
Professor; ENT Surgeon, Service d'O.R.L., Hôpital de Hautepierre, Strasbourg, France

JOOST DELANOTE, MD
Department of Radiology, AZ St-Jan Brugge AV, Brugge, Belgium

JACQUELINE DELAVELLE, MD
Chief, Neuroradiology Unit, Department of Radiology, Geneva University Hospital; Chargé de Cours, Faculty of Medicine, University of Geneva, Geneva, Switzerland

DAVIDE FARINA, MD
Department of Radiology, University of Brescia, Brescia, Italy

ERNST GARCON, MD
Assistant Professor of Neuroradiology, Department of Radiology, University of Arkansas Medical Science, Little Rock, Arkansas

ENZA GATTI, MD
Department of Radiology, University of Brescia, Brescia, Italy

JOHAN GHEKIERE, MD
Department of Radiology, AZ St-Jan Brugge AV, Brugge, Belgium

VOLKER GUDZIOL, MD
Smell and Taste Clinic, Department of Otorhinolaryngology, Technical University of Dresden Medical School, Dresden, Germany

THOMAS HUMMEL, MD
Smell and Taste Clinic, Department of Otorhinolaryngology, Technical University of Dresden Medical School, Dresden, Germany

HANS ROLF JÄGER, MD, FRCR
Reader in Neuroradiology; Consultant Neuroradiologist, Lysholm Department of Neuroradiology, The National Hospital for Neurology and Neurosurgery, London, United Kingdom

RANDY KARDON, MD, PhD
Professor of Neuro-Ophthalmology, Department of Ophthalmology and Visual Sciences, University of Iowa Hospitals and Clinics and Veterans Administration, Iowa City, Iowa

ROMAIN KOHLER, MD
Head and Neck and Maxillofacial Radiology, Department of Radiology, Geneva University Hospital, Geneva, Switzerland

TIMO KRINGS, MD, PhD
Bicêtre Hospital, Department of Neuroradiology, National Center for Malformative Neurovascular Diseases, Le Kremlin-Bicêtre, France

PIERRE LASJAUNIAS, MD, PhD
Bicêtre Hospital, Department of Neuroradiology, National Center for Malformative Neurovascular Diseases, Le Kremlin-Bicêtre, France

JENNIFER LINN, MD
Klinikum Grosshadern, Department of Neuroradiology, Munich, Germany

ANNA MARCONI, MD
Department of Radiology, University of Brescia, Brescia, Italy

ROBERTO MAROLDI, MD
Professor of Radiology, Department of Radiology, University of Brescia, Brescia, Italy

KOEN MERMUYS, MD
Department of Radiology, AZ St-Jan Brugge AV, Brugge, Belgium

KATHERINE ANNE MISZKIEL, BM(Hons), MRCP, FRCR
Consultant Neuroradioogist, Lysholm Department of Neuroradiology, The National Hospital for Neurology and Neurosurgery; Honorary Consultant Neuroradiologist, Moorfields Eye Hospital, London, United Kingdom

AUGUSTIN OZANNE, MD
Bicêtre Hospital, Department of Neuroradiology, National Center for Malformative Neurovascular Diseases, Le Kremlin-Bicêtre, France

VITOR PEREIRA, MD
Bicêtre Hospital, Department of Neuroradiology, National Center for Malformative Neurovascular Diseases, Le Kremlin-Bicêtre, France

BRUNO A. POLICENI, MD
Assistant Professor, Department of Radiology, University of Iowa Hospitals and Clinics, Iowa City, Iowa

DEBORAH L. REEDE, MD
Associate Professor of Clinical Radiology, State University of New York Health Science Center; Department of Radiology, Long Island College Hospital, Brooklyn, New York

S. RIEHM, MD
Service de Radiologie I, Hôpital de Hautepierre, Strasbourg, France

P. SCHULTZ, MD
Service d'O.R.L., Hôpital de Hautepierre, Strasbourg, France

WENDY R.K. SMOKER, MS, MD, FACR
Professor and Director of Neuroradiology, Department of Radiology, University of Iowa Hospitals and Clinics, Iowa City, Iowa

JOEL D. SWARTZ, MD
President, Germantown Imaging Associates, Gladwyne, Pennsylvania

L. RAMOS TABOADA, MD
Service de Radiologie I, Hôpital de Hautepierre, Strasbourg, France

FRÉDÉRIQUE TOULGOAT, MD
Bicêtre Hospital, Department of Neuroradiology, National Center for Malformative Neurovascular Diseases, Le Kremlin-Bicêtre, France

MARIA ISABEL VARGAS, MD
Neuroradiology Unit, Department of Radiology, Geneva University Hospital, Geneva, Switzerland

MAGALIE VIALLON, PhD
Clinical Physicist, Department of Radiology, Geneva University Hospital, Geneva, Switzerland

F. VEILLON, MD
Professor of Medical Imaging, Service de Radiologie I, Hôpital de Hautepierre, Strasbourg, France

INDRA YOUSRY, MD, PhD
Klinikum Grosshadern, Department of Neuroradiology, Munich, Germany

Contents

Foreword

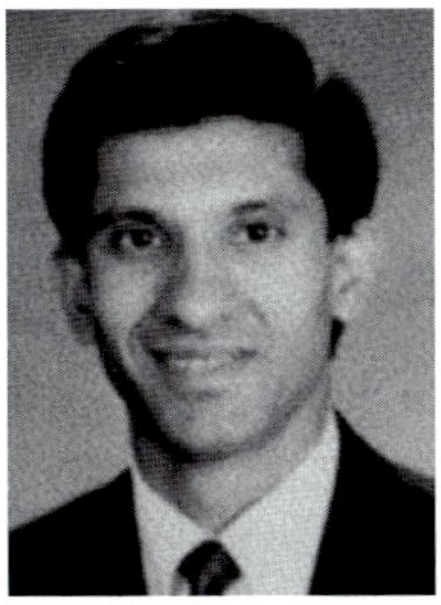

Suresh K. Mukherji, MD
Consulting Editor

Anatomy is the universal language of all physicians. Cranial nerves are the common lexicon for neuroradiologists, neurologists, neurosurgeons, ENT-surgeons, maxillofacial surgeons, and ophthalmologists. We learned about the cranial nerves in medical school through schematic diagrams and dissections in gross anatomy. Now we must apply this anatomy to our daily practice, as the individual cranial nerves can be routinely seen on properly performed imaging studies. Historically, our referring physicians could determine that a patient had a cranial nerve palsy based on physical examination. However, the referring physician could not determine the extent of the abnormality based on physical exam alone. This has all changed as the cranial nerves can now be routinely seen on cross-sectional imaging. It is now incumbent on the neuroradiologist to be familiar with the anatomy and pathology of the cranial nerves because identifying the cause of a cranial nerve palsy and determining the extent of disease is a routine part of the neuroradiologist's job!

When we first entertained this subject as a potential topic for *Neuroimaging Clinics of North America*, we faced the challenge of distinguishing this issue from previously published material on this topic. We felt that the first step was to find a world expert on this matter, and were delighted when Jan Casselman accepted our invitation. Dr. Casselman is a recognized world authority on Head and Neck Radiology and Past President of the European Society of Head and Neck Radiology. One of his primary areas of expertise is on cranial nerve imaging, and has published extensive research on this subject matter. Dr. Casselman has assembled an international group of experts and created a comprehensive, yet succinct, issue on cranial nerve imaging. The content includes articles on anatomy and pathology of the individual cranial nerves, Horner's syndrome, and the vexing topic of denervation atrophy. All of the authors are recognized experts in their fields. I would like to personally thank Jan Casselman and all the authors for their extraordinary contributions to this issue of *Neuroimaging Clinics of North America*.

Suresh K. Mukherji, MD
Neuroradiology and Head and Neck Radiology
Radiology, Otolaryngology Head Neck Surgery
and Radiation Oncology
University of Michigan Health System
1500 E. Medical Center Drive
Ann Arbor, MI 48109-0030, USA

E-mail address:
mukherji@med.umich.edu (S.K. Mukherji)

Neuroimag Clin N Am 18 (2008) xiii
doi:10.1016/j.nic.2008.03.001
1052-5149/08/$ – see front matter

Preface

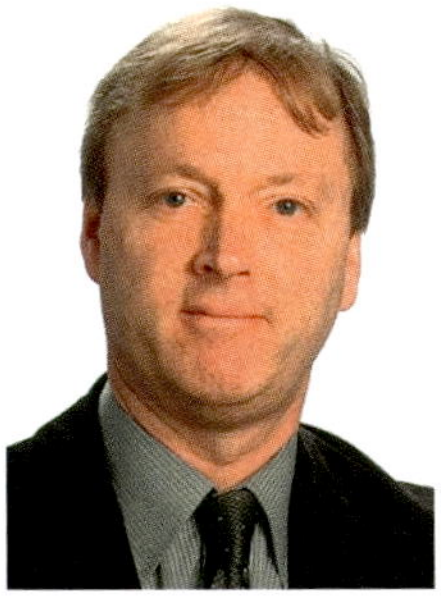

Jan Casselman, MD, PhD
Guest Editor

The 12 cranial nerve pairs are fascinating in many ways. The olfactory bulb and tract are extensions of the brain and are not segments of a real cranial nerve. The function of a cranial nerve can be simple (eg, motor, trochlear nerve) or complex (eg, motor-sensory–parasympathetic, facial nerve). The trochlear nerve is the only cranial nerve that exits the brainstem posteriorly and crosses the midline; the abducens nerve is the only ascending cranial nerve; and the accessory nerve has bulbar and spinal parts. These are only a few examples of the anatomical and functional diversity of the cranial nerves. All this anatomical and functional information is needed if one wants to visualize these nerves and understand which pathology will develop from which nerve.

Neurologists, neurosurgeons, ENT-surgeons, maxillofacial surgeons, and ophthalmologists detect cranial nerve deficits when they examine patients. The clinicians can often predict which nerve segment is causing the symptoms when they analyze the clinical findings, but they cannot confirm if a lesion is, indeed, present or, if any, which kind of lesion. Thus, the cranial nerve symptoms can be seen as the "external mirror" of intracranial problems, leading to earlier diagnosis of intracranial lesions or cranial nerve lesions.

CT was the first technique that could show cranial nerve lesions, though usually in an indirect way. Enlargement or destruction of skull base neuroforamina, fissures, and canals could be seen, and direct depiction of very large cranial nerve tumours also became possible. However, it remained impossible to depict smaller lesions and subtle involvement of the cranial nerves.

MR revolutionized cranial nerve imaging and made visualisation of all cranial nerves and all cranial nerve segments possible. As a consequence, MR is, today, the undisputed technique of choice to image the cranial nerves. Nevertheless, it took several years before the right MR equipment and sequences were developed. Therefore, radiologists in this field do not only have to learn the anatomy of the cranial nerves in detail again but also have to closely follow the evolution of the MR technique. Once the clinical symptoms are know, a tailored study is required to demonstrate or exclude cranial nerve pathology. A global brain study is most often not detailed enough. When non-tailored MR studies of different patients with cranial nerve problems do not provide the clinicians with the expected answers, they will start to believe that MR is a dead end and will no longer refer them. This stresses why MR studies of the cranial nerves must be detailed and tailored for specific nerves or nerve segments.

In this issue of *Neuroimaging Clinics of North America*, the MR technique is discussed, and the normal cranial nerve anatomy (particularly branches or nerve segments that only recently could be imaged) is briefly illustrated. Many works on anatomy exist already, but an overview of pathology of the 12 cranial nerves is more difficult to find.

Neuroimag Clin N Am 18 (2008) xv–xvi
doi:10.1016/j.nic.2008.03.002
1052-5149/08/$ – see front matter

That's why I decided to ask all authors to focus on pathology and to produce some specific articles on perineural tumour spread, denervation atrophy, Horner's syndrome, and vascularisation of the cranial nerves. It goes without saying that very specialized and experienced radiologists were needed for the job. Over many years, I have met several colleagues (and friends) who also became impassioned by the cranial nerves, and I'm very proud that I could bring them together for this project. I want to thank them for accepting the job and for their willingness to share their experience with you. And maybe, while reading this issue, you might get infected by their "cranial nerve passion" as well.

Jan Casselman, MD, PhD
AZ St-Jan Brugge AV
Department of Radiology
Ruddershove 10
Brugge B-8000
Belgium

E-mail address:
jan.casselman@azbrugge.be (J. Casselman)

MRI of the Cranial Nerves—More than Meets the Eye: Technical Considerations and Advanced Anatomy

Jan Casselman, MD, PhD*, Koen Mermuys, MD, Joost Delanote, MD, Johan Ghekiere, MD, Kenneth Coenegrachts, MD

KEYWORDS

- Cranial Nerves • Cranial Nerves, anatomy
- Magnetic Resonance Imaging
- Magnetic Resonance Imaging, anatomy
- Anatomy, Cross-Sectional • Skull Base

Magnetic resonance (MR) imaging is the method of choice to evaluate the cranial nerves. Although the skull base foramina can be seen on CT, the nerves themselves can only be visualized in detail on MR. To see the different segments of nerves I to XII, the right sequences must be used. It goes without saying that detailed clinical information is needed by the radiologist so that a tailored MR study can be performed. In this article, the MR principles for imaging of the cranial nerves are discussed. The anatomy of the 12 cranial nerves will be addressed but it is not possible to describe all of the anatomy in one article. Therefore, the basic anatomy of the cranial nerves and the cranial nerve nuclei as well as their central connections are discussed and illustrated briefly while the emphasis is on less known or more advanced extra-axial anatomy, illustrated with high-resolution MR images. For more complete anatomic descriptions and anatomic and/or MR illustrations the reader is referred to dedicated already existing complete works.[1–4]

MR TECHNIQUE

The MR technique must be pushed to its limits to see all 12 cranial nerves and especially some of the segments or branches of these nerves that are more difficult to depict. Imaging plane, coil and sequence choice, slice thickness and in-plane resolution, use of special techniques like parallel imaging, asymmetric k-space, fat suppression, and so forth will all influence the final image quality.[5]

Imaging Plane

All cranial nerves are paired and therefore it is wise to compare size and signal intensity of both nerves. The coronal plane is best suited to study the cranial nerves I to VI, as they have a dominant postero-anterior course. Cranial nerves VII to XII run in an antero-lateral-caudal direction but the lateral component is dominant. Hence the best plane will be the axial plane. Nevertheless it is always safe to perform for all cranial nerves at least one sequence in a second plane (additional axial or coronal plane).

Coil Choice

A phased array (synergy) head coil can be used for all cranial nerves. The advantage of a head coil is that it can cover all 12 cranial nerves and that it provides images with good signal-to-noise ratio (S/N) even on the midline and especially in the deepest regions: the cavernous sinus and prepontine cistern. A head coil also allows excellent evaluation of the brainstem (cranial nerve nuclei)

Department of Radiology, AZ St-Jan Brugge AV, Ruddershove 10, B-8000 Brugge, Belgium
* Corresponding author.
E-mail address: jan.casselman@azbrugge.be (J. Casselman).

Neuroimag Clin N Am 18 (2008) 197–231
doi:10.1016/j.nic.2008.02.002
1052-5149/08/$ – see front matter

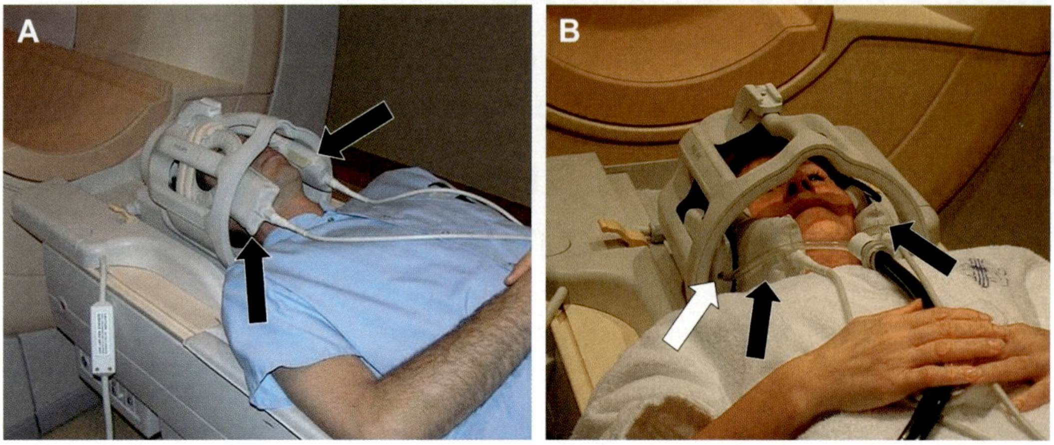

Fig. 1. Concentric coil technique applied for anterior skull base (*A*) and temporal bone (*B*) imaging. (*A*) The two coil elements of the synergy Flex S coil (*black arrows*) are put inside the eight-element synergy head-coil. To visualize the anterior skull base and olfactory nerves in detail, the small Flex S coils are positioned high and toward the midline. The coils must keep a more or less parallel position if a significant gain from parallel imaging is expected. The cables of the Flex S coils should not cross on the body of the patient. (*B*) The Flex S coils are now centered on the ears (*black arrows*). A headphone (*white arrow*) is put between the head-coil and the Flex S coils to push the surface coils even closer to the skin and to the inner ear.

and brain (eg, olfactory cortex, auditory cortex). Some very small nerves or branches can only be seen when very high resolution is available. This high resolution in combination with enough S/N is especially at 1.5 Tesla often only achievable when synergy surface coils are used. As mentioned above, these coils will only improve the results when one is imaging the more peripherally located nerves (I, II, VII, VIII). These coils can be put inside the head coil, the "concentric coil technique," so that the head coil can still be used to visualize the deeper structures and complete brain (**Fig. 1**). At 3 Tesla, the higher S/N often allows production of better images with higher resolution without the need of these surface coils. This also allows the use of different sequences and on 1.5 Tesla, two-dimensional (2D) sequences are still frequently used, at 3 Tesla today nearly all sequences are three-dimensional (3D) sequences and cover all cranial nerves. Finally, microscopic coils can be used (**Fig. 2**) when very small superficial nerve branches must be visualized. These coils can produce images with extremely high resolution; however, this is only possible when the MR unit is equipped with very strong gradients.

Sequences

The choice of the sequence will depend on the tissue or fluid that is surrounding the nerve.

In the brain stem, the cranial nerve nuclei and fascicular segment (nerve segment inside the brain stem) of the nerve cannot be visualized but their location can be deduced when the surrounding myelinated structures are recognized. These are best seen on T2-weighted (T2W), proton-density and especially multi-echo fast field echo (m-FFE) (**Fig. 3**) or T2*W 2D spoiled gradient echo multiecho sequence (MEDIC) images. In case of pathology the Flair sequences seem to be the most sensitive and a diffusion sequence is needed to exclude acute infarctions.

Heavily T2W sequences are used once the cisternal segment of the nerve, the segment that is surrounded by cerebrospinal fluid (CSF), is examined. The sequences that are available or

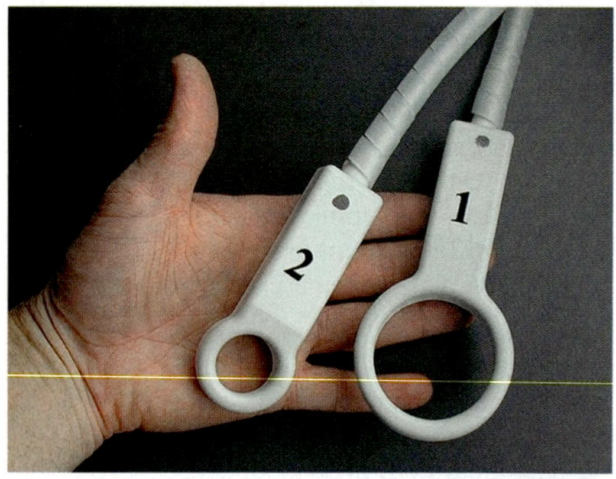

Fig. 2. Microscopic coils. A microscopic coil with a diameter of 4.7 mm (1) can be used to visualize very small superficial nerves. This coil will reach a depth of 2.35 mm and therefore nerves beyond this depth cannot be imaged with this coil. This coil will only provide higher resolution than a routine coil when strong gradients are available.

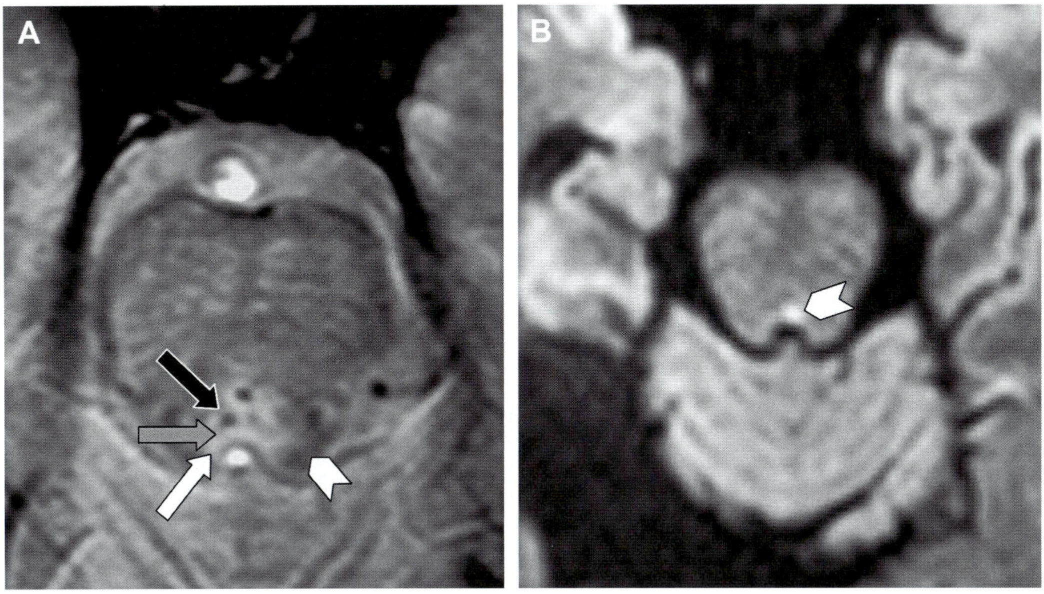

Fig. 3. Patient with right fourth nerve palsy and internuclear ophthalmoplegia, axial m-FFE (*A*) and b-1000 DWI (*B*) images at the level of the inferior colliculus–medullary velum. (*A*) The myelinated structures like the MLF (*black arrow*) and superior cerebellar peduncle (*white arrowhead*) are black on this image. The trochlear nucleus (*gray arrow*) must be located between the periaqueductal gray (*white arrow*) and the MLF. The signal intensity of the left MLF is increased. (*B*) Diffusion restriction can be seen on the diffusion image indicating acute infarction in the area of the left trochlear nucleus and MLF (*white arrowhead*), causing a right superior oblique muscle palsy.

used depend highly on the type of MR unit. Typically CISS,[6,7] 3D-TSE,[8] b-FFE,[9,10] DRIVE,[8,10] 3D-FSE,[11] FIESTA,[12] 3D FSE XETA,[13] and so forth sequences are used. All these sequences are heavily T2W 3D-sequences and provide images with very high resolution. However, these sequences should be carefully chosen. Some of these sequences are based on "steady state" (eg, CISS, b-FFF) and produce artifacts at the periphery of the image, especially when a higher spatial resolution is used. Hence, these sequences should be reserved for imaging around the

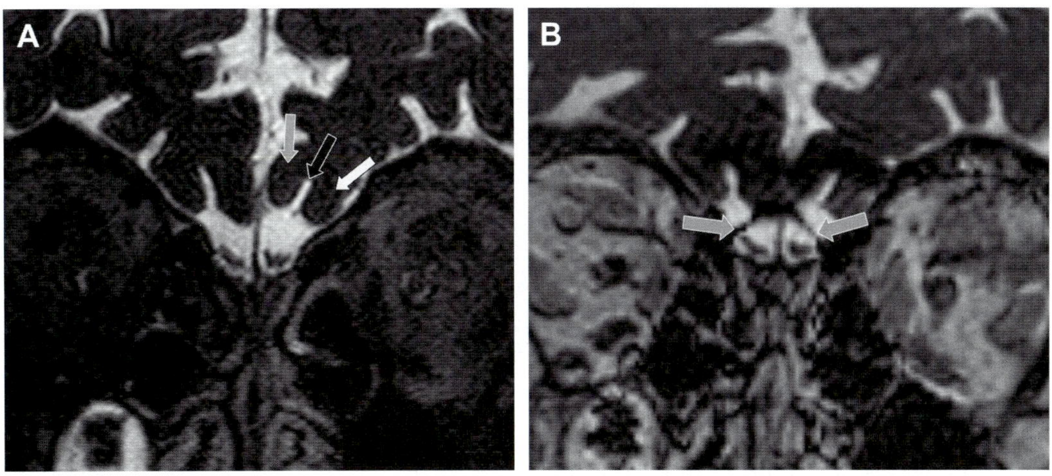

Fig. 4. DRIVE turbo spin-echo (*A*) versus balanced-FFE gradient-echo (*B*) heavily T2W coronal image through the olfactory bulbs. (*A*) The olfactory bulbs are surrounded by CSF and no artifacts are seen. Further posteriorly the olfactory tract can always be found under the olfactory sulcus (*black arrow*) situated between the medial orbital gyrus (*white arrow*) and rectus gyrus (*gray arrow*). (*B*) Image made in the same patient at the same level showing the typical phase artifacts, seen as black curved lines crossing the CSF (*gray arrows*), on this gradient-echo image.

brainstem, in the center of the image. These sequences are better replaced by other type of sequences (3D-TSE, DRIVE) for high resolution imaging of more superficially located nerves (eg, nerves I, VII, VIII) (**Fig. 4**).

Once the nerves are surrounded by a venous plexus (III to VI in the cavernous sinus, VI behind the clivus in the basilar plexus, IX to XI in the jugular foramen, XII in the hypoglossal canal) they are best seen on high resolution contrast-enhanced Time-Of-Flight MRA images or high resolution 2D (SE or TSE) or 3D (TSE or FFE) T1W images. On these images, the cranial nerves are seen as black structures surrounded by high signal intensity gadolinium-filled venous structures (**Fig. 5**).

The peripheral segments and branches of the cranial nerves are surrounded by soft tissues and especially fat in the neck and face. High-resolution T1W SE and TSE sequences are in this region best suited to visualize the nerves. The use of fat saturation will make the fat disappear and makes visualization of normal nerves difficult or impossible. Fat saturation has additional value only when an abnormal enhancement of the nerve is expected or must be excluded.

Slice Thickness, In-Plane Resolution

The T2W and proton density SE images through the brainstem have a thickness of 4 mm, to avoid partial volume effect. The in-plane resolution of these images is 0.9 × 0.9 mm.

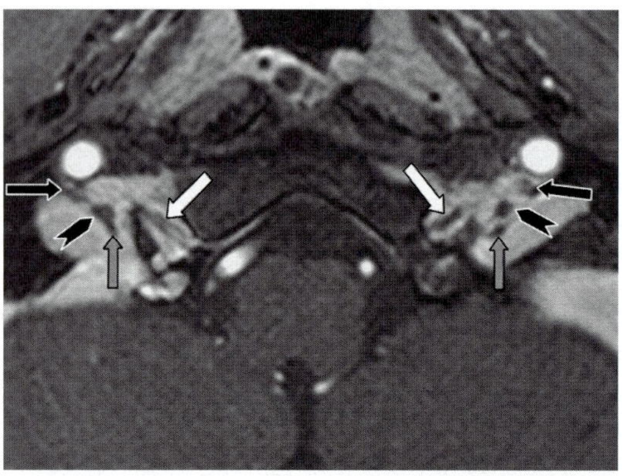

Fig. 5. Axial high resolution contrast-enhanced 3D-FFE image through the jugular foramina. This image has a resolution of 0.71 × 0.71 mm and a thickness of 0.6 mm. The hypoglossal nerves are seen as gray structures surrounded by contrast-enhanced surrounding venous structures (*white arrows*). This technique allows visualization of the glossopharyngeal nerves (*black arrows*) located close to the internal carotid artery and of the vagus nerves (*black arrowheads*) and accessory nerves (*gray arrows*), which at this level are crossing the center of the jugular foramen.

Coronal 2D T1 SE images can be thicker as there is no risk for partial volume problems as the nerves run antero-posterior and will be visualized anyway. Therefore, for this sequence, all energy is put in in-plane resolution, 0.58 × 0.64 mm while the slice thickness is 4 mm.

Selective contrast-enhanced T1-weighted FFE images through the cerebellopontine angle (CPA) and jugular foramen (JF) have a slice thickness of 0.625 mm and an in-plane resolution of 0.71 × 0.71 mm. This very thin slice thickness is needed to distinguish the different nerves.

The heavily T2W b-FFE (imaging around brainstem) and DRIVE (imaging more peripherally) have the highest resolution. The b-FFE images are 0.5 mm thick and have an in-plane resolution of 0.5 × 0.5. At 3 Tesla they have a 0.4^3 or even 0.35^3 mm isotropic voxel size. The DRIVE images are 0.35 mm thick and have an in-plane resolution of 0.33 × 0.30, but the 3D slab has only 48 partitions (covers a distance of 17 mm in cranio-caudal direction) while the b-FFE has a somewhat lower spatial resolution but covers a total cranio-caudal distance of up to 12 cm.

Special Techniques/Software

The nerves can be visualized only when the spatial resolution is very high or the voxel size is very small. The time needed to acquire such images is very long with the use of routine sequences. Therefore, any MR technique that speeds up the sequence, without or with minimal loss of S/N, can be used to shorten the examination time and to reduce movement/swallowing/breathing artifacts or can be invested to get even higher resolution in the same time.

Parallel imaging (eg, SENSE) is therefore used in most of the above-mentioned sequences and also helps to reduce susceptibility artifacts in sequences sensitive to this type of artifact (eg, DRIVE, b-FFE). However the maximal SENSE factor that can be used is equal to the number of coil elements used in the phased array coil (if there are only two coil elements, like for the flex S surface coils used for temporal bone imaging, then the acquisition time can maximal be reduced to ½ (1/N° coil elements) with a S/N reduction of the square root of 2 (N° coil elements). This maximal SENSE factor is already causing too much S/N loss when very high resolution imaging of the CPA nerves is performed and that is why routinely a parallel imaging factor of 1.7 is preferred. SENSE is avoided for midline imaging, even when the head coil is used, as the resulting signal drop will immediately degrade the contrast resolution quality of these very high resolution images and consequently make it more difficult to visualize the nerves.[14]

The use of an asymmetric k-space, only possible when TSE types of sequences are used, can reduce the examination time easily by 30%, without the penalty of S/N loss. Hence, this is an ideal technique to increase resolution in the same imaging time or to stick to the same resolution in a shorter examination time.

CRANIAL NERVE ANATOMY

The Olfactory Nerve or Cranial Nerve I

Olfactory epithelium

The olfactory epithelium is located in the upper one fifth of the nasal cavity and covers the septal and lateral surface of this cavity, including the upper part of the superior turbinate (**Fig. 6**).

Transethmoidal segment

Bipolar olfactory neurons connect the olfactory epithelium with the olfactory bulbs. These neurons experience a continuous cycle of growth, degeneration, and replacement, which make them "unique" neurons. The dendrites of these olfactory neurons reach the surface of the olfactory epithelium while the unmyelinated axons, about 3 million on each side, run upwards through the openings of the cribriform plate. These axons are grouped in bundles, called filia, which are invested by Schwann cells. This explains why olfactory schwannomas can develop. These filia enter the olfactory bulb and these filia together constitute the real "olfactory nerve." Some of these filia between the cribriform plate and olfactory bulb can sometimes be seen on high-resolution T2W images (**Fig. 7**).

Olfactory bulb and tract—intracranial

The olfactory bulb and tract (intracranial) are extensions of the brain and are not a real cranial nerve. The olfactory nerve fibers are received in about 50,000 mitral cells inside the olfactory bulbs. The olfactory bulbs have a convex ovoid shape and can easily be recognized on coronal T2W or T1W images (see **Figs. 4, 6, and 7**). The axons of the olfactory bulb mitral cells are located centrally in the olfactory tract and run from their paramedian origin in the olfactory bulbs posterolaterally toward the anterior border of the anterior perforated substance. Along this course, the olfactory tract follows the inferior border of the olfactory sulcus, located between the gyrus rectus and medial orbital gyrus. The olfactory tract is flatter and more difficult to visualize but its constant position under the olfactory sulcus helps to track this structure (**Fig. 8**).[15] The olfactory tract divides in lateral, medial, and intermediate stria in front of the anterior perforated substance. This division can be depicted on (para)-axial high-resolution T2W images (**Fig. 8**B).

Olfactory pathways—intracranial

Damage to the olfactory pathway on one side will cause ipsilateral anosmia. Olfaction, and taste are actually the only uncrossed sensations.[3] Some axons in the medial stria reach the septal area via the diagonal band, others cross the midline via

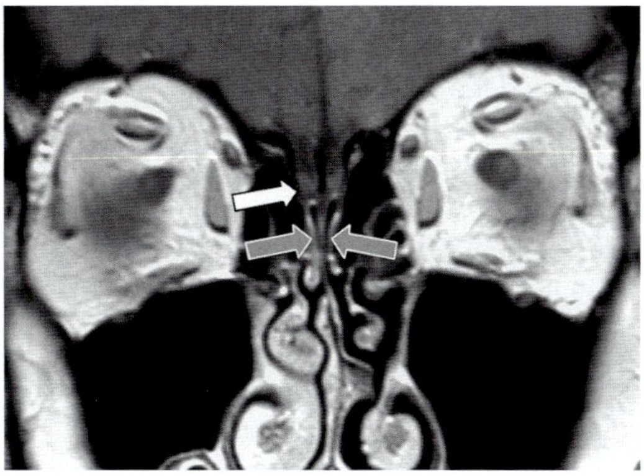

Fig. 6. Olfactory bulbs—coronal contrast-enhanced high-resolution T1W image. The olfactory bulbs (*white arrow*) are isointense with brain and are located just above the cribriform plate. Notice the enhancing olfactory mucosa located high in the nasal cavity on the medial surface of the superior turbinates and in the mucosa of the upper part of the septum (*gray arrows*).

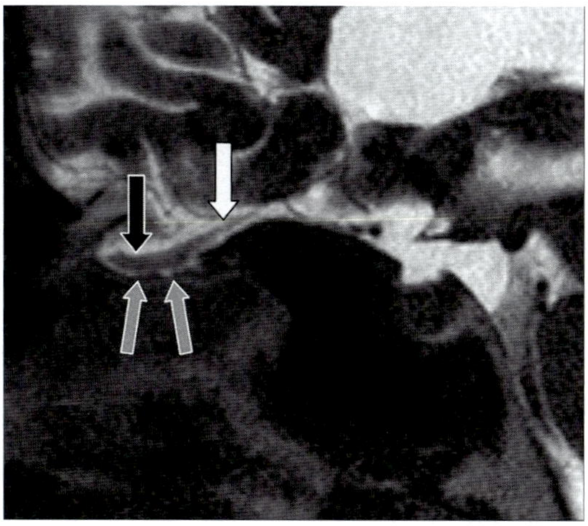

Fig. 7. Olfactory filia (nerves)—high-resolution parasagittal reformatted b-FFE image. The olfactory bulb (*black arrow*) can be seen as an ovoid dark structure surrounded by white CSF. The olfactory tract (*white arrow*) is emerging from the bulb. Some of the filia can be followed through the cribriform plate into the inferior surface of the bulb (*gray arrows*).

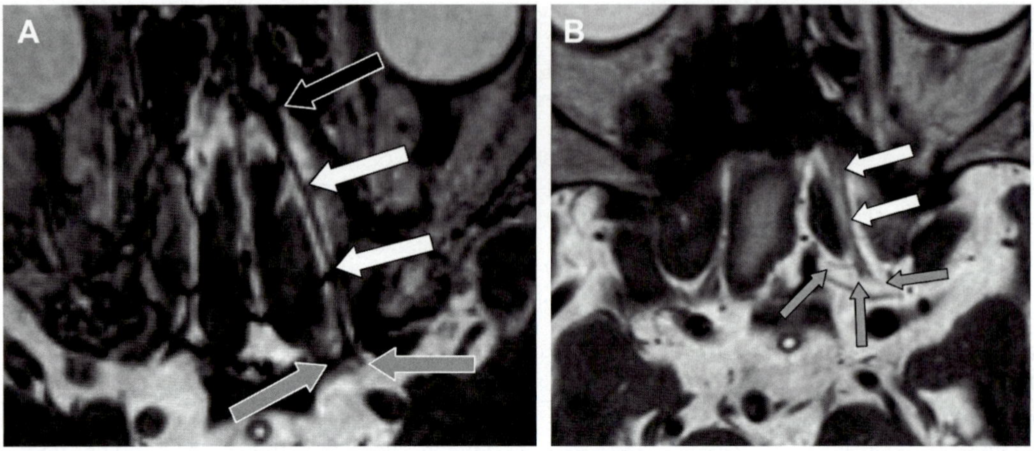

Fig. 8. Olfactory bulb-tract-striae—axial high-resolution (0.35 × 0.35 × 0.35 isotropic voxels) b-FFE image through the olfactory bulb-tract-striae (*A*) and para-axial reformatted image through the tract and striae (*B*). (*A*) The left olfactory bulb (*black arrow*), tract (*white arrows*), and division in lateral and medial striae (*gray arrows*) just anterior to the anterior perforated substance can be seen in and under the olfactory sulcus. Notice the oblique course of the olfactory tract from anteromedial to posterolateral. (*B*) The olfactory tract (*white arrows*) can be followed and splits in lateral, intermediate, and medial striae (*gray arrows*). Notice the acute medial angulation of the medial stria.

the anterior commissure to reach the contralateral olfactory tract. The lateral stria terminates in the piriform lobe (uncus, anterior part of the parahippocampal gyrus, cortical part of the amygdala) and connects through the thalamus (mediodorsal nucleus) with the orbital frontal cortex, which is the highest center for olfactory discrimination.[3] The intermediate stria reach the intermediate cortical olfactory area, a small zone of gray matter at the level of the anterior perforated substance.[16]

The Optic Nerve or Cranial Nerve II

The optic nerve is just like the olfactory bulb and tract; not a true cranial nerve but rather an extension of the brain. The optic nerve can be divided in several segments: intraocular, intraorbital,[17] intracanalicular, and intracranial.[18] The optic pathway then continues in the optic chiasm and optic tracts. The optic radiation and visual cortex are beyond the scope of this chapter.

Intraocular segment

The axons of the retinal ganglion cells form the intraocular optic nerve. This intraocular segment as well as the retina, where the ganglion cells are located, is difficult to visualize. Some of this anatomy can, however, be visualized when microscopic coils and very high resolution are used (**Fig. 9**). These axons get myelinated by oligodendrocytes as they leave the optic disc.

Intraorbital segment

The intraorbital segment runs through the intraconal space of the orbit, from the globe to the orbital apex and is at that level already surrounded by meninges, explaining the development of many intraorbital meningiomas. The subarachnoid CSF space, located between the pia mater and arachnoid/dura, is surrounding the intraorbital optic nerve and this CSF space is actually in continuity with the CSF of the suprasellar cistern. The nerve and surrounding CSF are best seen on heavily T2W or STIR images. This segment should be imaged with minimal water-fat chemical shift as the nerve-CSF-fat interfaces are otherwise artifacted and difficult to delineate (**Fig. 10**). The central retinal artery, a branch of the ophthalmic artery, enters the optic nerve with its accompanying vein only in the distal part of the intraorbital segment over a nerve length of 1 cm in the area just behind the globe.

Intracanalicular segment

This segment of the optic nerve inside the optic canal is best seen on MR images (**Fig. 11**); the bone fragments that can damage the nerve at this site caused by a trauma are of course better seen on CT. Inside this canal the nerve is positioned above the ophthalmic artery.

Intracranial segment

The intracranial segment bridges the gap between the optic canal anterolaterally and optic chiasm posteromedially over a distance of about 10 mm. This nerve segment is covered only by pia mater.

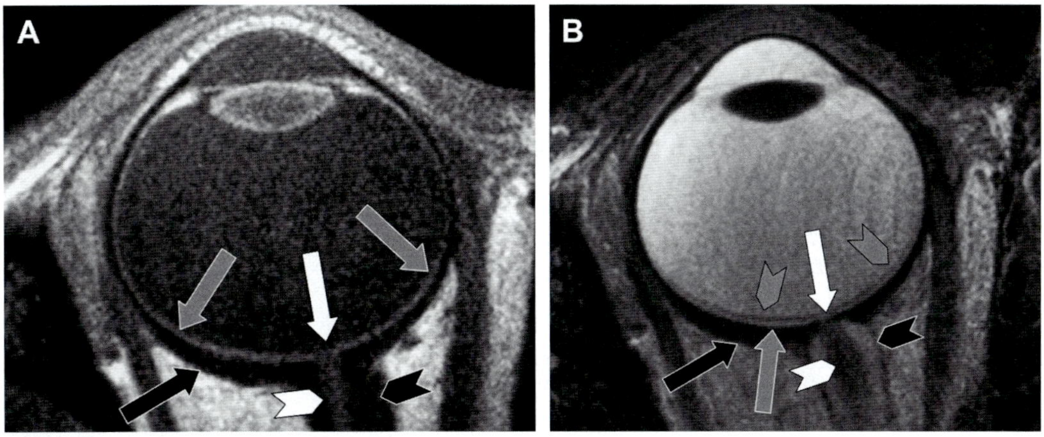

Fig. 9. Intraocular (+ retina) and orbital segment of the optic nerve—axial high-resolution contrast-enhanced T1W image (*A*) and TSE T2W image (*B*) acquired with a 4.7-mm-diameter microscopic coil using strong gradients. (*A*) The intraorbital segment (*white arrowhead*) and intraocular segment (*white arrow*) can be seen at the level of the lamina cribrosa of the sclera. The enhancing choroid (*gray arrows*) and dark sclera (*black arrow*) can be distinguished. CSF is in the subarachnoid space around the intraorbital segment (*black arrowhead*). (*B*) The choroid is now seen as a white area (*gray arrow*) between the dark thick sclera (*black arrow*) and a thin black line inside the globe, the retina (*gray arrowheads*). Intraocular (*white arrow*) and intraorbital (*white arrowhead*) optic nerve, CSF in the subarachnoid space (*black arrowhead*).

Optic chiasm

At the optic chiasm, fibers from the temporal hemiretina remain uncrossed and continue in the ipsilateral optic tract. Fibers from the nasal hemiretina cross and continue in the contralateral optic tract. This explains the X-shaped morphology of the chiasm, located just anterior to the pituitary stalk, which is best appreciated on reformatted 3D-T1W images (eg, 3D-FFE, 3D-MPRAGE) or 3D-T2W images (eg, DRIVE, b-FFE) (**Fig. 12**).

Optic tracts

The continuation of the chiasm in the left and right optic tract can also be visualized. These tracts divide in a smaller medial (containing only 10%

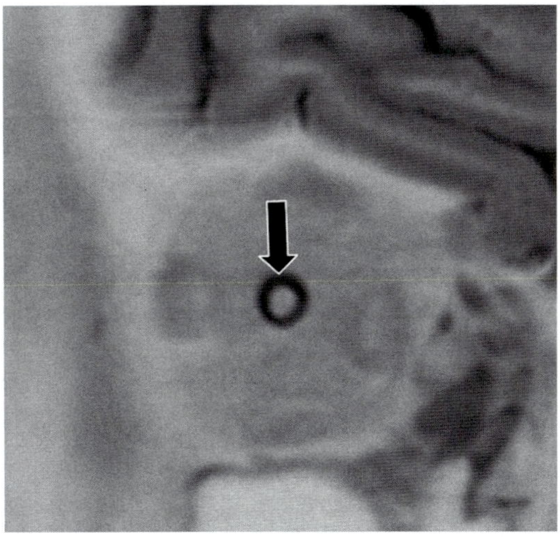

Fig. 10. Intraorbital optic nerve—para-coronal STIR image perpendicular on the course of the nerve. The CSF in the subarachnoid space (*black arrow*) around the intraorbital optic nerve segment is seen as a symmetric hypointense ring, showing that there are no deformations or chemical shift artifacts on this image. The optic nerve in the center of the CSF has a high signal intensity, isointense with white matter.

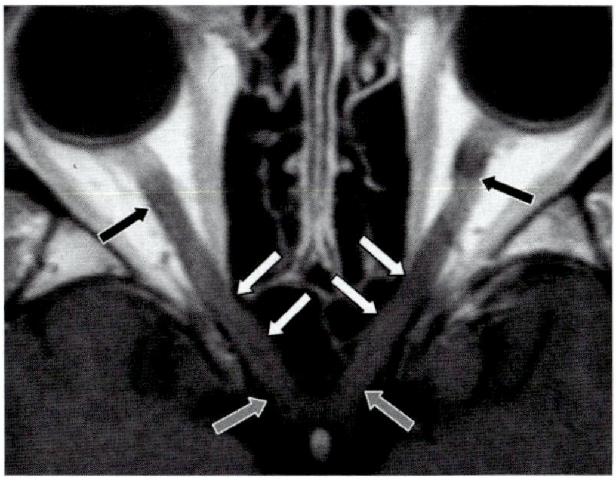

Fig. 11. Intracanalicular optic nerve—axial contrast-enhanced high resolution T1W image. The intracanalicular segment of the optic nerve can be seen in the optic canal (*white arrows*) which is far more difficult on CT because of the artifacts produced by the bony walls of the optic canal on CT. Intraorbital segment (*black arrows*) and intracranial segment (*gray arrows*) are shown.

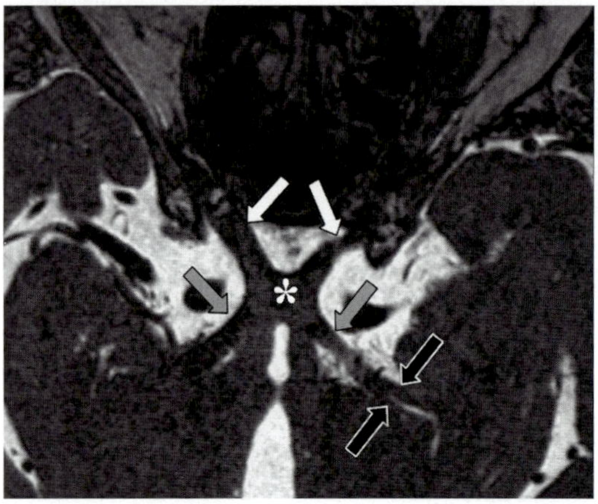

Fig. 12. Optic chiasm—axial reformatted high-resolution T2W balanced-FFE image. Para-axial reformation allows visualization of the intracranial segments of the optic nerves (*white arrows*), "X" shaped optic chiasm (*), optic tracts (*gray arrows*) and the medial and lateral root of the optic tract on the left side (*black arrows*).

of the fibers) and larger lateral root of the optic tract terminating in the medial geniculate body (see **Fig. 12**). These tracts are best distinguished on high-resolution T2W or FLAIR images.

The Oculomotor Nerve or Cranial Nerve III

The oculomotor nerve has a motor function (innervation of five of the extraocular muscles) and a parasympathetic function (innervation of the ciliaris and sphincter pupillae).

Oculomotor nuclear complex

The oculomotor nuclear complex is composed of five individual motor nuclei supplying the extraocular muscles and a more dorsal parasympathetic nucleus of Edinger-Westphal and is located at the level of the superior colliculus. The complex lies between the aqueduct and the red nucleus and is partially embedded in the periaqueductal gray. The structures are best visualized on multiecho FFE (m-FFE) images (**Fig. 13**) and the location of the nuclear complex can be deduced from it. The fascicular segment of the oculomotor nerve has an anterolateral course through the midbrain and crosses the medial longitudinal fasciculus (MLF), red nucleus, substantia nigra, and the medial part of the cerebral peduncle.

Cisternal segment

The cisternal segment starts once the nerve leaves the brainstem and enters the interpeduncular cistern. This segment is best seen on high-resolution heavily T2W images (**Fig. 14**); however, this nerve segment is also large enough to be depicted on T1W images. The nerve passes under the posterior cerebral and above the superior cerebellar artery, continues anteriorly below the posterior communicating artery, and pierces the dural roof of the cavernous sinus.[19]

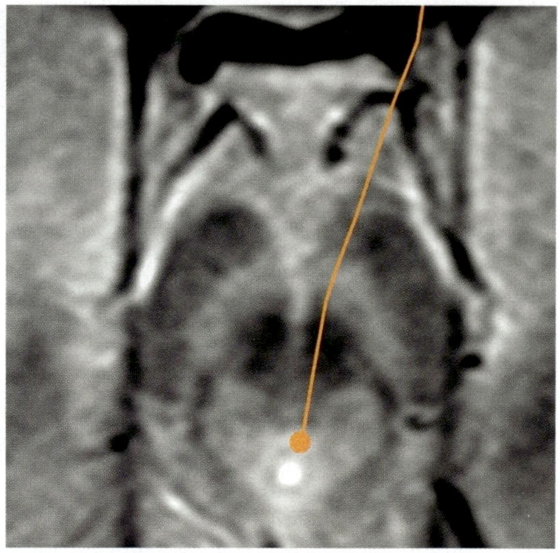

Fig. 13. The oculomotor nuclear complex—axial m-FFE image at the level of the superior colliculus. The oculomotor nuclear complex (*dot*) can be found at this level close to the midline, embedded in the periaqueductal gray anterolateral to the aqueduct and posterior to the red nucleus. The fascicular segment courses through the MLF, red nucleus, substantia nigra, and medial part of the cerebral peduncle (*line*).

Cavernous segment

This segment of the third nerve runs in the lateral wall of the cavernous sinus, superolateral to the cavernous internal carotid artery. This segment can best be seen in detail on coronal gadolinium-enhanced high-resolution T1W images through the cavernous sinus but nerve visualization on contrast-enhanced heavily T2W images has also be reported.[20,21] The third nerve is the nerve with the highest position in the wall of the cavernous sinus. However, just before entering the superior orbital fissure (SOF), the trochlear nerve ascends along the lateral wall of the third nerve and eventually even lies superolateral to the third nerve as they enter the SOF (**Fig. 15**).

Extracranial segment

The third cranial nerve divides in a superior and inferior branch within the SOF and enters the orbit through this SOF and the annulus of Zinn. The superior branch innervates the superior rectus muscles and levator palpebrae superioris

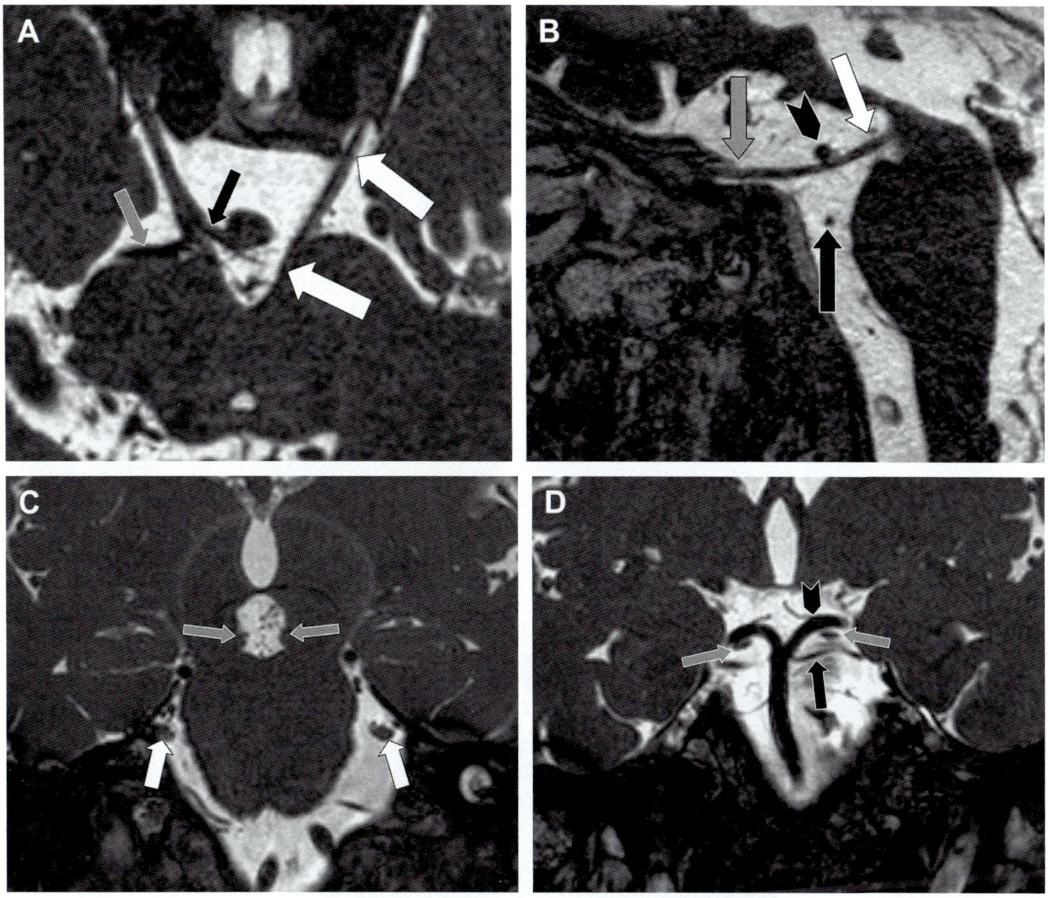

Fig. 14. Cisternal segment of the oculomotor nerve—high-resolution (0.4 mm^3) axial (*A*) and sagittal (*B*) and moderate resolution (0.6 mm^3) coronal (*C, D*) T2W FFE images through the cisternal segment of the oculomotor nerve. (*A*) The oculomotor nerve enters the prepontine cistern once it leaves the brainstem. The cisternal segment (*white arrows*) courses anterolaterally and passes through the space between the posterior cerebral artery (PCA) (*gray arrow*) above and superior cerebellar artery (SCeA) below (*black arrow*). (*B*) The third nerve can be followed from the interpeduncular cistern (*white arrow*) to the parasellar area (*gray arrow*) and passes between the PCA (*black arrowhead*) and SCeA (*black arrow*). (*C*) In the coronal plane the third nerves (*gray arrows*) can be seen inside the interpeduncular cistern and are in contact with the medial wall of the cerebral peduncles. Cisternal or preganglionic segment of the trigeminal nerves (*white arrows*) are shown. (*D*) More anteriorly in the prepontine cistern both third nerves (*gray arrows*) are seen in the space between the PCA (*black arrowhead*) and SCeA (*black arrow*).

muscles, while the inferior branch innervates the inferior rectus, medial rectus, and inferior oblique muscles.[18] These branches can again be depicted on high-resolution coronal T1W images (**Fig. 16**). Preganglionic parasympathetic fibers follow the cranial nerve III into the orbit and then exit the branch to the inferior oblique muscle to synapse in the ciliary ganglion. Postganglionic parasympathetic fibers continue as short ciliary nerves and enter the globe by piercing the lamina cribrosa of the sclera. They reach the ciliary body and iris, controlling the papillary sphincter and ciliary muscle.

The Trochlear Nerve or Cranial Nerve IV

The fourth cranial nerve provides motor innervation to only a single muscle, the superior oblique muscle.

Trochlear nucleus

The trochlear nucleus is situated at the level of the inferior colliculus, just ventral to the aqueduct, posterior to the MLF and just inferior to the oculomotor nerve complex. The localization of the nucleus very close to the MLF explains why lesions that involve the trochlear nucleus most often cause

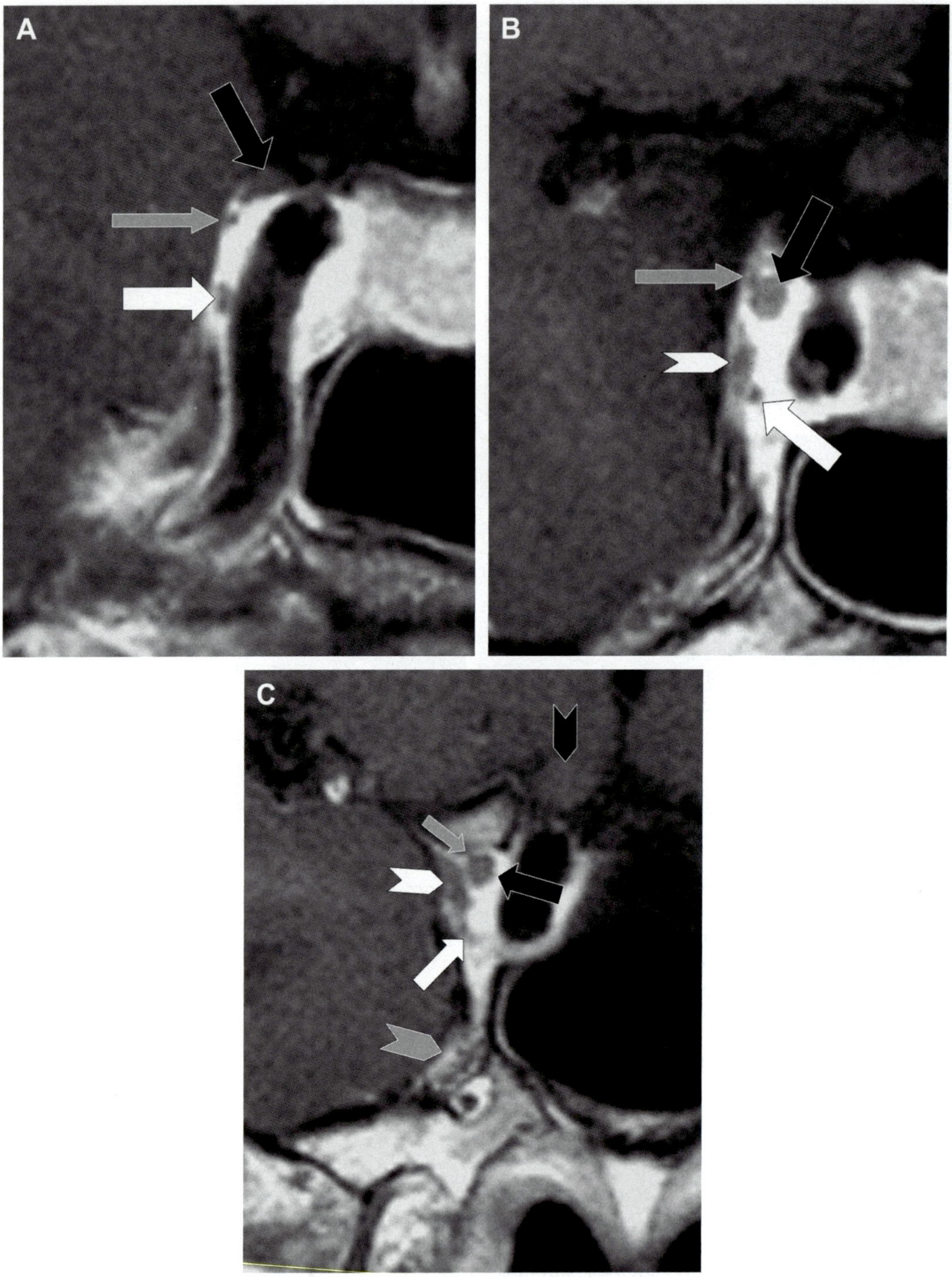

Fig. 15. Cavernous segment of the third nerve—coronal contrast-enhanced T1W images through the posterior (*A*), middle (*B*), and anterior (*C*) part of the cavernous sinus. (*A*) The third nerve is the largest nerve coursing in the wall of the cavernous sinus (*black arrow*); the trochlear nerve (*gray arrow*) is the smallest nerve, located just below the third nerve. The abducens nerve (*white arrow*) is located deep in the cavernous sinus, not in the wall, and enters the cavernous sinus just above Meckel's cave. (*B*) More anteriorly the ophthalmic nerve emerges from the Gasserian ganglion and is seen as an ovoid hypointensity (*white arrowhead*). The trochlear nerve (*gray arrow*) already ascended up to the superolateral border of the third nerve (*black arrow*). Abducens nerve (*white arrow*) is seen. (*C*) At the level of the entrance to the superior orbital fissure, the trochlear nerve (*gray arrow*) is seen above the oculomotor nerve (*black arrow*). The optic nerve (*black arrowhead*), ophthalmic nerve (*white arrowhead*), abducens nerve (*white arrow*), and maxillary nerve (*gray arrowhead*) are located just above the vidian canal and nerve.

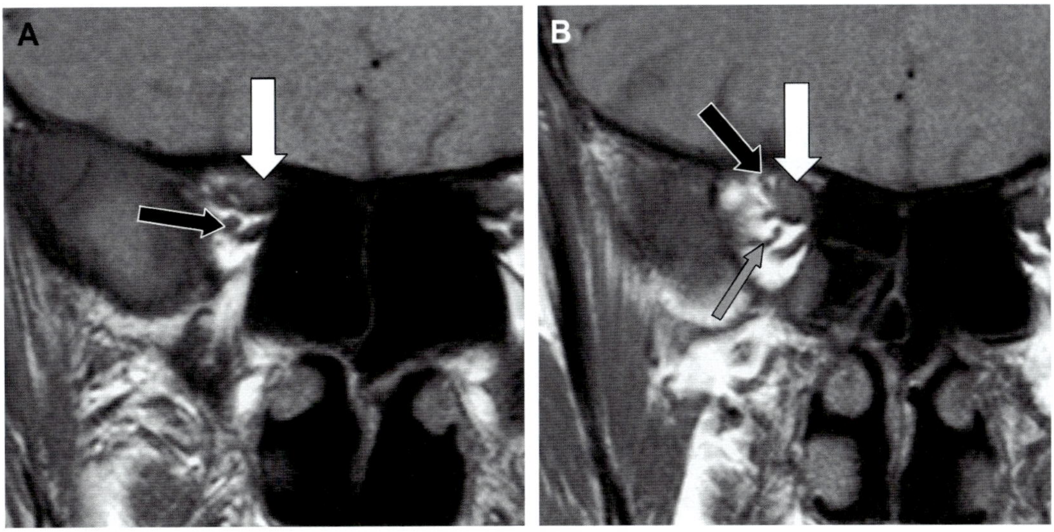

Fig. 16. Extracranial segment of the third nerve—coronal high-resolution T1W images through the superior orbital fissure (*A*) and orbital apex (*B*). (*A*) The oculomotor nerve (*black arrow*) and optic nerve (*white arrow*) enter the superior orbital fissure and orbit. (*B*) Once in the orbital apex the oculomotor nerve divides in a superior (*black arrow*) and inferior (*gray arrow*) branch. Also visible is the optic nerve (*white arrow*).

both a fourth nerve palsy and an internuclear ophthalmoplegia (INO). Axons leaving the nucleus course dorsally around the aqueduct and the left and right fascicular segments cross each other at the level of the superior medullary velum before exiting the midbrain at its posterior surface, just caudal to the inferior colliculus (**Fig. 17**). These are two unique features of the fourth cranial nerve: (1) it is the only cranial nerve crossing the midline, hence a superior oblique muscle is always innervated by the contralateral trochlear nucleus and (2) it is the only cranial nerve exiting the brainstem at its dorsal surface.

Cisternal segment

Once outside the brainstem, the nerve is best visualized on heavily T2W images in the axial plane.[10] The nerve is extremely small and is therefore sometimes difficult to find. The trick is to look for the superior medullary velum, a small flat band at the back of the superior part of the fourth ventricle. At that level, the nerves exit the brainstem in a nearly horizontal mediolateral direction until they reach the free edge of the tentorium (**Fig. 18**).[22] They then course anteriorly around the brainstem and pass through the gap between the superior cerebral artery and superior cerebellar artery, lateral to the oculomotor nerve. Because the nerves have to turn around the complete brainstem, they are the cranial nerves with the longest intracranial segment.

Cavernous segment

The trochlear nerve then enters the lateral wall of the cavernous sinus below the oculomotor nerve (**Fig. 19**).[21] As already mentioned, the cavernous segment of the trochlear nerve initially is situated

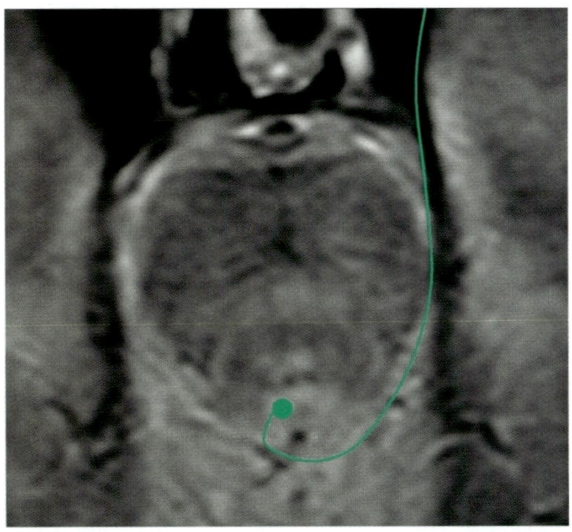

Fig. 17. Trochlear nucleus—axial m-FFE image at level of inferior colliculus. The trochlear nucleus (*dot*) is located posterolateral to the MLF and anterolateral to the aqueduct. The fascicular segment (*line*) then courses posteriorly to exit the midbrain just below the inferior colliculus. The contralateral nerve is crossed at this point and the cisternal segment of the nerve (*line outside brainstem*) then follows the lateral border of the brainstem until it reaches the cavernous sinus.

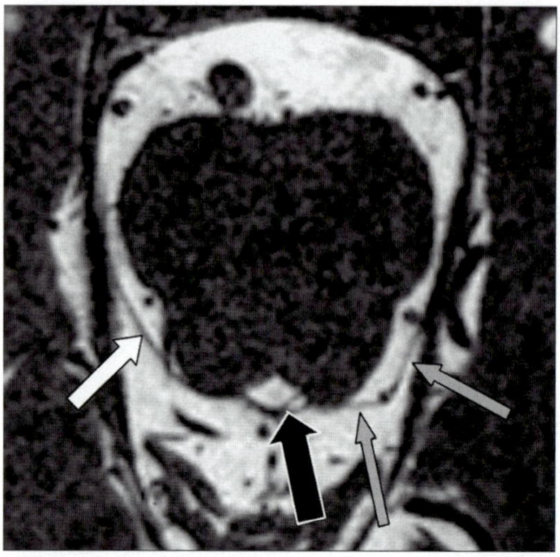

Fig. 18. Cisternal segment of the trochlear nerve—axial DRIVE image at level of medullary velum. The left (*gray arrows*) and right (*white arrow*) trochlear nerves exit the brainstem at the level where the medullary velum (*black arrow*) is seen. Note the displacement of the nerve on the left caused by a vessel.

below the third nerve but then gradually ascends along the lateral border of the third nerve as the nerves approach the SOF and once in the SOF the trochlear nerve can be found at the superolateral border of the third nerve.

Extracranial segment

The trochlear nerve then crosses over the superior border of the third nerve to run medially toward the superior oblique muscle. This nerve courses above the annulus of Zinn and does not pass through the annulus like the oculomotor and abducens nerve. The cavernous and extracranial segments are again best seen on coronal high resolution T1W images.

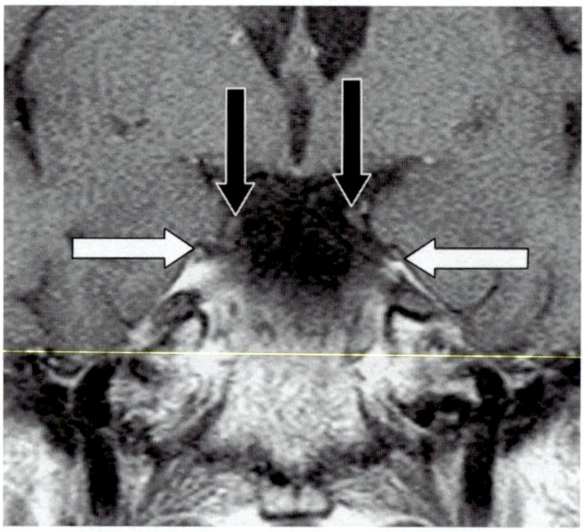

Fig. 19. Cavernous segment of the trochlear nerve—coronal contrast-enhanced T1W image. Both trochlear nerves (*white arrows*) are entering the wall of the cavernous sinus. At that level the oculomotor nerves are still seen in the prepontine cistern (*black arrows*).

The Trigeminal Nerve or Cranial Nerve V

The trigeminal nerve is both motor and sensory to the muscles of mastication and of course also has a large sensory territory.

Trigeminal nuclei—intra-axial segment

Four nuclei, 1 motor and 3 sensory, are located in the brainstem (**Fig. 20**). The "motor nucleus" is located in the lateral pontine tegmentum and supplies the muscles of mastication and the tensor veli palatini and tensor tympani muscle. The "pontine" or "principal" sensory nucleus (PSN), which can be found lateral to the motor nucleus and anterolateral to the fourth ventricle at the level of the root entry zone (REZ), processes discriminative tactile sensation from the skin of the face. The "mesencephalic nucleus" is a superior extension of the PSN in the midbrain up to the level of the inferior colliculus. It is the only nucleus in the CNS composed of unipolar neurons. It receives afferent fibers for facial proprioception (teeth, hard palate, temporomandibular joint [TMJ]). Their peripheral processes supply stretch receptors in the muscles of mastication and periodontal ligaments of the

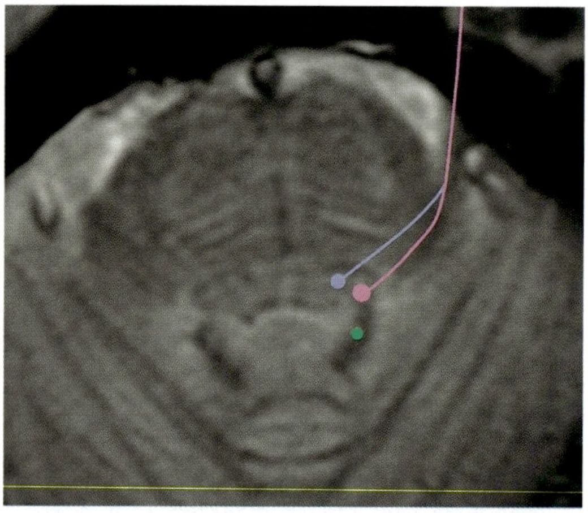

Fig. 20. Trigeminal nuclei—axial m-FFE through the mid pons. The motor nucleus (*blue dot*) is located in the lateral pontine tegmentum. The principal sensory nucleus (*dark pink dot*) can be found just lateral to the motor nucleus. The mesencephalic nucleus, a superior extension of the principal sensory nucleus, can be found more posteriorly toward the superior cerebellar peduncle (*green dot*). The fascicular segments connected with the first two nuclei (*blue and pink line*) form one single nerve at the REZ.

teeth. The spinal nucleus is a caudal extension of the PSN and descends from the level of the lower pons down to spinal cord level C3. The nucleus merges with dorsal gray matter of the cord. This nucleus mainly receives tactile, nociceptive, and thermal information from the entire V1, V2, and V3 trigeminal areas.

Cisternal or preganglionic segment

The cisternal or preganglionic segment leaves the brainstem at the site where the pons is widest in the coronal and axial plane, also called the REZ.[23] The cisternal segment is composed of a sensory and motor root and courses anterosuperiorly through the prepontine cistern, passes over the tip of the petrous apex, and enters the CSF-filled Meckel's cave through an opening in the dura mater called "the porus trigeminus." This segment and the sensory fibers inside Meckel's cave are best seen on heavily T2W images (**Fig. 21**) but can also be seen on high-resolution T1W images (**Fig. 22**).

Meckel's cave—interdural segment

The preganglionic segment ends in the gasserian or semilunar sensory ganglion.[24] This ganglion always enhances as it has no blood-nerve barrier. The motor root passes under the gasserian ganglion and leaves the skull through the oval foramen. The sensory root divides in an ophthalmic (V1), maxillary (V2), and mandibular (V3) division at the anterior aspect of the Gasserian ganglion.[25]

The ophthalmic nerve—V1 division

The ophthalmic nerve courses in the wall of the cavernous sinus, just below the fourth nerve and lateral to the sixth nerve. This can be seen as a craniocaudal ovoid nerve, which is much larger than the adjacent fourth and sixth nerves. This nerve can only be depicted in a reliable way on coronal contrast-enhanced high-resolution T1W images through the cavernous sinus (**Fig. 23**). The nerve then leaves the skull through the SOF and enters the orbit, where it divides into a frontal, lacrimal, and nasociliary nerve providing sensory innervation to the globe, nose, forehead, and scalp (see **Fig. 23**; **Fig. 24**).

The maxillary nerve—V2 division

The maxillary nerve also courses in the wall of the floor of the cavernous sinus (see **Fig. 23**) and can sometimes even be found under the cavernous sinus in a dural sheath. The nerve exits the skull through the foramen rotundum and is there always clearly visible on coronal images. The nerve continues through the upper part of pterygopalatine fossa where it gives off several side branches: the posterior superior alveolar nerve, the zygomatic nerve (**Fig. 25**), and two pterygopalatine nerves, which will reach the pterygopalatine ganglion (**Fig. 26**). Through these two connecting branches and the Vidian nerve the trigeminal nerve and facial nerve territories are connected. The maxillary nerve has a bayonet course and then reaches the orbit through the inferior orbital fissure (IOF) (**Fig. 27**).

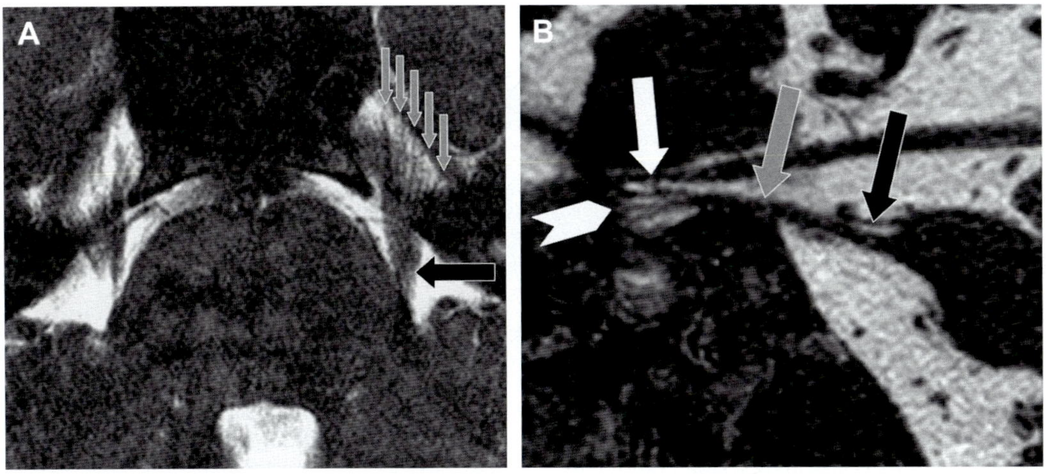

Fig. 21. Cisternal or preganglionic segment—axial CISS (*A*) and sagittal reformatted b-FFE image (*B*). (*A*) The preganglionic segment (*black arrow*) can be followed through the porus trigeminus into Meckel's cave where multiple nerve rootlets fan open (*gray arrows*) to end in the Gasserian ganglion. (*B*) The cisternal segment (*black arrow*) enters the porus trigeminus (*gray arrow*) and the multiple trigeminal nerve rootlets in Meckel's cave are again visible (*white arrow*) and end in the Gasserian ganglion (*white arrowhead*).

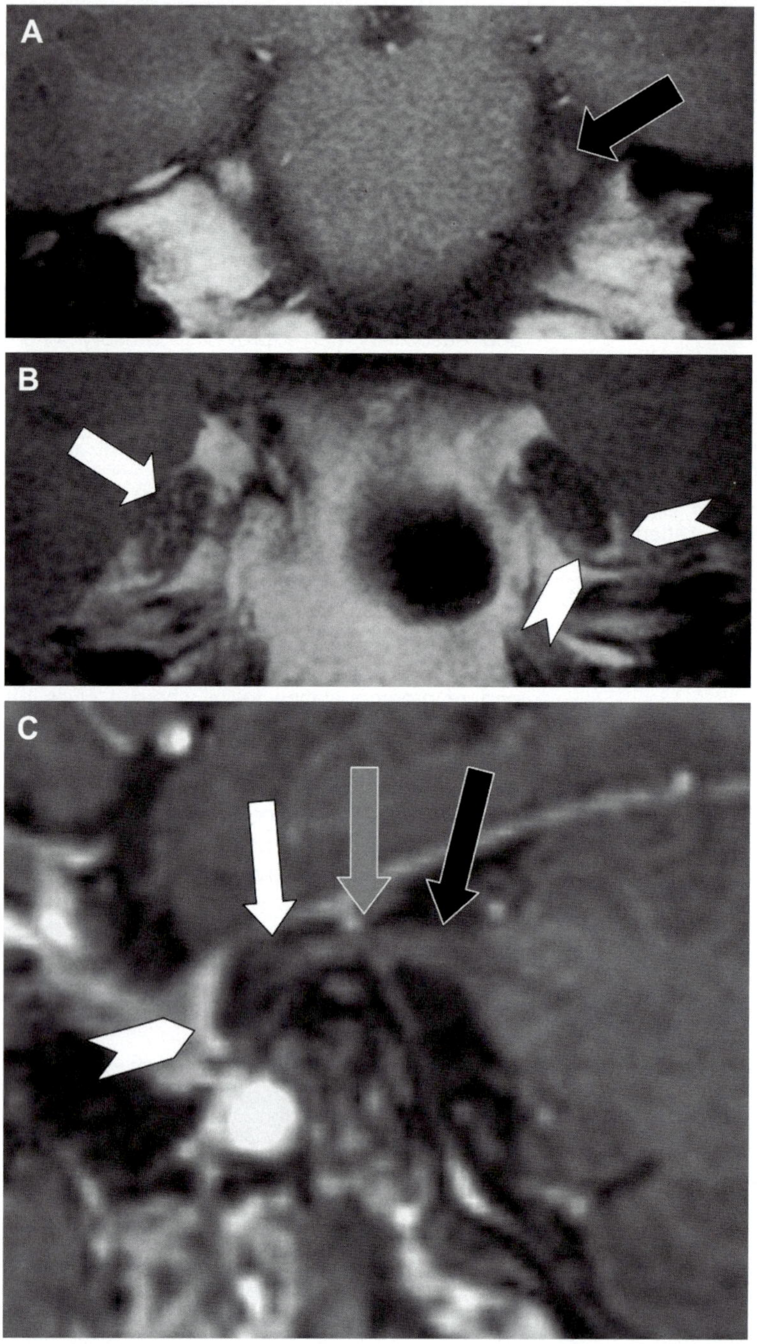

Fig. 22. Preganglionic segment—high resolution coronal contrast-enhanced T1W image through the preganglionic segment (*A*) and Meckel's cave (*B*) in a patient with trigeminal viral neuritis on the right side and para-sagittal reformatted image through the normal left nerve (*C*). A) The preganglionic segment can always be seen lateral to the widest part of the pons (*black arrow*). Notice the enhancing nerve on the right side. (*B*) The Gasserian ganglion can be seen as a V-shaped enhancement at the bottom of Meckel's cave (*white arrowheads*). Multiple trigeminal nerve rootlets inside Meckel's cave become visible because they enhance as a result of a viral infection (*white arrow*). These rootlets can hardly be recognized on the left side. (*C*) The preganglionic segment (*black arrow*), region of the porus trigeminus (*gray arrow*), trigeminal nerve rootlets in Meckel's cave (*white arrow*) and Gasserian ganglion (*white arrowhead*) can also be seen on this sagittal image.

There the nerve becomes the infraorbital nerve and follows the floor of the orbit. After giving off the anterior superior alveolar nerve, which can often be seen in the lateral nasal wall, the infraorbital nerve exits the infraorbital foramen and reaches the soft tissues of the midface. The V2 receives sensory information from the midface, cheek, and upper teeth (**Fig. 28**).

The mandibular nerve—V3 division

The mandibular nerve immediately leaves the skull inferiorly through the oval foramen, and does not run through the cavernous sinus (**Fig. 29**). In the oval foramen it is joined by the motor root and both nerves continue into the masticator space. The motor branch divides in two major nerves just beneath the skull base,

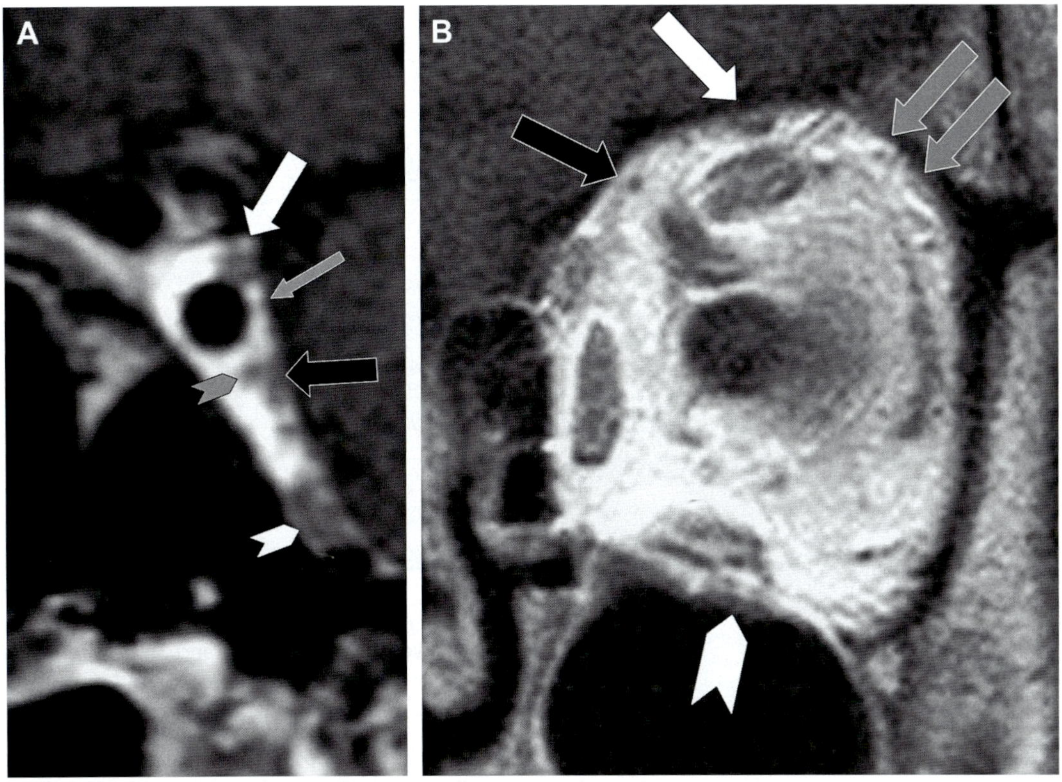

Fig. 23. V1 and V2 divisions of the trigeminal nerve—high-resolution coronal contrast-enhanced images through the left cavernous sinus (*A*) and orbit (*B*). (*A*) Image shows the oculomotor nerve (*white arrow*), trochlear nerve (*gray arrow*), ophthalmic nerve (*black arrow*), abducens nerve (only nerve deep in the cavernous sinus [*gray arrowhead*]), and maxillary nerve (*white arrowhead*) in bottom of cavernous sinus. (*B*) The frontal nerve already divided in a supraorbital (*white arrow*) and supratrochlear (*black arrow*) branch. The lacrimal vessels and nerves (*gray arrows*) course toward the lacrimal gland. Also visible is the infraorbital nerve (*white arrowhead*).

the masticator nerve, which innervates all the muscles of mastication, and the mylohyoid nerve, which innervates the mylohyoid muscle and anterior belly of the digastric muscle. The sensory branch divides into the inferior alveolar nerve, lingual nerve, auriculotemporal nerve, and a small buccal branch (**Fig. 30**). The auriculotemporal nerve will finally enter the parotid gland where it connects with branches of the facial nerve. The lingual nerve connects high in the masticator space with the chorda tympani, again a facial nerve branch. The otic ganglion, located just under the skull base, finally connects the mandibular nerve with the facial nerve via the lesser petrosal nerve. Hence there are four major connections between branches of the trigeminal and facial nerve. The alveolar nerve can be followed to the mandibular foramen on axial and coronal T1W images and then enters the inferior alveolar canal and innervates the teeth of the lower jaw. The nerve can again be seen in the canal (**Figs. 31 and 32**) and at the mental foramen, where the nerve leaves the mandible. The lingual nerve can be evaluated in a fat space, the pterygomandibular space, just before it enters the floor of the mouth, just posteromedial to the free edge of the mylohyoid muscle (see **Fig. 31**). Sensory information from the floor of the mouth, lower one third of the face, tongue, and jaw is transmitted through the sensory branches.

The Abducens Nerve or Cranial Nerve VI

The abducens is a pure motor nerve and innervates only the lateral rectus muscle, which abducts the eye.

Abducens nucleus

The nucleus of the abducens nerve is located at the level of the facial colliculus, in the middle of the pons, near the midline. The axons of the facial nerve, which loop around the abducens nucleus form this facial colliculus, which protrudes into the floor of the fourth ventricle. The axons of

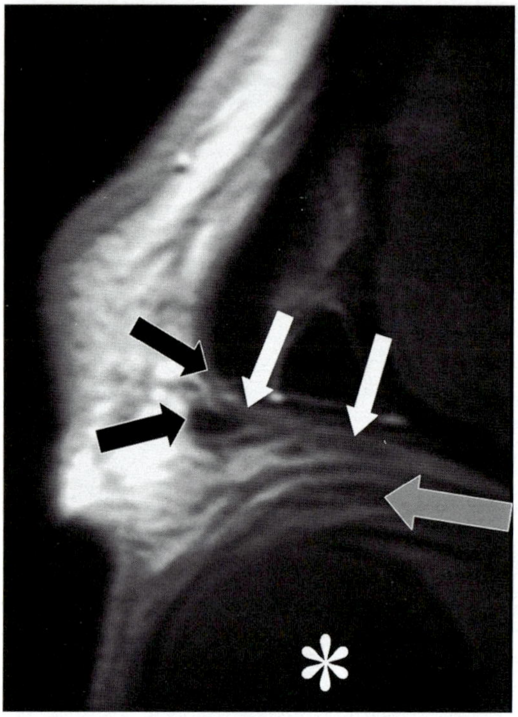

Fig. 24. V1 division, frontal nerve—sagittal high-resolution image acquired with a microscopic coil. The frontal nerve (*white arrows*) runs between the orbital roof and the levator palpebrae superioris/superior rectus muscles (*gray arrow*). The nerve exits the orbit through the supraorbital foramen (*black arrows*). *, Globe.

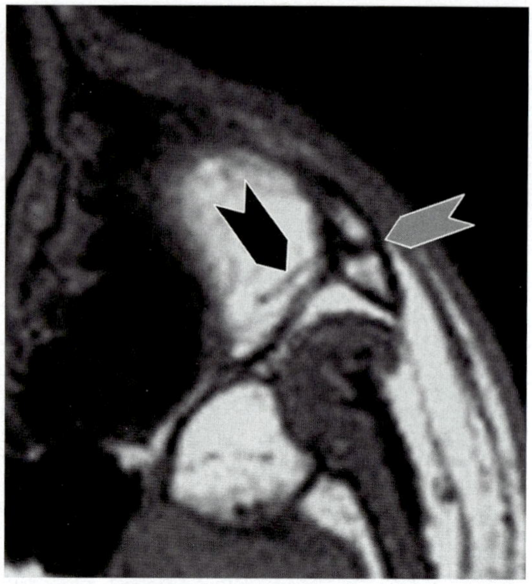

Fig. 25. V2 division, zygomatic nerve—axial T1W image through inferior part of the orbit. The zygomatic nerve leaves the main nerve branch in the pterygopalatine fossa, enters the orbit via the inferior orbital fissure, and can then be seen in the fat near the orbital floor (*black arrowhead*). A zygomaticoorbital and zygomaticotemporal branch of the nerve leave the orbit through foramina with the same name; one of these foramina is visualized (*gray arrowhead*).

the fascicular segment of the sixth nerve course anteroinferiorly through the pontine tegmentum and leave the brainstem anteriorly at the lower border of the pons or bulbopontine sulcus (**Fig. 33**). At this level, separate rootlets can be seen in more than 6% of the cases (**Fig. 34**).

Cisternal segment

This segment crosses the prepontine cistern and follows an antero-lateral-superior course until it reaches the back of the clivus. This segment is best seen in the axial plane on heavily T2W images[26,27] but can also be seen on coronal STIR (**Fig. 35**) and even T1W images. The cisternal segment of this nerve is unique as it represents the only intra-cranial segment of a cranial nerve, which runs upward.

Dorello's canal

The nerves then pierce the dura at the back of the clivus and enter Dorello's canal, which passes through the basilar venous plexus, and is located in a channel between two dural layers. On the T2W images one often sees how CSF can follow

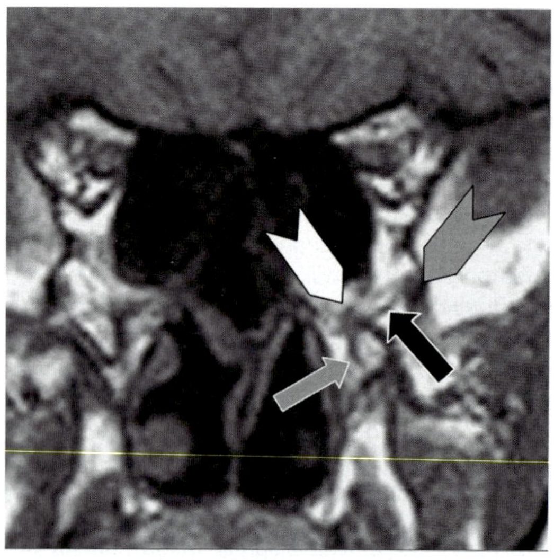

Fig. 26. V2 division, pterygopalatine nerve—2-mm-thick coronal T1W image. A connecting branch or a pterygopalatine nerve (*black arrow*) is connecting the maxillary nerve in the foramen rotundum (*gray arrowhead*) with the pterygopalatine ganglion (*white arrowhead*). The greater palatine nerve (*gray arrow*) emerges from the pterygopalatine ganglion.

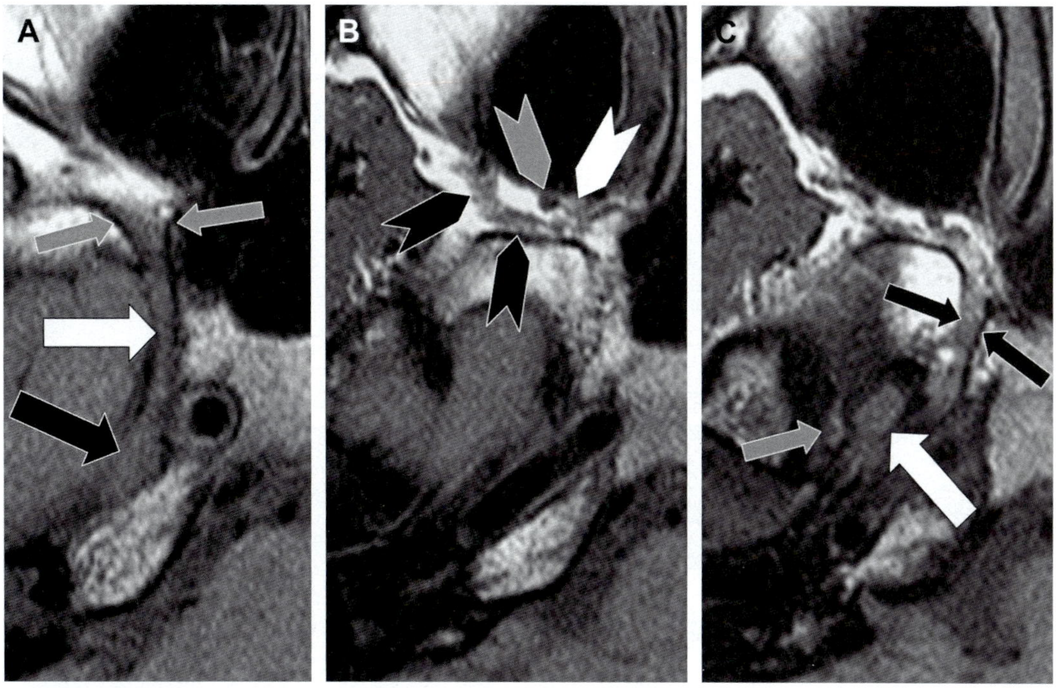

Fig. 27. V2 division—axial high-resolution contrast-enhanced T1W image at the level of the round foramen (*A*) and vidian canal (*C*) and in between (*B*). (*A*) Meckel's cave (*black arrow*), the maxillary nerve in the para-sellar region (*white arrow*), and the cortical bone at the foramen rotundum (*gray arrows*) can be recognized. (*B*) The maxillary nerve continues with a "bayonet" course high in the pterygopalatine fossa (*black arrows*). Pterygopalatine ganglion (*white arrowhead*) and branch of the internal maxillary artery are seen (*gray arrow*). (*C*) The Vidian nerve (*black arrows*) ends in the pterygopalatine ganglion. Also seen are the mandibular nerve in oval foramen (*white arrow*) and middle meningeal artery in spinous foramen (*gray arrow*).

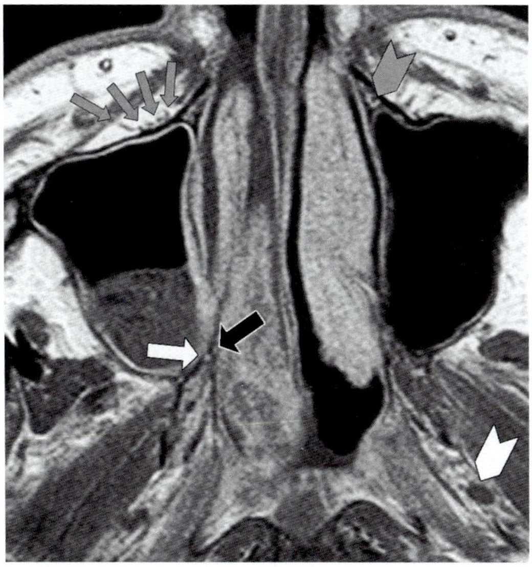

Fig. 28. V2 division, end branches—axial high-resolution T1W image at the level of the inferior turbinates. Shown are the greater (*black arrow*) and lesser (*white arrow*) palatine nerves, the cutaneous end branches of the infraorbital nerve (*gray arrows*), and the superoanterior alveolar branch (*gray arrowhead*), which detaches from the infraorbital nerve under the orbital floor. This alveolar branch then courses in the frontal process of the maxillary bone. The mandibular nerve in the masticator space (*white arrowhead*) is also seen.

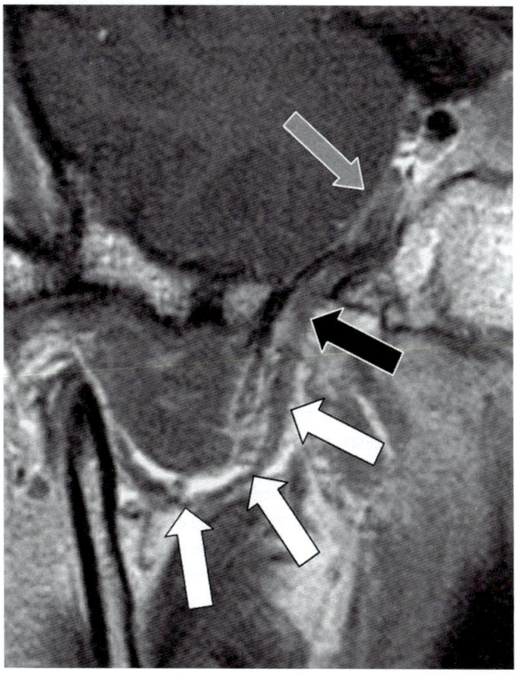

Fig. 29. V3 division, mandibular nerve—coronal T1W image. The mandibular nerve can be seen inside the oval foramen (*black arrow*) and its inferior alveolar branch can be followed toward the mandibular foramen (*white arrows*). Meckel's cave (*gray arrow*) can also be seen.

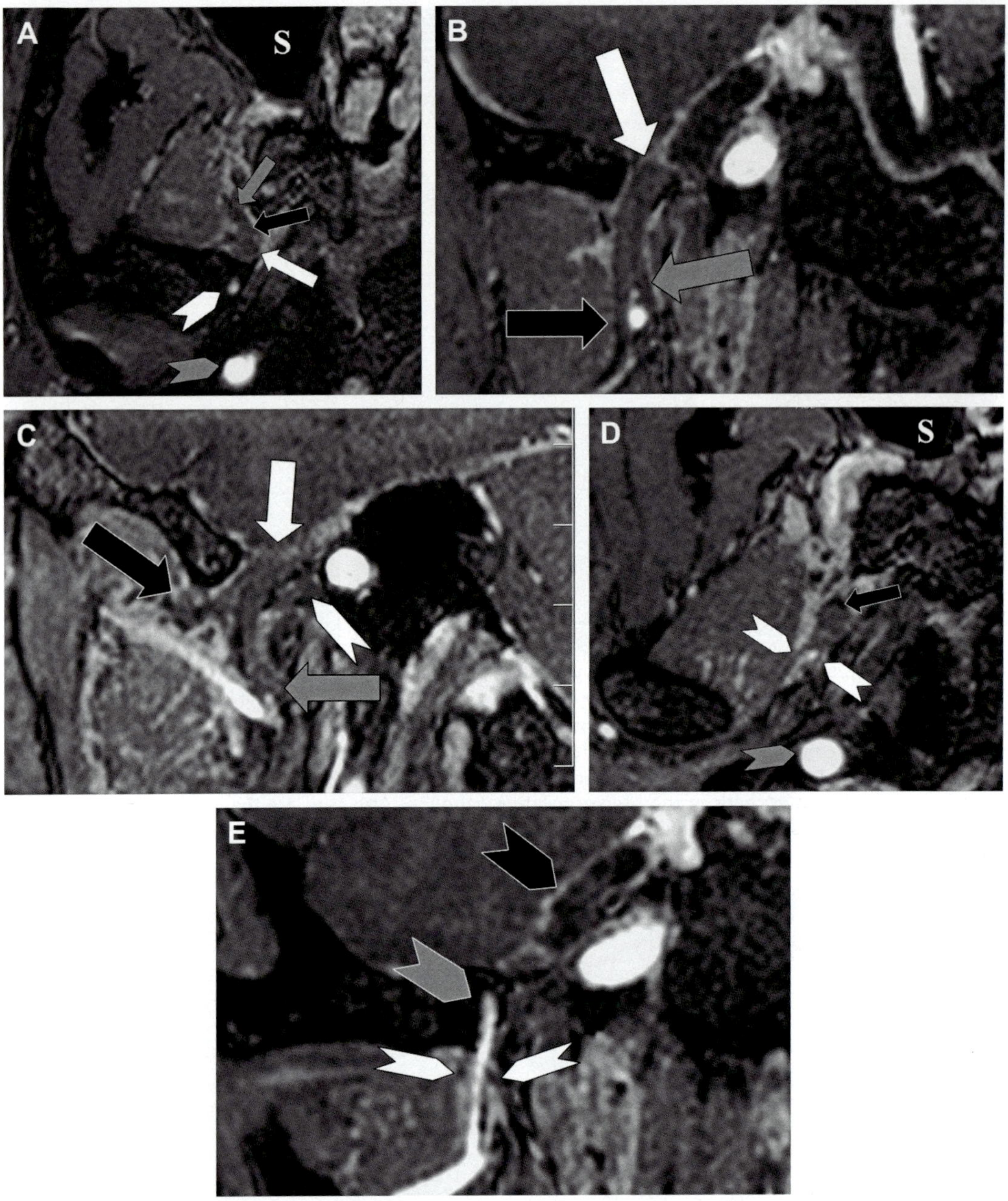

Fig. 30. V3 division, branches of the mandibular nerve—contrast-enhanced T1W 3D-FFE images with extreme high resolution (0.35 mm^3) through the oval foramen region in the axial (*A*), coronal (*B*), and sagittal (*C*) planes and axial (*D*) and coronal (*E*) similar images through the auriculotemporal nerve and the ring it forms around the middle meningeal artery. (*A*) The enhancing venous plexus around the trigeminal nerve just under the skull base makes it possible to distinguish the area of the buccal and anterior deep temporal nerve (*gray arrow*), major mandibular branch (*black arrow*), and the posterior extension of the nerve corresponds to the area of the otic ganglion, auricultotemporal nerve origin and meningeal branch (*white arrow*). The middle meningeal artery (*white arrowhead*) and internal carotid artery (*gray arrowhead*) are also seen. (*B*) The mandibular nerve (*white arrow*) is seen in the oval foramen and divides in a lingual (*gray arrow*) and inferior alveolar (*black arrow*) branch at the level of the internal maxillary artery branch. (*C*) Mandibular nerve in the oval foramen (*white arrow*), temporobuccal nerve (*black arrow*) and major mandibular branch (*gray arrow*), and the region of the auriculotemporal nerve and meningeal branch (*white arrowhead*) are seen. (*D*) Mandibular branch is just under the skull base (*black arrow*). The middle meningeal artery passes through an opening in the auriculotemporal nerve just below the skull base. At that level the hyperintense artery is surrounded by low-signal intensity nerve tissue (*white arrowheads*). The internal carotid artery (*gray arrowhead*) and maxillary sinus (*S*) are also visible. (*E*) Coronal reformatted image shows the enhancing middle meningeal artery even inside the spinous foramen (*gray arrowhead*). The hypointense auriculotemporal nerve, surrounding the artery, can again be seen (*white arrowheads*). Meckel's cave (*black arrowhead*) is also visible.

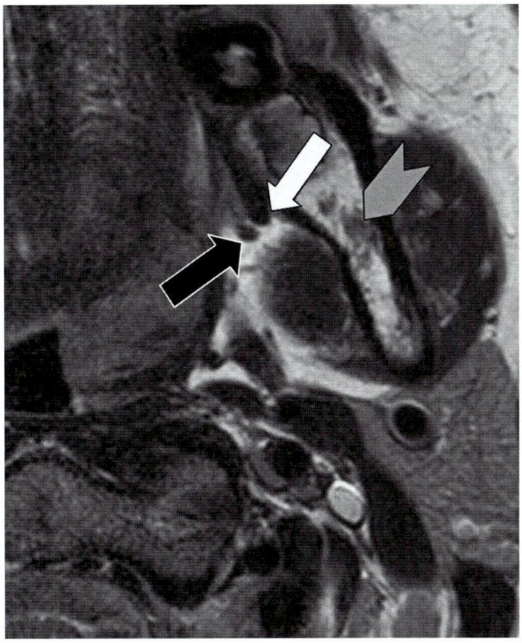

Fig. 31. V3 division, inferior alveolar and lingual nerve—axial T1W image through the retromolar region. The inferior alveolar nerve can be seen in its canal inside the mandible (gray arrowhead). The lingual nerve (black arrow) can always be checked in the pterygomandibular fat pad, located just behind and medial to the posterior free edge of the mylohyoid muscle (white arrow).

the nerve over a variable distance into Dorello's canal (**Fig. 36**).[28] Gadolinium-enhanced Time Of Flight (TOF) MRA images or 3D-FFE images are needed to visualize the sixth nerve as a black spot inside the enhancing venous plexus at the level of Dorello's canal (**Fig. 37**).[29] The segment in Dorello's canal is also called the interdural

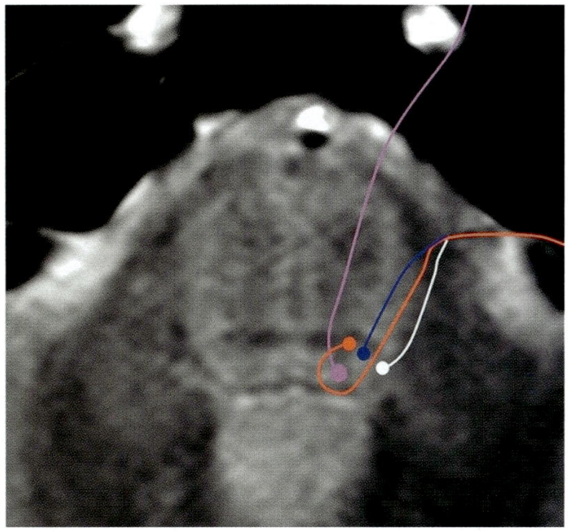

Fig. 33. Abducens nucleus—axial m-FFE image through the mid pons. The nucleus lies close to the fourth ventricle (*purple dot*). The axons of the facial nerve (*orange line*), which originate in the motor nucleus of the facial nerve (*orange dot*) loop posteriorly around the abducens nucleus and create an impression on the fourth ventricle, "the facial colliculus," and then travel lateral to leave the brainstem at the inferior border of the pons. The fascicular segment of the abducens nerve (*purple line*) continues anteroinferiorly to exit the brainstem at the bulbopontine sulcus. Shown are the superior salivary nucleus (*blue dot*), parasympathetic fibers to the salivary glands and lacrimal gland (*blue line*), and solitary tract nucleus (*white dot*) receiving sensory information arriving via the geniculate ganglion (*white line*). Parasympathetic and sensory information travel in the nervus intermedius.

segment. After passing through the basilar venous plexus, the sixth nerve turns over the petrous apex and enters the cavernous sinus in the area just above Meckel's cave.

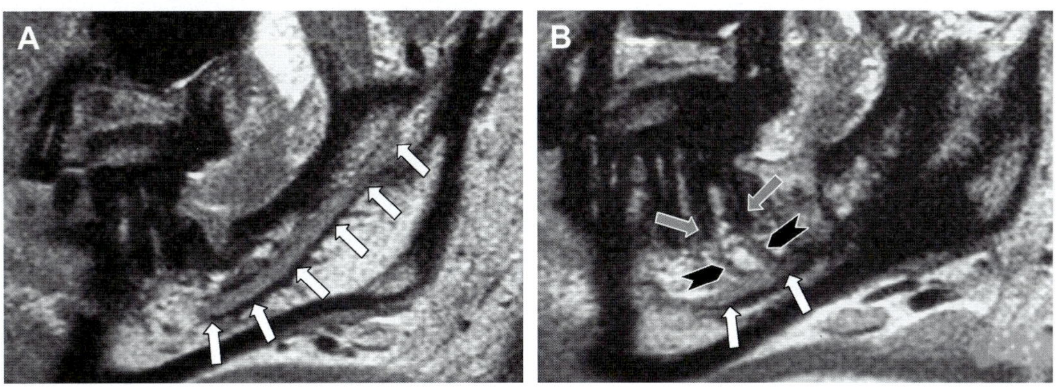

Fig. 32. V3 division, inferior alveolar nerve—parasagittal T1W images through the angle and body of the mandible. (*A*) The inferior alveolar nerve (*white arrows*) is seen in its canal. (*B*) Small nerves for the innervation of the above-lying teeth can be recognized on an adjacent slice (*black arrowheads*). Inferior alveolar nerve (*white arrows*) and roots of teeth (*gray arrows*) are seen.

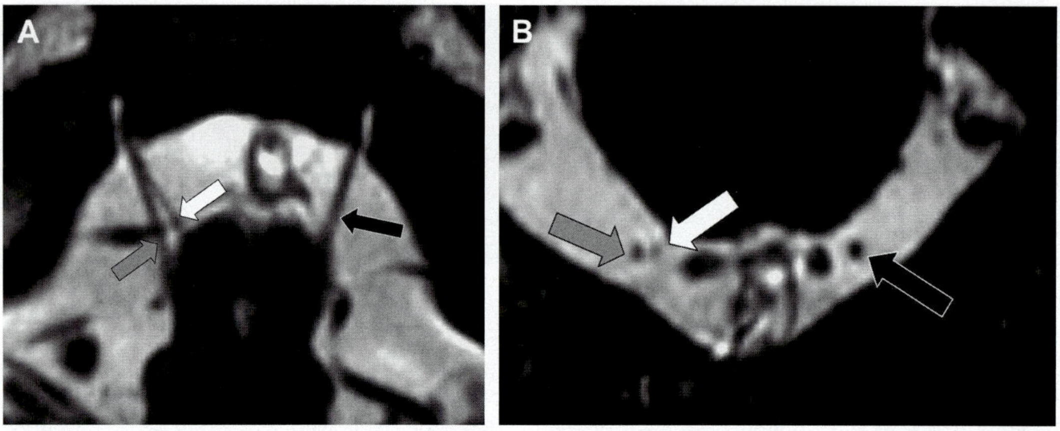

Fig. 34. Cisternal segment of the abducens nerve—para-axial (*A*) and coronal (*B*) b-FFE image of a double root nerve on the right and a normal nerve on the left. (*A*) The complete cisternal segment is seen on the left side on this T2W image (*black arrow*) until the nerve pierces the dura at the back of the clivus. Double root (*gray and white arrow*) abducens nerve on the right side, both roots fuse before the nerve eventually pierces the dura. (*B*) Coronal reformatted image showing both roots of the right abducens nerve (*gray and white arrow*) and the single normal root of the left abducens nerve (*black arrow*).

Cavernous segment

The nerve then courses within the cavernous sinus proper, medial to the ophthalmic branch of the trigeminal nerve (see **Fig. 15**), while all the other cranial nerves are located in the lateral wall of the cavernous sinus.

Intra-orbital segment

The nerve eventually reaches the SOF where the extra-cranial segment continues through the annulus of Zinn to finally reach the lateral rectus muscle. The cavernous and extra-axial segments are best seen on gadolinium-enhanced high-resolution T1W images (see **Fig. 15**).

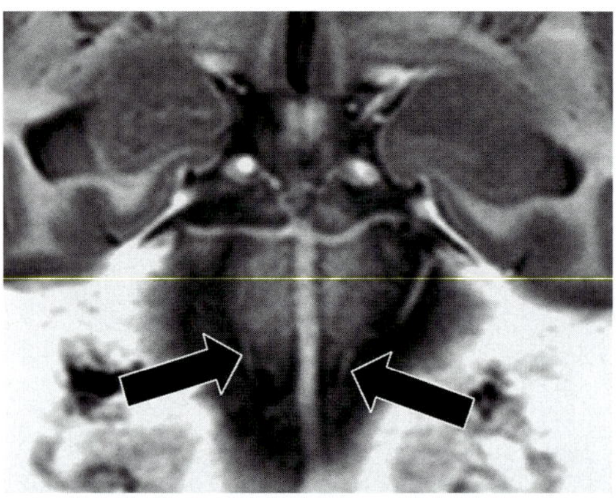

Fig. 35. Cisternal segment—coronal inversion recovery image. The proximal cisternal segments are typically seen as two ascending linear structures just lateral to the inferior pons (*black arrows*).

The Facial Nerve or Cranial Nerve VII

Facial nerve nuclei—intra-axial segment

The facial nerve consists of a motor (facial nerve proper) and sensory root (nervus intermedius) and has motor, sensory, and parasympathetic functions. The facial nerve proper supplies the muscles of facial expression, the stapedius and stylohyoid muscles, and the posterior belly of the

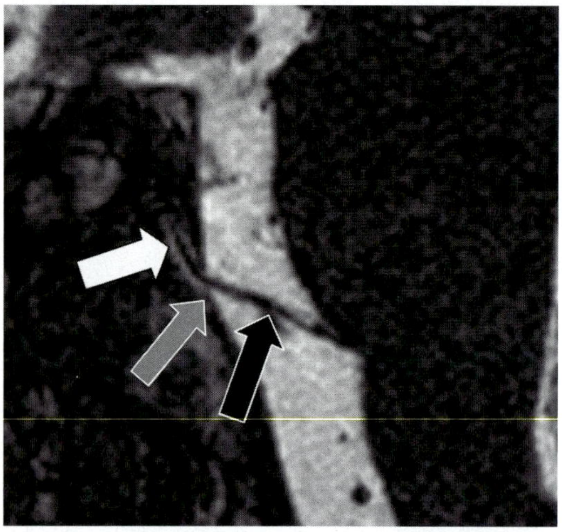

Fig. 36. Cisternal segment of the sixth nerve and Dorello's canal—sagittal reformatted high resolution b-FFE image. The cisternal segment (*black arrow*) can be followed from the inferior border of the pons to the back of the clivus where the nerve pierces the dura (*gray arrow*). Frequently CSF follows the nerve in Dorello's canal over a variable distance (*white arrow*).

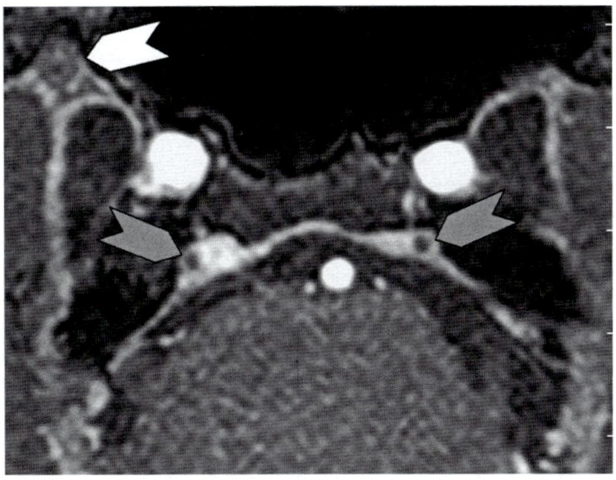

Fig. 37. Dorello's canal or interdural segment of the sixth nerve—axial high-resolution contrast-enhanced 3D-FFE image through the basilar venous plexus. Once the nerve is completely surrounded by the venous plexus the nerves can only be visualized after contrast administration. The nerves can then be seen as gray structures (*gray arrowheads*) surrounded by the enhancing high signal intensity plexus. Mandibular nerve emerges from the anteroinferior aspect of the Gasserian ganglion (*white arrowhead*).

digastric muscle. Its nucleus is located anterolateral in the tegmen of the lower pons.

The nerve then loops around the nucleus of the abducens nerve, creating the facial colliculus, a protrusion of the brainstem in the floor of the fourth ventricle. The nerve continues anterolaterally and exits the brainstem together with the intermediate nerve at the lower border of the pons (see **Fig. 33**). Sensory information, skin sensation of the ear, and taste sensation of the anterior two thirds of the tongue arrive via the geniculate ganglion in the nucleus solitarius, located posterolateral to the motor nucleus. The parasympathetic fibers, which supply the submandibular, sublingual, and lacrimal glands, have their origin in the superior salivary nucleus.

Cisternal segment

The cisternal segment starts once both nerves leave the brainstem and cross the cerebellopontine angle (CPA); they are best seen on heavily T2W images (**Fig. 38**).[30] The sensory and parasympathetic fibers travel in the nervus intermedius, which leaves the brainstem just posterior to the facial nerve proper.

Intratemporal segment

The facial nerve continues in the anterosuperior part of the internal auditory canal (IAC) (see **Fig. 38**). At the fundus of the IAC, the facial nerve enters the labyrinthine part of the facial nerve canal where the intratemporal segment starts.[16,31] On T2W images with very high resolution, especially at 3 Tesla, the facial nerve proper and intermedius nerve can be distinguished in the CPA and IAC with increasing frequency (**Fig. 39**).

The labyrinthine intratemporal segment turns anterior and reaches the geniculate ganglion. The greater superficial petrosal nerve (GSPN), carrying the parasympathetic fibers for lacrimation, is a branch that leaves the geniculate ganglion anteriorly. The canal for the GSPN can be short, long, or split (**Fig. 40**). The facial nerve proper continues posteriorly in the tympanic segment of the facial nerve canal, passes under the lateral semicircular canal, and then turns inferiorly at the level of the posterior genu (see **Fig. 40**; **Figs. 41 and 42**). The mastoid segment of the facial nerve continues inferiorly posterior to the pyramid eminence and external auditory canal (EAC) (see **Fig. 42**; **Fig. 43**) and provides motor innervation for the stapedius muscle (nerve or nerve canal—not visible on MR and CT) and also provides sensory fibers for taste from the anterior two thirds of the tongue via the chorda tympani. The chorda tympani and its canal can be seen just above the stylomastoid foramen and then courses from the mastoid segment of the facial nerve to the drum, where the nerve can again be seen on CT in a normally aerated middle ear (see **Fig. 43**). The normal chorda tympani is today not yet visible on MR. The chorda tympani then joins the lingual nerve (mandibular nerve branch) high in the masticator space.

Extracranial segment

Once the nerve leaves the stylomastoid foramen and enters the posterior parotid gland it is best visualized on high-resolution axial T1W images (**Fig. 44**). Soon the nerve is no longer visible but its course can be presumed, as it normally courses just lateral to the retromandibular vein. Nevertheless, if needed, even the intraparotid main branch can be followed over several centimeters when a microscopic coil and strong gradients are used (**Fig. 44**C).[32] Finally, the nerve divides in motor end branches supplying the muscles of facial expression, platysma, buccinator, stylohyoid, occipitalis muscles, and the posterior belly of the digastric muscle.

The Vestibulocochlear Nerve or Cranial Nerve VIII

The vestibulocochlear nerve is composed of a cochlear and vestibular nerve; both are sensory. Bipolar neurons connect the neuroepithelial cells in the cochlea and vestibular labyrinth with the nuclei in the brainstem and auditory and vestibular pathways.

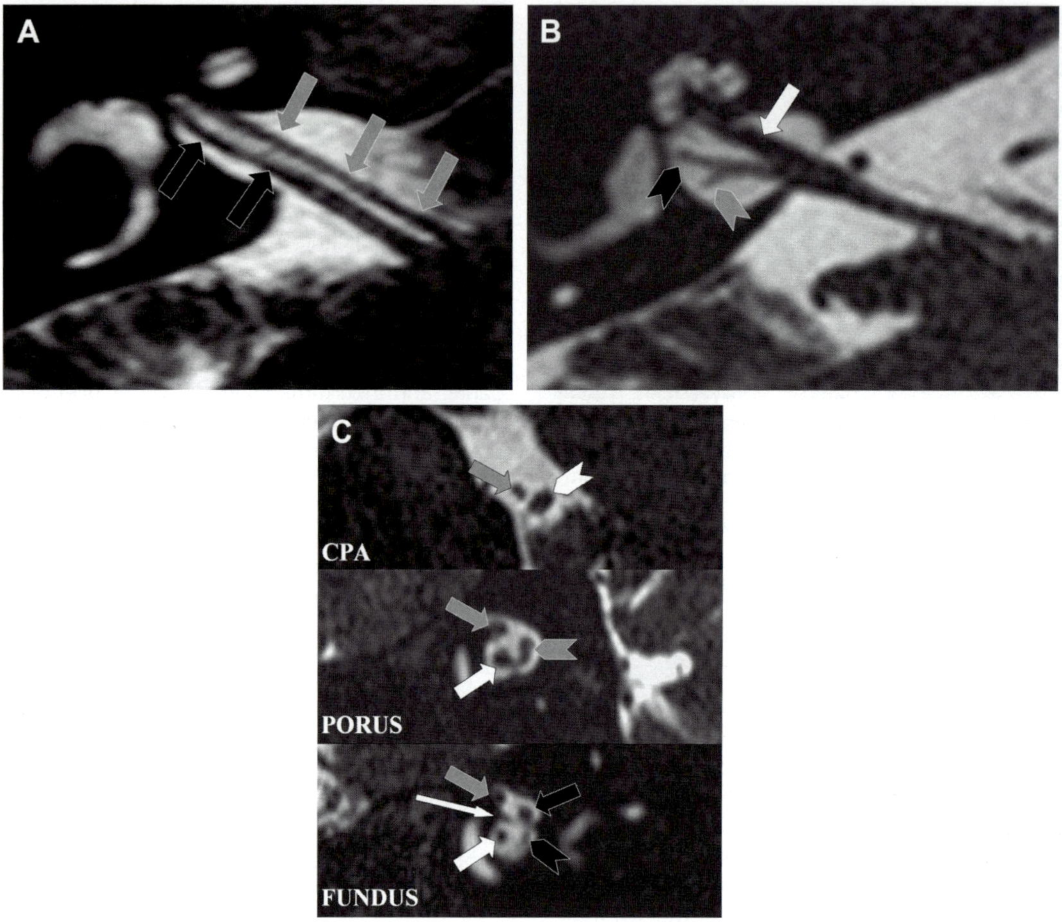

Fig. 38. Cisternal and intratemporal IAC segment of the facial nerve—axial high-resolution DRIVE images through the upper (*A*) and lower (*B*) part of the IAC and reformatted images (*C*) made perpendicular to the course of the facial and eighth nerve at the level of the CPA, PORUS, and FUNDUS of the IAC. (*A*) The facial nerve (*gray arrows*) and superior vestibular branch of the eighth nerve (*black arrows*) run parallel high in the IAC. (*B*) Near the floor of the IAC the VIII nerve bifurcates in an anterior cochlear branch (*white arrow*) and posterior inferior vestibular branch (*black arrowhead*). The posterior ampullar nerve (*gray arrowhead*) detaches from the inferior vestibular branch near the fundus of the IAC. (*C*) In the CPA the vestibulocochlear nerve (*white arrowhead*) is at least twice as thick as the facial nerve (*gray arrow*); the facial nerve is positioned more anteriorly. At the PORUS the vestibulocochlear nerve splits in a cochlear branch (*white arrow*) and a common vestibular branch (*gray arrowhead*). The facial nerve is found in the superoanterior quadrant of the IAC (*gray arrow*). Near the FUNDUS the common vestibular nerve divides in a superior (*black arrow*) and inferior (*black arrowhead*) vestibular branch. The falciform crest (*long white arrow*) can be seen as a black line between the facial nerve above (*gray arrow*) and the cochlear branch below (*white arrow*).

The cochlear nerve

Spiral ganglion The bipolar neurons are located in the spiral ganglion within the modiolus of the cochlea. The peripheral fibers are connected to the organ of Corti in the scala media of the cochlea. They leave the osseous spiral lamina at the habenula perforata where they are situated very close to the scala tympani. This explains why most of the schwannomas developing on these peripheral fibers develop in the scala tympani.[33]

Cochlear nerve in IAC and CPA The central fibers join to form the cochlear nerve, which enters the IAC through an opening in the anteroinferior part of the fundus of the IAC called the "cochlear aperture." This aperture has a maximum diameter of 2 mm and will be absent or small when the cochlear nerve is hypoplastic or absent. The cochlear nerve continues in the anteroinferior quadrant of the IAC and is joined by the superior and inferior vestibular nerve near the porus acusticus. From

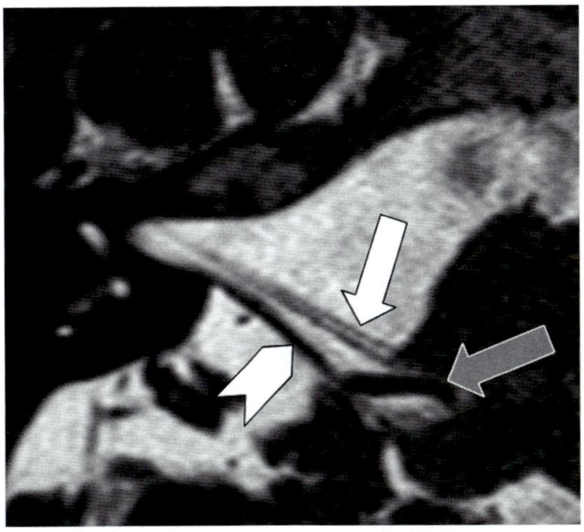

Fig. 39. Intermediate nerve—axial DRIVE image at 3 Tesla. The two roots of the facial nerve, facial nerve proper and intermediate nerve (posterior root), can be seen as two parallel nerves in the CPA (*white arrow*). Also visible are the vestibulocochlear nerve (*white arrowhead*) and posterior inferior cerebellar artery (*gray arrow*).

that point on the nerve is called the vestibulocochlear nerve or cranial nerve 8 and crosses the CPA posterior to the facial nerve (see **Figs. 38 and 39**).[34]

Cochlear nuclei The nerve enters the brainstem at the lateral pontomedullary junction where the nerve splits and ends in a dorsal and ventral cochlear nucleus (**Fig. 45**).

The vestibular nerve

Ganglion of Scarpa–maculae–cristae The bipolar neurons of the vestibular nerve are located in the ganglion of Scarpa. The peripheral fibers connect the maculae in the utricule (**Fig. 46**) and saccule (the static labyrinth which signals head position) and the three cristae in the three ampullae of the semicircular canals (the dynamic labyrinth which signals head movement) (**Fig. 47**) with the four vestibular nuclei in the brainstem. Multiple fibers pass the foramina in the cribriform plate in the fundus of the IAC and form the superior and inferior vestibular nerves, which course in the posterosuperior and posteroinferior quadrant of the IAC respectively. At this site, the superior and inferior vestibular nerve are separated from one another by the bony falciform crest (**Fig. 38**C), the superior vestibular nerve is separated from the facial nerve by the bony Bill bar. The ganglion of Scarpa can today often be seen as a thickening on the nerves near the fundus of the IAC (**Fig. 48**). The posterior ampullar nerve or singular nerve has its own canal and joins the inferior vestibular nerve in the IAC, some millimeters medial to the fundus of the IAC. Visualization of this nerve branch can be used as quality control and indicates high-quality imaging without movement artifacts (**Fig. 38**B). The superior and inferior vestibular nerves join to form a single vestibular nerve near the porus acusticus. A little more medially toward the porus acusticus the vestibular nerve will join with the cochlear nerve, forming the vestibulocochlear nerve.[30,34] The vestibular fibers follow this nerve in the CPA and enter the brainstem (see above).

The number of fibers in the facial nerve and vestibulocochlear nerve inside the CPA and IAC is also of particular interest. Normally the number of fibers in the facial nerve near the fundus of the IAC and near the brainstem and the number of fibers in the superior vestibular–inferior vestibular–cochlear nerve together and the vestibulocochlear nerve near the brainstem must be the same. Studies showed that this is not the case and that connecting fibers exist between the facial and vestibular nerves, causing a decrease in the number of facial nerve fibers and an increase in the vestibulocochlear fibers toward the brainstem. These connecting fibers can today often be visualized on high resolution images made at 3 Tesla (**Fig. 49**).

Vestibular nuclei Ascending and descending vestibular branches mainly connect with the four vestibular nuclei: lateral, medial, superior, and inferior nucleus. These nuclei are located in the lower pons along the lateral floor of the fourth ventricle (see **Fig. 45**). Axons from the nuclei have connections with many central structures but this is beyond the scope of this article.

The Glossopharyngeal Nerve or Cranial Nerve IX

Glossopharyngeal nuclei—intra-axial segment

The glossopharyngeal nerve has many functions and its nuclei are located in the upper and middle medulla. It innervates the stylopharyngeus muscle and the motor fibers originate in the nucleus ambiguus. This motor nucleus is shared by cranial nerves IX, X, and XI. Taste fibers from the posterior one third of the tongue follow the nerve and end in the solitary tract nucleus. Sensory information from the pharynx, tongue base, soft palate, and tympanic membrane arrives in the trigeminal spinal nucleus via sensory fibers of the ninth nerve. Parasympathetic fibers to the parotid gland have their origin in the inferior salivatory nucleus. Finally the ninth nerve

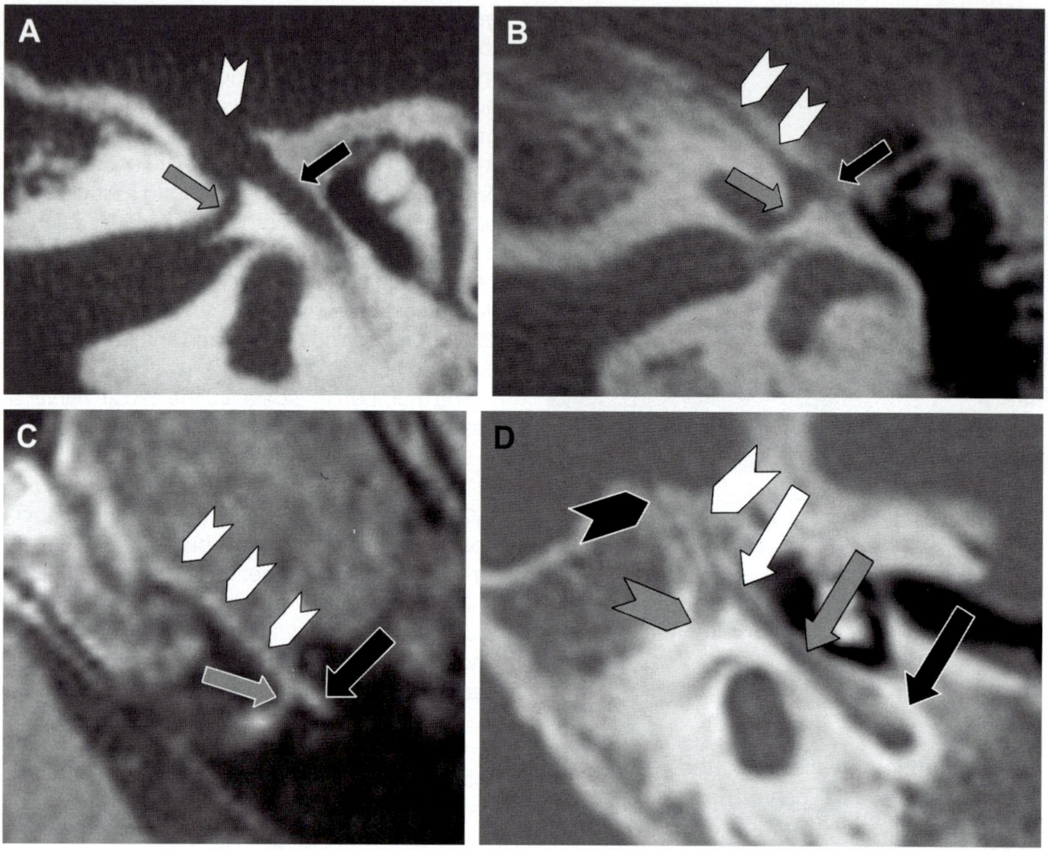

Fig. 40. Labyrinthine segment, GSPN—axial CT at the level of the geniculate ganglion in a patient with a short/absent GSPN canal (*A*), long GSPN canal (*B*) and in a patient where the canals of the greater and lesser superficial petrosal nerves could be distinguished (*D*) and axial contrast-enhanced T1W image through the facial nerve and GSPN in a patient with viral inflammation (*C*). (*A*) The canal of the labyrinthine segment (*gray arrow*) can be followed to the fossa for the geniculate ganglion. The hiatus of Fallopius, the opening where the GSPN leaves the temporal bone and enters the middle cranial fossa, is wide open (*white arrowhead*). Tympanic segment of the facial nerve canal (*black arrow*) is also seen. (*B*) Example of a long canal for the GSPN with a narrow hiatus of Fallopius (*white arrowheads*). Labyrinthine (*gray arrow*) and tympanic (*black arrow*) segment of the intratemporal facial nerve canal are seen. (*C*) The viral infection causes enhancement of the labyrinthine (*gray arrow*) and tympanic (*black arrow*) segment of the intratemporal facial nerve and also of the complete course of the GSPN, in its canal and along the superolateral border of the internal carotid artery (*white arrowheads*). (*D*) Small canals for the greater (*black arrowhead*) and lesser (*white arrowhead*) superficial petrosal nerves are seen, as are labyrinthine (*gray arrowhead*) and tympanic (*gray arrow*) segments of the facial nerve canal, geniculate ganglion fossa (*white arrow*), and posterior genu (*black arrow*).

also has a viscerosensory function to the carotid body and sinus (solitary tract nucleus) (**Fig. 50**).

Cisternal segment

The ninth nerve leaves the brainstem in the posterolateral sulcus or post-olivary sulcus, posterior to the medullary olive, and courses through the basal cistern in an anterolateral direction together with the vagus nerve and bulbar portion of the accessory nerve, which are located just caudal to the glossopharyngeal nerve. The three nerves are difficult to distinguish from one another but the lateral convexity of the pons and medulla, the thickness of the nerves, and MR imaging with very high resolution (0.35 mm^3) help to distinguish them on heavily T2W images (**Fig. 51**).[35,36]

Skull base segment

The ninth nerve then enters the pars nervosa of the jugular foramen where its superior and inferior ganglia are located as well. Cranial nerve X and XI travel in a common sheath through the pars vascularis of the jugular foramen. These nerves can only be distinguished inside the jugular foramen on axial and reformatted coronal high-resolution

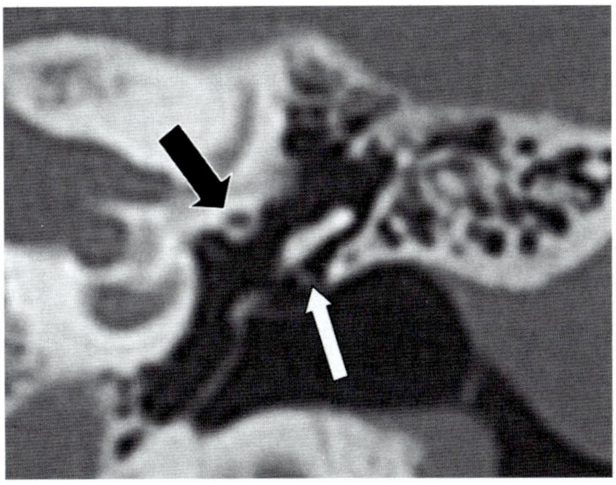

Fig. 41. Chorda tympani and tympanic segment of the facial nerve canal—coronal CT image through middle ear. The tympanic segment can be seen under the lateral semicircular canal (*black arrow*). The chorda tympani (*white arrow*) is see just medial to the tympanic membrane and close to the neck of the malleus and long process of the incus.

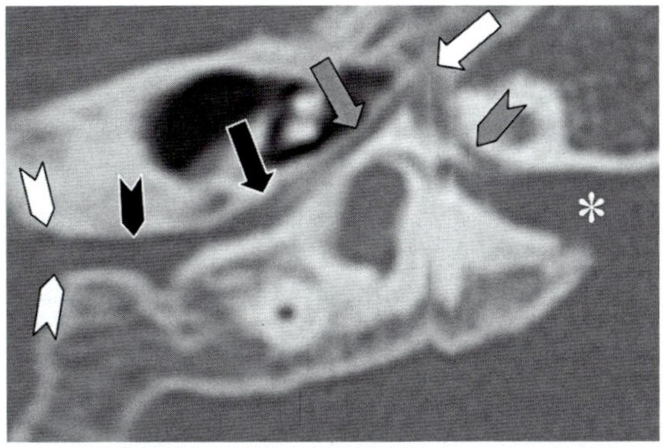

Fig. 42. Intratemporal facial nerve canal—curved reformatted CT image. Shown are IAC (*), labyrinthine segment (*gray arrowhead*), geniculate ganglion fossa (*white arrow*), tympanic segment (*gray arrow*), posterior genu (*black arrow*), mastoid segment (*black arrowhead*), and stylomastoid foramen (*white arrowheads*).

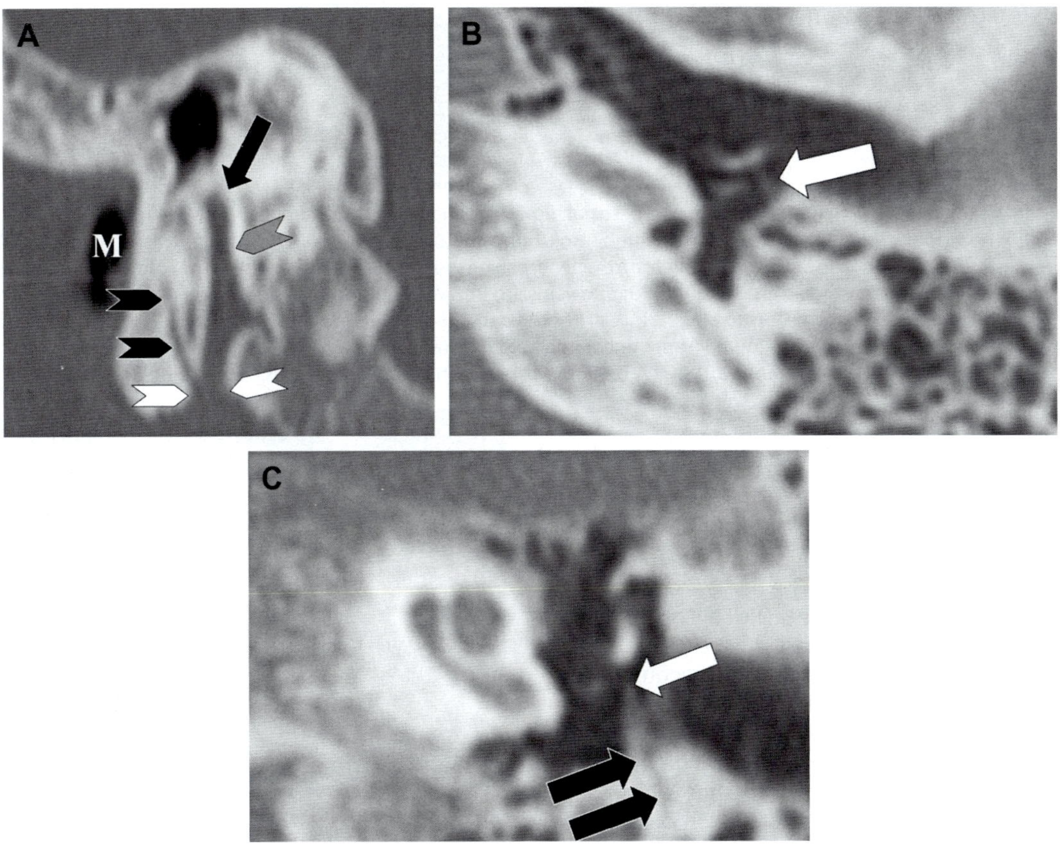

Fig. 43. Chorda tympani canal and nerve—coronal (*A*), axial (*B*), and para-axial reformatted (*C*) CT images. (*A*) The chorda tympani canal (*black arrowheads*) leaves the mastoid segment of the facial nerve canal (*gray arrowhead*) close to the stylomastoid foramen (*white arrowheads*). The canal then runs toward the posterior wall of the external auditory canal (M). Posterior genu of the facial nerve canal (*black arrow*). (*B*) Chorda tympani (*white arrow*) courses just deep to the tympanic membrane and near the neck of the malleus. (*C*) Reformatted image through the very thin distal chorda tympani canal (*black arrows*) with the nerve leaving the canal and entering the middle ear cavity (*white arrow*).

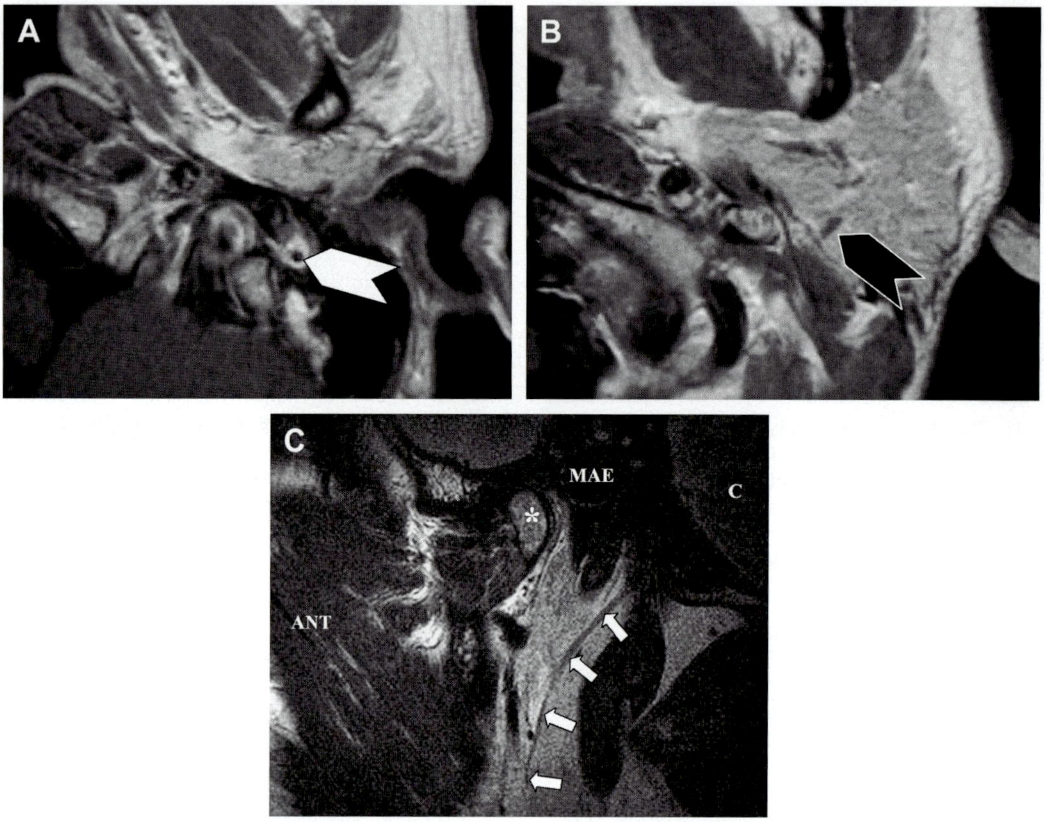

Fig. 44. Extracranial segment of the facial nerve—axial high-resolution contrast-enhanced T1W images at (*A*) and below (*B*) the stylomastoid foramen and sagittal high resolution TSE T2W image acquired with a microscopic coil (*C*). (*A*) The mastoid segment of the facial nerve (*white arrowhead*) can be seen as a black spot in the center of the stylomastoid foramen, surrounded by high signal intensity fat and veins. (*B*) Below the stylomastoid foramen the extracranial segment courses anteriorly and enters the posterior part of the parotid gland (*black arrowhead*). (*C*) The main intraparotid facial nerve branch can be followed from the stylomastoid foramen into the parotid gland over a distance of more than 3 cm (*white arrows*). ANT, anterior; C, cerebellum; MAE, externa auditory meatus; *, mandibular condyle.

gadolinium-enhanced FFE or TOF images (see **Fig. 5**; **Fig. 52**).

Extracranial segment and branches

The ninth nerve exits the jugular foramen and enters in the carotid space. The nerve then turns lateral to the carotid artery and stylopharyngeal muscle and continues lateral to the palatal tonsil area to finally end in the posterior sublingual space in the floor of the mouth as the lingual branch where it innervates the posterior one third of the tongue (taste and sensory). Other side branches of the extracranial segment are the pharyngeal branches (sensation from posterior oropharynx and soft palate), sinus nerve (parasympathetic supply to carotid body and sinus), stylopharyngeus branch (motor innervation to the stylopharyngeus muscle), and tympanic branch or Jacobson nerve. Jacobson nerve has its origin in the inferior sensory ganglion of the ninth nerve in the jugular foramen and passes through the

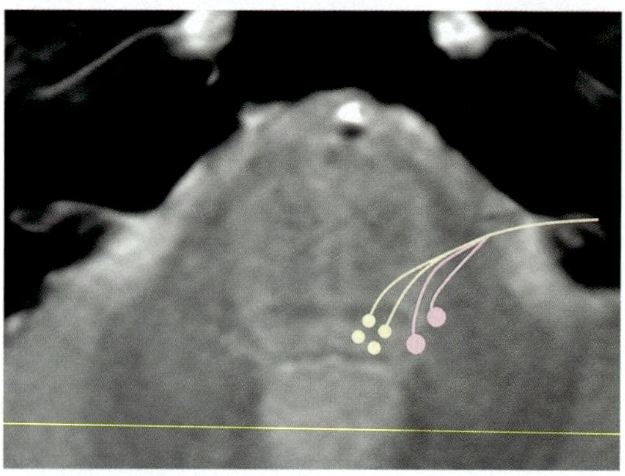

Fig. 45. Cochlear and vestibular nuclei—axial m-FFE image at the level of the lower pons. The dorsal and ventral cochlear nucleus (*pink dots*) are located in the lower pons, anterolateral to the inferior cerebellar peduncle. The four vestibular nuclei are located more medially, along the lateral floor of the fourth ventricle (*yellow dots*). The fascicular segments of the cochlear (*pink lines*) and vestibular nerves (*yellow lines*) join at the lateral border of the lower pons to form the vestibulocochlear nerve.

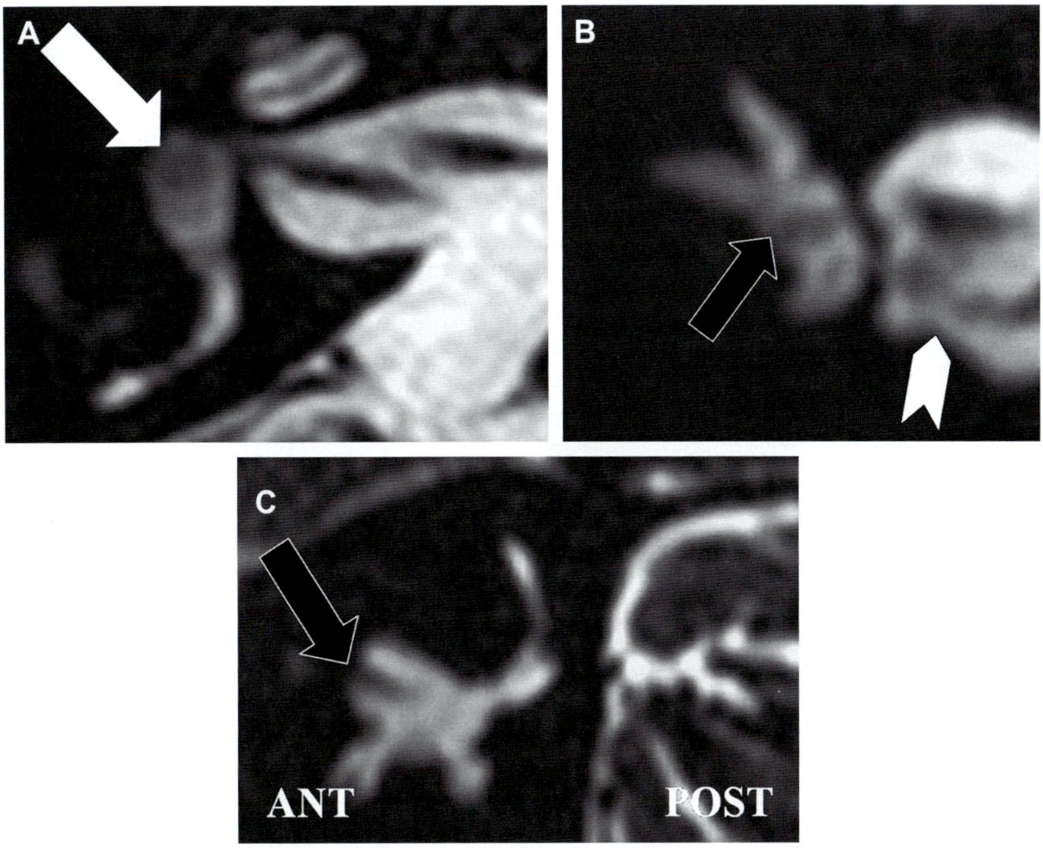

Fig. 46. Macula utriculi—axial DRIVE image through the right vestibule (*A*) and sagittal (*B*) and coronal (*C*) reformatted image. (*A*) An ovoid black structure can be seen on a 0.35-mm-thick DRIVE image through the anterior right vestibule: the macula of the utricle (*white arrow*). (*B*) On the coronal image the macula is seen as a horizontal hypointense linear structure in the lateral part of the utricle (*black arrow*). The IAC (*white arrowhead*) is seen. (*C*) The macula utriculi is seen as a horizontal low intensity line attached to the anterior wall of the utricle on coronal images (*black arrow*). ANT, anterior; POST, posterior.

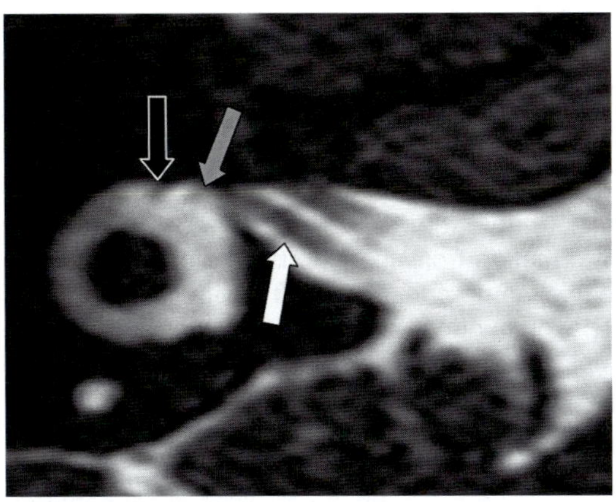

Fig. 47. Crista ampullaris and ampullar nerves—axial DRIVE image through IAC and lateral semicircular canal. The superior vestibular branch of the eighth nerve (*white arrow*) receives fibers from the superior ampullar nerve (*gray arrow*) and the area of the crista and corresponding ampullar nerve of the lateral semicircular canal (*black arrow*).

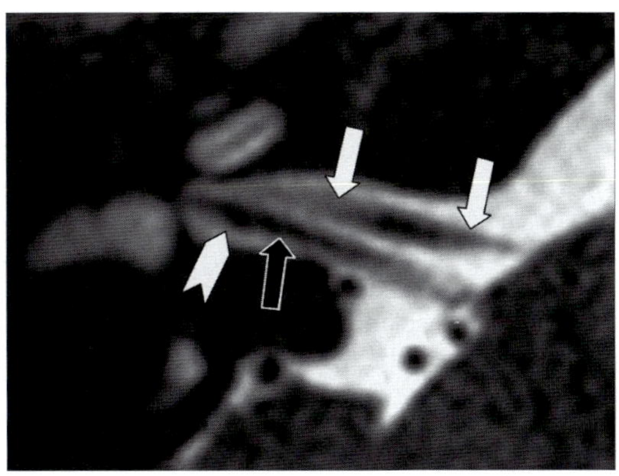

Fig. 48. Ganglion of Scarpa—high-resolution axial DRIVE image through the IAC fundus made at 3 Tesla. A subtle thickening can often be seen on the vestibular nerves in the region where the common vestibular branch splits into a superior and inferior branch. This thickening corresponds with the ganglion of Scarpa (*white arrowhead*). Also visible are the superior vestibular branch (*black arrow*) and facial nerve (*white arrows*).

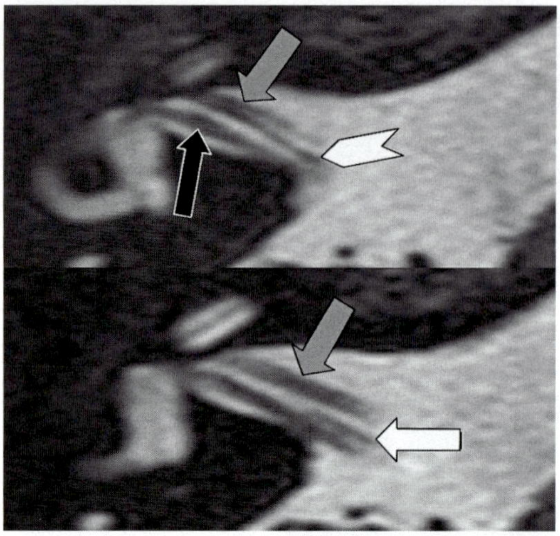

Fig. 49. Connecting fibers between facial and vestibular nerve—high resolution axial DRIVE images made at 3 Tesla. Connecting fibers (*white arrowhead*) are leaving the facial nerve (*gray arrows*) near the fundus of the IAC. These fibers run toward the superior vestibular branch of the eighth nerve (*black arrow*). These fibers join the vestibular branch in the CPA (*white arrow*).

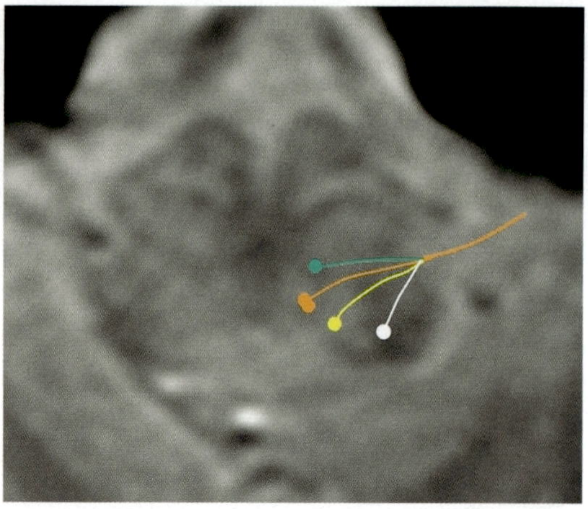

Fig. 50. Glossopharyngeal nuclei, intra-axial segment—axial m-FFE through upper/middle medulla. The nucleus ambiguus (*blue dot*), inferior salivatory nucleus (*orange dot*), solitary tract nucleus (*yellow dot*), spinal nucleus of the trigeminal nerve (*white dot*), and their corresponding fascicular nerve segments (*colored lines*) are located posteriorly in the medulla.

inferior tympanic canaliculus into the middle ear where the nerve fans open on the promontory (**Fig. 53**). The Jacobson nerve carries sensory information from the middle ear and is parasympathetic to the parotid gland.[4,37]

The Vagus Nerve or Cranial Nerve X

Vagal nuclei—intra-axial segment

The vagus nerve is a parasympathetic nerve supplying the head and neck region and thoracic and abdominal viscera, the parasympathetic fibers project from the dorsal vagal nucleus. It also has a motor function to the soft palate, pharyngeal constrictor muscle, larynx, and palatoglossus muscle of the tongue and these fibers originate in the nucleus ambiguus. It carries visceral sensory information from the esophagus, larynx, trachea, and thoracic and abdominal viscera, which terminate in the dorsal vagal nucleus. The tenth nerve also receives taste from the epiglottis, which is directed to the solitary tract nucleus. The nerve is also sensory to the tympanic membrane, EAC, and external ear. This information arrives in the spinal nucleus of the trigeminal nerve (**Fig. 54**).[2,3]

Cisternal segment

The vagus nerve exits the brainstem just below the ninth nerve and courses with this nerve through the basal cistern (see **Fig. 51**).[38]

Skull base segment

Its course in the jugular foramen was also already described together with the glossopharyngeal nerve. The superior vagal ganglion is also located in the jugular foramen; the inferior vagal ganglion is located just below the skull base. The nerve can be seen in the jugular foramen on contrast-enhanced FFE or TOF images (**Fig. 55**).

Extracranial segment and branches

The vagal nerve then follows the posterolateral wall of the internal carotid artery down to the anterior wall of the carotid arch on the left and the anterior wall of the subclavian artery on the right (**Fig. 56**).

The first branch of the ninth nerve, Arnold nerve or auricular branch, leaves the nerve inside the jugular foramen and has its origin in the superior vagal ganglion, travels through the mastoid canaliculus, and reaches the mastoid segment of the facial nerve (**Fig. 57**). This nerve carries sensory information from the external surface of the tympanic membrane, EAC, and external ear centrally. The pharyngeal branches exit the vagus nerve just below the skull base and are responsible for the motor innervation of the soft palate and pharyngeal constrictor muscles and receive sensory information from the epiglottis, trachea, and esophagus. The superior laryngeal nerve divides into a sensory internal branch transmitting sensory information from the hypopharynx, larynx, and true vocal cords and a motor external branch supplying the inferior constrictor muscle and cricothyroid muscle. The recurrent laryngeal nerve ascends in the tracheoesophageal groove

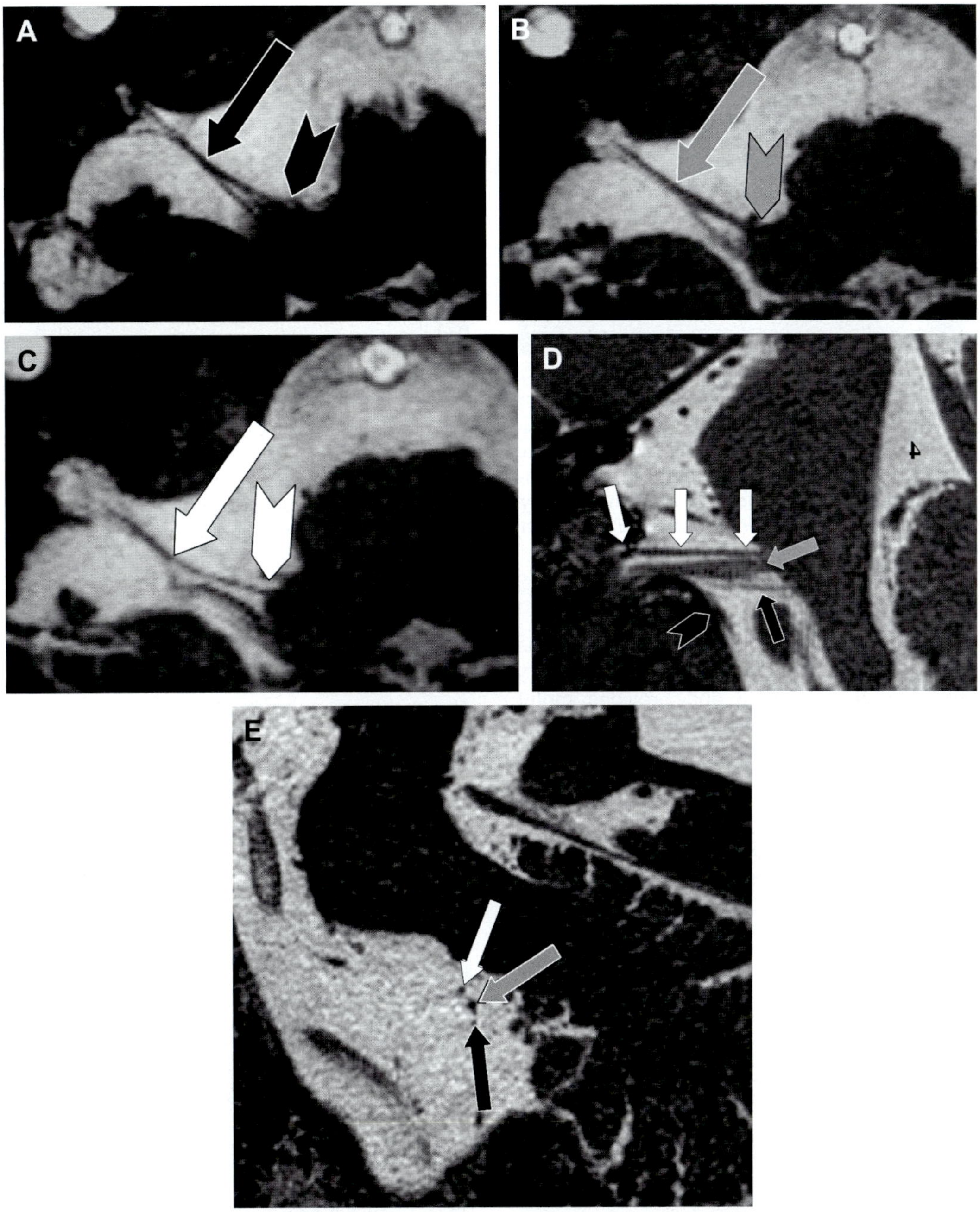

Fig. 51. Cisternal segment—axial 0.6-mm DRIVE images through the cisternal segment of nerve IX (*A*), X (*B*), and XI (*C*) and para-coronal (*D*) and para-sagittal (*E*) 0.35-mm-thick reformatted b-FFE images. (*A*) At the transition area pons-medulla the brainstem has still a pronounced lateral protrusion (*black arrowhead*), indicating the place where the ninth nerve crosses the basal cistern (*black arrow*). (*B*) The lateral protrusion of the upper medulla is less pronounced (*gray arrowhead*) at the level where the tenth nerve (*gray arrow*), the thickest of the three, exits the brainstem. (*C*) There is no longer a clear lateral protrusion of the upper/middle medulla (*white arrowhead*) at the level where the smallest of the three nerves, the bulbar cisternal segment (*white arrow*) crosses the basal cistern. (*D*) The complete cisternal segment of the glossopharyngeal nerve (*white arrows*) from the medulla to the jugular foramen can be seen. Also visible are the thicker vagus nerve (*gray arrow*), thinner bulbar portion (*black arrow*), and spinal portion (*black arrowhead*) of the accessory nerve. (*E*) These three nerves can be seen as hypointense dots in the high signal intensity CSF of the basal cistern: glossopharyngeal nerve (*white arrow*), thicker vagus nerve (*gray arrow*), and thinner bulbar portion of the accessory nerve (*black arrow*).

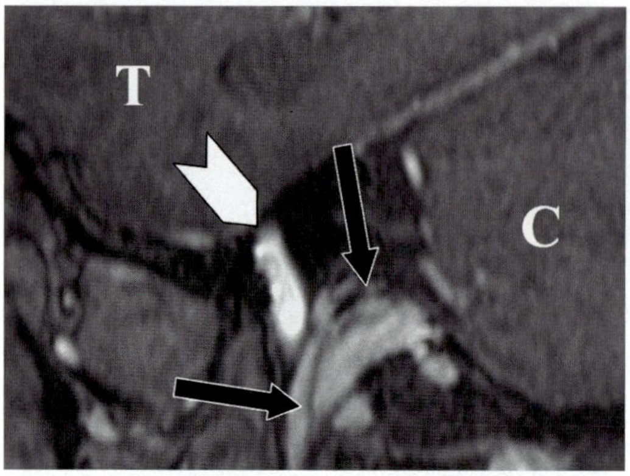

Fig. 52. Skull base segment of ninth nerve—para-coronal reformatted contrast-enhanced 0.4-mm^3-thick FFE image through the pars nervosa of the jugular foramen. The glossopharyngeal nerve can be seen as a hypointense thin arc (*black arrows*) surrounded by the enhancing venous structures. Also seen are the internal carotid artery (*white arrowhead*), temporal lobe (T), and cerebellum (C).

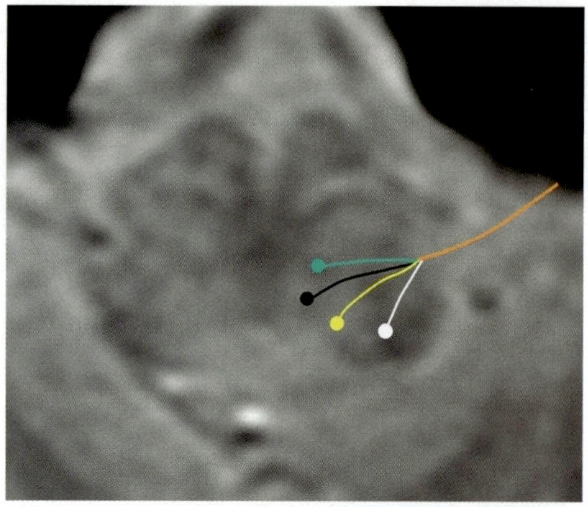

Fig. 54. Vagal nuclei, intra-axial segment—axial m-FFE through upper/middle medulla. The nucleus ambiguus (*blue dot*), dorsal vagal nucleus (*black dot*), solitary tract nucleus (*yellow dot*), spinal nucleus of the trigeminal nerve (*white dot*) and their corresponding fascicular nerve segments (*colored lines*) are located posteriorly in the medulla.

after looping around the subclavian artery on the right and passing through the aortopulmonary window on the left side and provides motor innervation to all laryngeal muscle except the cricothyroid muscle.[1,2,4]

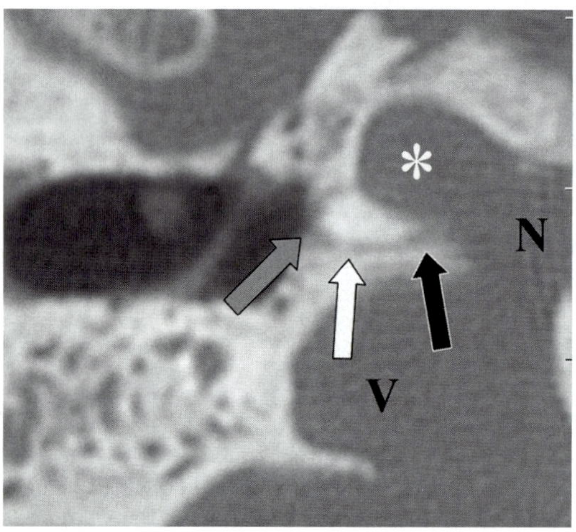

Fig. 53. Inferior tympanic canaliculus for Jacobson nerve or tympanic branch of the ninth nerve—para-axial reformatted CT image through the carotidojugular crest. At the jugular foramen side of this canal a depression for the inferior ganglion of the IXth nerve is seen in the bone: the fossula petrosa (*black arrow*). The inferior tympanic canaliculus can then be followed (*white arrow*) until it reaches the hypotympanum (*gray arrow*). N, pars nervosa of the jugular foramen; V, pars vascularis of the jugular foramen; *, carotid canal.

The Accessory Nerve or Cranial Nerve XI

The accessory nerve nuclei—intra-axial segment

The accessory nerve is a pure motor nerve, innervating the sternocleidomastoid and trapezius muscle. The bulbar motor fibers have their origin in the nucleus ambiguous; the spinal motor fibers in the spinal nucleus of the accessory nerve. The

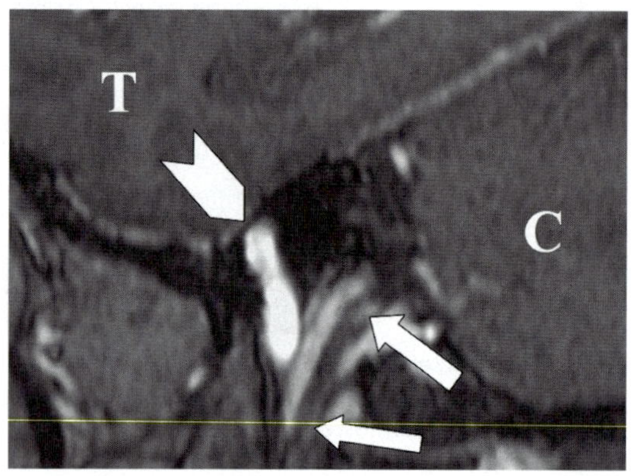

Fig. 55. The vagus and bulbar accessory nerve—para-coronal reformatted contrast-enhanced 3D-FFE image. The tenth and eleventh nerves travel through the jugular foramen together and cannot be distinguished from one another. Both nerves are seen as a low signal intensity thick arch (*white arrows*) surrounded by enhancing venous structures. Also visible are the internal carotid artery (*white arrowhead*), temporal lobe (T), and cerebellum (C).

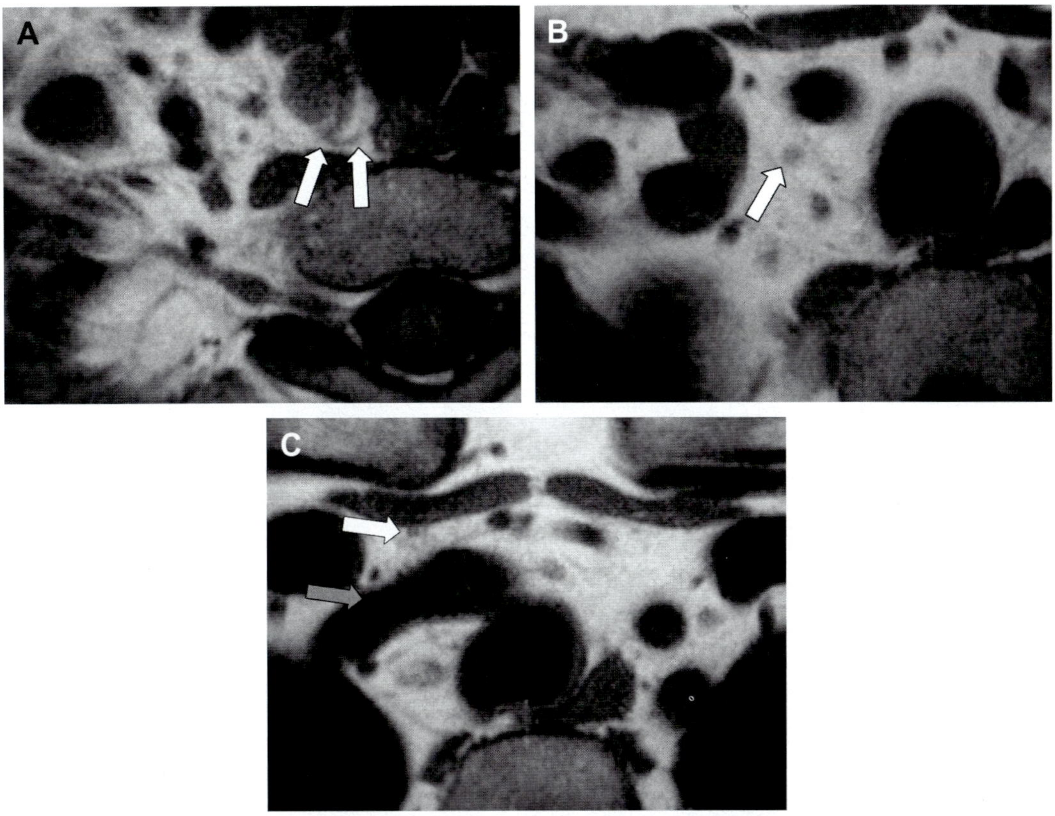

Fig. 56. Extracranial vagus nerve and recurrent laryngeal nerve—axial high-resolution T1W images at the level of the right tracheoesophageal groove (*A*), lower neck (*B*), and retroclavicular region (*C*). (*A*) The recurrent laryngeal nerve can be seen in the tracheoesophageal groove (*white arrows*). (*B*) The vagus nerve descends in the neck and travels toward the anterior border of the subclavian artery (*white arrow*). (*C*) The vagus nerve (*white arrow*) can be followed anterior to the subclavian artery (*gray arrow*).

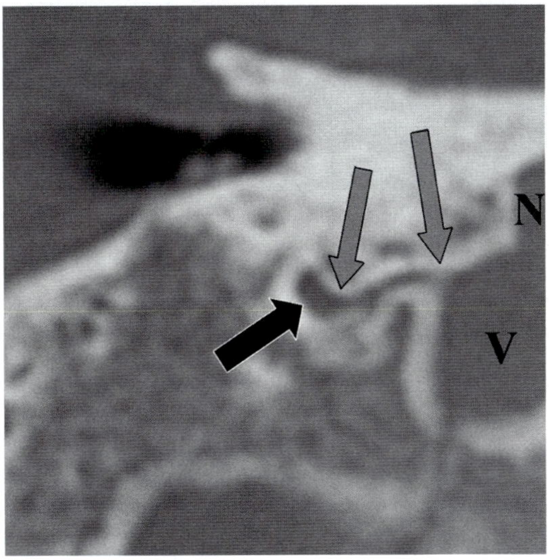

Fig. 57. Canal for Arnold nerve or auricular branch—axial CT scan through this canal. Arnold nerve is a branch of the vagus nerve, which leaves the pars vascularis of the jugular foramen and travels through Arnold's canal (*gray arrows*) to reach the mastoid segment of the facial nerve (*black arrow*) in its canal. N, pars nervosa of the jugular foramen; V, pars vascularis of the jugular foramen.

spinal nucleus is located lateral to the anterior horns at levels C1 to C5 and the fibers exit the cervical spinal cord on its lateral surface, in the area between the anterior and posterior roots (**Fig. 58**).[2,3]

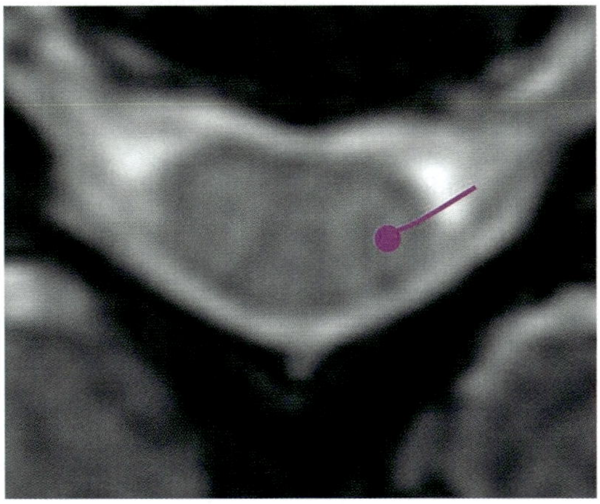

Fig. 58. The spinal nucleus of the accessory nerve—axial m-FFE image through the upper cervical medulla. Position of the spinal nucleus of the accessory nerve in the brain stem (*purple dot*) and of the spinal rootlets.

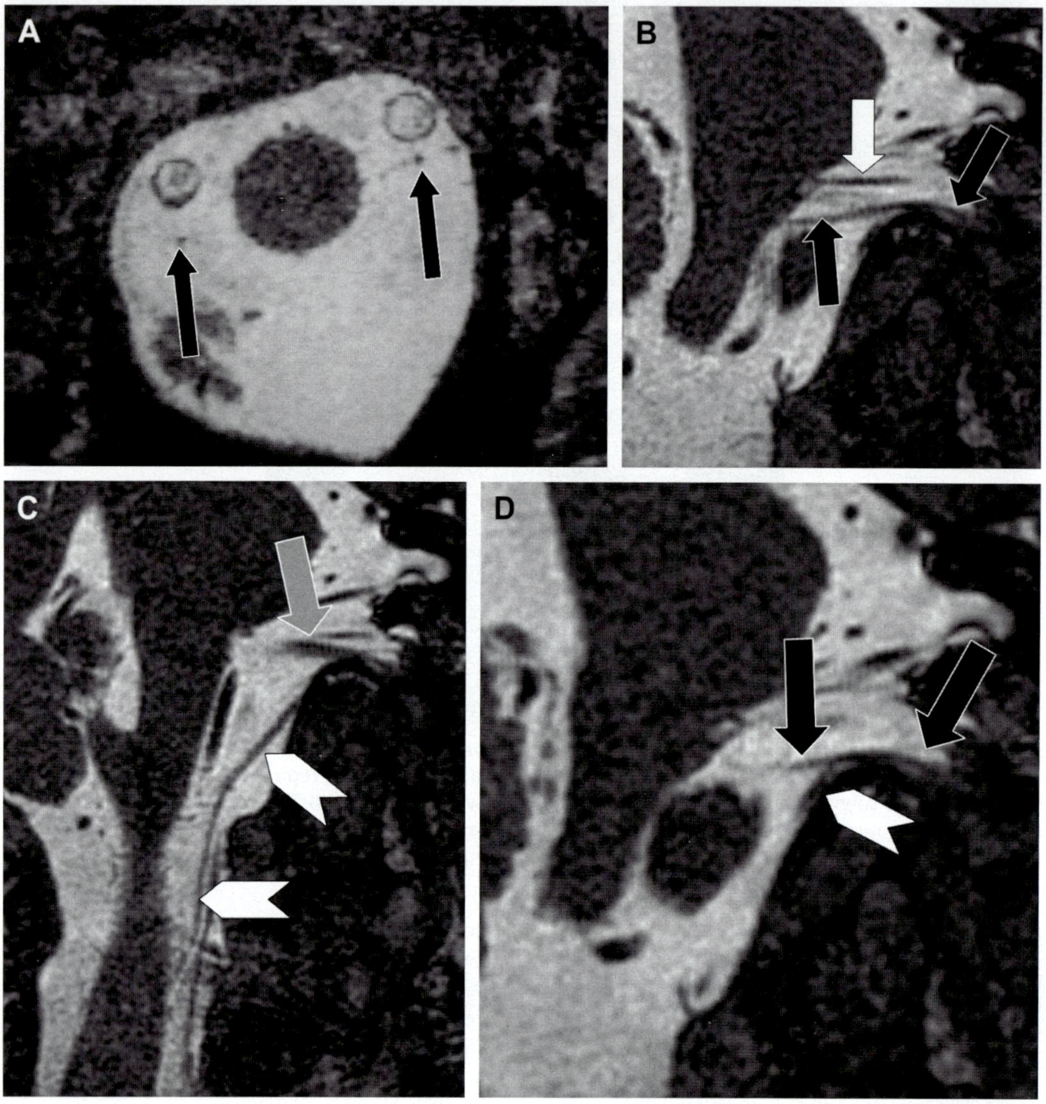

Fig. 59. Bulbar and spinal accessory nerve—axial DRIVE image through the upper medulla (*A*) and para-sagittal images through the bulbar segment of the eleventh nerve (*B–D*). (*A*) The spinal accessory nerves can be recognized as two black dots located just posterior to the vertebral arteries (*black arrows*). (*B*) Parasagittal reformatted image showing the complete cisternal segment of the bulbar XI (*black arrows*). The glossopharyngeal nerve (*white arrow*) is also seen. (*C*) Parasagittal reformatted image showing the spinal accessory nerve, ascending in the CSF and basal cistern (*white arrowheads*). The vagus nerve (*gray arrow*) is also seen. (*D*) On this reformatted image the confluence of the bulbar (*black arrows*) and spinal (*white arrowhead*) accessory nerve can be seen.

Cisternal segment

The nerve fibers then form an ascending nerve that reaches the jugular foramen after passing through the foramen magnum. The bulbar cisternal segment is located just below the tenth nerve. The bulbar and spinal portions of the nerve join in the lateral part of the basal cistern (**Fig. 59**).[39]

Skull base segment

The accessory nerve then passes through the pars vascularis of the jugular foramen and arrives beneath the skull base in the carotid space. The fibers follow the tenth nerve and eventually innervate the muscles of the larynx and pharynx. Fibers from the spinal portion continue posteralaterally to the carotid space and innervate the sternocleidomastoid muscle and trapezius muscle.[40]

The Hypoglossal Nerve or Cranial Nerve XII

Hypoglossal nucleus—intra-axial segment

The hypoglossal nerve is a motor nerve, innervating the intrinsic and extrinsic tongue musculature. The nucleus is located in the lower medulla, medial

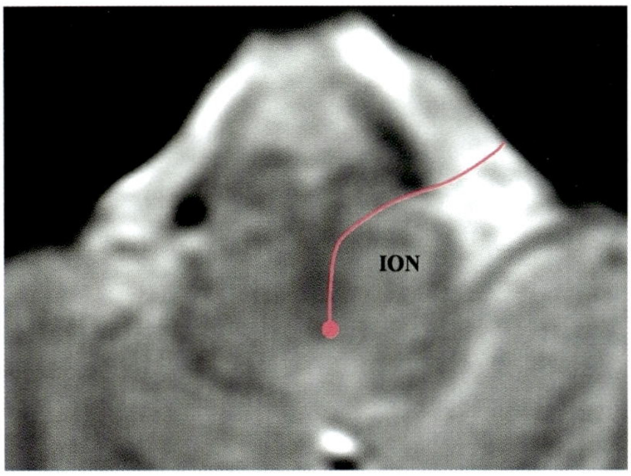

Fig. 60. Hypoglossal nucleus—axial m-FFE images through the lower half of the medulla. The hypoglossal nucleus has a paramedian location, against the floor of the fourth ventricle (*red dot*). The efferent axons (*red line*) travel through the medullary tegmentum, pass between the pyramid and inferior olivary nucleus (ION) to enter the subarachnoid CSF space at the pre-olivary sulcus.

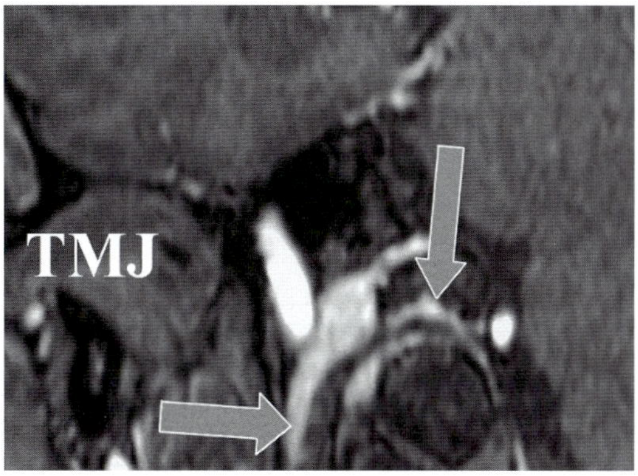

Fig. 62. Skull base segment of the hypoglossal nerve—para-coronal reformatted contrast-enhanced T1W 3D-FFE image (0.35 mm^3) through the hypoglossal canal. The hypoglossal nerve can be seen as a gray arch (*gray arrows*) from its entrance in the hypoglossal canal down to the inferior part of the jugular foramen and upper carotid space. The nerve can only be visualized because the surrounding venous structures enhance and become hyperintense. TMJ, temporomandibular joint.

to the dorsal nucleus of the vagus nerve, close to the midline in the floor of the fourth ventricle. It produces a slight bulge into the fourth ventricle called the "hypoglossal eminence" and extends the full length of the medulla. Axons travel anterolaterally through the medullary tegmentum and pass between the olivary nucleus and pyramid, where they exit the brainstem in the ventrolateral or pre-olivary sulcus. This is different from nerves IX, X, and XI, which exit the brainstem in the post-olivary sulcus (**Fig. 60**).[4]

Cisternal segment

The nerve emerges as a series of rootlets that converge to form a single- and sometimes a double-root hypoglossal nerve. The segment is best seen on heavily T2W images; however, the slices must be very thin, 0.4 mm or less, to visualize this nerve in a reliable way (**Fig. 61**).[41]

Skull base segment

After crossing the subarachnoid space, the nerve leaves the skull via the hypoglossal canal, located

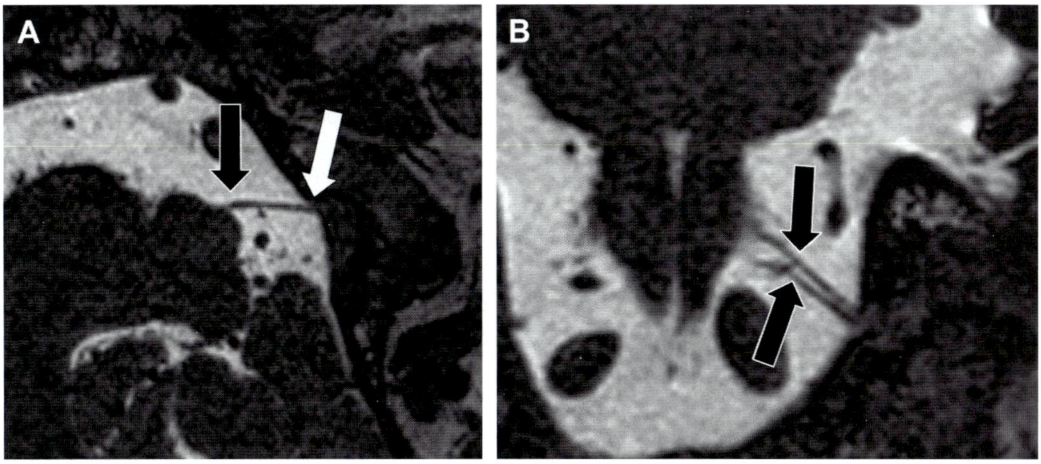

Fig. 61. Cisternal segment of the hypoglossal nerve—axial balanced-FFE image showing a single root (*A*) and coronal image showing a double root hypoglossal nerve (*B*). (*A*) The hypoglossal nerve becomes visible in the pre-olivary sulcus (*black arrow*) and crosses the CSF space to enter the hypoglossal canal in the occipital bone (*white arrow*). (*B*) Sometimes not all rootlets converge in one single hypoglossal nerve and then two or more roots cross the CSF space (*black arrows*).

below the jugular foramen in the inferior occipital bone. At this level the nerve is only visible following intravenous contrast administration when the veins around the nerve enhance and the nerve becomes visible inside the hypoglossal canal as a gray arch, surrounded by the hyperintense venous plexus (**Fig. 62**).

Extracranial segment

The hypoglossal nerve joins nerves X and XI in the carotid space once it has left the hypoglossal canal. The nerve leaves the carotid space at the level of the inferior margin of the posterior belly of the digastric muscle and then runs inferolaterally toward the hyoid bone where the nerve passes lateral to the carotid bifurcation. The muscular branch then enters the tongue on the lateral margin of the hyoglossus muscle in the posterior sublingual space from where the end branches for the intrinsic and extrinsic muscles of the tongue leave.

REFERENCES

1. Leblanc A. Encephalo-peripheral nervous system. Berlin: Springer-Verlag; 2001.
2. Harnsberger HR. Brain: cranial nerves. In: Harnsberg HR, Osborn AG, Macdonald AJ, editors. Diagnostic and surgical imaging anatomy of brain-head & neck-spine. Salk Lake City (UT): Amirsys Inc.; 2006. p. 173–259.
3. FitzGerald MJTF. Neuroanatomy, basic and clinical. 3rd edition. London: Saunders Inc.; 1996.
4. Laine FJ, Smoker WRK. Anatomy of the cranial nerves. Neuroimaging Clin N Am 1998;8(1): 69–100.
5. Borges A, Casselman J. Imaging the cranial nerves: part I: methodology, infectious and inflammatory, traumatic and congenital lesions. Eur Radiol 2007; 17:2112–25.
6. Casselman JW, Kuhweide R, Deimling M, et al. Constructive interference in steady state-3DFT MR imaging of the inner ear and cerebellopontine angle. AJNR Am J Neuroradiol 1993;14:47–57.
7. Lane JI, Ward H, Witte RJ, et al. 3-T imaging of the cochlear nerve and labyrinth in cochlear-implant candidates: 3D fast recovery fast spin-echo versus 3D constructive interference in the steady state techniques. AJNR Am J Neuroradiol 2004;25(4): 618–22.
8. Cifti E, Anik Y, Arslan A, et al. Driven equilibrium (drive) MR imaging of the cranial nerves V-VIII: comparison with the T2-weighted 3D-TSE sequence. Eur J Radiol 2004;51(3):234–40.
9. Tsuchiya K, Aoki C, Hachiya J. Evaluation of MR cisternography of the cerebellopontine angle using a balanced fast-field-echo sequence: preliminary findings. Eur Radiol 2004;14(2):239–42.
10. Jung NY, Moon WJ, Lee MH, et al. Magnetic resonance cisternography: comparison between 3-dimensional drive equilibrium with sensitivity encoding and 3-dimensional balanced fast-field echo sequences with sensitivity encoding. J Comput Assist Tomogr 2007;31(4):588–91.
11. Tsuchiya K, Yamakami N, Hachiya J, et al. MR cisternography using a three-dimensional half-fourier single-shot fast spin-echo sequence. Eur Radiol 1998;8(3):424–6.
12. Mikami T, Minamida Y, Yamaki T, et al. Cranial nerve assessment in posterior fossa tumors with fast imaging employing steady-state acquisition (FIESTA). Neurosurg Rev 2005;28(4):261–6.
13. Vertinsky A, Krasnokutsky M, Augustin M, et al. Cutting-edge imaging of the spine. Neuroimaging Clin N Am 2007;17(1):117–36.
14. van den Brink JS, Watanabe Y, Kuhl CK, et al. Implications of SENSE MR in routine clinical practice. Eur J Radiol 2003;46:3–27.
15. Castillo M, Mukherji SK. Magnetic resonance imaging of the olfactory apparatus. Top Magn Reson Imaging 1996;8(2):80–6.
16. Castillo M. Imaging of the upper cranial nerves I, III-VIII, and the cavernous sinuses. Neuroimaging Clin N Am 2004;14(4):579–93.
17. Tamraz JC, Outin-Tamraz C, Saban R. MR imaging of the optic pathways. Radiol Clin North Am 1999; 37(1):1–36.
18. Aviv RI, Casselman J. Orbital imaging: part 1. Normal anatomy. Clin Radiol 2005;60(3):279–87.
19. Eisenkraft B, Ortiz AO. Imaging evaluation of cranial nerves 3, 4 and 6. Semin Ultrasound CT MR 2001; 22(6):488–501.
20. Castillo M. Imaging of the upper cranial nerves I, III-VIII, and the cavernous sinuses. Magn Reson Imaging Clin N Am 2002;10(3):415–31.
21. Yagi A, Sato N, Takemura A, et al. Normal cranial nerves in the cavernous sinuses: contrast-enhanced three-dimensional constructive interference in the steady state MR imaging. AJNR Am J Neuroradiol 2005;26(4):946–50.
22. Yousry I, Moriggl B, Dieterich M, et al. MR anatomy of the proximal cisternal segment of the trochlear nerve: neurovascular relationships and landmarks. Radiology 2002;223(1):31–8.
23. Anderson VC, Berryhill PC, Sandquist MA, et al. High-resolution three-dimensional magnetic resonance angiography and three-dimensional spoiled gradient-recalled imaging in the evaluation of neurovascular compression in patients with trigeminal neuralgia: a double-blind pilot study. Neurosurgery 2006;58(4):666–73.
24. Williams LS, Schmalfuss IM, Sistrom CL, et al. MR imaging of the trigeminal ganglion, nerve, and the

perineural vascular plexus: normal appearance and variants with correlation to cadaver specimens. AJNR Am J Neuroradiol 2003;24(7):1317–23.
25. Yousry I, Moriggl B, Schmid UD, et al. Trigeminal ganglion and its divisions: detailed anatomic MR imaging with contrast-enhanced 3D constructive interference in the steady state sequences. AJNR Am J Neuroradiol 2005;26(5):1128–35.
26. Alkan A, Sigirci A, Ozveren MF, et al. The cisternal segment of the abducens nerve in man: three-dimensional MR imaging. Eur J Radiol 2004;51(3):218–22.
27. Lemmerling M, De Praeter G, Mortelé K, et al. Imaging of the normal pontine cisternal segment of the abducens nerve, using three-dimensional constructive interference in the steady state MRI. Neuroradiology 1999;41(5):384–6.
28. Ono K, Arai H, Endo T, et al. Detailed MR imaging anatomy of the abducent nerve: evagination of CSF into Dorello canal. AJNR Am J Neuroradiol 2004;25(4):623–6.
29. Yousry I, Camelio S, Wiesmann M, et al. Detailed magnetic resonance imaging anatomy of the cisternal segment of the abducent nerve: Dorello's canal and neurovascular relationships and landmarks. J Neurosurg 1999;91(2):276–83.
30. Naganawa S, Koshikawa T, Fukatsu H, et al. MR cisternography of the cerebellopontine angle: comparison of three-dimensional fast asymmetrical spin-echo and three-dimensional constructive interference in the steady-state sequences. AJNR Am J Neuroradiol 2001;22(6):1179–85.
31. Yetiser S, Kazkayas M, Altinok D, et al. Magnetic resonance imaging of the intratemporal facial nerve in idiopathic peripheral facial palsy. Clin Imaging 2003;27(2):77–81.
32. Takahashi N, Okamoto K, Ohkubo M, et al. High-resolution magnetic resonance of the extracranial facial nerve and parotid duct: demonstration of the branches of the intraparotid facial nerve and its relation to parotid tumours by MRI with a surface coil. Clin Radiol 2005;60(3):349–54.
33. Tieleman A, Casselman JW, Somers T, et al. Imaging of intralabyrinthine schwannomas: a retrospective study of 52 cases with emphasis on lesion growth. AJNR Am J Neuroradiol 2008, Epub ahead of print.
34. Mark AS, Casselman JW. Diseases of the temporal bone. In: Atlas S, editor. Magnetic resonance imaging of the brain and spine. 3rd edition. Philadelphia: Lippincott Williams & Wilkins; 2002. p. 1363–423.
35. Seitz J, Held P, Fründ R, et al. Visualization of the IXth to XIIth cranial nerves using 3-dimensional constructive interference in steady state, 3-dimensional magnetization-prepared rapid gradient echo and T2-weighted 2-dimensional turbo spin echo magnetic resonance imaging sequences. J Neuroimaging 2001;11(2):160–4.
36. Okumura Y, Suzuki M, Takemura A, et al. Visualization of the lower cranial nerves by 3D-FIESTA. Nippon Hoshasen Gijutsu Gakkai Zasshi 2005;61(2):291–7.
37. Laine FJ, Underhill T. Imaging of the lower cranial nerves. Magn Reson Imaging Clin N Am 2002;10(3):433–49.
38. Castillo M, Mukherji SK. Magnetic resonance imaging of cranial nerves IX, X, XI and XII. Top Magn Reson Imaging 1996;8(3):180–6.
39. Larson TC III, Aulino JM, Laine FJ. Imaging of the glossopharyngeal, vagus, and accessory nerves. Semin Ultrasound CT MR 2002;23(3):238–55.
40. Laine FJ, Underhill T. Imaging of the lower cranial nerves. Neuroimaging Clin N Am 2004;14(4):595–609.
41. Yousry I, Moriggl B, Schmid UD, et al. Detailed anatomy of the intracranial segment of the hypoglossal nerve: neurovascular relationships and landmarks on magnetic resonance imaging sequences. J Neurosurg 2002;96(6):1113–22.

Pathology of the Olfactory Nerve

Nasreddin Abolmaali, MD[a], Volker Gudziol, MD[b], Thomas Hummel, MD[b,*]

KEYWORDS

• Olfactory nerves • Olfactory bulb • Imaging

The olfactory nerve (ON) is the sum of the axons of all olfactory receptor neurons that are located in the nasal mucosa on both sides of the nasal cavity. The ganglion of the ON collects all these sensory afferents and is called the olfactory bulb (OB) or, less frequently, olfactory peduncle. It constitutes the primary olfactory cortex.

The OB is located bilaterally above the cribriform plate of the anterior skull base, the perforations of which let pass the ON. The OB is aligned in a strict ventrodorsal orientation and has an average volume of 125 ± 17 (mean $\pm$ standard deviation) mm^3.[1] The olfactory sulcus (OS) of the frontal lobe is visible above the OB and the olfactory tract (OT). The morphology of the OS seems dependent on the presence of the OB.[1] The OT connects the OB with the perforate substance. It runs from anteromedial (OB) to posterolateral (perforate substance) and its cross-sectional area is approximately one tenth of the cross-sectional area of the OB. Adding up the volumes of OB and OT results in an average of up to 160 mm^3. This volume showed a considerable variation depending on age.[2]

In vivo evaluation of the ON in humans and its functional characterization are possible using nasal endoscopy,[3] electrophysiologic recordings like the electro-olfactogram,[4] or biopsies in concert with immunohistochemical investigations[5] but not with currently available routine imaging methods. Because first brain images of living humans have been acquired by MRI at very high field strengths (ie, 9.4 T, with high spatial resolution [voxel size: 0.048 mm^3]), visualization of the ON seems foreseeable. The evaluation of the nasal mucosa preferably is done using MRI with T2-weighted sequences in a coronal image orientation.[6] In many centers, the nasal mucosa is investigated by CT, especially before surgery,[7] because this method provides additional information on bony nasal structures. With respect to the radiation exposure of CT (effective dose approximately 3 to 10 mSv) and the clinical question, MRI should be considered in every patient, because this method generates images without radiation exposure.

Perforations of the cribriform plate (with an average diameter of a single perforation well below 1 mm) may be visualized using recent CT systems, although as yet this is not shown convincingly. Such images are not possible with 1.5-T MRI systems but may be achieved using field strengths above 3 T, although susceptibility artifacts are a major concern.

Adequate visualization of human OB and OT in vivo is accessible only with MRI (**Fig. 1**). Because of the size and orientation of these structures, however, they often are not visible on routine clinical imaging of the brain and skull. Pathologies affecting the ON, OB, and OT are given in **Table 1**.

TECHNICAL CONSIDERATIONS (MRI)

Field Strength

MRI requires signals from hydrogen atoms. The amount of hydrogen atoms contributing to an MRI signal can be increased at higher field

[a] Radiation Research in Oncology, Technical University of Dresden Medical School, Fetscherstrasse 74, 01307 Dresden, Germany
[b] Smell and Taste Clinic, Department of Otorhinolaryngology, Technical University of Dresden Medical School, Fetscherstrasse 74, 01307 Dresden, Germany
* Corresponding author. Smell and Taste Clinic, Department of Otorhinolaryngology, Technical University of Dresden Medical School, Fetscherstrasse 74, 01307 Dresden, Germany.
E-mail address: thummel@mail.zih.tu-dresden.de (T. Hummel).

Neuroimag Clin N Am 18 (2008) 233–242
doi:10.1016/j.nic.2007.10.002
1052-5149/08/$ – see front matter

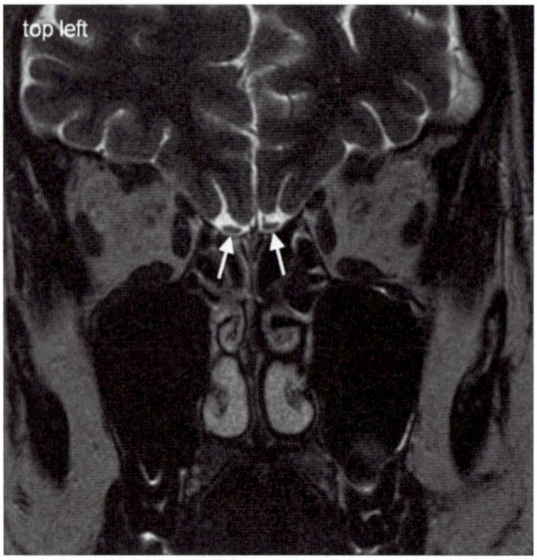

Fig. 1. Mildly T2-weighted TSE sequence (in plane resolution, 0.45 mm × 0.45 mm; slice thickness, 2 mm; voxel size, 0.405 mm^3) in coronal slice orientation of a healthy subject. OB (*arrows*) is surrounded by CSF and is situated above the cribriform plate and below the OS.

strengths. Therefore, visualization of small structures, such as OB and OT, should be done at 3 to 7 T. Because these systems are not widely available, the imaging technique at 1.5 T was optimized, using advanced receiver coil techniques or by selected imaging sequences. The techniques discussed herein were used at 1.5 T.

Receiver Coils

When MRI first was used to visualize the OB, mostly small loop coils were used, which were placed on the nasion and enabled comparatively high-resolution images of the OB.[8,9] Because of the limited field of view (depth penetration) of these coils, the OT and the posterior parts of the olfactory system could not be visualized. New head coils (eg, multichannel head array coils) allow a comparable or even better spatial resolution and provide information from the entire brain. Furthermore, these coils allow morphologic and functional imaging (functional MRI) without new positioning of patients. Most of the images shown herein were acquired with an eight-channel head array coil.

Sequence Techniques

The discussion of sequence techniques focuses on methods applied to imaging of the OB and OT. Two tissue characteristics may be elaborated, the T1 time, using T1-weighted sequences, and the T2 time, using T2-weighted sequences. Different sequence types (eg, turbo spin echo [TSE], constructive interference in steady state precession [CISS], and turbo fast low-angle shot [TFL]) are capable of generating different contrasts between tissues. Depending on the desired tissue contrast, some sequences may be optimized for 3-D imaging, whereas other sequences preferably are used for 2-D imaging.

For high-resolution imaging of the OB and OT, 2-D data acquisition preferably is done using TSE techniques, which generate a voxel size of 0.405 mm^3. Thus, accurate volumetry of the OB is feasible. 2-D TSE sequences should be acquired in coronal slice orientation (maximum slice thickness 2 mm) covering the entire anterior skull base and the pituitary gland. To visualize pathology within the OB, a sequence with stronger T2 weighting (eg, CISS)[10] seems advantageous (**Figs. 2 and 3**). This technique generates bright signals from cerebralspinal fluid (CSF) and very low signal intensities from all other tissues and structures (ie, high contrast for the sensitive visualization of structures surrounded by CSF). The disadvantage of this sequence is the poor contrast between OB, OT, gray matter, air, and bone. Consequently, it

Table 1
Examples of pathologies affecting the olfactory nerve, olfactory bulb, and olfactory tract

Congenital	Inflammation	Tumor, Benign	Tumor, Malignant
Aplasia of OB	Acute and chronic rhinosinusitis	Papilloma	Squamous cell carcinoma
Kallmann's syndrome	Mucor mycosis	Osteoma	Adenoidcystic carcinoma
Cyclops	Aspergillosis	Neurogenic tumor	Aesthesioneuroblastoma
	Cystic fibrosis	Meningioma	Rhabdomyosarcoma
	Mucocele	Giant cell tumor	Metastases
	Tuberculosis	Fibrous dysplasia	Lymphoma
		Nerve sheath tumor	Osteosarcoma
		Adenoma	PNET

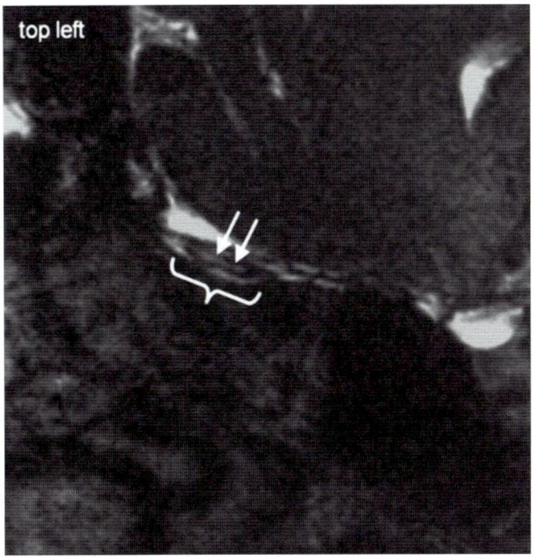

Fig. 2. Oblique sagittal multiplanar reformation of a strongly T2-weighted CISS sequence in a patient who had anosmia. Within the OB (*bracket*), a structure with pronounced T2 prolongation is visualized (*arrow*), which might be related to atrophy or, more likely, small dysontogenetic cysts.

may not be ideal for volumetric purposes, because the differentiation of the cribriform plate, the OB and OT, and the brain is difficult.

In cases where the entire olfactory system, including nasal cavity and posterior structures, is investigated, 3-D imaging with isotropic voxels (isotropic voxels reveal identical lengths of the margins of every voxel in all three spatial orientations) covering the entire cranium is preferred. The acquired data sets allow for multiplanar reformation in any orientation. **Table 2** shows important technical parameters of recommended sequence designs.

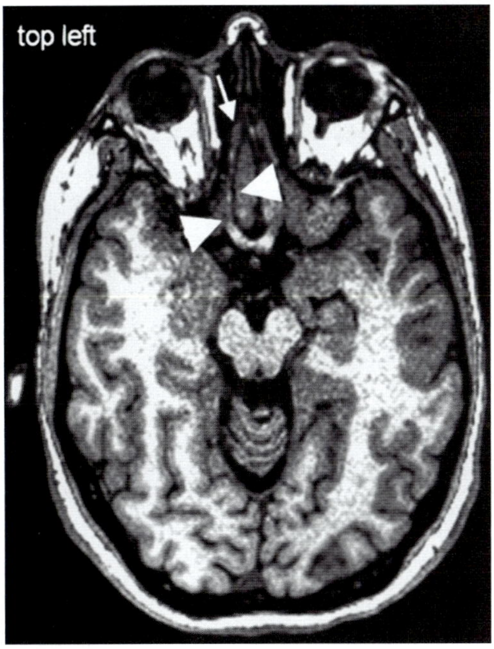

Fig. 3. Oblique axial multiplanar reformation of a T1-weighted TFL sequence along the right-sided OB (*arrow*) and OT (*arrowheads*). Note tissue contrast between gray and white matter for volumetry.

For clinical purposes (eg, excluding a frontal meningeoma or other tumors), the imaging protocol includes T1-weighted 2-D imaging before and after intravenous application of contrast material. Imaging should be done using axial, coronal, and sagittal planes to provide sufficient information for preoperative planning. The application of fat suppression techniques creates improved delineation of tumors that expanded beyond the cranium and invaded the subcutaneous fat. Diffusion-weighted imaging should be done before application of contrast material and might provide additional information on the microstructure of tumors, hence narrowing the differential diagnosis.

OLFACTORY NERVES

The nasal cavity harbors the olfactory neurons. From the roof of the nasal cavity they send their axons in bundles (called the ONs) through the cribriform plate to the OB, where they synapse with mitral cells. In the nasal cavity, the most frequent cases of olfactory loss are inflammatory disorders (eg, sinonasal disease [SND] with and without polyposis) (**Fig. 4**).[11–14] In addition, respiratory problems may prevent airflow to the olfactory cleft, thus producing olfactory loss. More recently, localized inflammation of the olfactory cleft with consecutive thickening of the mucosa is described as a possible cause of olfactory loss.[15]

Acute obstructions of the nasal cavity may result from acute trauma and may modify olfactory sensations temporarily or permanently. Bleedings after midfacial fractures may obstruct the nasal cavity, but causative fractures of the anterior skull base may cause permanent injuries of the ON, OB, and OT (**Fig. 5**).

IMAGING OF THE OLFACTORY BULB

Congenital Anosmia

Largely based on the work by Yousem and colleagues, magnetic resonance–based imaging of the OB has found its way into clinical practice (**Fig. 6**). Today the diagnosis of isolated congenital anosmia or Kallmann's syndrome centers on MRI.[1,9,16–25] In addition, assessment of OB volume is applied in subjects who have CHARGE syndrome[26–28] where the olfactory system is compromised.

Table 2
Characteristic features of MRI sequences for application in the olfactory system

	T1 TSE (2-D)	T1 TFL (3-D) (MP-RAGE)	T2 TSE (2-D)	T2 TSE (3-D)	CISS (3-D)
TR (ms)	400	2180	4800	2500	12.2
TE (ms)	14	3.2	148	354	6.1
TI (ms)	—	1100	—	—	—
Bandwidth (Hz/pixel)	70	160	130	930	130
Slice thickness (mm)	2	0.8	2	0.8	0.7
In plane resolution (mm^2)	0.45 × 0.45	0.8 × 0.8	0.45 × 0.45	0.8 × 0.8	0.7 × 0.7
Voxel size (mm^3)	0.405	0.512	0.405	0.512	0.343
Acquisition time (min)	14	6 (PAT factor 2)	8	11	6

Abbreviations: MP-RAGE, magnetization prepared rapid acquisition gradient echo; PAT, parallel acquisition technique; TE, echo time; TI, inversion time; TR, repetition time.

The flattening of the olfactory sulcus in the plane of the posterior tangent through the eyeballs can be used as an additional criterion to separate patients who have isolated congenital anosmia from normosmic controls.[1] This might be important when the OBs are difficult to identify in subjects moving during the image acquisition.

Tumors Affecting Olfactory Bulb Function

Tumors of the anterior skull base commonly induce alterations of the olfactory sense, such as hyposmia, anosmia, or parosmia. Most commonly, meningiomas (**Figs. 7 and 8**) affect the OB and OT.[29,30] Esthesioneuroblastomas typically involve the frontal skull base and grow along the cranial nerves into and out of the skull base. Therefore, the ON, OB, and OT commonly are affected by such tumors (**Fig. 9**). In rare cases, other tumors, such as olfactory ensheathing cell tumor[31] or primitive neuroectodermal tumors (PNETs) in children (**Fig. 10**), affect the olfactory system.

The Volume of the Olfactory Bulb Changes

Morphologic imaging in healthy, normosmic subjects suggests that the volume of the OB is highly variable, especially in relation to aging.[26,32,33] Such variability makes it problematic to come up

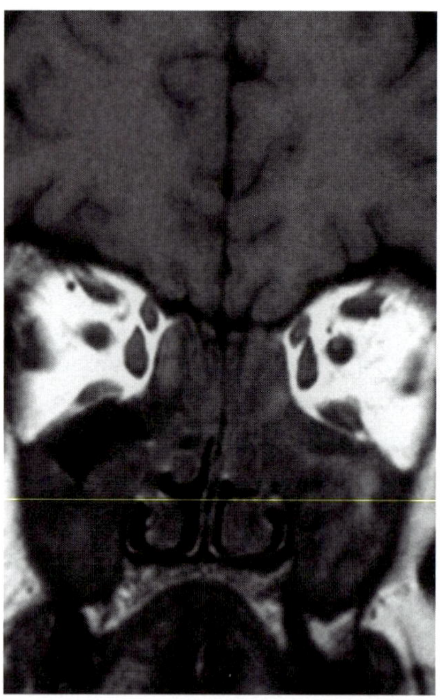

Fig. 4. Coronal T1-weighted TSE sequence acquired behind the eyeballs to depict the OB. Mucinous secretions and polyps obstruct the airways of the nose and the sinuses, causing anosmia.

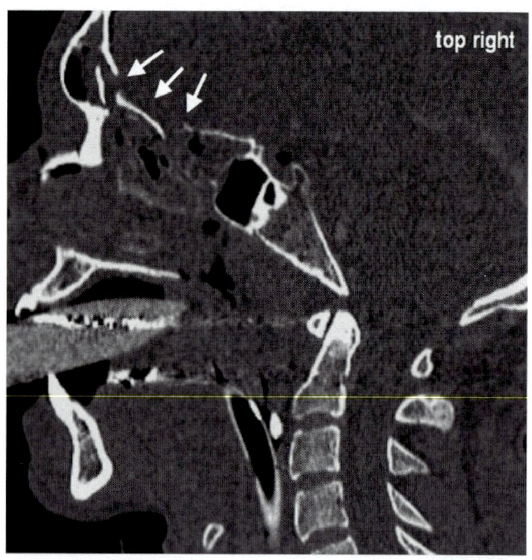

Fig. 5. Sagittal multiplanar reformation of a CT of the head of a patient who had a car accident. Multiple fractures of the posterior wall of the frontal sinuses and the frontal skull base (*arrows*). Bleeding into the sinuses and the nasal cavity.

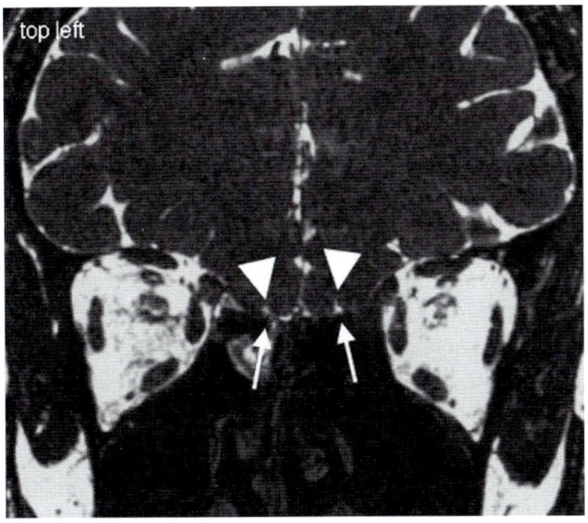

Fig. 6. Coronal CISS in a patient who had congenital anosmia. The OBs and OTs are not developed and not visible (*arrows*). Additionally, the OS are undersized (*arrowheads*), which is a frequent finding in aplastic OBs.

with normative data.[2] As indicated by the authors' preliminary work, however, it seems likely that, on individual levels, changes of the OB provide a measure of the prognosis of olfactory dysfunction (**Fig. 11**). Reliability of measures of OB volume does not contribute to this variability, as high interobserver reliability is reported in many studies.[1,2,34]

The reason for the high plasticity of the OB volume can be found in the continuing synaptogenesis in the OB, which remains highly plastic throughout adult life, reflecting to some degree the level of afferent neural activity.[35,36] In animals, one of the most pronounced effects of olfactory deprivation is the reduction in OB size[37,38] as a result of a decreased number of cells. These changes are based additionally on the OB as one of the few brain areas to replace its neuronal populations continuously.[39] These bulbar changes are related to the sensory input from the olfactory epithelium.[40,41] Such neuronal recruitment may, in turn, lead to an improvement of sensory abilities.[42] In addition to the continuous replacement of gamma amino butyric

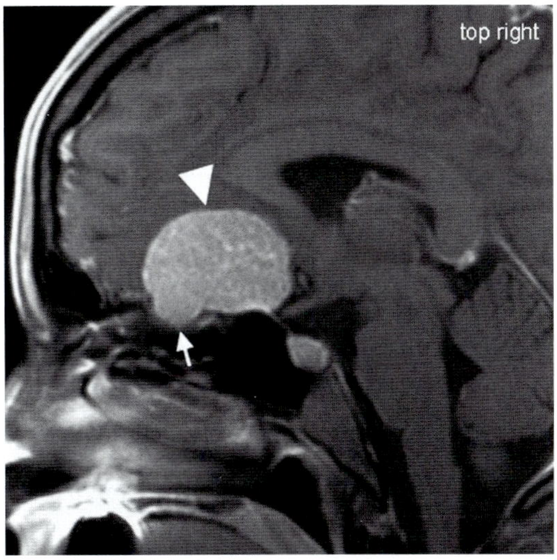

Fig. 8. Sagittal T1-weighted TSE after intravenous application of a contrast agent. This patient suffers from a markedly contrast enhancing frontobasal meningioma (*arrowhead*) that destroyed the cribriform plate and grows into the nasal cavity (*arrow*). OBs and OTs are not visible.

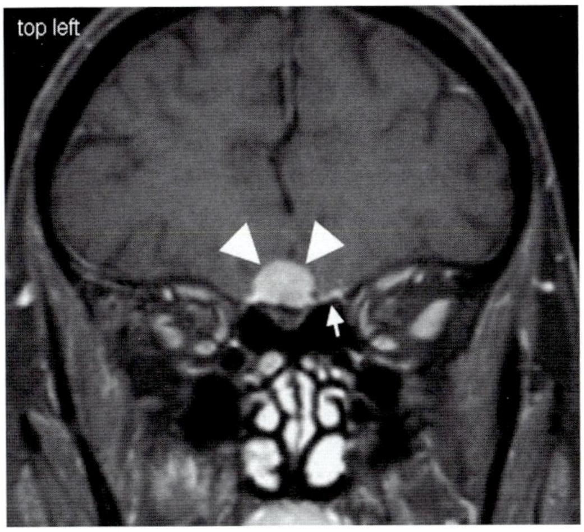

Fig. 7. Coronal fat-suppressed, T1-weighted TSE after intravenous application of a contrast agent. This patient suffers from a markedly contrast-enhancing, medium-sized frontobasal meningioma (*arrowheads*). Neither OBs nor OTs are visible. Typically, meningiomas show a shallow contrast enhancement in the adjacent meninges, referred to as dural tail (*small arrow*).

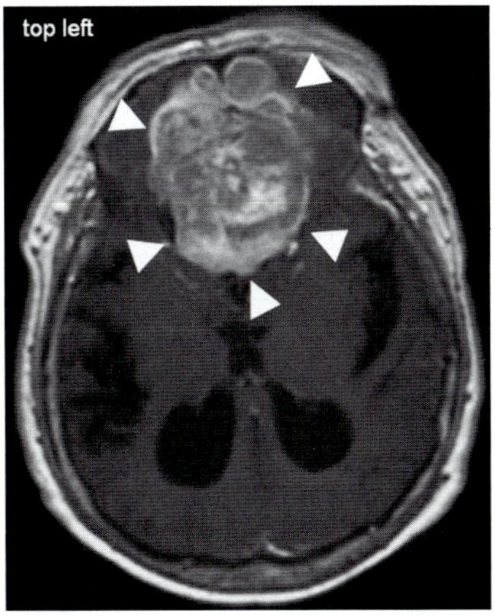

Fig. 9. Axial T1-weighted TSE with intravenous application of a contrast agent. This frontobasal tumor (esthesioneuroblastoma) shows inhomogeneous, partly septated enhancement, and a severe mass effect.

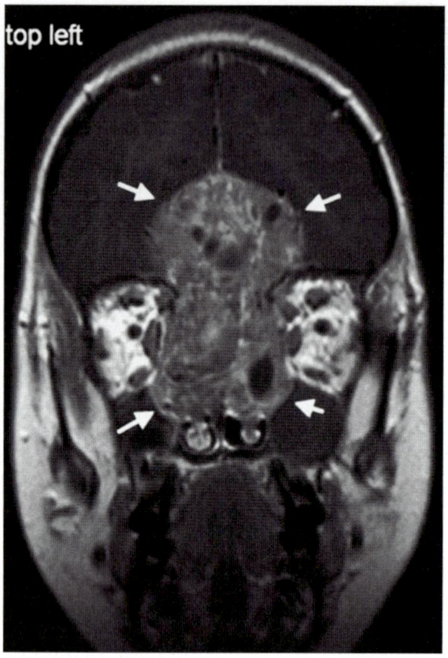

Fig. 10. Coronal contrast-enhanced, T1-weighted sequence in a young patient suffering from a PNET (*arrows*) with cystic transformations. The ONs, OB, and OT are destroyed.

acid (GABA)-ergic neurons, plasticity of mitral/tufted cells in OB recently has been reported.[43] Further, apoptosis seems an important mechanism of plasticity by which the olfactory system is able to adjust the number of neurons in the OB.[44]

Olfactory Bulb Volume Correlates with Olfactory Function and May be of Prognostic Value

In patents who have olfactory loss, OB volume correlates with decreased olfactory sensitivity regardless of the cause of olfactory loss;[45] it varies with regard to olfactory function and decreases with duration of olfactory loss.[46,47] Although awaiting further confirmation, some research is demonstrating a correlation between olfactory function and OB volume, which was more pronounced for retronasal than for orthonasal olfactory function.[48] The data confirm that OB volume is an indicator of olfactory function, but in this study, it largely is determined by retronasal olfactory sensitivity.

Regarding the possible predictive value of volumetric measures of the OB, in a more recent study (Rombaux, personal communication, 2007), patients who had SND were compared with healthy controls. Orthonasal olfactory testing did not yield significant differences between the two groups. Patients who had more pronounced signs of a nasal sinusitis, however, had significantly smaller OB volumes than patients who had less pronounced inflammatory signs. Even when controlling for the subjects' ages, a significant correlation was present between OB volume and the degree of sinusitis ($r = -0.52$), with smaller OB volumes associated with a higher degree of sinunasal pathology. Thus, SND patients who had a slight decrease or even normal olfactory function already may exhibit changes in their OB volume, which clearly emphasizes that OB volume changes are sensitive to subtle changes in the olfactory system. In turn, on an intra-individual level, OB volume could be used as a predictor of the change of olfactory function in the future.

Olfactory Bulb Volume is Decreased in Patients Who Have Parosmia

Other work indicates[45,46] that patients who have parosmia exhibit smaller OB volumes compared

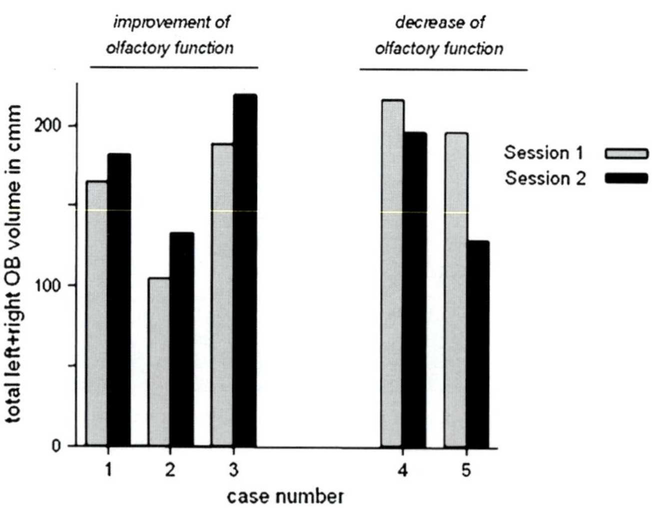

Fig. 11. Changes of OB volume over time in patients who have olfactory loss resulting from chronic rhinosinusitis before (Session 1) and approximately 60 days after sinus surgery. In patients 1 to 3, olfactory function improved (*left*), whereas it became worse in patients 4 and 5. The total volume of the left plus right OBs (in mm^3) changed accordingly.

with those who do not have parosmia. The molecular mechanisms leading to parosmia are unknown. Even the site of the generation of parosmia (olfactory epithelium, OB, or higher central olfactory structures) is not clear.[49,50] Based on current findings, it may be hypothesized that a decrease in the number of OB neurons is associated with generation of parosmia. A mechanism behind this could be that a decreased number of OB interneurons results in a decrease of lateral inhibition.[51] In turn, this may allow olfactory activation to produce an irregular pattern, which may result in a "parosmic odor." If this mechanistic idea is true, future investigations should be able to show an inverse correlation between the degree of parosmia and the size of the OB.

Olfactory Bulb Volume in Parkinson's Disease

OB volume also may explain/question the background of olfactory loss in patients who have Parkinson's disease,[52] where hyposmia typically is observed even years before onset of the motor symptoms.[53,54] Specifically, results from a pilot study suggest there is little or no difference between patients who have idiopathic Parkinson's disease (IPD) and healthy controls in terms of OB volume.[55] Based on the relation between loss of olfactory input to the OB and consecutive decrease in volume, these data support the idea that olfactory loss in IPD is not a primary consequence of damage to the olfactory epithelium but results from central-nervous alterations. This is backed up by reports from Huisman and coworkers,[56] indicating that the number of dopaminergic neurons is increased by 100% in patients who have Parkinson's disease compared with controls, which may translate into a normal volume of the OB. As dopaminergic neurons mostly are inhibitors, this may suggest that olfactory input is inhibited at the level of OB despite the fact that the number of neurons in the anterior olfactory nucleus decreases with duration of disease. This idea also is supported by findings of a normal olfactory epithelium in patients who have Parkinson's disease as compared with healthy controls.[57]

IMAGING OF THE OLFACTORY TRACT

The OT has a small cross-sectional area (ie, it is a thin structure) and runs from the OB to the perforate substance. The course of the OT is oblique with respect to all routinely acquired imaging planes and, therefore, the OT is difficult to visualize on standard MRI. Alternatively, processes invading or infiltrating the OT may be visualized easily (eg, small meningiomas affecting only one OT) (**Fig. 12**). Systemic diseases with meningeal metastases can be visualized with T1-weighted images after application of contrast material (**Fig. 13**).

IMAGING OF OLFACTORY ELOQUENT BRAIN STRUCTURES

Brain structures of high significance in the processing of olfactory information involve the piriform cortex, perirhinal cortex, entorhinal cortex, amygdala, periamygdaloid cortex, hippocampus, mediodorsal thalamus, ventral pallidum, ventral striatum (or nucleus accumbens), orbitofrontal cortex, insula, and hypothalamus[58] Primary olfactory cortex includes the anterior olfactory nucleus (in humans integrated into the OB/OT), the pririform cortex, the periamygdaloid cortex, the amygdala, the entorhinale cortex, and the olfactory tubercle. All other areas (discussed previously) can be regarded as secondary or tertiary olfactory projection areas. Among other processes, tumors,[59] infarctions,[60] hemorrhage,[61] or changes in blood perfusion[62] may affect olfactory function.

Tumors of mesial temporal structures, especially the amygdala, seem to play important roles in the genesis of olfactory auras.[63] Work in a sample size of 10 patients indicated that only right-sided tumors of the frontal or temporal lobe produced a more bilateral decrease of olfactory function compared with left-sided tumors,[64] possibly highlighting a higher significance of the right hemisphere in the processing of olfactory

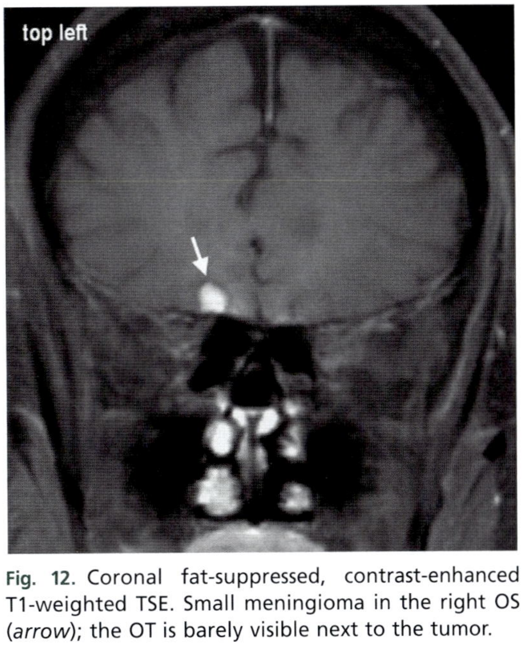

Fig. 12. Coronal fat-suppressed, contrast-enhanced T1-weighted TSE. Small meningioma in the right OS (*arrow*); the OT is barely visible next to the tumor.

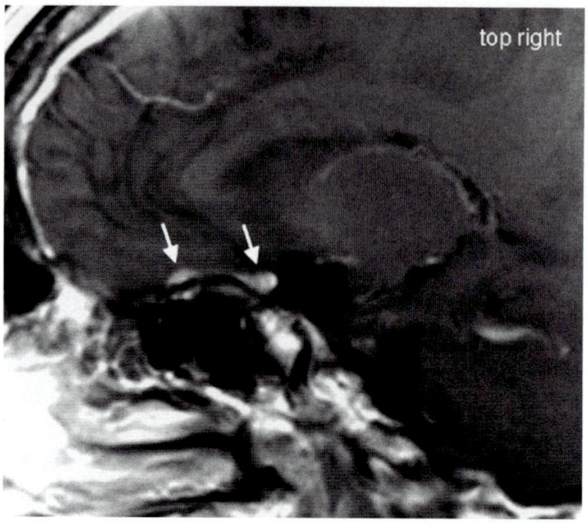

Fig. 13. Sagittal T1-weighted TSE after intravenous application of a contrast agent. This patient suffered from metastasizing breast carcinoma. Two markedly contrast enhancing metastases (*arrows*) in the meninges have destroyed olfactory structures.

information.[65] Other work in patients who have brain surgery also indicates the role of the temporal lobe and the orbitofrontal cortex in the execution of various olfactory functions (eg, odor identification, odor discrimination, or odor memory).[66–69] Thus, there is ample evidence that brain lesions can affect olfactory function even when they are not associated directly with the OB or OT. In turn, when using MRI as a diagnostic tool, the whole brain of patients who have olfactory dysfunction needs to be investigated thoroughly.

SUMMARY

In conclusion, olfactory dysfunction may be caused at various levels during the processing of olfactory information. Olfactory function seems accessible through measures of the volume of the OB. It can be expected that techniques with higher resolution will provide even better insights in the structural and functional organization of the olfactory system.

ACKNOWLEDGMENT

The authors thank Prof. Rüdiger von Kummer, Chairman of the Department for Neuroradiology, and Dr. Gabriele Hahn, Pediatric Radiology, from the Medical Faculty Carl Gustav Carus, Dresden University of Technology, for their support with some of the images shown in this article.

REFERENCES

1. Abolmaali ND, Hietschold V, Vogl TJ, et al. MR evaluation in patients with isolated anosmia since birth or early childhood. AJNR Am J Neuroradiol 2002;23:157–64.
2. Yousem DM, Geckle RJ, Bilker WB, et al. Olfactory bulb and tract and temporal lobe volumes. Normative data across decades. Ann N Y Acad Sci 1998;855:546–55.
3. Leopold DA, Bartels S. Evaluation of olfaction. J Otolaryngol 2002;31(Suppl 1):S18–23.
4. Knecht M, Hummel T. Recording of the human electro-olfactogram. Physiol Behav 2004;83:13–9.
5. Jafek BW, Murrow B, Michaels R, et al. Biopsies of human olfactory epithelium. Chem Senses 2002;27:623–8.
6. Abolmaali N, Kantchew A, Hummel T, et al. Evaluation of the "nasal cycle" using MR-imaging. Eur Radiol 2003;13:C2.
7. Mueller C, Temmel AFP, Toth J, et al. Computed tomography scans in the evaluation of patients with olfactory dysfunction. Am J Rhinol 2006;20:109–12.
8. Suzuki M, Takashima T, Kadoya M, et al. MR imaging of olfactory bulbs and tracts. Am J Neuroradiol 1989;10:955–7.
9. Yousem DM, Turner WJD, Li C, et al. Kallmann Syndrome: MR evaluation of olfactory system. Am J Neuroradiol 1993;14:839–43.
10. Casselman JW, Kuhweide R, Deimling M, et al. Constructive interference in steady state-3DFT MR imaging of the inner ear and cerebellopontine angle. Am J Neuroradiol 1993;14:47–57.
11. Jafek BW, Murrow B, Linschoten M. Evaluation and treatment of anosmia. Curr Opin Otol Head Neck Surg 2000;8:63–7.
12. Kern RC. Chronic sinusitis and anosmia: pathologic changes in the olfactory mucosa. Laryngoscope 2000;110:1071–7.
13. Seiden AM. Olfactory loss secondary to nasal and sinus pathology. In: Seiden AM, editor. Taste and smell disorders. New York: Thieme; 1997. p. 52–71.
14. Seiden AM, Duncan HJ. The diagnosis of a conductive olfactory loss. Laryngoscope 2001;111:9–14.
15. Trotier D, Bensimon JL, Herman P, et al. Inflammatory obstruction of the olfactory clefts and olfactory loss in humans: a new syndrome? Chem Senses 2007;32:285–92.
16. Aiba T, Inoue Y, Matsumoto K, et al. Magnetic resonance imaging for diagnosis of congenital anosmia. Acta Otolaryngol Suppl 2004;554:50–4.
17. De Bellis A, Sinisi AA, Conte M, et al. Antipituitary antibodies against gonadotropin-secreting cells in adult male patients with apparently idiopathic hypogonadotropic hypogonadism. J Clin Endocrinol Metab 2007;92:604–7.
18. Gasztonyi Z, Barsi P, Czeizel AE. Kallmann syndrome in three unrelated women and an association with femur-fibula-ulna dysostosis in one case. Am J Med Genet 2000;93:176–80.
19. Ghadami M, Majidzadeh AK, Morovvati S, et al. Isolated congenital anosmia with morphologically

normal olfactory bulb in two Iranian families: a new clinical entity? Am J Med Genet A 2004;127:307–9.
20. Ho TP, Carrie S. Congenital anosmia. Int J Clin Pract 2001;55:418–9.
21. Ishman SL, Loehrl TA, Smith MM. Calcification of the olfactory bulbs in three patients with hyposmia. AJNR Am J Neuroradiol 2003;24:2097–101.
22. Madan R, Sawlani V, Gupta S, et al. MRI findings in Kallmann syndrome. Neurol India 2004;52:501–3.
23. Massin N, Pecheux C, Eloit C, et al. X chromosome-linked Kallmann syndrome: clinical heterogeneity in three siblings carrying an intragenic deletion of the KAL-1 gene. J Clin Endocrinol Metab 2003;88: 2003–8.
24. Vagenakis GA, Hyphantis TN, Papageorgiou C, et al. Kallmann's syndrome and schizophrenia. Int J Psychiatry Med 2004;34:379–90.
25. Yousem DM, Geckle RJ, Bilker W, et al. MR evaluation of patients with congenital hyposmia or anosmia. AJR Am J Roentgenol 1996;166:439–43.
26. Azoulay R, Fallet-Bianco C, Garel C, et al. MRI of the olfactory bulbs and sulci in human fetuses. Pediatr Radiol 2006;36:97–107.
27. Chalouhi C, Faulcon P, Le Bihan C, et al. Olfactory evaluation in children: application to the CHARGE syndrome. Pediatrics 2005;116:E81–8.
28. Pinto G, Abadie V, Mesnage R, et al. CHARGE syndrome includes hypogonadotropic hypogonadism and abnormal olfactory bulb development. J Clin Endocrinol Metab 2005;90:5621–6.
29. Obeid F, Al-Mefty O. Recurrence of olfactory groove meningiomas. Neurosurgery 2003;53:534–42 [discussion: 42–3].
30. Welge-Luessen A, Temmel A, Quint C, et al. Olfactory function in patients with olfactory groove meningioma. J Neurol Neurosurg Psychiatry 2001;70:218–21.
31. Yasuda M, Higuchi O, Takano S, et al. Olfactory ensheathing cell tumor: a case report. J Neurooncol 2006;76:111–3.
32. Yousem DM, Geckle RJ, Bilker W, et al. Olfactory bulb and tract and temporal lobe volumes. Ann N Y Acad Sci 1998;855:546–55.
33. Yousem DM, Oguz KK, Li C. Imaging of the olfactory system. Semin Ultrasound CT MR 2001;22:456–72.
34. Yousem DM, Geckle RJ, Doty RL, et al. Reproducibility and reliability of volumetric measurements of olfactory eloquent structures. Acad Radiol 1997;4:264–9.
35. Baker H, Kawano T, Albert V, et al. Olfactory bulb dopamine neurons survive deafferentation-induced loss of tyrosine hydroxylase. Neuroscience 1984; 11:605–15.
36. Margolis FL, Roberts N, Ferriero D, et al. Denervation in the primary olfactory pathway of mice: biochemical and morphological effects. Brain Res 1974;81:469–83.
37. Cummings DM, Knab BR, Brunjes PC. Effects of unilateral olfactory deprivation in the developing opossum, Monodelphis domestica. J Neurobiol 1997;33:429–38.
38. Korol DL, Brunjes PC. Unilateral naris closure and vascular development in the rat olfactory bulb. Neuroscience 1992;46:631–41.
39. Curtis MA, Kam M, Nannmark U, et al. Human neuroblasts migrate to the olfactory bulb via a lateral ventricular extension. Science 2007;315: 1243–9.
40. Lledo PM, Gheusi G. Olfactory processing in a changing brain. Neuroreport 2003;14:1655–63.
41. Lledo PM, Gheusi G, Vincent JD. Information processing in the mammalian olfactory system. Physiol Rev 2005;85:281–317.
42. Lledo PM, Saghatelyan A, Lemasson M. Inhibitory interneurons in the olfactory bulb: from development to function. Neuroscientist 2004;10:292–303.
43. Fletcher ML, Wilson DA. Olfactory bulb mitral-tufted cell plasticity: odorant-specific tuning reflects previous odorant exposure. J Neurosci 2003;23: 6946–55.
44. Najbauer J, Leon M. Olfactory experience modulated apoptosis in the developing olfactory bulb. Brain Res 1995;674:245–51.
45. Mueller A, Rodewald A, Reden J, et al. Reduced olfactory bulb volume in post-traumatic and post-infectious olfactory dysfunction. Neuroreport 2005; 16:475–8.
46. Rombaux P, Mouraux A, Bertrand B, et al. Olfactory function and olfactory bulb volume in patients with postinfectious olfactory loss. Laryngoscope 2006; 116:436–9.
47. Rombaux P, Mouraux A, Bertrand B, et al. Retronasal and orthonasal olfactory function in relation to olfactory bulb volume in patients with posttraumatic loss of smell. Laryngoscope 2006;116:901–5.
48. Rombaux P, Weitz H, Mouraux A, et al. Olfactory function assessed with orthonasal and retronasal testing, olfactory bulb volume, and chemosensory event-related potentials. Arch Otolaryngol Head Neck Surg 2006;132:1346–51.
49. Frasnelli J, Landis BN, Heilmann S, et al. Clinical presentation of qualitative olfactory dysfunction. Eur Arch Otorhinolaryngol 2003;11:11–3.
50. Leopold D. Distortion of olfactory perception: diagnosis and treatment. Chem Senses 2002;27: 611–5.
51. Mori K, Nagao H, Yoshihara Y. The olfactory bulb: coding and processing of odor molecule information. Science 1999;286:711–5.
52. Doty RL, Deems D, Steller S. Olfactory dysfunction in Parkinson's disease: a general deficit unrelated to neurologic signs, disease stage, or disease duration. Neurology 1988;38:1237–44.
53. Haehner A, Hummel T, Hummel C, et al. Olfactory loss may be a first sign of idiopathic Parkinson's disease. Mov Disord 2007;22:839–42.

54. Ponsen MM, Stoffers D, Booij J, et al. Idiopathic hyposmia as a preclinical sign of Parkinson's disease. Ann Neurol 2004;56:173–81.
55. Mueller A, Abolmaali ND, Hakimi AR, et al. Olfactory bulb volumes in patients with idiopathic Parkinson's disease–a pilot study. J Neural Transm 2005;112:1363–70.
56. Huisman E, Uylings HB, Hoogland PV. A 100% increase of dopaminergic cells in the olfactory bulb may explain hyposmia in Parkinson's disease. Mov Disord 2004;19:687–92.
57. Witt M, Gudziol V, Haehner A, et al. Nasal mucosa in patients with Parkinson's disease. Chem Senses 2006;31:A31.
58. Gottfried JA. Smell: central nervous processing. Adv Otorhinolaryngol 2006;63:44–69.
59. Furukawa M, Kamide M, Miwa T, et al. Importance of unilateral examination in olfactometry. Auris Nasus Larynx (Tokyo) 1988;15:113–6.
60. Shelley WB, Shelley ED. The smell of burnt toast: a case report. Cutis 2000;65:225–6.
61. Reiter ER, DiNardo LJ, Costanzo RM. Effects of head injury on olfaction and taste. Otolaryngol Clin North Am 2004;37:1167–84.
62. Mann NM, Vento JA. A study comparing SPECT and MRI in patients with anosmia after traumatic brain injury. Clin Nucl Med 2006;31:458–62.
63. Chen C, Shih YH, Yen DJ, et al. Olfactory auras in patients with temporal lobe epilepsy. Epilepsia 2003;44:257–60.
64. Daniels C, Gottwald B, Pause BM, et al. Olfactory event-related potentials in patients with brain tumors. Clin Neurophysiol 2001;112:1523–30.
65. Doty RL, Bromley SM, Moberg PJ, et al. Laterality in human nasal chemoreception. In: Christman S, editor. Cerebral asymmetries in sensory and perceptual processing. Amsterdam: North Holland Publishing; 1997. p. 497–542.
66. Jones-Gotman M, Zatorre RJ. Odor recognition memory in humans: role of right temporal and orbitofrontal regions. Brain Cogn 1993;22:182–98.
67. Jones-Gotman M, Zatorre RJ, Cendes F, et al. Contribution of medial versus lateral temporal-lobe structures to human odour identification. Brain 1997;120:1845–56.
68. Jones-Gotman M, Zatorre RJ, Olivier A, et al. Learning and retention of words and designs following excision from medial or lateral temporal-lobe structures. Neuropsychologia 1997;35:963–73.
69. Zatorre RJ, Jones-Gotman M, Evans AC, et al. Functional localization and lateralization of human olfactory cortex. Nature 1992;360:339–40.

Pathology of the Optic Nerve

Hans Rolf Jäger, MD, FRCR[a,*],
Katherine Anne Miszkiel, BM(Hons), MRCP, FRCR[a,b]

KEYWORDS

- Trauma • Vascular lesions • Tumors
- Inflammation • Granulomatous lesions/infections
- External compression • Hypertension
- Degenerative conditions

CLINICAL SIGNS AND SYMPTOMS

Decrease in visual acuity and visual field defects are the cardinal symptoms of optic nerve lesions.[1] Their mode of onset depends on the underlying pathology: slowly growing compressive and infiltrative lesions lead to progressive visual loss, whereas ischemia, demyelinating lesions, trauma, and a sudden increase in orbital pressure can lead to rapid visual loss. The type of field defect depends on the location of the lesion. Lesions of the intraorbital portion of the optic nerves usually start with a central scotoma that may spread peripherally. Compression of the optic nerve at the level of the orbital apex may lead to abnormalities in a localized sector. Loss of color vision may be an early sign in several optic nerve pathologies, including demyelination, tumors, and toxic neuropathy. Intracranial compression of the optic chiasm classically leads to bitemporal hemianopia.

When examining patients who have suspected optic nerve lesions, it is important to have knowledge of visual field defects produced by postchiasmatic lesions. Selective involvement of the temporal fibers of the optic radiation (Meyer's loop), which may occur in tumors or infarctions confined to the temporal lobe, results in a homonymous superior quandrantanopia. Posterior lesions in the optic radiation produce a hemianopia with macular sparing.

Involvement of the entire striate cortex of the occipital lobe results in a contralateral homonymous hemianopia. Lesions involving the inferior lip of the striate cortex present with a contralateral upper quadrantanopia, and those involving the superior lip present with a contralateral lower quadrantanopia.

Other symptoms associated with optic nerve pathology include proptosis (with intraorbital mass lesions), strabismus, oculomotor nerve palsies (which may be a feature of optic nerve gliomas or other orbital mass lesions and of raised intracranial pressure), headaches (idiopathic intracranial hypertension [IIH]), and conjunctival injection (arteriovenous fistulae). Pituitary lesions compressing the optic nerves and chiasm can be associated with endocrine symptoms.

DEVELOPMENTAL AND INHERITED CONDITIONS

Colobomas

Colobomas are a developmental abnormality arising from failure of closure of the fetal intraocular fissure during gestation. The defect can affect the iris, lens, ciliary body, retina, choroid, sclera, and optic nerve; optic nerve involvement may result in visual field scotomas.

Colobomas account for approximately 2% of congenital malformations of the eye and may occur as an isolated anomaly or part of a multisystemic syndrome. The posterior globe and optic nerve are involved most commonly and the cleft often is in the inferonasal quadrant. Up to 60% may be bilateral (**Fig. 1**A) and inheritance may be autosomal dominant, with variable penetrance.

The shape of the globe and optic nerve coloboma depend on the extent of retinal inversion,

[a] Lysholm Department of Neuroradiology, The National Hospital for Neurology and Neurosurgery, 8-11 Queen Square, London WC1 3BG, United Kingdom
[b] Moorfields Eye Hospital, City Road, London, United Kingdom
* Corresponding author.
E-mail address: r.jager@ion.ucl.ac.uk (H.R. Jäger).

Neuroimag Clin N Am 18 (2008) 243–259
doi:10.1016/j.nic.2007.10.001

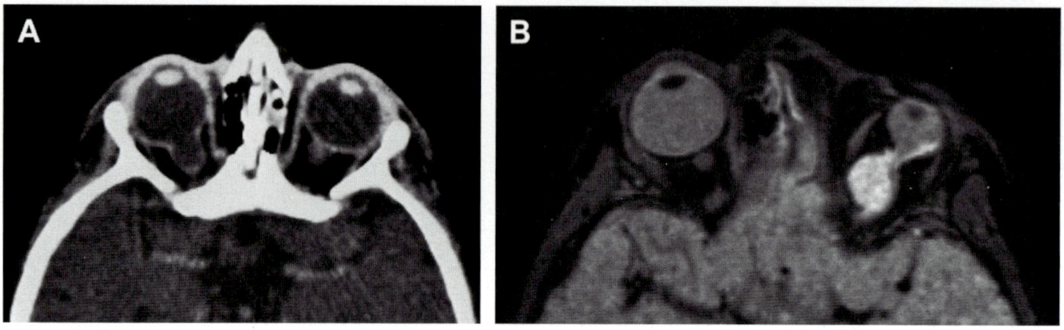

Fig. 1. (*A*) Axial CT showing a fluid density outpouching of the right optic nerve head, in keeping with a coloboma. (*B*) Axial proton density-weighted MRI demonstrating left micro-ophthalmos in association with a posterior cystic colobomatous defect.

and if there is extensive separation of the retinal layers in association with retinal proliferation, large cysts may form that have mass effect and are associated with micro-ophthalmos (**Fig. 1**B).[2]

Systemic abnormalities and syndromes associated with colobomas include trisomy 13 and 18, Potter's syndrome, CHARGE and VATER association, Joubert and Warburg syndromes, congenital heart disease, polydactyly, and holoprosencephaly.[3] The renal-coloboma syndrome is associated with a mutation of the PAX2 gene.[4]

Leber's Hereditary Optic Neuropathy

Leber's hereditary optic neuropathy, a hereditary condition resulting from degeneration of retinal ganglion cells and their axons, results in severe acute or subacute visual loss. It affects predominantly young men and is transmitted maternally. It is the result of several mutations in the mitochondrial genome with effects on the oxidative phosphorylation chain in mitochondria, but it remains unclear exactly how this causes death of cells in the optic nerve head.

Patients usually present with acute unilateral visual loss, followed by a similar event in the contralateral eye several weeks later, and the end result is severe optic atrophy and a permanent reduction in visual acuity. More than 50% of men and 85% of women who have the genetic mutations do not experience visual loss, however.

MRI of the anterior visual pathway in the acute stages may be normal, but in later stages, optic atrophy and increased T2 signal in the optic nerves are present.[5] Swelling and enhancement of the nerves is reported in the acute stage, and demyelinating/multiple sclerosis–like lesions are also encountered on cranial MRI.[6]

Other inherited optic neuropathies, such as dominant optic neuropathy, hereditary spastic paraparesis, and Friedreich's ataxia share the mechanism of mitochondrial dysfunction.

TRAUMA

Trauma of the anterior optic pathways includes direct and indirect injury to the optic nerve. Direct injury is caused most frequently by objects penetrating the orbit (**Fig. 2**) or by bone fragments at the orbital apex. Deceleration injury to the optic nerves and chiasm can be a feature of severe head trauma. The traumatic chiasmal syndrome frequently results in blindness in one eye and a temporal defect in the other or in bitemporal field defects.[7] Soft tissue injuries and bleeding can lead to a rapid rise in intraorbital pressure with secondary (indirect) compressive and ischemic injury to the optic nerve. Shearing forces also may lead to hemorrhage into the optic sheath, causing profound visual symptoms with minimal orbital signs.[7]

Traumatic injury of the globe and optic nerve is assessed best with CT, including multiplanar reformatted images. CT is able to demonstrate intraocular and intraorbital hemorrhage, foreign bodies, and bony fragments. MRI should be avoided if the injury involves metallic fragments, which may be deflected in a magnetic field, thereby causing further damage.

Trauma to the optic nerve also may result from thermal, chemical, or radiation injury. Damage to the optic nerve can occur after radiotherapy of sellar and parasellar tumors and of lymphoproliferative and leukemic disease of the orbit.

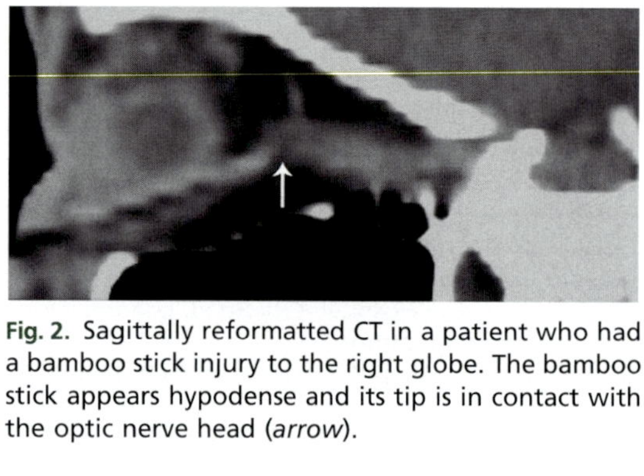

Fig. 2. Sagittally reformatted CT in a patient who had a bamboo stick injury to the right globe. The bamboo stick appears hypodense and its tip is in contact with the optic nerve head (*arrow*).

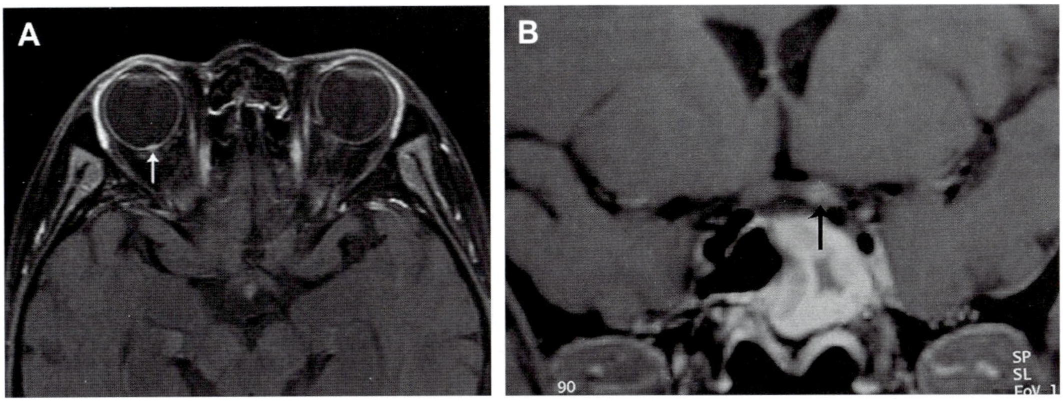

Fig. 3. (*A*) Postcontrast axial T1-weighted MRI with fat saturation showing a small area of enhancement at the optic nerve head (*arrow*) in a patient treated with radiotherapy for a nasopharyngeal carcinoma. The appearances are consistent with postradiation papillitis. (*B*) Postcontrast coronal T1-weighted, fat-saturated MRI in a patient who had received radiotherapy for orbital lymphoma, showing enhancement of the intracranial portion of the left optic nerve (*arrow*), indicating radiation-induced optic neuritis.

Radiation-induced optic neuropathy can involve any part of the optic nerve, including the optic nerve head (**Fig. 3**A), and, not infrequently, the intracranial portion of the optic nerve (**Fig. 3**B). The affected portions are T2 hyperintense and may show contrast enhancement.

VASCULAR LESIONS

Ischemia

The retina and optic nerve head are sensitive to ischemia, which may lead to transient monocular blindness (amaurosis fugax) or to a more permanent visual deficit.[8] In young patients, consider ophthalmic migraine, but in older patients, ischemic ocular symptoms usually are caused by a stenosis or occlusion of the internal carotid artery and retinal artery emboli. Retinal vein occlusion also may cause ischemic symptoms, predisposing conditions being lupus erythematosis or phospholipid syndrome.[9]

Caroticocavernous Fistulae

Caroticocavernous fistulae (CCF) cause raised pressure and enlargement of the ophthalmic veins (**Fig. 4**A, B), leading to proptosis and raised intraocular pressure. If sufficiently high, the raised intraocular pressure interferes with the vascular supply and function of the optic nerve and can

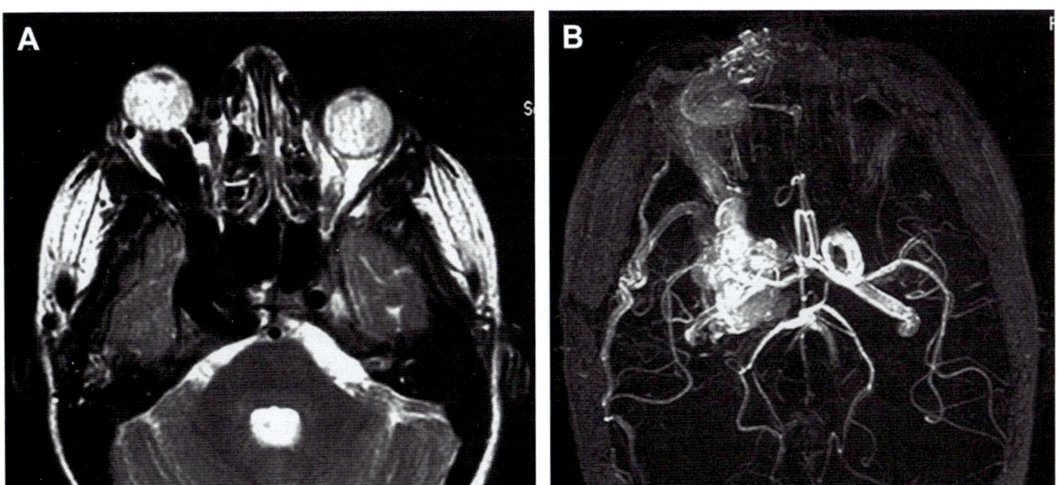

Fig. 4. (*A*) Axial T2-weighted MRI in a patient who had a CCF. There is right-sided proptosis. The right side of the cavernous sinus and right ophthalmic veins are dilated and flow void. (*B*) Axial maximum intensity projection image of a 3-D time-of-flight magnetic resonance angiogram in this patient demonstrating dilatation of the right side of the cavernous sinus and right-sided ophthalmic and superficial cerebral veins.

lead to monocular blindness if not treated in time. Direct CCF are the result of a tear in the wall of the cavernous portion of the internal carotid artery, which creates a direct communication with the cavernous sinus, and are post-traumatic in the majority of cases. Indirect CCF are the result of dural arteriovenous fistulae in the wall of the cavernous sinus, usually supplied by multiple feeders from the external or internal carotid arteries. Indirect CCF may develop spontaneously or secondary to cavernous sinus thrombosis. Direct and indirect CCF reverse the flow in the ophthalmic veins and increase the intraocular pressure. Both types of CCF can be treated by endovascular means. Direct CCF are treated most commonly with occlusion of the tear by balloons inserted from the arterial side, and indirect dural fistulae are treated most commonly with coil embolization of the cavernous sinus from the venous side.

Aneurysms

Aneurysms arising from the cavernous and supraclinoid segments of the internal carotid artery can present with visual symptoms resulting from their mass effect on the optic nerves and optic chiasm (**Fig. 5**). Giant aneurysms in this region are delineated best with contrast-enhanced magnetic resonance angiography[10] or CT angiography. Endovascular treatment options include occlusion of the parent artery (after a successful balloon test occlusion) and coiling. The former leads to a more immediate decrease in mass effect; the latter reduces the pulsatility of the mass in a first instance, which is associated with clinical improvement.

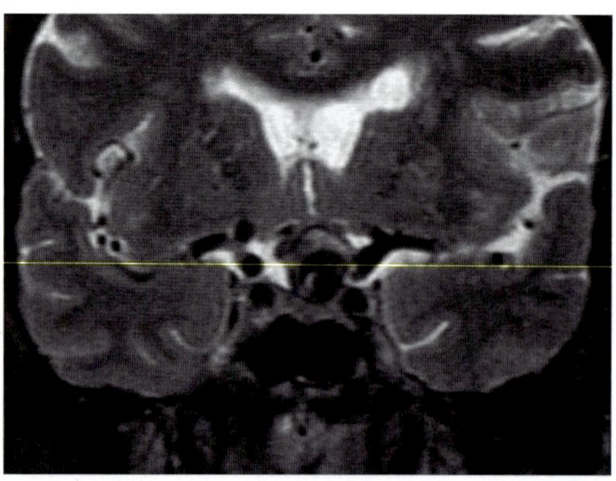

Fig. 5. Coronal T2-weighted MRI demonstrating a partially thrombosed aneurysm of the left internal cerebral artery, which extends medially to compress the optic chiasm.

Wyburn-Mason Syndrome

Wyburn-Mason syndrome is a rare congenital neurocutaneous disorder with facial nevi and ipsilateral arteriovenous malformations (AVMs), which can occur anywhere along the visual pathways from the occipital cortex to the orbit. A recent review of 27 cases found orbital AVMs in 17 cases and involvement of the optic chiasm in seven. Decrease in visual acuity is not uncommon in Wyburn-Mason syndrome, with optic nerve compromise caused by compression by an expanding AVM or ischemia.[11]

TUMORS OF THE OPTIC NERVE

Primary Tumors of the Optic Nerve

The most frequent primary tumors of the optic nerve are gliomas and optic nerve sheath meningiomas, the former four times more common. Other primary optic nerve tumors are rare and include hemangioblastomas, hemangiopericytomas, medulloepitheliomas, and gangliogliomas.[12]

Optic Nerve Gliomas

Optic nerve gliomas originate from astrocytes of the optic nerve and the majority of these tumors occur below age 20 with a peak incidence of from 2 to 8 years.[13] In children, these tumors have a benign histology (pilocytic astrocytomas) and slow growth rate. The more rare adult subgroup has a malignant histology with features of an anaplastic astrocytoma or glioblastoma mutliforme and rapidly may invade adjacent structures, such as the hypothalamus or temporal lobes.

Gliomas can occur anywhere along the optic pathway and present with loss of visual acuity or color vision, abnormal pupillary function, or painless proptosis, depending on their location.

Fusiform enlargement, kinking, and tortuosity of the optic nerve and enlargement of the optic canal are typical features on CT and MRI. Unlike optic nerve sheath meningiomas, gliomas do not show calcification on CT. On MRI, they appear hypo- or isointense on T1- and hyperintense on T2-weighted images and enhance to a variable degree (**Fig. 6**A, B).

Optic nerve gliomas also are a feature of neurofibromatosis 1 (NF1) and bilateral optic nerve gliomas virtually are diagnostic of this condition (**Fig. 7**A–C).[14] Patients who have NF1 may show other intracranial lesions, such as hyperintensities in the basal ganglia, brainstem, and cerebellum or astrocytomas. There is increasing evidence that optic pathway gliomas behave differently in patients who have and who do not have NF1.[15] In NF1 patients optic gliomas involve most frequently

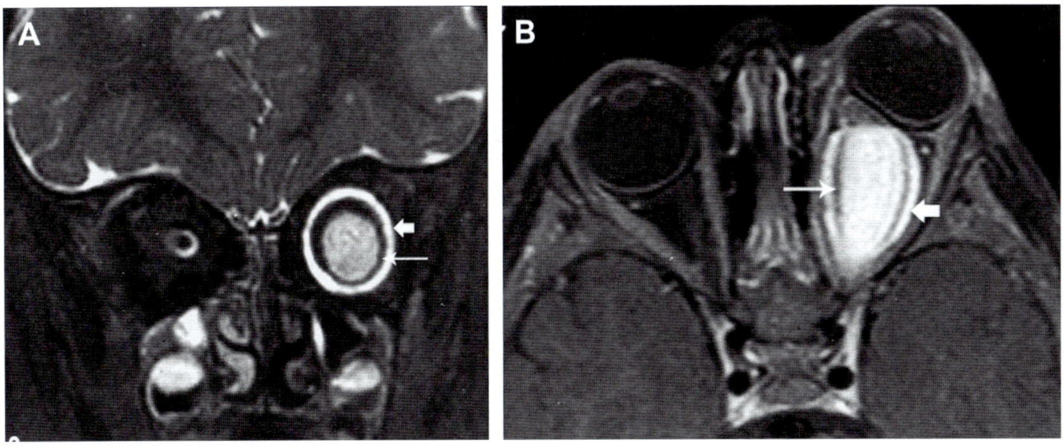

Fig. 6. (*A*) Coronal fat-saturated, contrast-enhanced, T1-weighted images in a child who had an optic nerve glioma. There is marked expansion and hyperintensity of the left optic nerve within the orbit, with a surrounding pseudocapsule (*long arrow*) and involvement of the dura of the optic nerve sheath (*short thick arrow*). (*B*) Axial fat-saturated, contrast-enhanced, T1-weighted images showing proptosis and deformity of the posterior globe and a small anterior tumor cyst. The pseudocapsule (*long arrow*) does not enhance, but there is enhancement of the optic nerve sheath (*short thick arrow*), indicating perineural extension of the tumor.

the optic nerve, whereas in patients who do not have NF1, the optic chiasm represents the most common site (**Fig. 8**A, B). In patients who do not have NF1, the tumors are less stable on follow-up imaging and more likely to extend outside the optic pathways. Visual loss is more common in patients who do not have NF1 (80%) compared with those who have NF1 (20%). There are many well-documented cases of spontaneous regression of optic nerve gliomas in NF1.[14]

Treatment options for optic nerve gliomas are subject to debate, and documentation of disease progression by imaging has an important influence on the decision-making process. Chemotherapy with carboplatin and vincristin now is advocated as first-line therapy for children who have progressive disease.[14] Surgery should be performed only for cosmetic reasons, such as disfiguring proptosis. Optic nerve gliomas that do not involve the chiasm at initial presentation tend not to "grow backward," so that removal of the optic nerve to prevent spread to the chiasm does not seem justified. Conventional radiotherapy has been advocated in the past but has significant side effects, including secondary brain tumors, occlusive cerebral vasculopathy, and pituitary gland malfunction. Fractionated stereotactic radiotherapy has fewer side effects and shows promising results.[14]

The differential diagnosis of optic nerve gliomas includes perioptic meningioma, demyelinating optic neuritis, lymphoma, and idiopathic orbital inflammation (discussed later). The optic chiasm also may be involved in multifocal cerebral glioma (**Fig. 9**A–C).

Optic Nerve Sheath Meningioma

Optic nerve sheath meningiomas are seen most commonly in women between ages 30 and 50. Bilateral tumors are associated with neurofibromatosis 2. Primary optic nerve sheath meningiomas arise from the arachnoid cap cells of the arachnoid sheath; secondary tumors represent an extension of intracranial meningiomas into the orbit via the optic canal, superior orbital fissure, or bone.[16] Optic nerve sheath meningiomas impair the vascular supply and axonal transport of the optic nerve, thereby comprising its function.

These tumors present with slowly progressive visual loss and painless proptosis. Transient visual obscurations may be one of the initial symptoms. Ophthalmoscopic examination shows disc pallor and retinochoroidal shunts.

MRI and CT features are fusiform or eccentric thickening of the optic nerve sheath complex.[16,17] CT frequently shows calcification within the tumor (**Fig. 10**A). MRI provides better detail of the tumor extension than CT and contrast-enhanced, fat-suppressed, T1-weighted images are particularly useful. MRI typically shows a hypodense optic nerve surrounded by a fusiform or globular rim of enhancing tissue with very fine extensions into the orbital fat (**Fig. 10**B). The tram-track sign is typical but not specific for meningiomas.[18] It is the result of the relative hypointensity or hypodensity of the optic nerve, compared with the surrounding tumor, which enhances strongly and may be hyperdense on CT because of calcification.

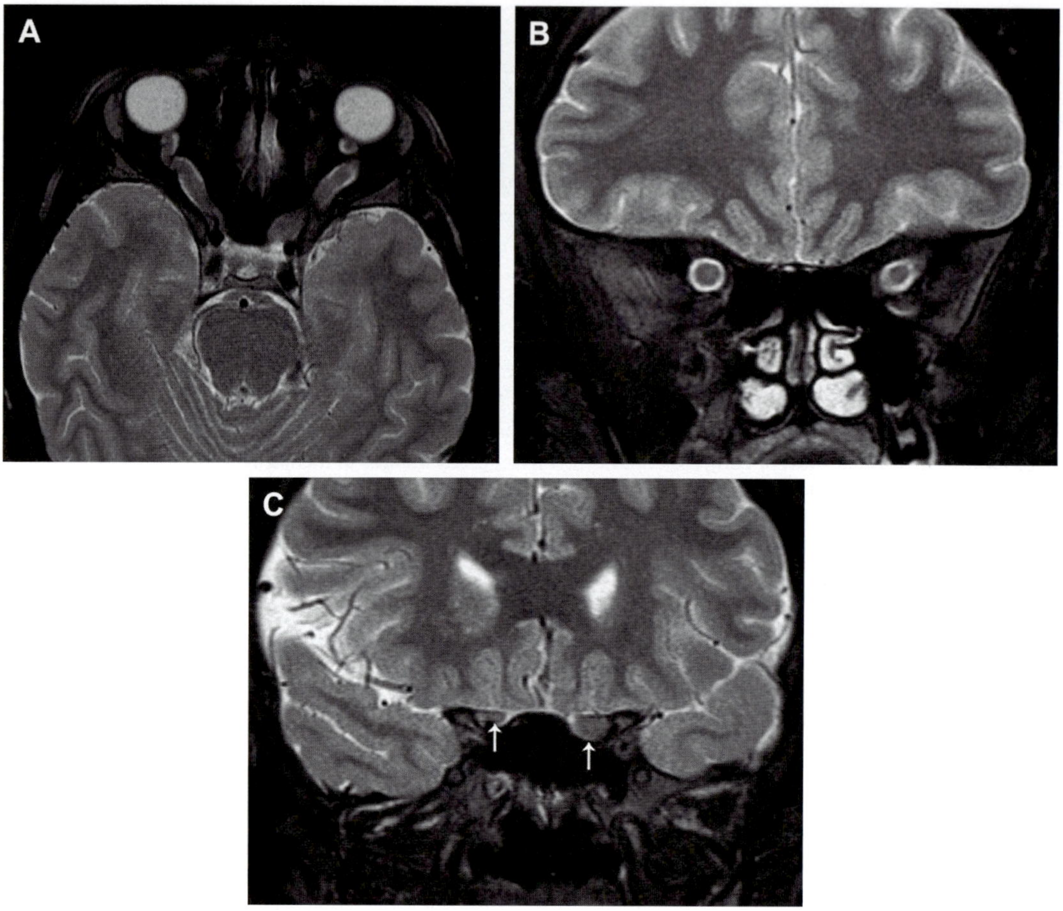

Fig. 7. (*A*) Axial T2-weighted images showing dilatation, tortuosity, and kinking of both optic nerves in a patient who had NF1 and bilateral optic nerve gliomas, the left side affected more severely with dilatation of the optic canal. (*B*, *C*) Coronal T2-weighted images showing dilated intraorbital and intracranial (*arrows*) portions of the optic nerves.

Once the meningioma has extended through the optic canal, it spreads along the intracranial meninges and can endanger the contralateral optic nerve, if it crosses the midline at the level of the planum sphenoidale, which is appreciated best on coronal MRI.

Assessment of tumor extension and progression with imaging is relevant to clinical management. Optic nerve sheath menigiomas are slowly progressive and do not metastasize, so that observation without invasive treatment is an option. In conservatively treated menigiomas, MRI studies at 6-month intervals in the first 2 years followed by yearly studies for 2 to 3 years are recommended.[19]

Recent evidence suggests that patients treated with radiotherapy alone have a better long-term visual outcome compared with patients who have optic nerve sheath meningioma who are managed conservatively and surgically.[20] A major concern with radiotherapy is its toxicity to the optic nerve, retina, and pituitary gland. Stereotactic fractionated radiotherapy can deliver a sufficient dose to the optic nerve while minimizing the exposure to adjacent structures. Stereotactic fractionated radiotherapy requires complex planning based on pretreatment CT and MRI and has emerged as the primary treatment option for optic nerve sheath meningiomas after several published series demonstrated disease control in more than 90% and visual improvement in more than 50% of patients.[19]

Secondary Tumors of the Optic Nerve

Secondary tumors of the optic nerve originate either from contiguous spread of neoplasms in adjacent structures, distant spread of solid tumor metastasis, or infiltration by hematopoietic malignancies.

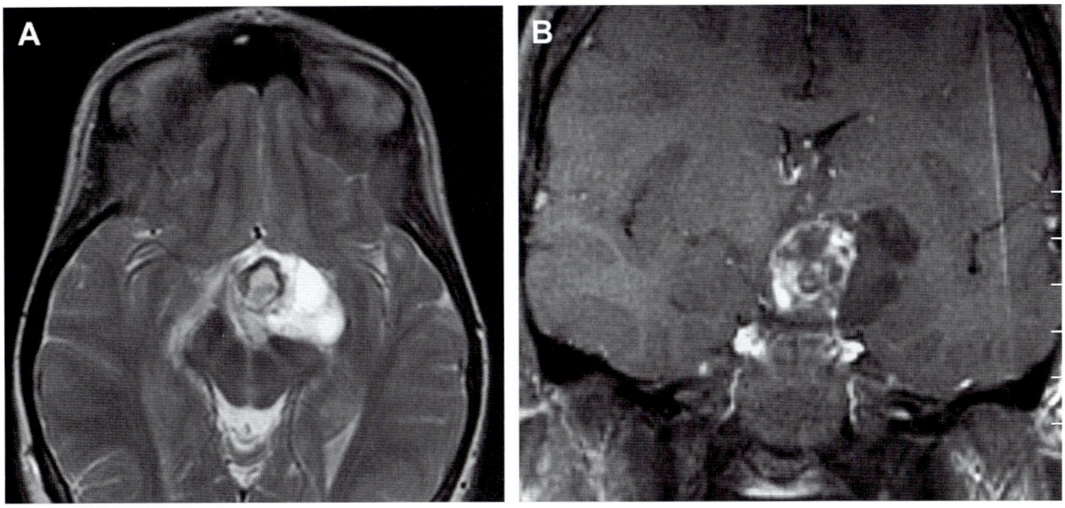

Fig. 8. (*A*) Axial T2-weighted images in a chiasmatic optic nerve glioma, which is of mixed signal intensity with solid and cystic components, occupying the chiasmatic cistern and indenting the left temporal lobe and cerebral peduncle. (*B*) Coronal contrast-enhanced, T1-weighted images showing patchy enhancement of the solid portions and invasion of the medial temporal lobe on the left.

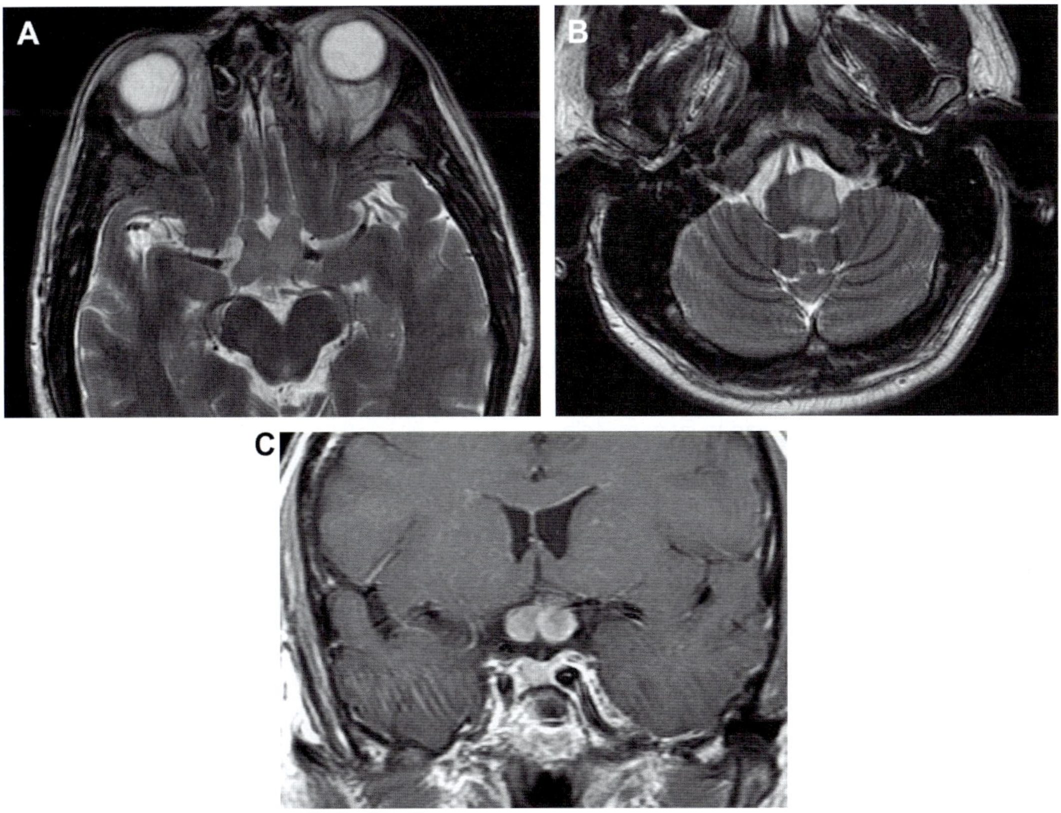

Fig. 9. (*A*, *B*) Axial T2-weighted images in a patient who had multifocal glioma showing thickening and hyperintensity of the optic nerves, chiasm, and optic tracts (*A*) and a T2 hyperintense mass in the medulla oblongata. (*C*) Coronal-enhanced T1-weighted images showing marked enhancement of the optic chiasm.

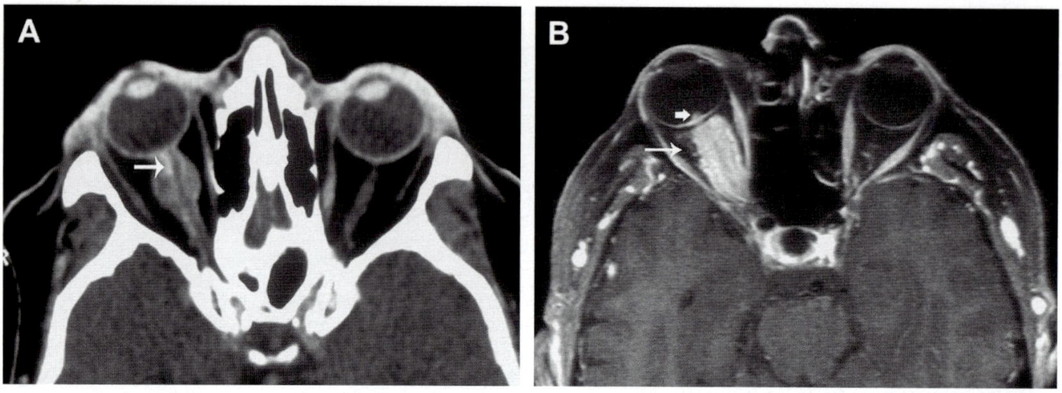

Fig. 10. (*A*) Axial contrast-enhanced CT in a patient who had a right optic nerve sheath meningioma exhibiting fusiform dilatation of the optic nerve sheath with a tram-track sign and focal calcification (*arrow*). (*B*) Axial contrast-enhanced, fat-saturated, T1-weighted image in a different patient who had a right optic nerve sheath meningioma. There is an enhancing tumor surrounding the right optic nerve, which extends into the globe (*short arrow*) and has fine extensions into the orbital fat (*long arrow*).

Direct Invasion of the Optic Nerve

The optic nerve may be invaded by intraocular neoplasms, such as retinoblastomas and uveal melanomas. Retinoblastoma is a common malignant intraocular tumor in childhood and in approximately a third of cases the optic nerve is invaded.[12] Uveal melanoma represents the most common intraocular neoplasm in adults and may invade the optic nerve, which is particularly seen with juxtapapillary primary tumors. Optic nerve invasion may indicate a more malignant subcategory of uveal melanomas.

Direct invasion of the optic nerve by intracranial neoplasms also is possible (**Fig. 11**A–C) but less common.[12]

Metastases

Most orbital metastases spread to bone, fat, or muscles, and can lead to optic nerve compression. The optic nerve also may be infiltrated by metastases that have initially spread to fat or muscle. Direct metastases to the optic nerve are rare and occur predominantly in breast carcinoma.

Lymphoproliferative Disorders

In leukemia, diffuse infiltration of the optic nerve can lead to rapid loss of vision, which represents a clinical emergency, requiring treatment with radiotherapy.[21]

The spectrum of orbital disease in non-Hodgkin's lymphoma is wide. It includes well-defined mass lesions in the extraconal or intraconal space, lacrimal gland masses, and diffusely infiltrative lesions.[21] Visual loss is a feature of infiltrative retrobulbar lesions, which may resemble idiopathic orbital inflammation.

INFLAMMATORY CONDITIONS

Optic Neuritis

Optic neuritis is one of the most common causes of acute visual loss in young adults in temperate climates and occurs with an incidence of 1 to 5 per 100,000 per year and most cases are the result of idiopathic inflammatory demyelination. It usually presents as a painful subacute unilateral loss of vision over a few days to 2 weeks, usually associated with decreased color vision and contrast sensitivity.[22] At least partial recovery of vision is the norm but progression to monocular blindness is possible and 10% to 15% of individuals are left with severe visual impairment. In the acute phase, MRI shows swelling, T2 hyperintensity, and contrast enhancement of the optic nerve (**Fig. 12**A, B). This may involve segments or the entire length of the optic nerve and extend posteriorly to involve the optic chiasm. Enhancement of the nerve sheath also can be seen in up to 75% of cases if triple-dose gadolinium contrast agent is used, and interruption of cerebrospinal fluid (CSF) flow can result in some distension of the nerve sheath, seen anteriorly in up to 45% of cases.[23] Serial MRI has shown continued atrophy of the optic nerve over months and years after optic neuritis.[24] A recent study[25] showed that in patients who have optic neuritis, 77% have one or more asymptomatic T2 lesions on their baseline cranial MRI scan, with 26% having active intracranial lesions showing contrast enhancement; 26% also have spinal cord lesions. The risk for developing multiple sclerosis after an episode of optic neuritis is approximately 40% at 10 years' and 50% at 20 years' follow-up.[22] Clinically silent demyelinating lesions on an MRI of the brain represent a strong indicator of multiple sclerosis. In cases

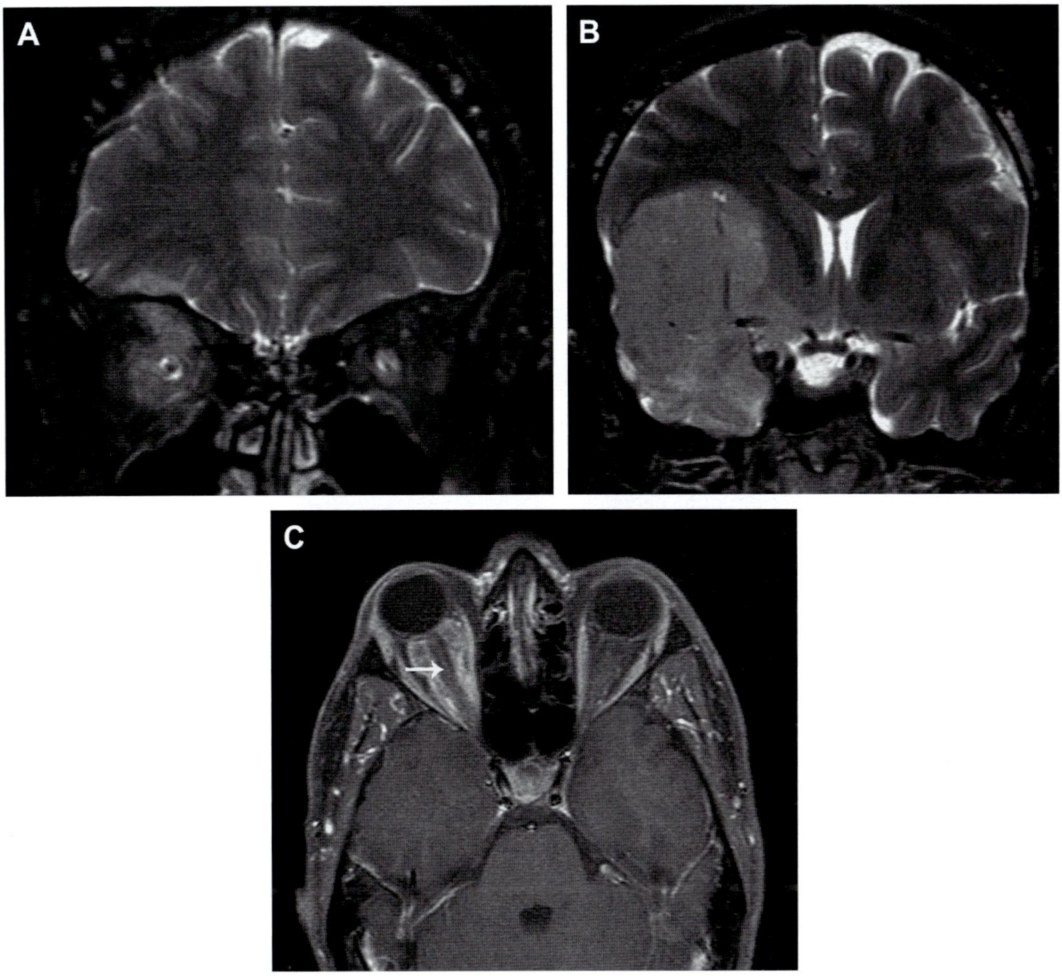

Fig. 11. (*A, B*) Axial fat-saturated, T2-weighted images of a patient who had a primitive neuroectodermal tumor (PNET) of the right hemisphere, which extends into the orbit, invading the orbital fat and optic nerve sheath. (*C*) Axial contrast-enhanced, fat-saturated T1-weighted image shows an enhancing mass surrounding the right optic nerve sheath complex (*arrow*).

of a clinically isolated syndrome with optic neuritis, the appearance of new T2 lesions on a 3-month follow-up MRI also is suggestive of multiple sclerosis.[26] Acute optic neuritis associated with transverse myelitis is known as neuromyelitis optica or Devic's syndrome.[27]

Optic neuritis also may occur in isolation or secondary to sarcoidosis, viral infection (including patients who have AIDS [HIV-related optic neuropathy]), vasculitides, ischemia, toxins, and radiation.

Idiopathic Orbital Inflammation

Idiopathic orbital inflammation is a steroid-responsive inflammatory condition, which can affect any orbital compartment and extend intracranially. Visual deficits are produced by direct infiltration of the optic nerve sheath complex (perineuritis) (**Fig. 13**) or compression of the optic nerve by inflammatory masses at the orbital apex.

GRANULOMATOUS LESIONS/INFECTIONS

Granulomatous diseases, such as sarcoidosis, Wegener's granulomatosis, tuberculosis, and eosinophilic granulomas, can affect the anterior optic pathways. There may be primary involvement or secondary infiltration of the optic chiasm with enhancing lesions in the chiasmatic cistern, enhancement of the basal meninges, and thickening of the pituitary infundibulum. Posterior extension of these lesions may involve the optic tracts. Wegener's granulomatosis is associated with destruction of the paranasal sinuses (**Fig. 14**A, B).

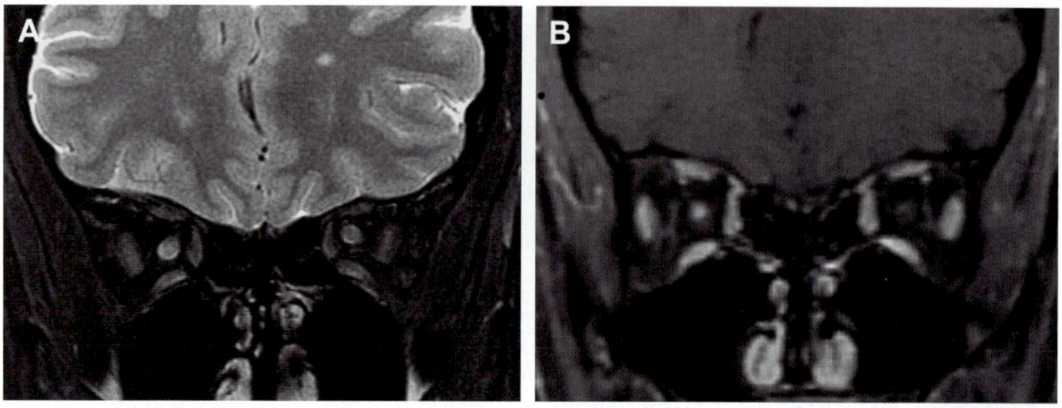

Fig. 12. (*A*) Coronal fat-saturated T2-weighted image in a patient who had multiple sclerosis. There is enlargement and hyperintensity of the right optic nerve consistent with optic neuritis. In addition, there is a left frontal hyperintense white matter lesion. (*B*) Coronal contrast-enhanced, fat-saturated, T1-weighted image demonstrates enhancement of the enlarged right optic nerve.

Sarcoidosis is an inflammatory disorder, which may involve any part of the optic pathways, most commonly the optic nerves and optic chiasm (**Fig. 15**A, B).[28] The anterior optic pathways are involved in approximately 1% to 5% of cases of sarcoidosis. Occult sarcoidosis may present with an isolated optic neuropathy and can be confused with other conditions, such as an optic nerve meningioma. Establishing a suspected diagnosis of optic nerve sarcoidosis by careful examination of systemic signs rather than by optic nerve biopsy, which carries a risk of blindness, is strongly recommended. Up to 80% of patients have abnormal pulmonary function tests and raised serum angiotensin-converting enzyme levels, and 40% show evidence of past or active uveitis.[28] The imaging appearance also can give a clue: bilateral optic nerve involvement is found in a third of patients, and pathologic enhancement of the optic nerve from the globe to the chiasm is strongly suggestive of sarcoidosis. Enhancement of the frontobasal meninges and enlargement of the lacrimal glands are other features indicative of sarcoidosis.[28]

EXTERNAL COMPRESSION OF OPTIC NERVE

Intraorbital Compressive Lesions

The orbital apex and optic canal represent the narrowest part of the optic pathway. Any additional narrowing caused by soft tissue or bone in that region can lead to compression of the optic nerve with visual symptoms. This occurs most frequently with thyroid eye disease where the optic nerve is compressed by enlarged extraocular muscles. This can lead to bilateral or asymmetric compression depending on the muscle groups affected.

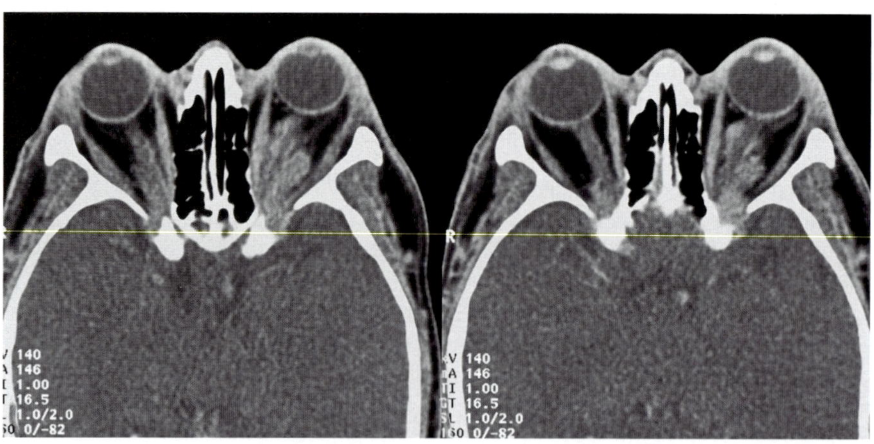

Fig. 13. Axial postcontrast CT images showing asymmetric infiltrative soft tissue masses within both orbits around the optic nerve sheath complexes. The changes are more extensive on the left and there is early intracranial extension through both superior orbital fissures. Biopsy confirmed idiopathic orbital inflammation.

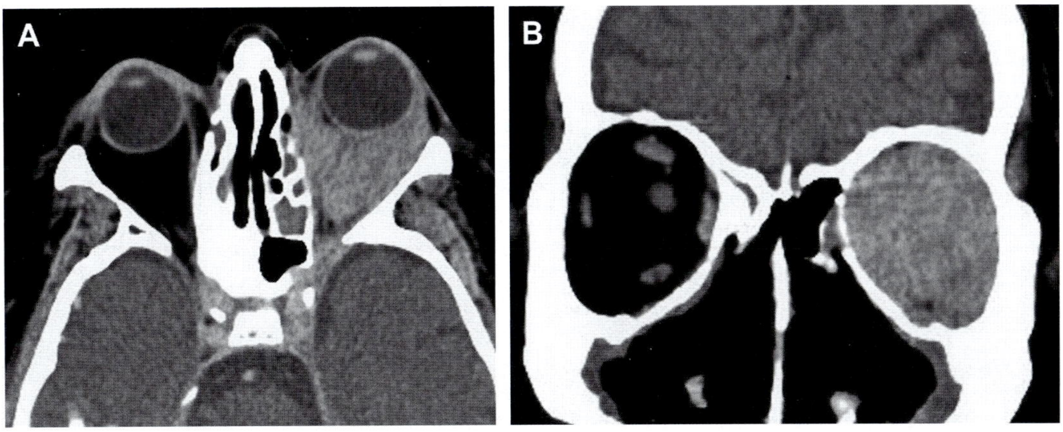

Fig. 14. (*A*) Axial CT in a patient who had Wegener's granulomatosis showing a diffuse infiltrative soft tissue mass within the left orbit involving the orbital apex and ethmoid sinuses. (*B*) Coronal reformatted images show complete infiltration of the left orbit by soft tissue and extensive loss of normal bony anatomy in the maxillary antra.

Other intraorbital soft tissue masses that can cause optic nerve compression include cavernomas (**Fig. 16**A, B), neuroma, and idiopathic orbital inflammation. Bony narrowing of the optic canal is seen in fibrous dysplasia of the skull base.

Intracranial Compressive Lesions

Tumors of the sellar region can lead to compression of the intracranial portions of the optic nerve and optic chiasm, and pituitary adenomas are the most common neoplasms in this region.

Macroadenomas expand the sella turcica and can present with visual symptoms if they have significant suprasellar extension, bitemporal hemianopia being the hallmark of symmetric optic chiasm compression. Pituitary adenomas can produce several other visual defects when compressing predominantly the optic nerves or tracts. The position of the optic chiasm with respect to the tumor is important for surgical planning and is assessed best with sagittal and coronal MRI. The optic chiasm sometimes may be inseparable or indistinguishable from the pituitary tumor. The onset of visual symptoms usually is gradual, and a recent study demonstrated that T2 hyperintensity of the optic nerves ventral to compressive pituitary tumors correlated well with visual acuity disturbance.[29]

Acute deterioration of vision can occur with pituitary apoplexy, an intratumoural hemorrhage, possibly the result of hemorrhagic infarction in a tumor outgrowing its blood supply. The hemorrhage can lead to rapid enlargement of the tumor and

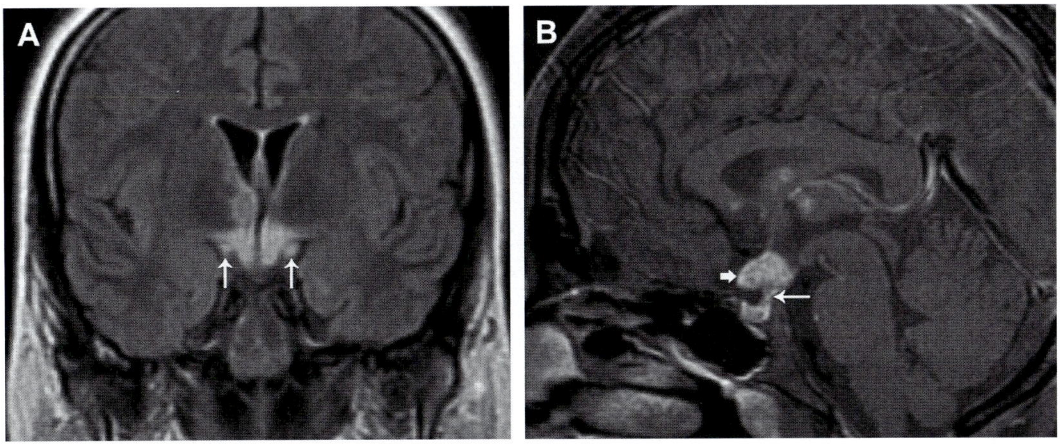

Fig. 15. (*A*) Coronal fluid-attenuated inversion recovery image in a patient who had neurosarcoidosis demonstrating bilateral hyperintense hypothalamic and optic tract (*arrows*) lesions. (*B*) Sagittal contrast-enhanced, T1-weighted image in this patient shows thickening and enhancement of the optic chiasm (*short thick arrow*) and pituitary infundibulum (*long arrow*). There also are several enhancing intracerebral lesions.

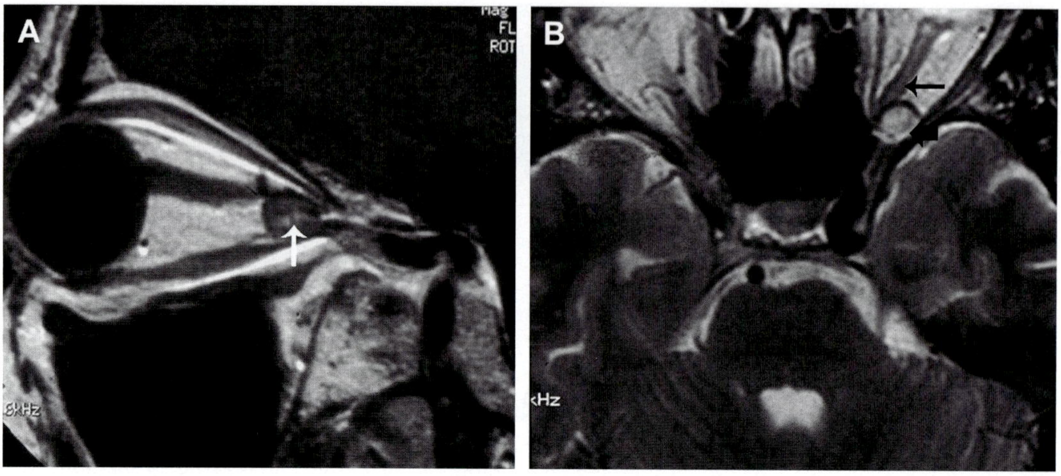

Fig. 16. (*A*) Sagittal contrast-enhanced, T1-weighted image in a patient presenting with compressive left optic neuropathy shows a small rounded T1 hypointense mass at the left orbital apex which enhances patchily (*arrow*). (*B*) Axial T2-weighted image shows a T2 hyperintense mass (*short thick arrow*) compressing the left optic nerve (*long arrow*). The mass was confirmed to be a cavernous hemangioma. Patchy enhancement frequently is seen in these lesions.

appears as high density on CT and as T1 hyperintensity on MRI (**Fig. 17**A, B).

Meningiomas arising from the diaphragma sellae or adjacent meningeal surfaces can compress the optic chiasm. They may cause expansion (blistering) of the sphenoid sinus and hyperostosis but usually do not expand the sella turcica. Coronal and sagittal MRI images often demonstrate the pituitary gland as a separate structure form the tumor (**Fig. 18**).

Craniopharyngiomas are the most frequent chiasmatic tumor in children but have a second incidence peak in adults at approximately the fifth decade. Craniopharyngiomas arise from squamous epithelial cell rests of Rathke's pouch. Cystic tumor components and calcification, best appreciated on CT, are common features.[30] Craniopharyngiomas may be associated with perilesional edema extending into the optic tracts, a feature usually absent in pituitary tumors or meningiomas.[31]

Large intracranial aneurysms are another cause of anterior optic pathway compression (discussed previously).

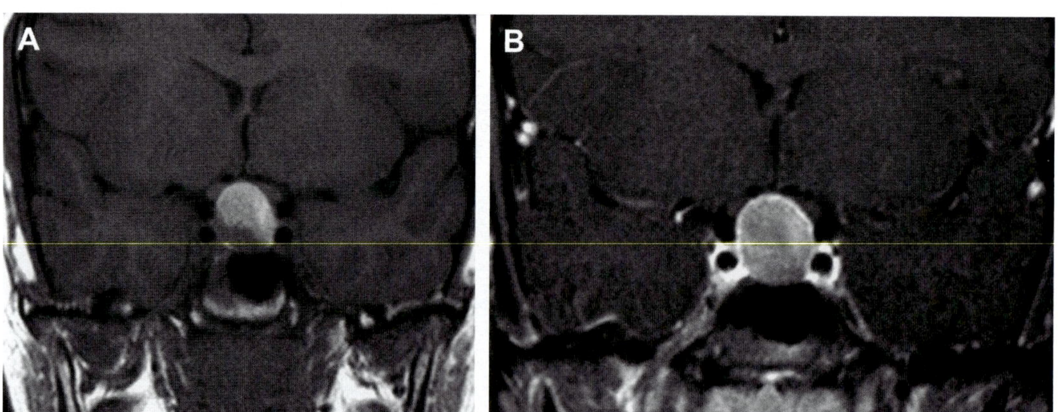

Fig. 17. (*A*) Coronal T1-weighted images in a patient who had pituitary apoplexy demonstrating a sellar and suprasellar mass splaying the optic chiasm. The left and superior portions of the mass are T1 hyperintense, consistent with blood products (methemoglobin) from hemorrhage into a pituitary adenoma. (*B*) The contrast-enhanced, fat-saturated T1-weighted image shows enhancement of the nonhemorrhagic part and periphery of the mass.

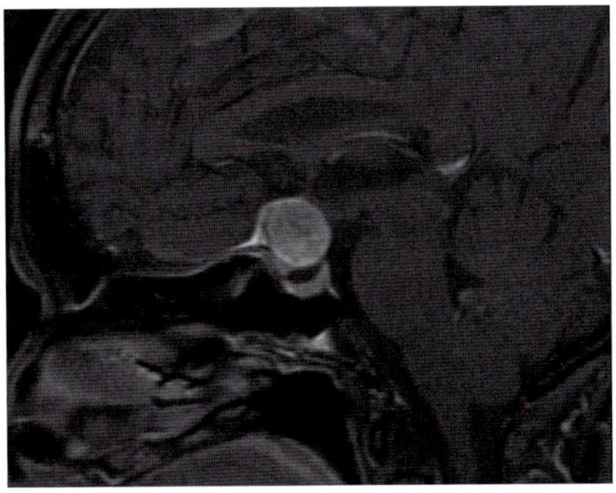

Fig. 18. Sagittal contrast-enhanced, T1-weighted image of a suprasellar meningioma compressing the optic chiasm. There is blistering of the sphenoid sinus and a dural tail along the planum sphenoidale (*long arrow*), and the pituitary gland (*short thick arrow*) is identified as separate structure inferior to the enhancing suprasellar mass.

IDIOPATHIC INTRACRANIAL HYPERTENSION

IIH is a syndrome of signs and symptoms of increased intracranial pressure, including headaches and visual disturbance. In the past, this condition was called pseudotumour cerebri and benign intracranial hypertension. The latter is a misnomer, as it can lead to blindness resulting from raised intraocular pressure and, therefore, is not "benign".[32] Intracranial hypertension also may be secondary to dural sinus thrombosis or medication, such as doxycycline.

Imaging features include a large CSF-filled (empty) sella and a patulous optic nerve sheath with CSF tracking between the optic nerve and sheath (**Fig. 19**A, B). In severe cases, the optic nerve head protrudes into the globe. None of these imaging features, however, is specific for IIH.

Narrowing of the transverse sinus frequently is demonstrated in patients who have IIH. A recent study, however, demonstrates that transverse

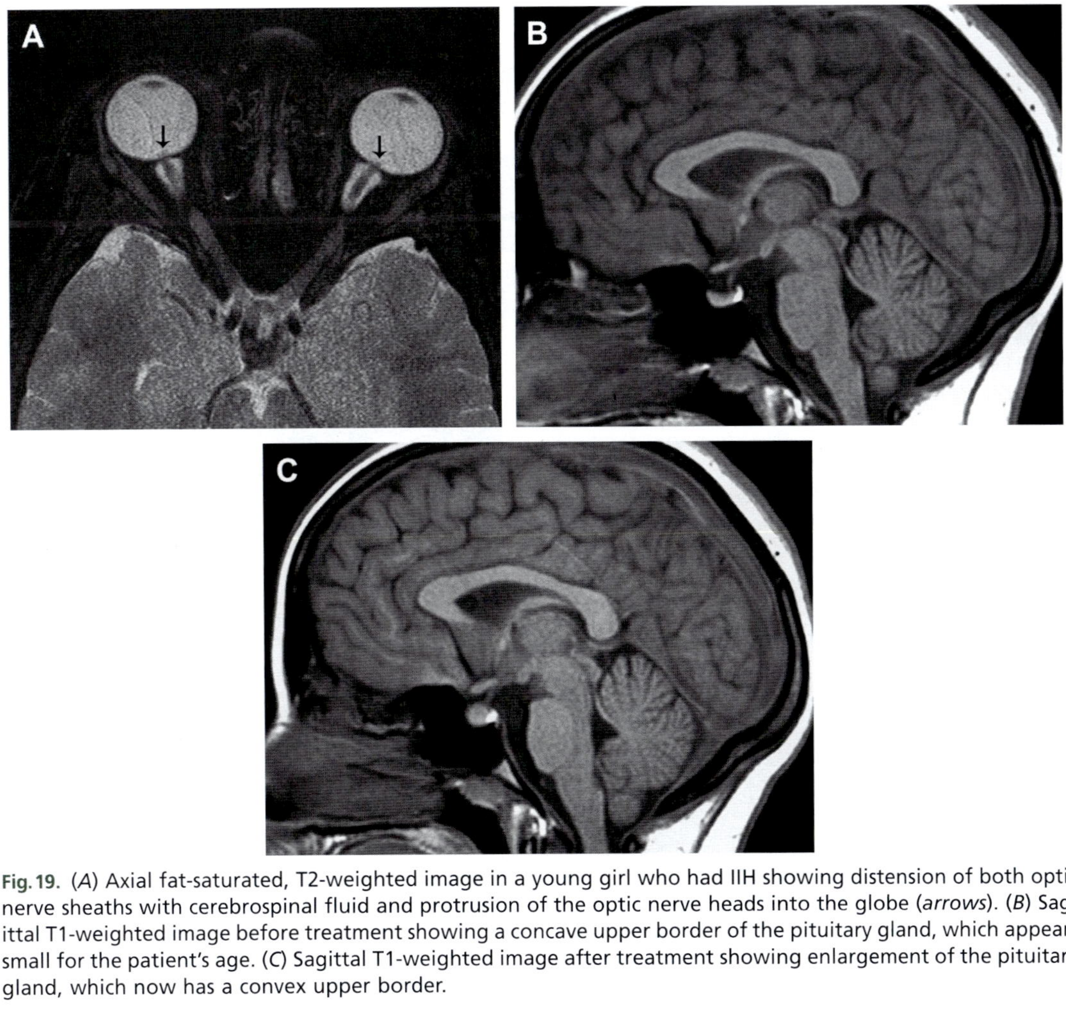

Fig. 19. (*A*) Axial fat-saturated, T2-weighted image in a young girl who had IIH showing distension of both optic nerve sheaths with cerebrospinal fluid and protrusion of the optic nerve heads into the globe (*arrows*). (*B*) Sagittal T1-weighted image before treatment showing a concave upper border of the pituitary gland, which appears small for the patient's age. (*C*) Sagittal T1-weighted image after treatment showing enlargement of the pituitary gland, which now has a convex upper border.

sinus narrowing is reversible after CSF diversion, suggesting that it represents a secondary phenomenon.[33] Treatment of IIH and CSF diversion also can result in a change of shape of the pituitary gland (**Fig. 19**C).

DEGENERATIVE CONDITIONS

Drusen

Optic nerve head drusen are seen in approximately 1% of the population and may be bilateral in 70% of cases; caucasians are affected preferentially, and inheritance may be autosomal dominant, with incomplete penetrance. They occur as a result of retained hyaline bodies in the optic nerve head and often become calcified after adolescence and then are detected easily with ultrasound or CT (**Fig. 20**). Patients often are asymptomatic, and they may be an incidental finding but are a major cause of psuedopapilloedema.

Some patients, however, may experience mild reduction in visual acuity and arcuate scotomas, sectoral field loss, and altitudinal defects. Patients also may be at increased risk for developing nonarteritic anterior ischemic optic neuropathy or branch and central retinal vein occlusion. Occasionally, a small new area of blood vessels develops as a choroidal neovascular membrane adjacent to the optic disc, which can bleed and result in visual loss. Patients who have optic nerve head drusen need clinical follow-up.

Toxic Amblyopia and Other Acquired Optic Neuropathies

As in Leber's hereditary optic neuropathy, mitochondrial dysfunction is the presumed pathophysiologic mechanism of several nutritional and toxic neuropathies.[34] This results in degeneration of the fibers of the papillomacular bundle with central or cecocentral visual field defects. Excess alcohol intake and smoking can lead to tobacco-alcohol amblyopia, characterized by a central loss of vision for colors. Poor diet, in particular a deficiency of thiamine, is a recognized cause of amblyopia, particularly in developing countries. Adequate nutrition with supplements of thiamine, folic acid, and vitamin B_{12} may reverse nutritional amblyopia. Methanol is the cause of toxic neuropathy that is recognized most widely and it can also be caused by several drugs, including ethambutol, amiodorone, and tamoxifen.

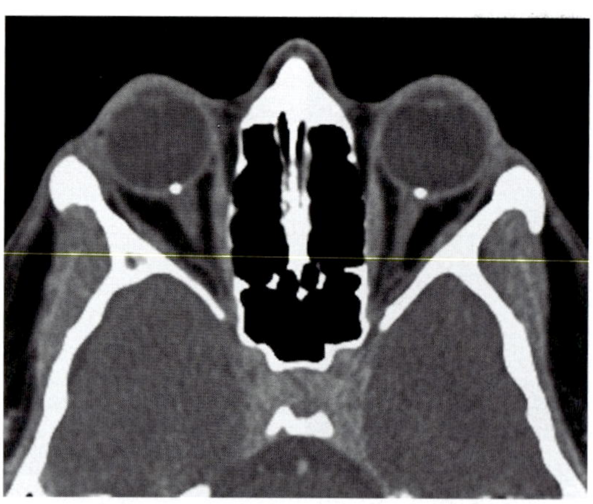

Fig. 20. Axial CT. Small bilateral hyperdense lesions at the optic nerve heads are shown incidentally and are typical of calcified drusen.

VISUAL PATHWAYS POSTERIOR TO THE CHIASM

Lateral Geniculate Bodies

Isolated lesions of the lateral geniculate bodies are rare, the most frequent pathology being infarctions in the anterior or lateral posterior choroidal arteries. They may be involved in inflammatory and neoplastic processes extending along the optic tracts or originating in the thalamus.

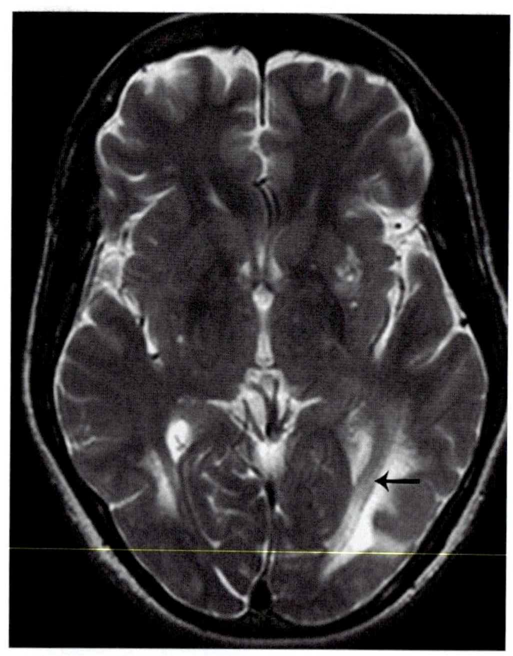

Fig. 21. Axial T2-weighted MRI T2-hyperintense white matter lesions extending into the subcortical U fibers are seen in both occipital lobes, surrounding the optic radiations, which appear as hypointense structures running through the center of the lesions (*arrow*). This patient had AIDS and the lesions were confirmed as progressive multifocal leukoencephalopathy.

Optic Radiation

The optic radiation may be affected by any disease process involving white matter. This includes subcortical infarctions, demyelinating lesions, progressive multifocal leukoencephalopathy (**Fig. 21**), radiation-induced leukoencephalopathy, gliomas, or metastases.[35]

Visual Cortex

Infarctions and tumors are the most common type of pathology found in the occipital cortex. Acute occipital infarctions can exert mass effect and subacute infarction may show enhancement. Diffusion-weighted MRI allows easy distinction between acute/subacute infarction and glial tumors. Bilateral occipital infarctions secondary to emboli from the distal basilar artery territory may lead to cortical blindness.

Thrombosis of the posterior part of the superior sagittal sinus can lead to venous infarctions of the occipital cortex, which frequently are hemorrhagic. Sinus thrombosis should be included in the differential diagnosis of patients who have prothrombotic conditions and visual symptoms.

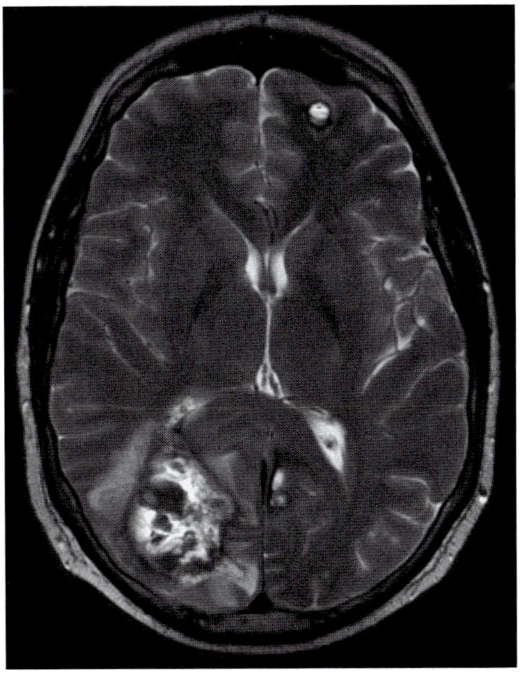

Fig. 22. Axial T2-weighted MRI showing bilateral occipital mass lesions in a patient who had a known melanoma and visual loss. The larger metastasis in the right occipital is surrounded by vasogenic edema and there is a further metastasis in the right frontal lobe. The T2 hypointense rim is typical of melanoma metastases.

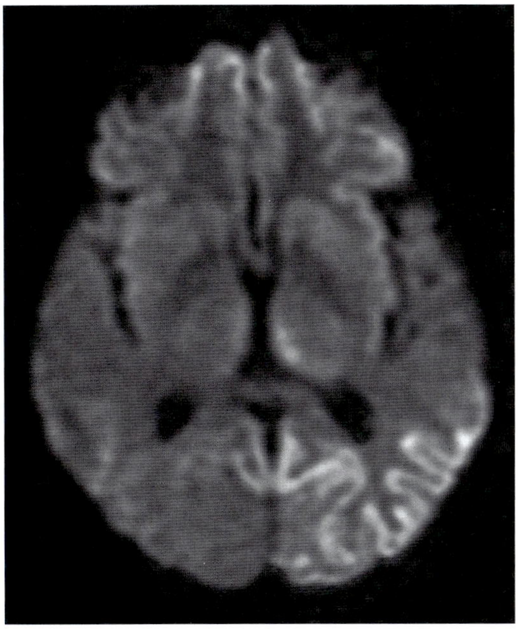

Fig. 23. Axial diffusion-weighted image in a patient who had sporadic Creutzfeldt-Jakob disease 2 weeks after onset of symptoms showing hyperintensity of several cortical regions, including the visual cortex on both sides. The corresponding T2-weighted images were normal.

AVMs fed by occipital artery branches that are large enough to cause visual symptoms can be detected easily with MRI.

The differential diagnosis of malignant mass lesion in the occipital region includes primary brain tumors, lymphoma, and metastases (**Fig. 22**), as elsewhere in the brain.

Another condition that can affect the visual cortex and subcortical occipital white matter is posterior reversible leukoencephalopathy syndrome. This is a clinicoradiologic entity associated with several conditions, including hypertensive encephalopathy, eclampsia, and cytotoxic or immunosuppressive drugs, such as cyclosporine.[36] MRI shows increased T2 signal intensity of the posterior white matter with variable involvement of the overlying cortex. The presumed etiology is failure of the autoregulation and endothelial function of the posterior cerebral circulation.

Diffusion-weighted MRI and apparent diffusion coefficient measurements may reveal involvement of the visual cortex in sporadic Creutzfeldt-Jakob disease despite normal conventional MRI (**Fig. 23**).

REFERENCES

1. Rootman J. Confirmatory investigation of orbital disease and effect on function. In: Rootman J, editor. Diseases of the orbit: a multidisciplinary approach. 2nd edition. Philadelphia: Lippincott Williams & Wilkins; 2002. p. 97–120.
2. Schubert HD. Structural organization of choroidal colobomas of young and adult patients and mechanism of retinal detachment. Trans Am Ophthalmol Soc 2005;103:457–72.
3. Berk AT, Yaman A, Saatci AO. Ocular and systemic findings associated with optic disc colobomas. J Pediatr Ophthalmol Strabismus 2003;40:272–8.
4. Cunliffe HE, McNoe LA, Ward TA, et al. The prevalence of PAX2 mutations in patients with isolated colobomas or colobomas associated with urogenital anomalies. J Med Genet 1998;35:806–12.
5. Mashima Y, Oshitari K, Imamura Y, et al. Orbital high resolution magnetic resonance imaging with fast spin echo in the acute stage of Leber's hereditary optic neuropathy. J Neurol Neurosurg Psychiatry 1998;64:124–7.
6. Kovacs GG, Hoftberger R, Majtenyi K, et al. Neuropathology of white matter disease in Leber's hereditary optic neuropathy. Brain 2005;128:35–41.
7. Rootman J. Structural lesions—trauma. In: Rootman J, editor. Diseases of the orbit: a multidisciplinary approach. 2nd edition. Philadelphia: Lippincott Williams & Wilkins; 2002. p. 437–53.
8. Mead GE, Lewis SC, Wardlaw JM, et al. Comparison of risk factors in patients with transient and prolonged eye and brain ischemic syndromes. Stroke 2002;33:2383–90.
9. Au A, O'Day J. Review of severe vaso-occlusive retinopathy in systemic lupus erythematosus and the antiphospholipid syndrome: associations, visual outcomes, complications and treatment. Clin Experiment Ophthalmol 2004;32:87–100.
10. Jäger HR, Ellamushi H, Moore EA, et al. Contrast-enhanced magnetic resonance angiography in intracranial giant aneurysms. AJNR Am J Neuroradiol 2000;21:1900–7.
11. Dayani PN, Sadun AA. A case report of Wyburn-Mason syndrome and review of the literature. Neuroradiology 2007;49:445–56.
12. Lindegaard J. Primary and secondary tumours of the optic nerve, with emphasis on invasion of uveal malignant melanoma. Acta Ophthalmol Scand 2007;85:347–8.
13. Dutton JJ. Gliomas of the anterior visual pathway. Surv Ophthalmol 1994;38:427–52.
14. Listernick R, Ferner RE, Liu GT, et al. Optic pathway gliomas in neurofibromatosis-1: controversies and recommendations. Ann Neurol 2007;61:189–98.
15. Kornreich L, Blaser S, Schwarz M, et al. Optic pathway glioma: correlation of imaging findings with the presence of neurofibromatosis. AJNR Am J Neuroradiol 2001;22:1963–9.
16. Mafee MF, Goodwin J, Dorodi S. Optic nerve sheath meningiomas. Role of MR imaging. Radiol Clin North Am 1999;37:37–58, ix.
17. Ortiz O, Flores RA. Clinical and radiologic evaluation of optic pathway lesions. Semin Ultrasound CT MR 1998;19:225–39.
18. Kanamalla US. The optic nerve tram-track sign. Radiology 2003;227:718–9.
19. Miller NR. New concepts in the diagnosis and management of optic nerve sheath meningioma. J Neuroophthalmol 2006;26:200–8.
20. Turbin RE, Thompson CR, Kennerdell JS, et al. A long-term visual outcome comparison in patients with optic nerve sheath meningioma managed with observation, surgery, radiotherapy, or surgery and radiotherapy. Ophthalmology 2002;109:890–9 [discussion 899–900].
21. Valvassori GE, Sabnis SS, Mafee RF, et al. Imaging of orbital lymphoproliferative disorders. Radiol Clin North Am 1999;37:135–50, x–xi.
22. Hickman SJ, Dalton CM, Miller DH, et al. Management of acute optic neuritis. Lancet 2002;360:1953–62.
23. Hickman SJ, Miszkiel KA, Plant GT, et al. The optic nerve sheath on MRI in acute optic neuritis. Neuroradiology 2005;47:51–5.
24. Hickman SJ, Brierley CM, Brex PA, et al. Continuing optic nerve atrophy following optic neuritis: a serial MRI study. Mult Scler 2002;8:339–42.
25. Swanton JK, Fernando K, Dalton CM, et al. Is the frequency of abnormalities on magnetic resonance imaging in isolated optic neuritis related to the prevalence of multiple sclerosis? A global comparison. J Neurol Neurosurg Psychiatry 2006;77:1070–2.
26. Dalton CM, Brex PA, Miszkiel KA, et al. New T2 lesions enable an earlier diagnosis of multiple sclerosis in clinically isolated syndromes. Ann Neurol 2003;53:673–6.
27. Cree BA, Goodin DS, Hauser SL. Neuromyelitis optica. Semin Neurol 2002;22:105–22.
28. Frohman LP, Guirgis M, Turbin RE, et al. Sarcoidosis of the anterior visual pathway: 24 new cases. J Neuroophthalmol 2003;23:190–7.
29. Tokumaru AM, Sakata I, Terada H, et al. Optic nerve hyperintensity on T2-weighted images among patients with pituitary macroadenoma: correlation with visual impairment. AJNR Am J Neuroradiol 2006;27:250–4.
30. Smith MM, Strottmann JM. Imaging of the optic nerve and visual pathways. Semin Ultrasound CT MR 2001;22:473–87.
31. Hirunpat S, Tanomkiat W, Sriprung H, et al. Optic tract edema: a highly specific magnetic resonance

imaging finding for the diagnosis of craniopharyngiomas. Acta Radiol 2005;46:419–23.
32. Digre KB. Not so benign intracranial hypertension. BMJ 2003;326:613–4.
33. Rohr A, Dorner L, Stingele R, et al. Reversibility of venous sinus obstruction in idiopathic intracranial hypertension. AJNR Am J Neuroradiol 2007;28:656–9.
34. Kesler A, Pianka P. Toxic optic neuropathy. Curr Neurol Neurosci Rep 2003;3:410–4.
35. Jager HR. Loss of vision: imaging the visual pathways. Eur Radiol 2005;15:501–10.
36. Lamy C, Oppenheim C, Meder JF, et al. Neuroimaging in posterior reversible encephalopathy syndrome. J Neuroimaging 2004;14:89–96.

Pathology of the Ocular Motor Nerves III, IV, and VI

Matthew E. Adams, MD[a,*], Jennifer Linn, MD[b], Indra Yousry, MD, PhD[b]

KEYWORDS

- Oculomotor nerve • Abducent nerve • Ischemia
- Aneurysms, neurovascular conflicts, and fistulas
- Trauma • Neoplasia • Inflammatory • Infection

The ocular motor nerves are cranial nerves three (CNIII), four (CNIV), and six (CNVI), also known as the oculomotor, trochlear, and abducent nerves, respectively. Collectively they supply motor fibers to the extraocular muscles of the globe and levator muscle of the eyelid and parasympathetic pupillomotor fibers to the ciliary ganglion.

Lesions of the ocular motor nerves are classified according to the anatomic location at which they occur: nuclear, fascicular, cisternal, cavernous, or orbital apex. The course each nerve follows influences the sites at which it is most vulnerable to damage and the range of pathologies to which it is exposed. Although cranial nerve palsies may occur in isolation, they frequently are associated with additional neurologic deficits that may assist in localizing the lesion anatomically.

This article provides an overview of the pathology of the ocular motor nerves with an emphasis on lesion localization and the associated imaging findings.

OCULOMOTOR NERVE

The oculomotor nerve (CNIII) innervates the superior, medial, and inferior recti, inferior oblique, and levator palpebrae superioris muscles. In addition, the nerve carries preganglionic parasympathetic pupillomotor fibers to the ciliary ganglion. In two large series,[1,2] the most common identifiable causes of CNIII palsy in order of frequency were ischemia (predominantly microvascular), trauma, aneurysm, and neoplasia.

Nuclear Lesions

The nuclear complex of CNIII lies within the periaqueductal midbrain at the level of the superior colliculus. Complete nuclear injuries result in contralateral superior rectus paresis, bilateral ptosis, ipsilateral dilatation of the pupil (mydriasis), and ipsilateral paresis of inferior oblique and the medial and inferior recti. Lesions also may be incomplete with sparing of pupil function in caudal lesions and absence of ptosis in rostral lesions.

Fascicular Lesions

Axons projecting from the nuclear complex coalesce to form fascicles that pass anteriorly through the midbrain. Fascicular lesions usually involve adjacent structures, and the association of third nerve palsies with additional neurologic signs gives rise to several eponymous syndromes. Injury to the cerebral peduncle produces a contralateral hemiparesis (Weber's syndrome); injury to the red nucleus produces a contralateral tremor (Benedikt's syndrome); and damage to the superior cerebellar peduncle gives rise to ipsilateral ataxia (Nothnagel's syndrome).[3]

[a] Lysholm Department of Neuroradiology, The National Hospital for Neurology and Neurosurgery, Queen Square, London, WC1N 3BG, UK
[b] Klinikum Grosshadern, Department of Neuroradiology, Marchioninistrasse 15, 81377 Munich, Germany
* Corresponding author.
E-mail address: matt@adams888.freeserve.co.uk (M.E. Adams).

Neuroimag Clin N Am 18 (2008) 261–282
doi:10.1016/j.nic.2007.11.001
1052-5149/08/$ – see front matter

Cisternal Lesions

After emerging from the ventral surface of the midbrain, CNIII passes between the posterior cerebral artery (PCA) and the superior cerebellar artery (SCA). It then courses inferior to the posterior communicating artery (PcomA) and inferomedial to the uncus of the temporal lobe to enter the cavernous sinus. Complete peripheral CNIII palsy manifests clinically as ptosis, mydriasis, and deviation of the eye downwards and outwards. Injury to the nerve also may result in partial dysfunction, sparing pupil function or affecting only a single extraocular muscle.

Cavernous Sinus and Orbital Apex Lesions

Within the cavernous sinus, CNIII lies superiorly and laterally, just deep to the dura propria, adjacent to CNIV. It passes anteriorly and exits the cavernous sinus at the orbital apex. Pathologies affecting the cavernous sinus and orbital apex commonly give rise to multiple cranial nerve palsies, often in combination with dysfunction of the traversing vascular structures. At the extreme end of this spectrum are cavernous sinus syndrome and orbital apex syndrome. Cavernous sinus syndrome is characterized by ophthalmoplegia, chemosis, proptosis, Horner's syndrome (due to involvement of occulosympathetic fibers around the internal carotid artery [ICA]), and trigeminal pain or sensory loss. Orbital apex syndrome is characterized by ophthalmoplegia, optic neuropathy, and involvement of the ophthalmic division of the trigeminal nerve (CNV).[4] As the cavernous sinus and orbital apex are continuous, the etiologies of the syndromes are similar and clinical features may overlap.

TROCHLEAR NERVE

The trochlear nerve (CNIV) innervates the superior oblique muscle. Lesions of the nerve present clinically with vertical diplopia that worsens in downgaze. The most common identifiable cause of CNIV palsy is trauma, followed by ischemia and neoplasia.[1,2]

Nuclear Lesions

The nucleus of CNIV lies within the midbrain at the level of the inferior colliculus, caudal to the nuclear complex of CNIII. Nuclear lesions give rise to contralateral superior oblique weakness. Isolated nuclear lesions are rare, however, and associated findings include ipsilateral internuclear ophthalmoplegia (injury to the medial longitudinal fasciculus [MLF]), ipsilateral Horner's syndrome (injury to sympathetic fibers within the periaqueductal gray matter), and contralateral afferent papillary defect (injury to the superior colliculus).[4] More extensive lesions may result in signs of dorsal midbrain (Parinaud's) syndrome.

Fascicular Lesions

The fascicles run posteriorly, decussate within the superior medullary velum, and exit the dorsal midbrain immediately below the inferior colliculus.[5] Fascicular lesions arising after the decussation result in an ipsilateral superior oblique weakness.

Cisternal Lesions

The cisternal segment courses around the lateral midbrain within the quadrigeminal and ambient cisterns. Because of its long course and relation to the edge of the tentorium, the cisternal segment of CNIV is particularly vulnerable to injury. Lesions may be associated with contralateral hemiparesis resulting from compression of the cerebral peduncle or contralateral ataxia resulting from compression of the superior cerebellar peduncle.

Cavernous Sinus and Orbital Apex Lesions

CNIV lies within the lateral wall of the cavernous sinus inferior to CNIII and superior to the ophthalmic division of CNV. In common with the other ocular motor nerves, lesions of CNIV frequently are associated with multiple cranial nerve palsies as part of the spectrum of cavernous sinus and orbital apex syndromes.

ABDUCENT NERVE

The abducent nerve (CNVI) innervates the ipsilateral lateral rectus muscle, which serves to abduct the globe, and palsies present clinically with horizontal diplopia. It is the ocular motor nerve that is injured most frequently. The most common identifiable cause of CNVI palsy is ischemia, followed by trauma, neoplasia, and aneurysm.[1]

Nuclear Lesions

The nucleus of CNVI lies just beneath the floor of the fourth ventricle in the dorsal pons. It lies close to the MLF and the fascicles of the facial nerve (CNVII) course around its dorsal aspect producing a protruberance, known as the facial colliculus. Lesions of CNVI nucleus produce a conjugate horizontal gaze palsy toward the side of the lesion. Lesions usually are associated with additional neurologic signs, the most common of which is an ipsilateral CNVII palsy resulting from facial colliculus injury. Injury to the MLF results in a one-and-a-half syndrome characterized by loss of conjugate gaze toward the lesion and reduced adduction away from the lesion.[3]

Fascicular Lesions

The fascicles pass anteriorly through the pons to emerge from its caudal aspect. Lesions affecting CNVI fascicles usually are associated with features reflecting more widespread pontine injury. Lesions of the anterior paramedian pons result in Millard-Gubler syndrome characterized by ipsilateral CNVI and CNVII palsies and contralateral hemiplegia. Ischemic lesions in the territory of the anterior inferior cerebellar artery (AICA) may result in a combination of ipsilateral CNV, CNVI, and CNVII palsies with deafness and Horner's syndrome (Foville's syndrome).

Cisternal Lesions

The cisternal portion of the nerve passes rostrally, paralleling the clivus ventrally. It then passes into the fibro-osseous tunnel, known as Dorello's canal, passing over the petrous apex to enter the cavernous sinus. This segment of CNVI is particularly vulnerable to pathologies arising from the skull base or from compression against the clivus or basilar artery (BA) and to pathologies affecting the petrous apex.

Cavernous Sinus Lesions

Because of its close contact with the internal carotid artery and surrounding sympathetic plexus, the combination of a CNVI palsy with occulosympathetic dysfunction should localize the lesion to the cavernous segment of the nerve.

ISCHEMIA

Ischemia, including diabetic ophthalmoparesis, is the most common identifiable cause of CNIII and CNVI palsies and is second only to trauma in CNIV palsies. Overall, ischemia accounts for approximately a quarter of cases of ocular motor nerve palsy in which underlying cause can be identified.[1,2]

Nuclear/Fascicular

The mesencephalon is supplied by branches of the upper BA, SCA, and PCA. It frequently is affected by posterior circulation embolic stroke but usually with simultaneous involvement of the pons, thalamus, or cerebellum. Isolated infarctions of the midbrain are unusual, but when they occur, ocular motor disturbance, usually in the form of CNIII palsy, is the second most common feature after ataxia. As expected, such infarctions usually are localized to the anteromedial part of the brainstem where the nucleus and fascicles of CNIII are situated.[6] Occasionally, infarctions may be localized enough to result in isolated ocular motor nerve palsies (**Fig. 1**). As discussed previously, AICA territory infarctions may result in Foville's syndrome.

Extra-Axial

Microvascular infarction of the cisternal segments of CNIII, CNIV, and CNVI, secondary to systemic vascular diseases, such as diabetes and

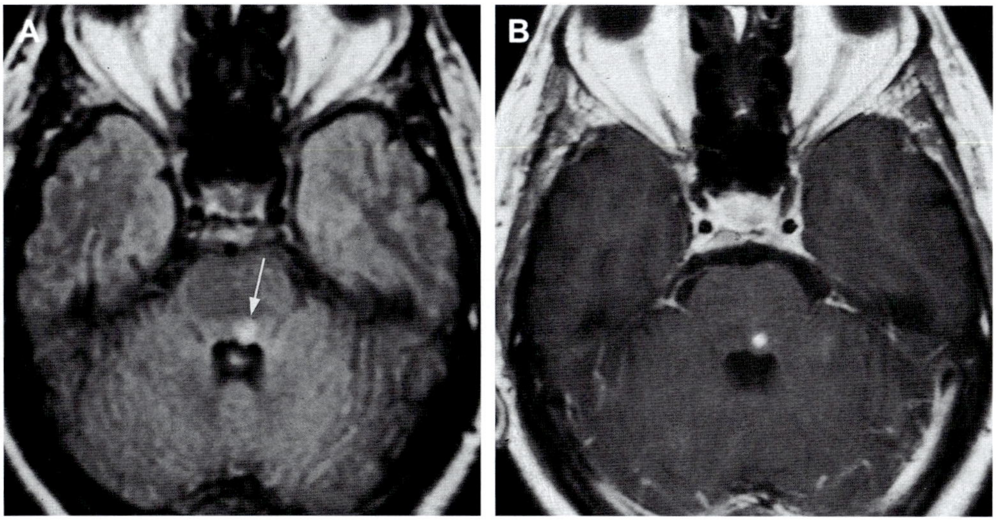

Fig. 1. Acute ischemic lesion. (*A*) Axial FLAIR and (*B*) postgadolinium T1-w images of a patient presenting with an isolated CNVI palsy. Images demonstrate a hyperintense, enhancing lesion within the dorsal pons at the level of the facial colliculus representing an acute ischemic lesion of the CNVI nucleus (*white arrow*).

hypertension, is the most common overall cause of ocular motor nerve dysfunction.[1,7]

Involvement of CNIII usually results in a pupil sparing palsy. This can be explained by the parasympathetic pupilloconstrictor fibers distributed in an arc sited dorsomedially within the periphery of the nerve; it is the more central neurons supplied by end arteries from the vasa vasorum that are most vulnerable to ischemia.[3,7,8]

MRI appearances of the nerve after microvascular infarction almost always are normal,[7] although moderate enhancement of the cisternal portion has been described.[9,10]

ANEURYSMS, NEUROVASCULAR CONFLICTS, AND FISTULAS

In addition to lesions resulting from ischemic vascular disease, ocular motor nerve dysfunction may arise because of compression by vascular structures, in particular intracranial aneurysms, or secondary to carotid-cavernous fistulas.

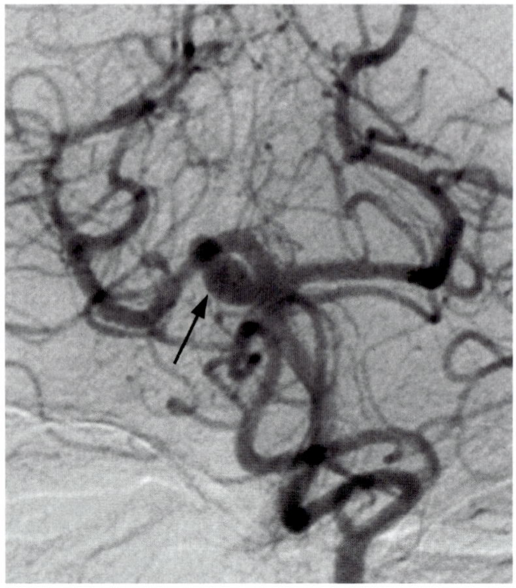

Fig. 2. SCA aneurysm. DSA of the left VA demonstrating an aneurysm of the right SCA (*black arrow*) in a patient presenting with a complete right CNIII palsy.

Cisternal

Intracranial aneurysms and dolichoectatic vessels

Intracranial aneurysms and dolichoectatic vessels account for up to 14% of CNIII palsies overall and a much higher proportion of isolated peripheral palsies. CNIV and CNVI are affected less frequently accounting for approximately 2% and 4% of cases, respectively.[1,2] The vascular structures that potentially may give rise to ocular motor dysfunction are determined by the anatomic course of the cisternal segments of each nerve.

On route to the cavernous sinus, CNIII first passes between the PCA and SCA and then inferior to the PcomA. Although palsies related to aneurysms of the SCA are well recognized (**Fig. 2**), aneurysms of the PcomA (**Fig. 3**) are the most common culprit, with the incidence of a CNIII deficit at presentation ranging from 34% to 61%.[8] In cases of ruptured aneurysm, neural injury occurs secondary to direct hemorrhagic dissection of the nerve or uncal herniation. In cases of unruptured aneurysms, localized extravasation leading to intraneural fibrosis or acute dilatation of the aneurysm sac leading to mechanical distortion and edema of the nerve are the proposed mechanisms.[8]

Most series demonstrate that a high proportion of isolated CNIII palsies secondary to PcomA aneurysms are associated with disturbance of pupillomotor function.[8,11] Anatomically, this is explained by the aneurysms tending to point posteriorly, inferiorly, and laterally, making the peripheral, dorsomedially sited parasympathetic pupillomotor fibers most vulnerable to impingement.

The discrimination between an acute onset of isolated CNIII palsy resulting from aneurysm and resulting from other causes, principally microvascular infarction, is critical. Microvascular infarction follows a benign self-limiting course with almost 100% recovery. In contrast, nerve dysfunction secondary to aneurysm may herald a more sinister outcome and it is shown that the rupture rate of aneurysms associated with CNIII palsy is 2.4 times that of aneurysms without.[11] Most studies concur that the most important discriminatory feature clinically is the presence or absence of pupillary involvement. Between 68% and 80% of CNIII palsies resulting from microvascular infarction spare the pupil compared with 4% to 14% of those resulting from aneurysm.[3,8] Another potentially useful discriminatory feature is the presence of aberrant CNIII innervation resulting from misdirected regrowth of fibers to an inappropriate target structure. This process takes at least 8 weeks and suggests a compressive lesion, such as an unruptured aneurysm or tumor, almost never occurring after microvascular infarction.[3] Retro- or periorbital pain is associated with both causes and is not a useful discriminatory feature.[3]

As CNIV passes anteriorly between the lateral midbrain and tentorial edge, it also passes between the PCA and SCA. In contrast to CNIII, CNIV nerve palsy secondary to aneurysms of these vessels is rare.

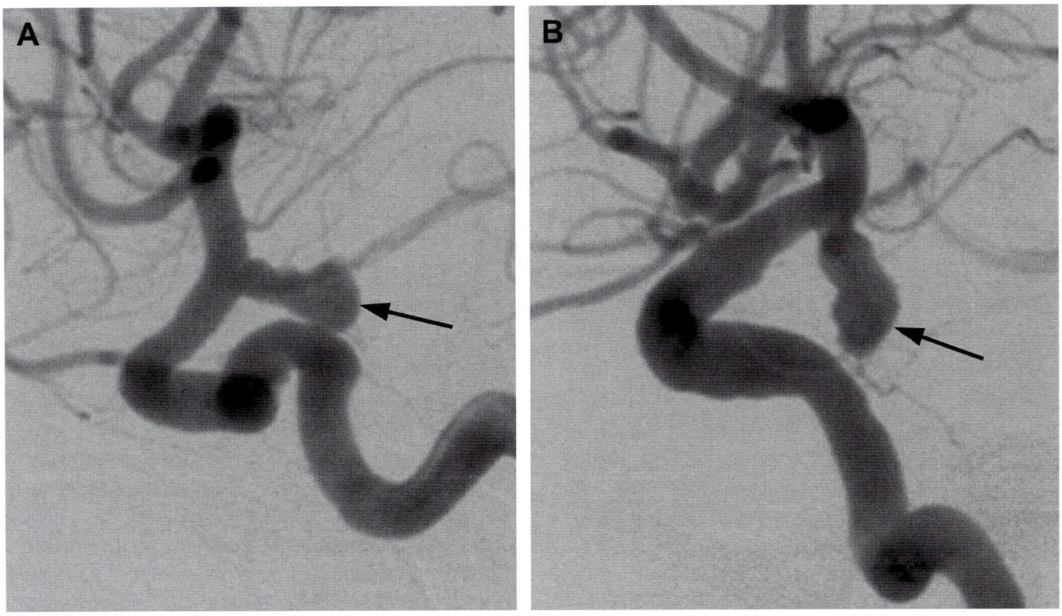

Fig. 3. Posterior communicating artery aneurysms. Lateral projection DSA of the ICA of two separate patients (*A*, *B*) presenting with complete CNIII palsy. Aneurysms of the posterior communicating segment of the supraclinoid ICA are demonstrated pointing posteriorly and inferiorly (*black arrows*). (*Courtesy of* Dr. F. Robertson, National Hospital for Neurology and Neurosurgery, London.)

CNVI courses through the prepontine cistern in close proximity to the vertebral artery (VA) and BA. As a result, the most common vascular causes of cisternal segment dysfunction are dissecting aneurysms of the VAs or dolichoectatic vessels.[12]

Although digital subtraction angiography (DSA) remains the gold standard investigation, CT angiography and magnetic resonance angiography (MRA) are demonstrated as having sensitivities approaching that of DSA for detecting aneurysms 5 mm or more in diameter.[13,14] In the context of aneurysms presenting with CNIII palsy, it is estimated that MRA detects 98% of aneurysms and overlooks only 1.5% of those that subsequently rupture.[11,14]

Neurovascular conflicts

Neurovascular conflicts are disorders believed to arise from vascular impingement and are characterized by hyperactive nerve dysfunction rather than nerve palsy. This group includes disorders, such as trigeminal neuralgia (CNV), hemifacial spasm (CNVII), and superior oblique myokymia (SOM) (CNIV). A proposed common mechanism for the neurovascular conflicts group is vascular compression at a specific portion of the cisternal segment of the nerve known as the root exit zone (RExZ). The cisternal portion of the ocular motor nerves can be divided into a central (glial) segment sheathed in myelin derived from oligodendrocytes and a peripheral segment sheathed in myelin derived from Schwann cells.[15] The RExZ refers to this central portion and is less stable anatomically and electrophysiologically because it lacks perineurium and epineurium.[16] It is proposed that the region of transition between oligodendrocyte and Schwann cell–derived myelin is particularly vulnerable to continued pulsatile pressure, which may result in focal demyelination and short-circuiting of impulses. The length of the RExZ differs for each nerve, measuring up to 4 mm for CNIII, 1 mm for CNIV, and 1 mm for the CNVI.[15]

Neurovascular conflicts involving CNIII usually are the result of atherosclerotic, dolichoectatic, or abnormally positioned PCA or SCA.[17] Neurovascular conflicts of CNIV occur because of the SCA or its branches lying in close contact with the nerve within the ambient cistern.[18] Compression of the CNIV RExZ may lead to a rare recurring disorder of ocular motility, called SOM (**Fig. 4**). SOM is characterized by unilateral paroxysmal oscillopsia and microtremor resulting from intermittent contractions of the superior oblique muscle.[19]

In microsurgical and radiologic studies the vessels that are identified as having a close relationship with CNVI are the AICA, posterior inferior cerebellar artery (PICA), BA, VA, SCA, and the petrosal vein.[20,21] The VA, in particular, is reported as causing CNVI compression.[22]

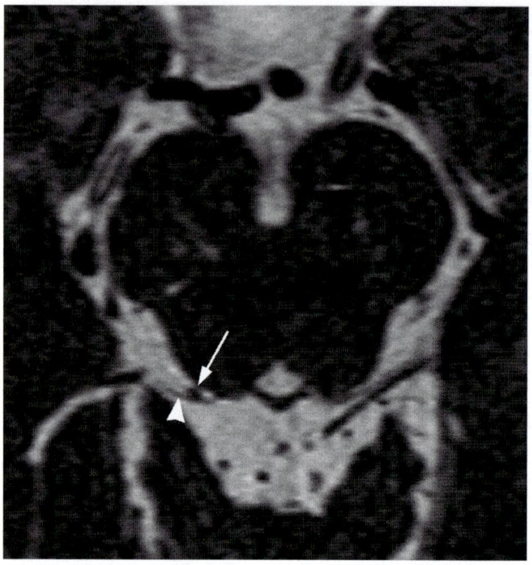

Fig. 4. A 54-year-old female patient who had right-sided SOM. High resolution 3-D–CISS MRI reveals a neurovascular contact between the RExZ of the right trochlear nerve (*arrowhead*) and a branch of the right SCA (*arrow*).

Neurovascular contacts within the central segment of the ocular motor nerves, however, commonly occur in asymptomatic individuals,[21,23] and arteries may even penetrate the nerve without clinical consequences.

MRI is the most useful imaging tool for imaging neurovascular conflict syndromes. Although imaging of CNIII is relatively easy because of its larger diameter (2.5 to 3 mm), CNIV and CNVI are smaller (diameter 0.75 to 1 mm for CNIV and 0.43 to 1.85 for CNVI), and imaging the cisternal segments is more challenging. Furthermore, CNIV lies in close proximity to vessels of similar course and caliber in the ambient cistern, making depiction particularly difficult. The ocular motor nerves are identified best using high-resolution imaging techniques, such as the 3-D constructive interference in steady state (CISS) sequence, 3-D T2-weighted (T2-w) fast spin-echo, or 3-D fast imaging employing steady-state acquisition sequences.[21,23–25] The 3-D datasets of these sequences allow reconstructions along each individual nerve course and very thin slices (down to 0.6 mm). The problem of misinterpretation of a vascular structure as a nerve can be overcome by adding a 3-D time-of-flight sequence, with and without administration of gadolinium-DTPA.[23,25,26] Furthermore, this technique allows differentiation of arteries and veins.

Cavernous

Aneurysms

Aneurysms of the distal ICA may occur extradurally within the cavernous sinus (**Fig. 5**). The most common symptom associated with such

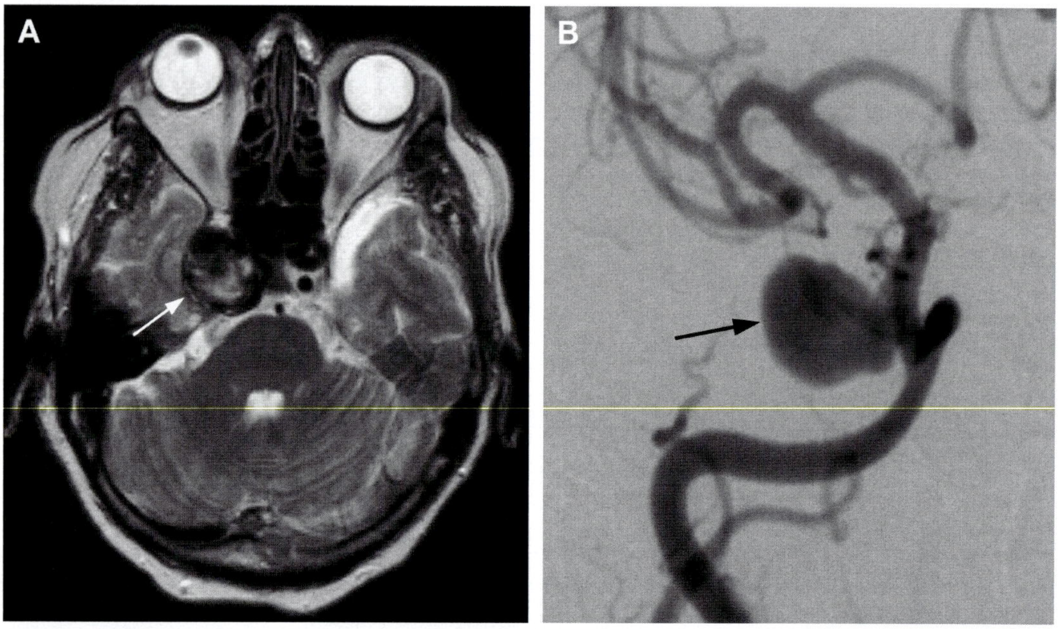

Fig. 5. Cavernous ICA aneurysm. Axial T2-w images (*A*) and DSA (*B*) of the right ICA of a patient presenting with a right CNIII palsy demonstrating a large intracavernous aneurysm expanding the right cavernous sinus (*white and black arrows*, respectively).

aneurysms is ocular motor dysfunction.[27] Unlike intradural aneurysms, the nerve affected most commonly is CNVI, possibly related to its anatomic location within the central venous portion of the sinus tethered to the ICA. Frequently, there is evidence of a more extensive cavernous sinus syndrome with multiple ocular motor palsies, trigeminal pain, and Horner's syndrome.[27]

Carotid-cavernous fistulas

Carotid-cavernous fistulas represent abnormal shunting of arterial blood through the cavernous sinus and most commonly are secondary to rupture of extradural cavernous ICA aneurysms or trauma. They are categorized as direct or indirect depending on whether or not the arterial shunt is derived from the ICA itself or arteries supplying the dura of the cavernous sinus. Typically, patients who have the direct type present with chemosis, pulsatile exophthalmos, and ocular bruit, whereas those who have indirect type present with a more insidious onset of exophthalmos, glaucoma, and pain.[28] Ophthalmoplegia is a common finding in both types and in one series examining indirect fistulae, isolated ocular motor dysfunction was found the presenting feature in one third of patients. Moreover, recovery rate of ocular motor function after treatment of the fistula was more than 50% at 1 year.[29]

The sensitivity of CT in detecting carotid-cavernous fistulas is low,[29] but dilatation of the cavernous sinus and superior ophthalmic vein, proptosis, and expansion of the extraocular muscles may be demonstrated. MRI is more sensitive and, in addition to the CT features, flow-related enhancement of the cavernous sinus with abnormal flow voids within the superior ophthalmic vein or petrosal veins may be visible.[28] DSA is the most sensitive imaging modality and the diagnosis is made with visualization of arterial shunting to the cavernous sinus from the ICA or dural arteries (**Figs. 6 and 7**).

TRAUMA

Ocular motor nerve dysfunction is a common finding after severe head trauma [30] and may be seen after minor head injuries.[31] CNVI is the ocular motor nerve damaged most frequently, trauma being the second most common cause of injury to this nerve overall. In addition, trauma is the most common identifiable cause of CNIV palsy and the second most common cause of damage to CNIII.[1,2]

The ocular motor nerves may be damaged as part of the primary injury at the moment of the traumatic event or may be damaged secondarily by swelling and transcompartmental herniation of brain structures.

Nuclear/Fascicular

The pons and midbrain are susceptible to primary injury directly from impact against the tentorial incisura and indirectly from diffuse axonal injury.[32]

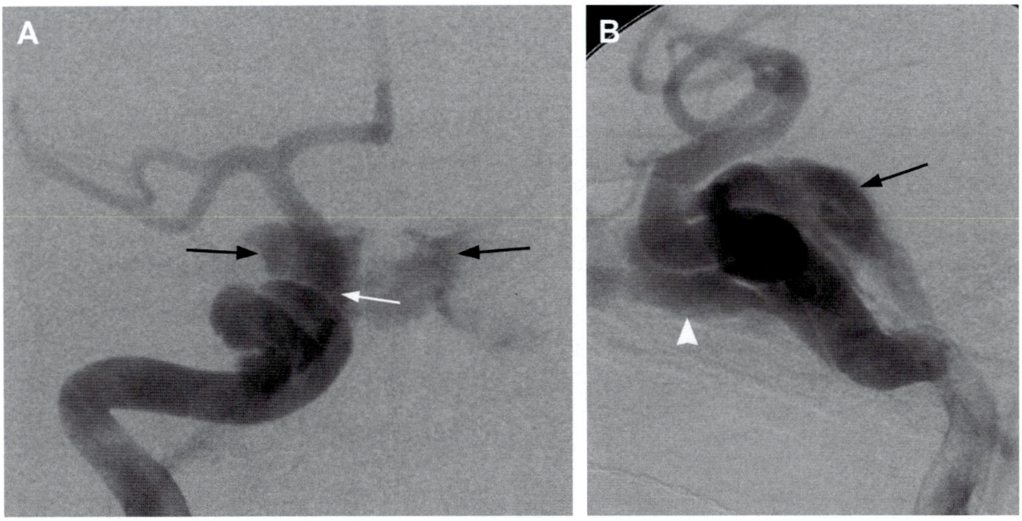

Fig. 6. Direct carotid cavernous fistula. A 30-year-old man presenting with proptosis, chemosis, and ophthalmoplegia after a head injury while snowboarding. Anteroposterior (*A*) and lateral (*B*) DSA projections of the right ICA demonstrate shunting of arterial contrast directly from the intracavernous ICA into the cavernous sinus (*white arrow*, intracavernous ICA; *black arrows*, contrast within the cavernous sinus bilaterally; and *white arrowhead*, contrast within dilated superior ophthalmic vein). (*Courtesy of* Dr. S. Brew, National Hospital for Neurology and Neurosurgery, London.)

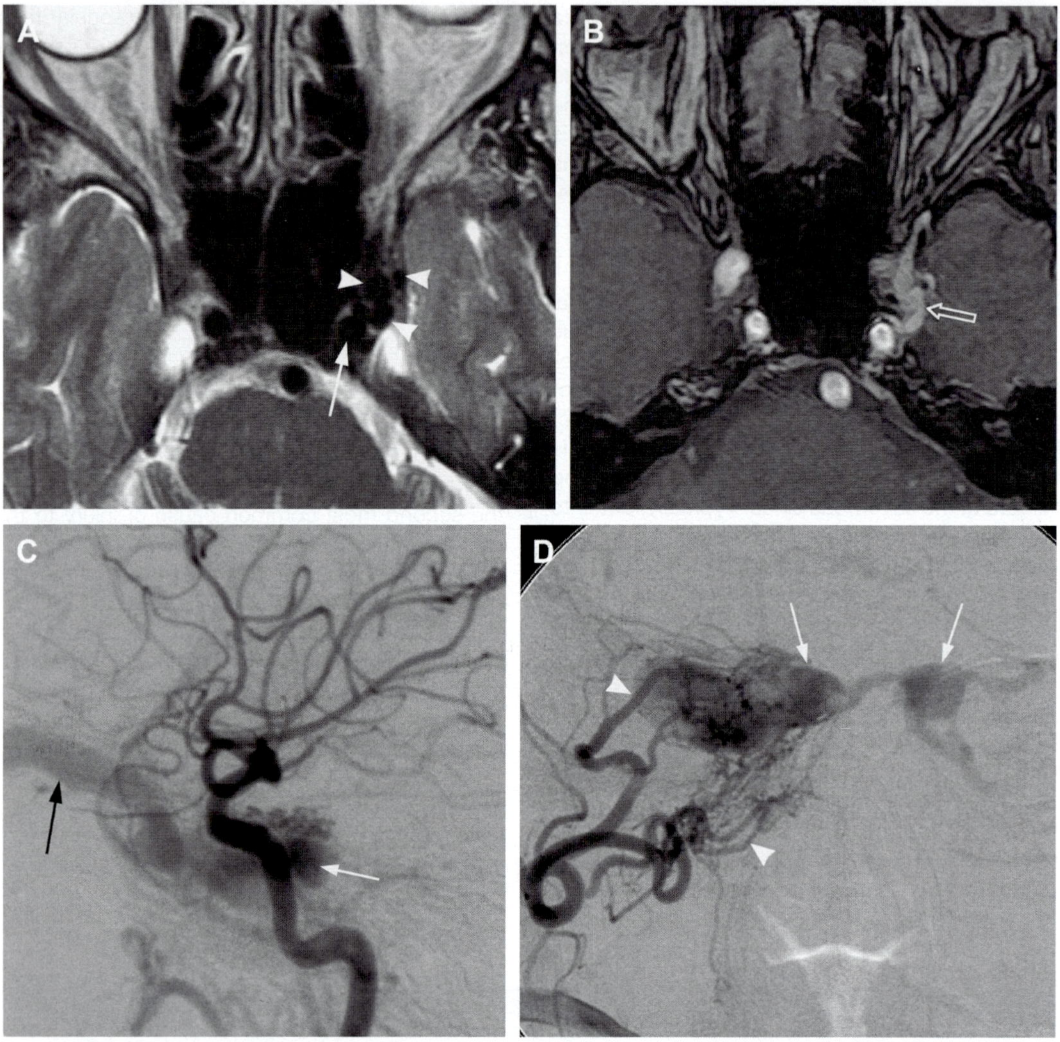

Fig. 7. Indirect carotid cavernous fistula. (*A*) Axial T2-w image showing expansion of the left cavernous sinus with multiple abnormal flow voids (*white arrowheads*) adjacent to the intracavernous ICA (*white arrow*). (*B*) Axial time-of-flight MRA image demonstrating increased signal within the cavernous sinus reflecting abnormally high flow (*open white arrow*). Lateral (*C*) and anteroposterior (*D*) projection DSA of a second patient who had an indirect fistula. (*C*) Demonstrates shunting of contrast into the cavernous sinus (*white arrow*) from dural branches of the ICA with drainage into the superior ophthalmic vein (*black arrow*). (*D*) Demonstrates shunting of contrast into the cavernous sinuses (*white arrows*) from dural branches of the external carotid artery (*arrowheads*). (*Courtesy of* Dr. F. Robertson, National Hospital for Neurology and Neurosurgery, London.)

The nucleus of CNIV is supplied by paramedian branches of the basilar bifurcation. These very fine vessels are susceptible to shearing forces leading to secondary ischemic infarction.[33]

Cisternal

Primary injuries

The cisternal portions of the ocular motor nerves are particularly vulnerable at points of relative fixation.

CNIII has the shortest cisternal course of the ocular motor nerves. Traumatic injury to this segment occurs as a result of differential movement between the brainstem and supratentorial structures or skull base leading to rootlet avulsion or stretching over the tough posterior petroclinoid ligament.[30,31,34]

CNIV has the longest cisternal course.[35] In addition to avulsion injuries at the point of emergence from the dorsolateral midbrain, damage may be caused by compression of the nerve against the rigid tentorial edge as it passes anteriorly through the ambient cistern.[36]

CNVI is tethered rostrally by Dorello's canal, where most traumatic injuries occur.[35,37]

The usefulness of CT and MRI is demonstrated in identifying blood within the ambient cistern in relation to avulsion injuries of CNIV.[36,38] MRI also demonstrates hemorrhage at the point of emergence of CNIII in similar injuries.[39] Fluid-attenuated inversion recovery (FLAIR) and gradient-echo sequences may be particularly sensitive in these scenarios.[36,39]

Secondary injuries

In addition to primary injuries, the ocular motor nerves are susceptible to secondary injury as a result of raised intracranial pressure (ICP) leading to transcompartmental herniation. This is true of any etiology of raised ICP, including supra- and infratentorial space-occupying lesions, idiopathic intracranial hypertension, and venosinus thrombosis. CNVI reportedly is the nerve affected most commonly.[35] In inferior transtentorial herniation, the proposed pathophysiology is descent of the brainstem resulting in necrosis of the nerve at Dorello's canal or compression of the nerve against the clivus or BA. CNVI also is vulnerable to shifts in intracranial contents resulting from low ICP for similar reasons. In CNIII palsy, the mechanism is believed the result of impingement on the free edge of the tentorium or kinking over the clivus. The peripherally distributed parasympathetic pupilloconstrictor fibers are most vulnerable and mydriasis may be the earliest manifestation.

Cavernous

Injuries to the cavernous portion of the ocular motor nerves may result directly from fractures of the skull base. As CNVI traverses the cavernous sinus, it is tethered to the lateral wall of the ICA and vulnerable to indirect traumatic injury.[37]

Orbital Apex

Traumatic orbital apex syndrome usually arises in the context of penetrating trauma and fractures[40] but may occur as a delayed phenomenon resulting from the retention of foreign bodies.[4] Iatrogenic injury also is described in the context of sinonasal and periorbital surgery.

NEOPLASIA

Nuclear/Fascicular

Any neoplasm involving the nuclear or fascicular component of the nerves within the midbrain and brainstem may give rise to ocular motor nerve dysfunction. Tumors recognized as causing nuclear palsies include metastases, brainstem and midbrain gliomas, medulloblastomas, and cavernous hemangiomas.[1,38] Although such lesions may produce multiple neurologic deficits,[38] some series report isolated ocular motor nerve palsies more commonly[1] and have described them as secondary to metastases,[41,42] gliomas,[1,43] and cavernous hemangiomas (**Fig. 8**).[44]

Cisternal

The cisternal segments may be affected by primary neoplastic processes of the nerves or by secondary mass effect, local invasion, or metastatic spread via the cerebrospinal fluid (CSF).

Primary

Schwannomas account for approximately 8% of all intracranial tumors.[45] They usually arise from sensory cranial nerves at the point at which the axonal sheath changes from glial to Schwann cells.[45–47] Schwannomas of mixed or purely motor cranial nerves usually are associated with neurofibromatosis type 2 or schwannomatosis. Tumors of CNIII (**Fig. 9**), CNIV, and CNVI arising outside of these syndromic associations are particularly rare, with only 32, 35, and 13 cases, respectively, reported in the literature.[46,48,49]

In cisternal schwannomas of CNIII and CNVI, paresis of the affected nerve usually is the only nerve deficit.[50] In contrast, schwannomas of CNIV are associated with paresis of the nerve in only 50% of cases and frequently are associated with hemiparesis (46%), ataxia (19%), or other cranial nerve palsies, in particular CNIII and CNII (optic nerve).[46] The reason for this difference in clinical presentation may be related to the location of the tumor. Although the glial-Schwann junction lies on average 0.6 mm from the dorsal midbrain origin,[51] tumors of this nerve usually occupy the ambient cistern lateral or anterolateral to the cerebral peduncle at the level of the tentorial notch. The tumor, therefore, may expand into the prepontine or interpeduncular cisterns, causing cranial nerve deficits, or compress the cerebral peduncle and midbrain, resulting in an ataxic hemiparetic syndrome.[50]

On CT, schwannomas generally are of lower attenuation than brain parenchyma and show moderate enhancement.[52] The MRI appearances of schwannomas are variable but generally of well-circumscribed lesions isointense or slightly hypointense to brain parenchyma on T1-weighted (T1-w) images and isointense or heterogeneously hyperintense on T2-w images.[32,47,52,53] The heterogeneity tends to increase with increasing tumor size and may be the result of regions of different histology (hypercellular Antoni A tissue appearing isointense and hypocellular Antoni B tissue appearing hyperintense) or cystic change. Regions of T2-w hypointensity also may be seen

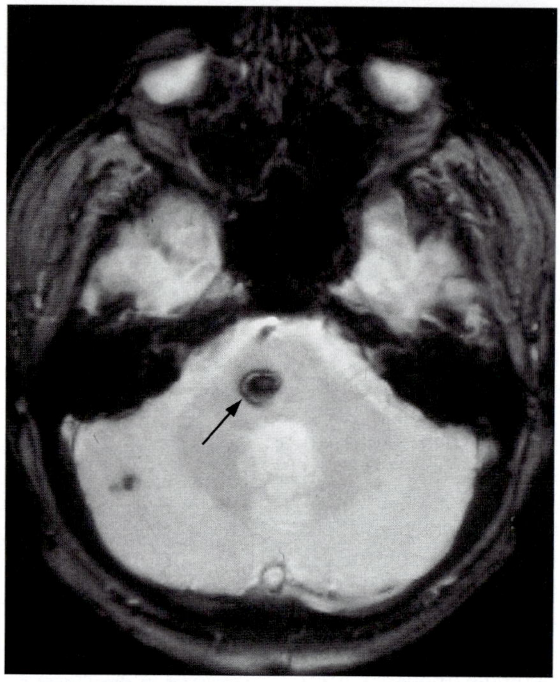

Fig. 8. Cavernous hemangioma. Axial T2 gradient-echo image of a patient presenting with right CNVI and CNVII palsy. Images demonstrate a circumscribed susceptibility artifact within the right CNVI nucleus (*black arrow*) reflecting blood products secondary to an underlying cavernous hemangioma.

corresponding to areas of calcification, hemorrhage, or hyalinized stroma. Contrast enhancement is avid but may be inhomogeneous with enhancement corresponding to isointense tissue on T2-w images.[32,54,55]

Other intrinsic tumors of the ocular motor nerves are described but are rare. Three cases of cavernous hemangiomas affecting CNIII are reported.[56] On MRI, these tumors are iso- or hyperintense on T1-w images and hyperintense on T2-w images

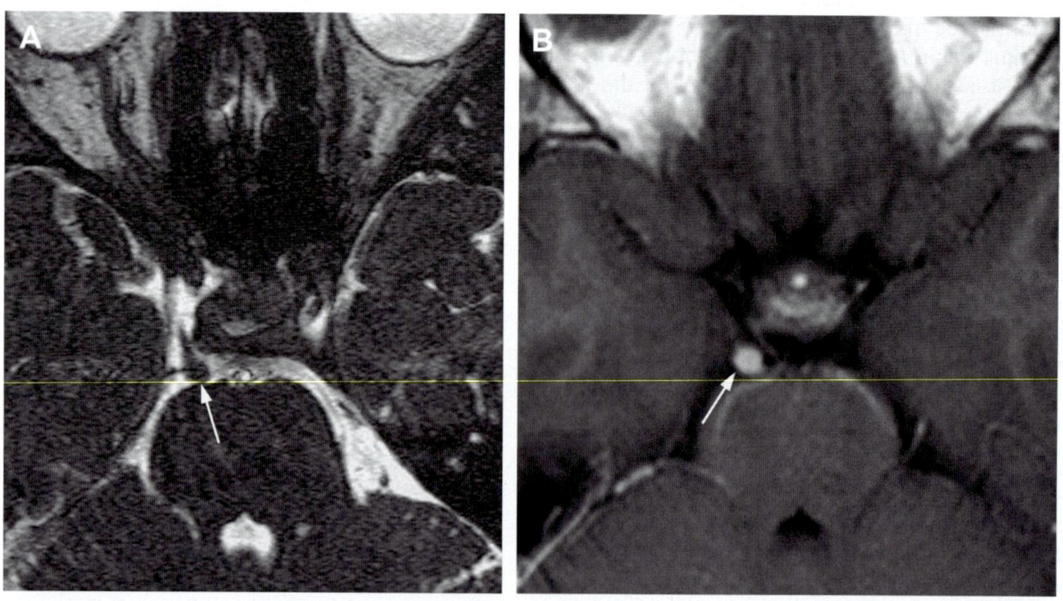

Fig. 9. Schwannoma of CNIII. Axial CISS (*A*) and postgadolinium T1-w (*B*) images of a patient presenting with right CNIII palsy. Images demonstrate focal fusiform thickening of the proximal cisternal portion of the right CNIII with homogeneous enhancement (*white arrows*).

with no enhancement post contrast. Rhabdomyoma (choristoma) of CNIII also is reported.[57] These tumors have imaging appearances identical to schwannomas.

Secondary

The cisternal segments of CNIII, CNIV, and CNVI are susceptible to local mass effect and local invasion from any tumor occupying the cisterns surrounding the brainstem and midbrain. In particular, ocular motor nerve palsies are described in relation to epidermoids (**Fig. 10**)[38] and arachnoid cysts.

Because of the ascending course of CNVI through the prepontine cistern, it is particularly vulnerable to pathologies affecting the clivus.[35] Neoplastic pathologies include chordoma, chondrosarcoma, meningioma, and metastasis.[58,59] In one series examining 60 patients who had skull-base chordoma or chondrosarcoma, CNVI was the cranial nerve affected most commonly, with dysfunction present in 45% of cases.[60]

In addition to mass effect and local invasion, cranial nerves may be affected by the seeding of malignant cells to the leptomeninges. On MRI, this may manifest as perineural enhancement or nodular masses after intravenous contrast. This often is appreciated best along the cisternal portions of the nerves, with the T1 shortening effects of the gadolinium contrasted against the CSF. Leptomeningeal seeding may be secondary to lymphomatous or leukemic infiltrates (**Fig. 11**) or leptomeningeal carcinomatosis secondary to solid tumors.[52]

Although lymphoma and leukemia are the most common malignancies seeding to the CSF, only a minority invokes a leptomeningeal reaction visible on imaging. The most common finding in childhood leukemia is enlargement of the ventricles, possibly representing hydrocephalus secondary to occult disease involvement.[61] Meningeal and parenchymal metastatic disease is much less common than ventricular enlargement; however, when the leptomeninges are involved, enhancement of the cranial nerves may be the only imaging finding.[7,61]

Leptomeningeal carcinomatosis most commonly is the result of metastasis of extracranial malignancy. The most common extracranial malignancies to involve the leptomeninges are breast (**Fig. 12**), lung, and melanoma.[62] Primary neoplasms of the central nervous system also may disseminate to the leptomeninges via the CSF. Tumors commonly spreading by this route include medulloblastomas (**Fig. 13**), other primitive neuroectodermal tumors, germ cell tumors, ependymomas (**Fig. 14**), high-grade astrocytomas, and choroid plexus carcinomas.[52] The basal and interpeduncular cisterns are characteristic locations for

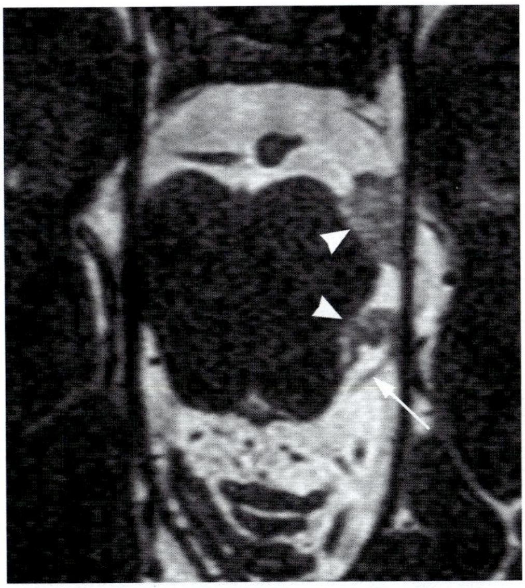

Fig. 10. Epidermoid. Axial CISS image of an epidermoid within the left ambient cistern displacing the midbrain and encasing CNIV, resulting in paresis of the left superior oblique muscle. The epidermoid is predominantly hyperintense and poorly contrasted against the surrounding CSF, although regions of lower signal due to internal architecture are evident (*white arrowheads*). CNIV is seen as a fine linear structure passing through the mass within the ambient cistern (*white arrow*).

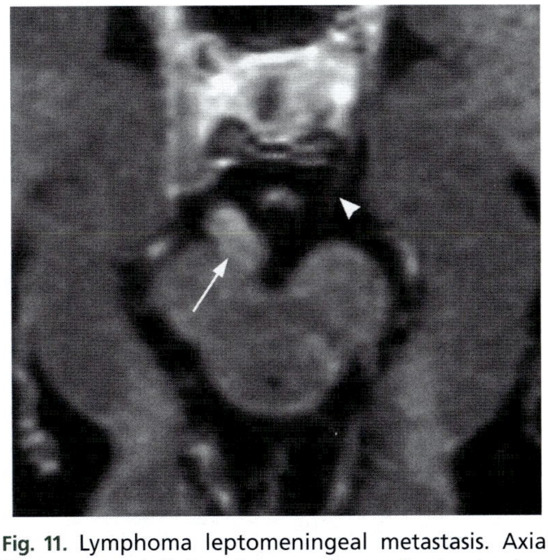

Fig. 11. Lymphoma leptomeningeal metastasis. Axial T1-w postgadolinium image of a patient who had right-sided ophthalmoplegia demonstrating an enhancing nodule (*white arrow*) adjacent to the anteromedial aspect of the right cerebral peduncle surrounding the cisternal portion of the right CNIII. A normal CNIII is seen on the left side (*arrowhead*).

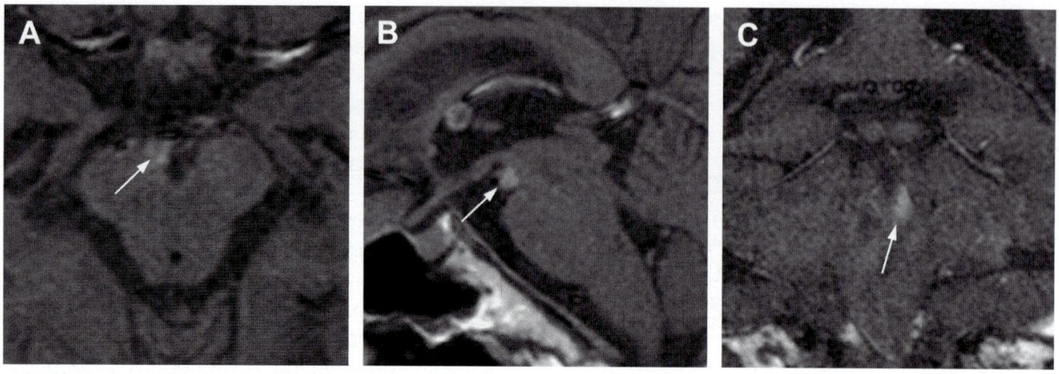

Fig. 12. Breast carcinoma leptomeningeal metastasis. A 79-year old female patient who had metastatic breast cancer and a right-sided paresis of the right CNIII. Axial (*A*), sagittal (*B*), and coronal (*C*) contrast-enhanced T1-w images depict a small metastasis at the point of exit of the right CNIII (*white arrows*).

leptomeningeal deposits, and involvement of the cranial nerves themselves may be seen on MRI as smooth or nodular perineural enhancement.

Cavernous

The cavernous segments of the nerves are susceptible to mass effect and direct invasion from tumors expanding outwards from the pituitary fossa or inwards from the parasellar region, skull base, or paranasal sinuses or from tumors arising from within the cavernous sinus itself. In addition, tumors may spread along branches of the nerves from distant compartments of the head and neck.

Meningiomas

Approximately 15% of meningiomas arise from parasellar locations,[28] including the medial sphenoid wing, posteromedial petrous bone, tuberculum sellae, Meckel's cave, and the cavernous sinus itself. In a large series examined by Richards and colleagues,[2] meningiomas were found the most common intracranial neoplasm, giving rise to ocular motor nerve palsy. Nerve dysfunction may result from invasion of the cavernous sinus or orbital apex.

CT typically demonstrates a mass of slightly increased attenuation compared with adjacent brain with avid enhancement. Associated hyperostosis or expansion of the adjacent paranasal sinuses also may be evident. On MRI, meningiomas are iso- or hypointense on T1-w images and isointense on T2-w images, although 30% may show hyperintensity on long TR sequences.[28] Intense enhancement after gadolinium is characteristic.

Pituitary tumors

The most common ophthalmologic presentation of pituitary tumors is with visual field defects. Ocular motor disturbance occurs less commonly with a prevalence of 1% to 14%. The most common scenario is isolated CNIII dysfunction.[1,63] The second most common scenario is a combination of CNIII palsy and dysfunction of at least one other

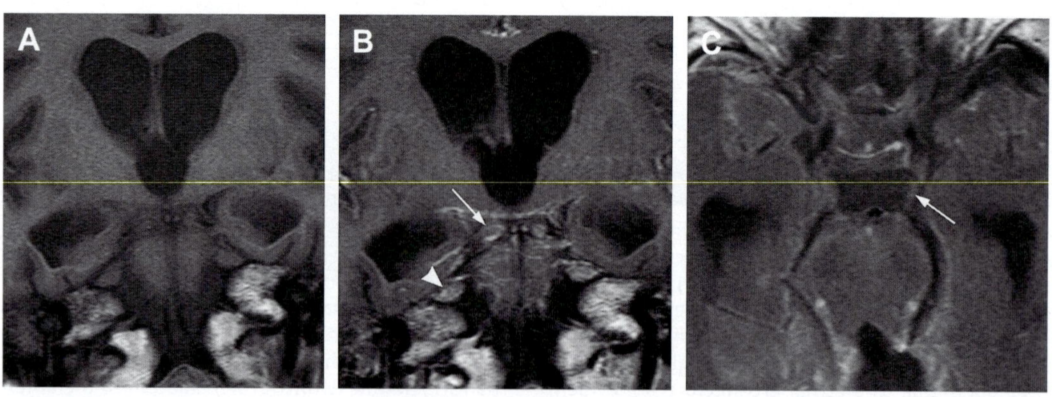

Fig. 13. Medulloblastoma leptomeningeal metastasis. Coronal precontrast T1-w (*A*) and coronal (*B*) and axial (*C*) postgadolinium images demonstrating widespread leptomeningeal enhancement, including perineural enhancement of CNIII (*white arrows*) and CNV (*white arrowhead*).

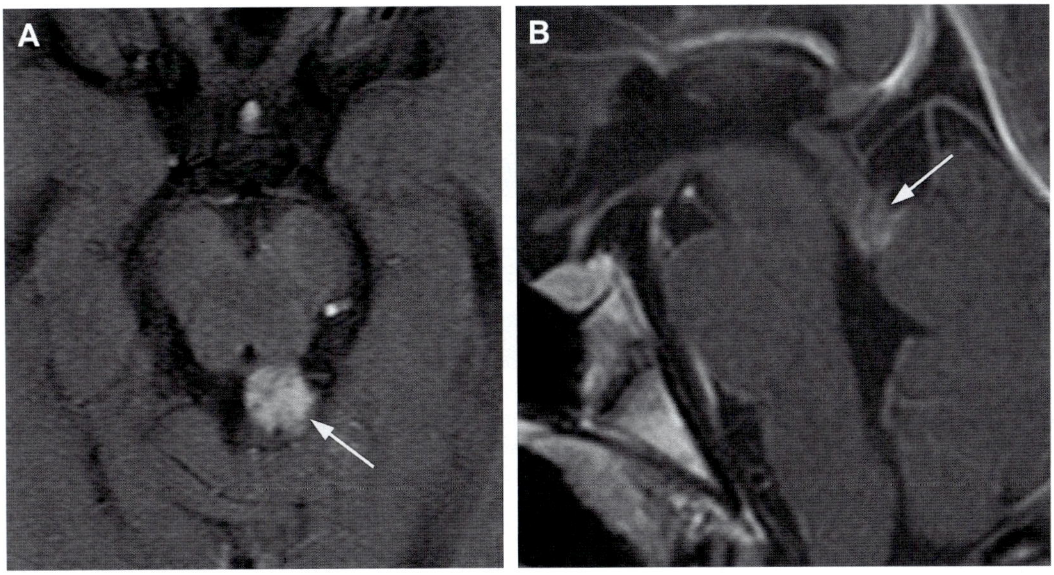

Fig. 14. Ependymoma leptomeningeal metastasis. Axial (*A*) and sagittal (*B*) postgadolinium images demonstrating a nodular metastasis adjacent to the left inferior colliculus and superior medullary velum at the origin of left CNIV (*white arrows*).

nerve. Isolated CNIV or CNVI palsies are described but are less common.[1,63]

On MRI, pituitary macroadenomas appear as T1-w hypointense masses compressing the adjacent higher signal normal pituitary tissue; and hyper- or isointense on T2-w images.[32] Invasion laterally into the cavernous sinus to involve the ocular motor nerves may be difficult to determine on imaging, as the lateral wall of the pituitary fossa is thin and poorly visualized. Methods described for using MRI to determine cavernous sinus invasion include extension of abnormal tissue lateral to the tangent between the intra- and supracavernous portions of the ICA in the coronal plane[64] and encasement of the intracavernous ICA by more than 67%.[65]

Pituitary apoplexy

Ocular paresis secondary to pituitary tumors usually occurs insidiously. In contrast, pituitary apoplexy is characterized by sudden onset of headache, visual symptoms, and hormonal dysfunction resulting from acute hemorrhage or infarction of the gland. In almost all cases, this occurs spontaneously within a pre-existing pituitary adenoma. Several predisposing factors, however, are identified, such as pregnancy, hormone administration, and open heart surgery; in these cases, pituitary apoplexy may occur in the absence of an underlying tumor.[66] Hemorrhage into adenomas is a common finding, although only a fraction presents with apoplexy.[32] In contrast to the more usual chronic ophthalmologic presentations of pituitary adenomas, the most common presenting symptom of pituitary apoplexy after headache is ophthalmoplegia (78%), with visual field defects present in 64%.[67] The nerve affected most commonly is CNIII and this may occur in isolation.[68,69]

The imaging findings of pituitary apoplexy usually include the presence of an expanded pituitary fossa. CT may demonstrate high attenuation within the pituitary gland representing hemorrhage, although this is visible in less than half of cases.[67] MRI is more sensitive and hemorrhage manifests as heterogeneity within the gland. If the scan is performed within the hyperacute phase, the most apparent change may be low signal on T2-w images. If the scan is acquired after more than 3 days, the hemorrhage usually is most evident as high signal intensity on T1-w images (**Fig. 15**).[32,66]

Schwannomas

Schwannomas occasionally may occur within the cavernous sinus itself. The most common origin is the trigeminal nerve, although primary intracavernous tumors of the ocular motor nerves and even the sympathetic plexus of the ICA are described.[70]

Cavernous hemangioma

Cavernous hemangioma of the cavernous sinus is a rare tumor that may cause ocular motor nerve palsy. These lesions are reported as characteristically well demarcated, T1-w hypointense,

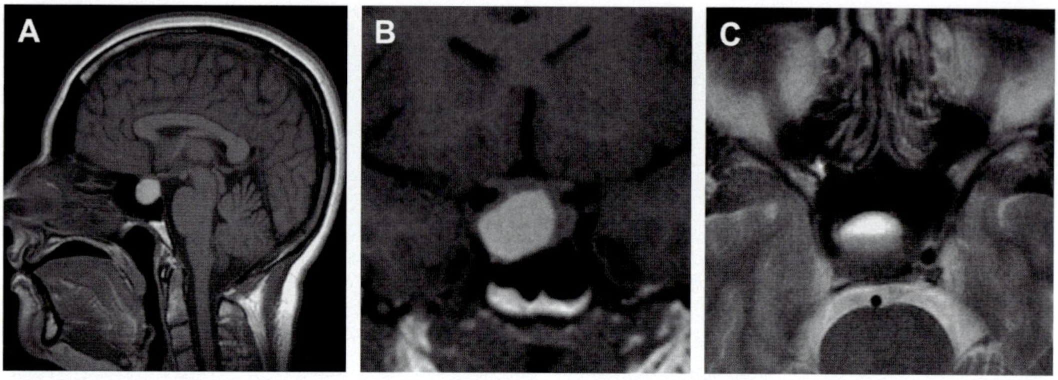

Fig. 15. Pituitary apoplexy. Patient presenting with headache and ophthalmoplegia. Sagittal (*A*) and coronal (*B*) T1-w noncontrast images demonstrating an enlarged pituitary fossa with homogeneous high signal representing blood products occupying most of the sella. A thin rim of isointense tissue is seen within the periphery of the sella on the left representing residual macroadenoma. (*C*) Axial T2-w image demonstrating layering of blood products within the expanded pituitary fossa.

markedly T2-w hyperintense, with avid homogeneous postcontrast enhancement, and often as having no tumor blush on DSA.[71,72]

Orbital Apex

The orbital apex may be involved in any primary orbital neoplasm or tumors of the head, neck, and paranasal sinuses.

Although schwannomas usually arise along the cisternal course of the cranial nerves, the orbital apex is a well-recognized site.[54] Orbital schwannomas arise most commonly from the supraorbital or supratrochlear branches of CNV; however, primary tumors of the ocular motor nerves are described.[55]

Primary tumors of the head, neck, and paranasal sinuses usually are associated with other findings; however, orbital apex syndrome resulting from local invasion is occasionally the presenting sign.[73–75] Malignancies also may metastasize hematogenously to the orbit, particularly secondary to breast, lung, kidney, and malignant melanoma primaries.

Perineural spread is another form of tumor dissemination characteristic of certain neurotropic malignancies, such as adenoid cystic carcinoma (**Fig. 16**), mucoepidermoid carcinoma,[76] malignant melanoma,[77] lymphoma, and squamous cell carcinoma of the skin.[78] The orbital apex and cavernous sinus commonly are involved as the nerves passing through the associated foramina and fissures provide a conduit to and from the orbit, nose, mouth, infratemporal fossa, and skin of the face. The nerves affected most commonly are CNV and CNVII,[76] although ophthalmoplegia may result from associated orbital apex and cavernous sinus syndromes, and direct spread along the ocular motor nerves is described.[78] The imaging correlate of perineural spread is thickening and enhancement of the nerve, often with corollary features reflecting denervation of the end organ, such as muscle atrophy.[77]

INFLAMMATORY

Nuclear/Fascicular

Demyelination

Demyelination is one of the most common inflammatory conditions affecting the nuclear and fascicular portions of the nerves. The most common ocular motor manifestations of multiple sclerosis are nystagmus or internuclear ophthalmoplegia. Focal lesions of the brainstem may result, however, in isolated ocular nerve palsies or complex dysfunctions, such as one-and-a-half syndrome.[79,80]

In reported cases, MRI has demonstrated focal T2-w hyperintense lesions with or without gadolinium enhancement (**Fig. 17**).[79]

Inflammatory vasculitides

Inflammatory vasculitides, such as systemic lupus erythematosis and Behçet's disease, may involve the midbrain and brainstem. Multiple large lesions often are present and ocular motor dysfunction is not uncommon.[81] Isolated pareses of the nerves are reported but rare.[82]

Behçet's disease in particular has a propensity to affect the brainstem.[81,83] In the acute phase, large confluent lesions extending from the brainstem to the basal ganglia, often with mottled enhancement, are characteristic.[81,83] In the chronic phase of the disease, atrophy of the brainstem frequently is observed and may help discriminate from other inflammatory conditions.[83]

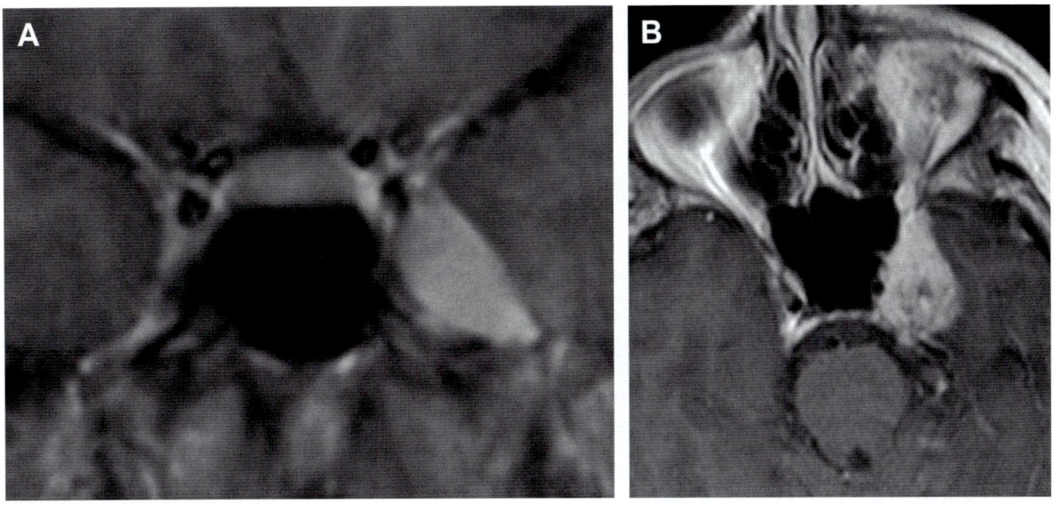

Fig. 16. Perineural spread of adenoid cystic carcinoma. A 65-year-old patient several years after resection of a left parotid gland adenoid cystic carcinoma developed ophthalmoparesis secondary to retrograde perineural spread into the cavernous sinus. Coronal (*A*) and axial (*B*) T1-w postgadolinium images showing expansion of the left cavernous sinus by abnormal enhancing soft tissue.

Cisternal

Inflammatory meningitis

Inflammatory diseases affecting the meninges may lead to palsies of the cisternal segments of the ocular motor nerves. Such conditions include Behçet's disease, sarcoid (**Fig. 18**), Wegener's granulomatosis, and systemic lupus erythematosis. These conditions all produce imaging appearances of nodular thickening and enhancement of the meninges with a predilection for the basal, perimesencephalic, and suprasellar regions.[84]

Miller Fisher syndrome

Miller Fisher syndrome (MFS) is a variant of Guillain-Barré syndrome characterized by an acute onset of ophthalmoplegia, ataxia, and areflexia with complete recovery over weeks to months. Classically, the ophthalmoplegia takes the form of bilateral abduction palsy, although isolated CNIII and CNIV palsies are described.[3] MRI may reveal neural enhancement that decreases with the resolution of symptoms.[85,86]

Ophthalmoplegic migraine

Another disease process involving the cisternal portions of the ocular motor nerves is ophthalmoplegic migraine. This entity typically occurs in children or young adults and is characterized by recurrent migraine-like headache with ocular motor nerve palsy following within 4 days of onset and

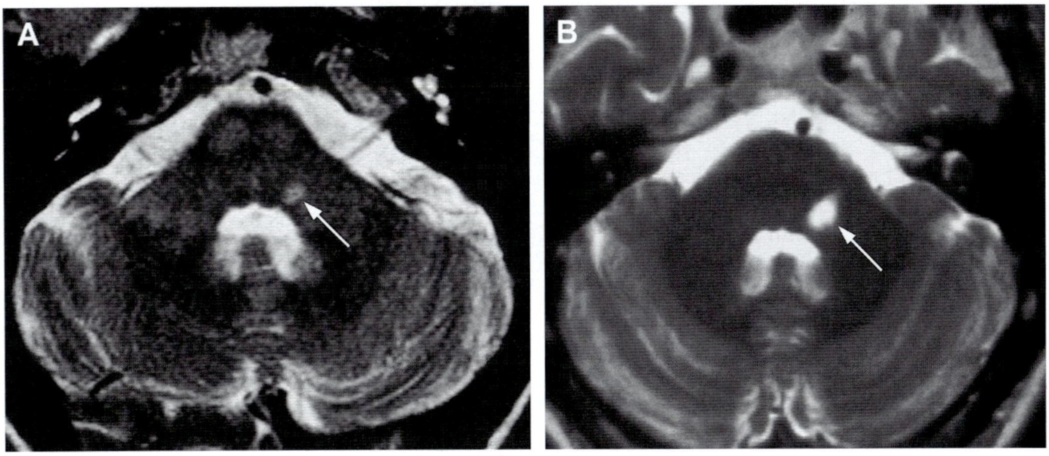

Fig. 17. Demyelination. Axial T2-w images of two different patients (*A, B*) who had multiple sclerosis presenting with diplopia. In both cases, images demonstrate focal T2-w hyperintense plaques adjacent to the CNVI nucleus (*white arrows*).

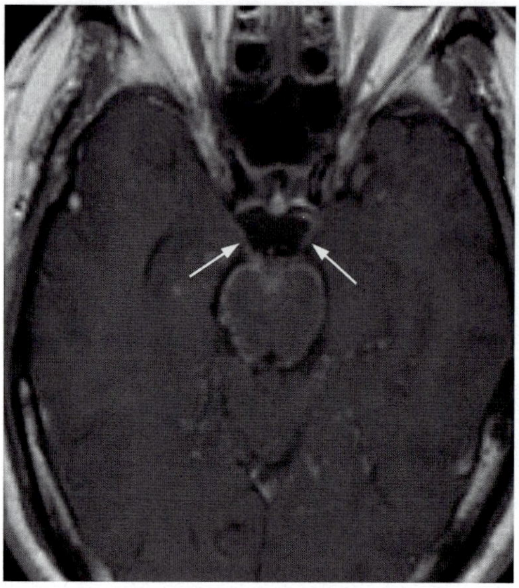

Fig. 18. Neurosarcoidosis. A 34-year-old patient who had known sarcoidosis of the lung and newly developed CNIII palsy. Axial T1-w postgadolinium images demonstrate nodular leptomeningeal enhancement with perineural enhancement of the oculomotor nerves bilaterally (*white arrows*).

lasting for days or weeks after headache cessation.[87] CNIII is by far the nerve affected most commonly although involvement of CNIV and CNVI is well described. On MRI, there is enhancement and thickening of the origin of the cisternal segment of the affected nerve that resolves with cessation of symptoms.[88] Enhancement is seen much less frequently when CNIV and CNVI are involved, raising speculation as to whether or not these cases represent different pathologic entities.[87,89]

Other conditions, in particular Tolosa-Hunt syndrome (THS), aneurysms, and diabetic ophthalmoparesis, may present with similar clinical features and should be excluded before a diagnosis of ophthalmoplegic migraine is made. Although enhancement of the cisternal portion of the ocular motor nerves is nonspecific, the absence of enhancement during symptom-free periods may assist in making the diagnosis. The cause of ophthalmoplegic migraine is unclear, although clinical and imaging similarities with Bell's palsy and trigeminal sensory neuropathy suggests a common inflammatory pathogenesis with the associated migrainous symptoms possibly representing a CNV epiphenomenon secondary to ocular motor nerve inflammation.[87,89]

Cavernous

Tolosa-Hunt syndrome

THS is a painful ophthalmoplegia secondary to nonspecific steroid-responsive granulomatous inflammation of the cavernous sinus.[28,90] It may extend to the orbital apex and is considered as part of a continuum with orbital pseudotumour (from which it is indistinguishable histopathologically). The key criteria in confirming diagnosis are prompt response to steroid treatment and imaging or histologic features compatible with granulomatous inflammation.[90] CNIII is the ocular motor nerve involved most commonly,[3] although THS commencing with CNIV and CNVI deficits is described. Additional features include paresthesias of the face and Horner's syndrome resulting from involvement of the cavernous segments of CNV and sympathetic nerves, respectively. CT may demonstrate an enlarged cavernous sinus or abnormal soft tissue at the orbital apex side but is relatively insensitive and often normal.[32,90,91] MRI is more sensitive and characteristically shows the cavernous sinus distended by abnormal soft tissue that is isointense to gray matter on T1-w images and iso- to hypointense on T2-w images with homogeneous avid enhancement after gadolinium (**Fig. 19**).[28,32,90,91] Imaging abnormalities characteristically improve with the administration of steroids.

Orbital Apex

As discussed previously, THS extending anteriorly and orbital pseudotumour extending posteriorly are considered parts of a continuum and both may lead to an orbital apex syndrome. Inflammatory processes within the orbit itself rarely result in islolated ocular motor palsies and ophthalmoplegia usually is the result of involvement of the muscles themselves.[3]

INFECTION

Nuclear/Fascicular

Isolated infection of the brainstem and midbrain is unusual. One such disease is mesenrhombencephalitis, an infective process selectively involving the midbrain, pons, and medulla, typically presenting with areflexia, ataxia, and ophthalmoplegia.[92] The infectious agent frequently remains undetermined although viruses are implicated in the majority of cases with herpes simplex the most common culprit. Bacteria also may be responsible, most commonly *Listeria monocytogenes.* MRI demonstrates brainstem swelling with areas of hyperintensity on T2-w images. Moderate, patchy contrast enhancement sometimes is seen.[92]

Cisternal

The cisternal portions of the ocular motor nerves may be infected directly, leading to neuronitis, or

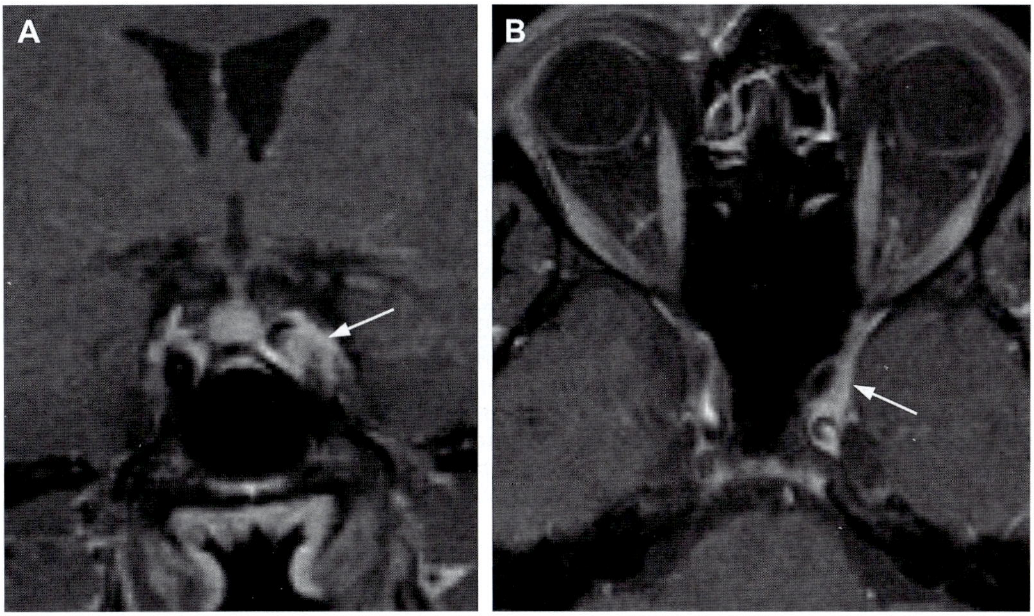

Fig. 19. Coronal (*A*) and axial (*B*) T1-w postgadolinium images of a 47-year-old man patient who had THS who presented with acute double vision. Arrows delineate the contrast-enhancing lesion within the left cavernous sinus.

may be involved secondarily by infection of the meninges or skull base.

Herpes zoster

The ocular motor nerves may be involved in herpes zoster ophthalmicus in which the ophthalmic division of CNV is infected by varicella zoster virus. Ophthalmoplegia occurs in 11% to 29% of patients,[93] most commonly the result of paresis of the muscles innervated by CNIII. Demyelination and microinfarction of the nerve are proposed as possible mechanisms, although the cause remains controversial and direct infiltration of the extraocular muscles also is suggested. MRI may demonstrate thickening and enhancement of the cavernous and cisternal portions of the affected nerves, often with an abnormal area of hyperintensity on FLAIR imaging in the region of the CNV nucleus.[94]

Lyme disease

Lyme disease is an infection involving multiple organ systems caused by the spirochete, *Borellia burgdorferi*. Involvement of the central nervous system is seen in 10% to 15% of cases usually as a combined cranial neuritis and meningitis.[95] CNVII is affected most commonly but palsies of CNIII and CNIV are not uncommon. MRI findings include brainstem leptomeningeal enhancement, thickening and enhancement of affected nerves, and hyperintense lesions within the cerebral white matter on T2-w images simulating demyelination.[95,96]

Meningitis

Agents that may cause ocular motor nerve palsies secondary to meningitis include tuberculosis and *Cryptococcus neoformans*. In tuberculous meningitis, the meninges of the basal cisterns are involved preferentially with formation of thick gelatinous exudates. Infection may spread to involve the cavernous sinus and orbital apex (**Fig. 20**). CT and MRI may demonstrate nodular lepto- and pachymeningeal thickening and enhancement.[32]

Gradenigo's syndrome

Because of its proximity to the petrous apex as it enters Dorello's canal, CNVI is susceptible to infections spreading medially from the middle ear cleft. The association of CNVI palsy with otitis media and facial pain in the distribution of CNV is known as Gradenigo's syndrome.[28,97] In the current antibiotic era, this is rare but still may be found in patients who have diabetes and those who are immunosuppressed. The most common causative agents are *Staphylococcus aureus* and *Pseudomonas aeruginosa*. CT using a bone algorithm may be useful particularly in demonstrating opacification and coalescence of the petrous apex air cells and expansile, subperiosteal lucency in the advent of abscess formation. On MRI, the petrous

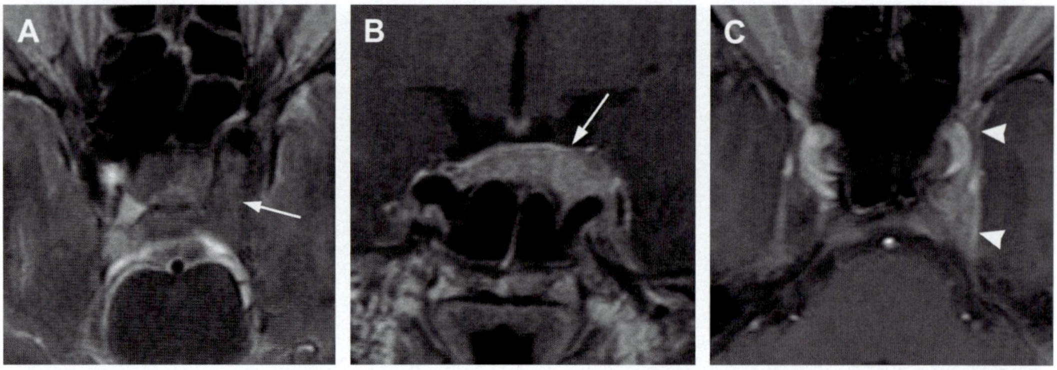

Fig. 20. Tuberculous meningitis. A 50-year-old woman presenting with ophthalmoplegia and reduced visual acuity. (*A*) Axial T2-w image demonstrating abnormal tissue, isointense to gray matter, expanding the left cavernous sinus (*white arrow*). Coronal (*B*) and axial (*C*) T1-w postgadolinium images demonstrating thickening and enhancement of the parasellar pachymeninges (*white arrow*). Abnormal enhancing tissue is seen expanding the left cavernous sinus and extending to the orbital apex (*white arrowheads*).

apicitis may appear as low signal on T1-w images with peripheral enhancement.[97]

Cavernous

Cavernous sinus thrombosis

The cavernous sinus may be involved by infections spreading from the paranasal sinuses, petrous apex, or retrogradely from the orbit or skin of the face and scalp. Cavernous sinus thrombosis is a potential complication and is seen most commonly as a sequel of sinusitis or infections of the midface.[28] *Staphylococcus aureus* accounts for approximately 70% of cases and fungi occasionally are implicated. Clinically, there usually is a history of midface infection followed by headache, periorbital swelling, chemosis, and ophthalmoplegia. CT and MRI appearances are variable but may demonstrate enlargement of the cavernous sinus with irregular filling defects post contrast. Corollary features of venous obstruction, such as dilatation of the superior ophthalmic vein, exophthalmos, and induration of orbital fat, frequently are evident and underlying sinusitis may be demonstrated.[28] Even with aggressive treatment, mortality remains at 30%.

Fungal infection

Fungal infection of the paranasal sinuses resulting from aspergillus or mucormycosis is seen in diabetic and immunocompromised patients and may spread to the cavernous sinus and orbit through destruction of intervening bony walls. Involvement of the ocular motor nerves is frequent, and wider involvement of the intracranial compartment may occur as a result of perineural spread.[84] The presence of metallic ions within the fungal balls causes characteristic very low signal intensity on T2-w images that may be mistaken for normal aerated sinus. T1-w images reveal iso- or hypointense masses with peripheral rim or homogeneous enhancement.[98]

Orbital Apex

Infections of the postseptal orbit may result in an orbital apex syndrome or may spread retrogradely into the cavernous sinus. As with inflammatory lesions of the orbit, isolated ocular motor nerve palsies are rare and ophthalmoplegia often is the result of direct involvement of the extraocular muscles.

SUMMARY

Palsies of CNIII, CNIV, and CNVI may arise secondary to a wide range of pathologies, and ocular motor nerve dysfunction may reflect the presence of an indolent self-limiting pathology or herald a life-threatening emergency. Lesions may be categorized according to the anatomic location in which they occur, and the presence of additional symptoms and signs frequently assist the localization of pathology to one of these segments. In addition, many pathologies exhibit a predilection for specific locations, assisting in reducing the number of potential diagnoses and prompting urgent investigation when specific combinations of clinical features are recognized. Knowledge of the anatomic basis for lesion localization and the pathologies to which each anatomic segment is predisposed is essential in developing an imaging strategy for the investigation of ocular motor nerve palsies.

ACKNOWLEDGMENTS

The authors thank Prof. Tarek Yousry for editorial assistance, Adrienne Wallis for assistance in gathering literature, and Dr. Stefan Brew and Dr. Fergus Robertson for the provision of images.

REFERENCES

1. Rush JA, Younge BR. Paralysis of cranial nerves III, IV, and VI. Cause and prognosis in 1,000 cases. Arch Ophthalmol 1981;99(1):76–9.
2. Richards BW, Jones FR, Younge BR. Causes and prognosis in 4,278 cases of paralysis of the oculomotor, trochlear, and abducens cranial nerves. Am J Ophthalmol 1992;113:489–96.
3. Bennett JL, Pelak VS. Palsies of the third, fourth, and sixth cranial nerves. Ophthalmol Clin North Am 2001;14(1):169–85.
4. Yeh S, Foroozan R. Orbital apex syndrome. Curr Opin Ophthalmol 2004;15(6):490–8.
5. Brazis PW. Palsies of the trochlear nerve: diagnosis and localization—recent concepts. Mayo Clin Proc 1993;68(5):501–9.
6. Kim JS, Kim J. Pure midbrain infarction: clinical, radiologic, and pathophysiologic findings. Neurology 2005;64(7):1227–32.
7. Blake PY, Mark AS, Kattah J, et al. MR of Oculomotor nerve palsy. AJNR Am J Neuroradiol 1995;16: 1665–72.
8. Kissel JT, Burde RM, Klingele TG, et al. Pupil-sparing oculomotor palsies with internal carotid-posterior communicating artery aneurysms. Ann Neurol 1983; 13(2):149–54.
9. Mark AS, Blake P, Atlas SW, et al. Gd-DTPA enhancement of the cisternal portion of the oculomotor nerve on MR imaging. AJNR Am J Neuroradiol 1992; 13(5):1463–70.
10. Hosoya T, Adachi M, Yamaguchi K, et al. Abducens nerve enhancement demonstrated by multiplanar reconstruction of contrast-enhanced three-dimensional MRI. Neuroradiology 2001;43(4): 295–301.
11. Jacobson DM, Trobe JD. The emerging role of magnetic resonance angiography in the management of patients with third cranial nerve palsy. Am J Ophthalmol 1999;128(1):94–6.
12. Zhu Y, Thulborn K, Curnyn K, et al. Sixth cranial nerve palsy caused by compression from a dolichoectatic vertebral artery. J Neuroophthalmol 2005;25(2):134–5.
13. Karamessini MT, Kagadis GC, Petsas T, et al. CT angiography with three-dimensional techniques for the early diagnosis of intracranial aneurysms. Comparison with intra-arterial DSA and the surgical findings. Eur J Radiol 2004;49(3):212–23.
14. Kupersmith MJ, Heller G, Cox TA. Magnetic resonance angiography and clinical evaluation of third nerve palsies and posterior communicating artery aneurysms. J Neurosurg 2006;105(2):228–34.
15. Lang J. Ueber Bau, Laenge und Gefaessbeziehungen der zentralen und peripheren Strecken der intrazisternalen Hirnnerven. Zentralbl Neurochir 1982;43:217–55 [in German].
16. Møller AR. The cranial nerve vascular compression syndrome. I. A review of treatment. Acta Neurochir 1991;113:18–23.
17. Albayram S, Ozer H, Sarici A, et al. Unilateral mydriasis without ophthalmoplegia—a sign of neurovascular compression? Case report. Neurosurgery 2006;58(3):582–3.
18. Marinkovic S, Gibo H, Zelic O, et al. The neurovascular relationships and the blood supply of the trochlear nerve: surgical anatomy of its cisternal segment. Neurosurgery 1996;38:161–9.
19. Leigh RJ, Tomask RL, Seidmann SH, et al. Superior oblique myokymia. Arch Ophthalmol 1991;109: 1710–3.
20. Marinkovic SV, Gibo H, Stimec B. The neurovascular relationships and the blood supply of the abducent nerve: surgical anatomy of its cisternal segment. Neurosurgery 1994;34:1017–26.
21. Yousry I, Camelio S, Wiesmann M, et al. Detailed magnetic resonance imaging anatomy of the cisternal segment of the abducent nerve: Dorello's canal and neurovascular relationship and landmarks. J Neurosurg 1999;91:276–83.
22. Narai H, Manabe Y, Deguchi K, et al. Isolated abducens nerve palsy caused by vascular compression. Neurology 2000;55(3):453–4.
23. Yousry I, Moriggl B, Dieterich M, et al. MR anatomy of the proximal cisternal segment of the trochlear nerve: neurovascular relationships and landmarks. Radiology 2002;223(1):31–7.
24. Casselman JW, Dehaene I. Imaging of the IIIrd, IVth, and VIth cranial nerves. Neuroophthalmology 1998; 19:63–8.
25. Yousry I, Dieterich M, Naidich TP, et al. Superior oblique myokymia: magnetic resonance imaging support for neurovascular compression hypothesis. Ann Neurol 2002;51:361–8.
26. Yousry I, Moriggl B, Schmid U, et al. Detailed MR anatomy of the motor and sensory roots of the trigeminal nerve and their neurovascular relationships. J Neurosurg 2004;101:427–34.
27. Field M, Jungreis CA, Chengelis N, et al. Symptomatic cavernous sinus aneurysms: management and outcome after carotid occlusion and selective cerebral revascularization. AJNR Am J Neuroradiol 2003;24(6):1200–7.
28. Larson TL. Petrous apex and cavernous sinus: anatomy and pathology. Semin Ultrasound CT MR 1993; 14(3):232–46.

29. Wu HC, Ro LS, Chen CJ, et al. Isolated ocular motor nerve palsy in dural carotid-cavernous sinus fistula. Eur J Neurol 2006;13(11):1221–5.
30. Mariak Z, Mariak Z, Stankiewicz A. Cranial nerve II-VII injuries in fatal closed head trauma. Eur J Ophthalmol 1997;7(1):68–72.
31. Muthu P, Pritty P. Mild head injury with isolated third nerve palsy. Emerg Med J 2001;18(4):310–1.
32. Gentry LR. Head trauma. In: Atlas SW, editor. Magnetic resonance imaging of the brain and spine. 3rd edition. Philadelphia: Lippincott, Williams and Wilkins; 2002. p. 1059–98.
33. Makki AA, Newman NJ. A trochlear stroke. Neurology 2005;65(12):1989.
34. Heinz J. Cranial nerve avulsion and other neural injuries. Med J Aust 1969;2:1246–9.
35. Hanson RA, Ghosh S, Gonzalez-Gomez I, et al. Abducens length and vulnerability? Neurology 2004; 62(1):33–6.
36. Hara N, Kan S, Simizu K. Localization of post-traumatic trochlear nerve palsy associated with hemorrhage at the subarachnoid space by magnetic resonance imaging. Am J Ophthalmol 2001;132(3): 443–5.
37. Sam B, Ozveren MF, Akdemir I, et al. The mechanism of injury of the abducens nerve in severe head trauma: a postmortem study. Forensic Sci Int 2004;140(1):25–32.
38. Keane JR. Fourth nerve palsy: historical review and study of 215 inpatients. Neurology 1993;43(12): 2439–43.
39. Balcer LJ, Galetta SL, Bagley LJ, et al. Localization of traumatic oculomotor nerve palsy to the midbrain exit site by magnetic resonance imaging. Am J Ophthalmol 1996;122(3):437–9.
40. Bater MC, Ramchandani PL, Ramchandani M, et al. An orbital apex fracture resulting in multiple cranial neuropathies. Br J Oral Maxillofac Surg 2007. [Epub ahead of print].
41. Mielke C, Alexander MS, Anand N. Isolated bilateral trochlear nerve palsy as the first clinical sign of a metastatic [correction of metastasic] bronchial carcinoma. Am J Ophthalmol 2001;132(4):593–4.
42. Modi M, Singla V, Bhatia R, et al. Isolated nuclear oculomotor nerve palsy due to a solitary midbrain metastasis: a rare presentation. Indian J Ophthalmol 2006;54:286–7.
43. Krohel GB, Mansour AM, Petersen WL, et al. Isolated trochlear nerve palsy secondary to a juvenile pilocytic astrocytoma. J Clin Neuroophthalmol 1982;2(2):119–23.
44. Leibovitch I, Pakrou D, Selva D, et al. Neuro-ophthalmic manifestations of intracranial cavernous hemangiomas. Eur J Ophthalmol 2006;16(1):148–52.
45. Russell DS, Rubinstein LJ. Tumours of the cranial, spinal and peripheral nerve sheaths. In: Russell DS, Rubinstein J, editors. Pathology of tumors of the nervous system. 5th edition. London: Edward Arnold; 1989. p. 533–89.
46. Ohba S, Miwa T, Kawase T. Trochlear nerve schwannoma with intratumoral hemorrhage: case report. Neurosurgery 2006;58(4):791.
47. Gentry LR, Mehta RC, Appen RE, et al. MR imaging of primary trochlear nerve neoplasms. AJNR Am J Neuroradiol 1991;12:707–13.
48. Tanriover N, Kemerdere R, Kafadar AM, et al. Oculomotor nerve schwannoma located in the oculomotor cistern. Surg Neurol 2007;67(1):83–8.
49. Acharya R, Husain S, Chabra SS, et al. Sixth nerve schwannoma: a case report with literature review. Neurol Sci 2003;24(2):74–9.
50. Celli P, Ferrante L, Acqui M, et al. Neurinoma of the third, fourth, and sixth cranial nerves: a survey and report of a new fourth nerve case. Surg Neurol 1992;38(3):216–24.
51. Ho SY, Kveton JF. Acoustic neuroma. Assessment and management. Otolaryngol Clin North Am 2002;35(2):393–404.
52. Borges A, Casselman J. Imaging the cranial nerves: part II: primary and secondary neoplastic conditions and neurovascular conflicts. Eur Radiol 2007;17(9): 2332–44.
53. Ginsberg F, Peyster RG, Rose WS, et al. Sixth nerve schwannoma: MR and CT demonstration. J Comput Assist Tomogr 1988;12:482–4.
54. Wang Y, Xiao LH. Orbital schwannomas: findings from magnetic resonance imaging in 62 cases. Eye 2007. [Epub ahead of print].
55. Shen WC, Yang DY, Ho WL, et al. Neurilemmoma of the oculomotor nerve presenting as an orbital mass: MR findings. AJNR Am J Neuroradiol 1993;14(5): 1253–4.
56. Deshmukh VR, Albuquerque FC, Zabramski JM, et al. Surgical management of cavernous malformations involving the cranial nerves. Neurosurgery 2003;53(2):352–7.
57. Kawamoto S, Matsuda H, Ueki K, et al. Neuromuscular choristoma of the oculomotor nerve: case report. Neurosurgery 2007;60(4):777–8.
58. Eisenkraft B, Ortiz AO. Imaging evaluation of cranial nerves 3, 4, and 6. Semin Ultrasound CT MR 2001; 22(6):488–501.
59. Harada T, Ohashi T, Ohki K, et al. Clival chordoma presenting as acute esotropia due to bilateral abducens palsy. Ophthalmologica 1997;211(2): 109–11.
60. Gay E, Sekhar LN, Rubinstein E, et al. Chordomas and chondrosarcomas of the cranial base: results and follow-up of 60 patients. Neurosurgery 1995; 36(5):887–96.
61. Barkovich AJ. Intracranial, orbital and neck masses of childhood. In: Barkovich AJ, editor. Pediatric neuroimaging. 4th edition. Philadelphia: Lippincott, Williams and Wilkins; 2005. p. 506–658.

62. Saremi F, Helmy M, Farzin S, et al. MRI of cranial nerve enhancement. AJR Am J Roentgenol 2005; 185(6):1487–97.
63. Petermann SH, Newman NJ. Pituitary macroadenoma manifesting as an isolated fourth nerve palsy. Am J Ophthalmol 1999;127:235–6.
64. Knosp E, Steiner E, Kitz K, et al. Pituitary adenomas with invasion of the cavernous sinus space: a magnetic resonance imaging classification compared with surgical findings. Neurosurgery 1993;33(4): 610–7.
65. Cottier J-P, Destrieux C, Brunereau L, et al. Cavernous sinus invasion by pituitary adenoma: MR imaging. Radiology 2000;215(2):463–9.
66. Riedl M, Clodi M, Kotzmann H, et al. Apoplexy of a pituitary macroadenoma with reversible third, fourth and sixth cranial nerve palsies following administration of hypothalamic releasing hormones: MR features. Eur J Radiol 2000;36(1):1–4.
67. Bills DC, Meyer FB, Laws ER Jr, et al. A retrospective analysis of pituitary apoplexy. Neurosurgery 1993; 33(4):602–9.
68. Chen Z, Murray AW, Quinlan JJ. Pituitary apoplexy presenting as unilateral third cranial nerve palsy after coronary artery bypass surgery. Anesth Analg 2004;98(1):46–8.
69. Rossitch E Jr, Carrazana EJ, Black PM. Isolated oculomotor nerve palsy following apoplexy of a pituitary adenoma. J Neurosurg Sci 1992;36(2):103–5.
70. Nakagawa T, Uchida K, Ozveren MF, et al. Abducens schwannoma inside the cavernous sinus proper: case report. Surg Neurol 2004;61(6): 559–63.
71. Shi J, Hang C, Pan Y, et al. Cavernous hemangiomas in the cavernous sinus. Neurosurgery 1999; 45(6):1308–13.
72. Sohn CH, Kim SP, Kim IM, et al. Characteristic MR imaging findings of cavernous hemangiomas in the cavernous sinus. AJNR Am J Neuroradiol 2003; 24(6):1148–51.
73. Srinivasan S, Fern AI, Wilson K. Orbital apex syndrome as a presenting sign of maxillary sinus carcinoma. Eye 2001;15:343–5.
74. Gore HL, Corin SM, Klussmann KG, et al. Mucoepidermoid carcinoma presenting as an orbital apex syndrome. Ophthalmic Surg 1992;23:59–61.
75. McDonald HR, Char DH. Adenoid cystic carcinoma presenting as an orbital apex syndrome. Ann Ophthalmol 1985;17:757–9.
76. Parker GD, Harnsberger HR. Clinical-radiologic issues in perineural tumor spread of malignant diseases of the extracranial head and neck. Radiographics 1991;11(3):383–99.
77. Chang PC, Fischbein NJ, McCalmont TH, et al. Perineural spread of malignant melanoma of the head and neck: clinical and imaging features. AJNR Am J Neuroradiol 2004;25:5–11.
78. Veness MJ, Biankin S. Perineural spread leading to orbital invasion from skin cancer. Australas Radiol 2000;44:296–302.
79. de Seze J, Vukusic S, Viallet-Marcel M, et al. Unusual ocular motor findings in multiple sclerosis. J Neurol Sci 2006;243(1–2):91–5.
80. Thomke F, Ringel K. Isolated superior oblique palsies with brainstem lesions. Neurology 1999; 53(5):1126–7.
81. Lee SH, Yoon PH, Park SJ, et al. MRI findings in neuro-Behçet's disease. Clin Radiol 2001;56(6): 485–94.
82. Aydin MD, Aydin N. A neuro-Behcet's lesion in oculomotor nerve nucleus. Acta Neurol Scand 2003; 108(2):139–41.
83. Coban O, Bahar S, Akman-Demir G, et al. Masked assessment of MRI findings: is it possible to differentiate neuro-Behcet's disease from other central nervous system diseases? Neuroradiology 1999;41(4): 255–60.
84. Borges A, Casselman J. Imaging the cranial nerves: part I: methodology, infectious and inflammatory, traumatic and congenital lesions. Eur Radiol 2007; 17(8):2112–25.
85. Garcia-Rivera CA, Rozen TD, Zhou D, et al. Miller Fisher syndrome: MRI findings. Neurology 2001; 57(10):1755.
86. Nagaoka U, Kato T, Kurita K, et al. Cranial nerve enhancement on three-dimensional MRI in Miller Fisher syndrome. Neurology 1996;47(6):1601–2.
87. Crevits L, Verschelde H, Casselman J. Ophthalmoplegic migraine: an unresolved problem. Cephalalgia 2006;26(10):1255–9.
88. Mark AS, Casselman J, Brown D, et al. Ophthalmoplegic migraine: reversible enhancement and thickening of the cisternal segment of the oculomotor nerve on contrast-enhanced MR images. AJNR Am J Neuroradiol 1998;19(10):1887–91.
89. Celebisoy N, Sirin H, Gokcay F. Ophthalmoplegic migraine: two patients, one at middle age with abducens palsy. Cephalalgia 2005;25(2): 151–3.
90. La Mantia L, Curone M, Rapoport AM, et al. International Headache Society. Tolosa-Hunt syndrome: critical literature review based on IHS 2004 criteria. Cephalalgia 2006;26(7):772–81.
91. de Arcaya AA, Cerezal L, Canga A, et al. Neuroimaging diagnosis of Tolosa-Hunt syndrome: MRI contribution. Headache 1999;39(5):321–5.
92. Wasenko JJ, Park BJ, Jubelt B, et al. Magnetic resonance imaging of mesenrhombencephalitis. Clin Imaging 2002;26(4):237–42.
93. Im M, Kim BJ, Seo YJ, et al. Complete ophthalmoplegia after herpes zoster. Clin Exp Dermatol 2007; 32(2):162–4.
94. Quisling SV, Shah VA, Lee HK, et al. Magnetic resonance imaging of third cranial nerve palsy and

trigeminal sensory loss caused by herpes zoster. J Neuroophthalmol 2006;26(1):47–8.
95. Lell M, Schmid A, Stemper B, et al. Simultaneous involvement of third and sixth cranial nerve in a patient with Lyme disease. Neuroradiology 2003;45(2):85–7.
96. Savas R, Sommer A, Gueckel F, et al. Isolated oculomotor nerve paralysis in Lyme disease: MRI. Neuroradiology 1997;39(2):139–41.
97. Sherman SC, Buchanan A. Gradenigo syndrome: a case report and review of a rare complication of otitis media. J Emerg Med 2004;27(3):253–6.
98. Siddiqui AA, Bashir SH, Ali Shah A, et al. Diagnostic MR imaging features of craniocerebral Aspergillosis of sino-nasal origin in immunocompetent patients. Acta Neurochir (Wien) 2006;148(2):155–66.

Pathology of the Trigeminal Nerve

Minerva Becker, MD[a,b,c,*], Romain Kohler, MD[a], Maria Isabel Vargas, MD[d], Magalie Viallon, PhD[e], Jacqueline Delavelle, MD[c,d]

KEYWORDS

- Imaging techniques • Clinical symptoms
- Pathologic conditions of the trigeminal nerve

Various benign and malignant conditions may affect the trigeminal nerve, resulting in trigeminal nerve dysfunction (trigeminal neuropathy). Trigeminal neuropathy may be the only, the first, or one of several clinical signs of an underlying disease, leading the patient to seek medical advice. Based on clinical examination alone, it is not always possible to locate a lesion along the course of the trigeminal nerve precisely, because the trigeminal nerve has complex branching and anastomotic patterns.[1–3] In addition, the underlying cause of trigeminal neuropathy cannot always be found based on clinical and laboratory findings alone. Therefore, trigeminal nerve dysfunction has become a common indication for imaging. The purpose of this article is to discuss the most common symptoms related to trigeminal pathology and their implications for imaging; to review the lesions involving the trigeminal nerve at specific levels, with special emphasis on clinical–radiologic correlation; and to demonstrate a spectrum of pathologic conditions, as observed on MR and CT images. Knowledge of the imaging features of these pathologic conditions can prevent their misinterpretation and facilitates therapeutic choice.

IMAGING TECHNIQUES

Although CT and MR imaging have a complementary role in the evaluation of trigeminal neuropathy, allowing evaluation of bony detail and soft tissues, respectively, MR imaging is, in many instances, the only imaging modality needed to provide the diagnosis. MR imaging is uniquely suited to image the entire course of the trigeminal nerve, from the brainstem nuclei, through the basal cisterns, within the skull base foramina, and in the suprahyoid neck. As suggested by several investigators,[2–7] the diagnostic yield of imaging mostly depends on the quality of the examination and on the appropriate tailoring.

To image trigeminal neuropathy, high-field units (1 T–3 T) are mandatory because they provide a better signal-to-noise ratio, a better spatial resolution, and a shorter examination time. When performing an MR imaging examination of the trigeminal nerve, the challenge consists of performing high-resolution studies with smaller fields of view on one hand and covering the entire presumptive anatomic area of interest on the other hand, while keeping the duration of the MR imaging study within a reasonable time frame. High-resolution MR images can be obtained using parallel imaging techniques, surface coils, thin slices (0.5–2.0 mm), and the highest matrix size (384–512) for a minimal field of view, resulting in an in-plane spatial resolution of 0.4 mm to 0.7 mm. The nuclear and supranuclear portion of the trigeminal nerve are imaged using a standard brain protocol, including T2-weighted (T2-w),

[a] Head and Neck and Maxillofacial Radiology, Department of Radiology, Geneva University Hospital, Rue Micheli-du-Crest 24, CH – 1211 Geneva 14, Switzerland
[b] Head and Neck Surgery Clinic, Department of Neurosciences, Geneva University Hospital, Geneva, Switzerland
[c] Faculty of Medicine, University of Geneva, Geneva, Switzerland
[d] Neuroradiology Unit, Department of Radiology, Geneva University Hospital, Geneva, Switzerland
[e] Department of Radiology, Geneva University Hospital, Geneva, Switzerland
* Corresponding author. Department of Radiology, Geneva University Hospital, Rue Micheli-du-Crest 24, CH – 1211 Geneva 14, Switzerland.
E-mail address: minerva.becker@hcuge.ch (M. Becker).

Neuroimag Clin N Am 18 (2008) 283–307
doi:10.1016/j.nic.2007.11.002
1052-5149/08/$ – see front matter

fluid-attenuated inversion recovery (FLAIR), diffusion-weighted, and T1-weighted (T1-w) images before and after intravenous administration of contrast material. The cisternal portion of the trigeminal nerve is best imaged using three-dimensional (3D) heavily T2-w sequences, such as 3D gradient-echo steady-state free precessing (SSFP) sequences, constructive interface in steady state (CISS) sequences, fast imaging employing steady-state acquisition [FIESTA], true fast imaging with steady-state precession [TrueFISP], balanced fast field echo [bFFE]) or, more recently, fast spin echo 3D sequences with optimized contrast using flip angle evolution (driven equilibrium [DRIVE], sampling perfection with application optimized contrasts [SPACE]). These techniques provide an excellent cerebral spinal fluid–nerve contrast and an excellent resolution because of thin slices (0.35–0.7 mm). Multiplanar reconstructions and 3D and virtual endoscopic views generated from these 3D data sets are extremely useful in assessing neurovascular conflicts in conjunction with 3D time of flight (TOF) MR angiography and contrast-enhanced MR angiography.[4–8] Recently, diffusion tensor imaging has been used to assess the tissue integrity of the trigeminal nerve, with diffusion tensor imaging–derived fractional anisotropy (FA) being calculated for the cisternal portion of the trigeminal nerve.[9] Meckel's cave, cavernous sinus, skull base, and extracranial portions of the trigeminal nerve are imaged using high-resolution 2 to 3-mm thin spin echo (SE) or fast spin echo T1-w images in the axial and coronal plane pre- and postcontrast, and 3D T1-w sequences with 1-mm thin slices, such as 3D spoiled gradient echo, Magnetized Prepared Rapid Gradient Echo (Ultrafast Gradient Echo 3D sequence with magnetization transfer), or 3D Volume Interpolation Breath hold Enhancement, which allow multiplanar reconstructions in any chosen plane. Fat saturation techniques after intravenous administration of contrast material are extremely useful in that they increase lesion conspicuity, allowing identification of subtle enhancement patterns along the course of the trigeminal nerve, especially in the cavernous and extracranial portions.

Volumetric acquisition achieved with 16, 32, or 64 multidetector CT scanners enhanced by various 3D volume rendering, virtual endoscopy, and two-dimensional (2D) multiplanar or curved reconstructions is capable of imaging most pathologic conditions of the trigeminal nerve. However, CT of the trigeminal nerve is not as sensitive as MR imaging in the brainstem, cisternal segments, and cavernous sinus. Nevertheless, CT is nearly equal to MR imaging at the level of the skull base foramina and in the suprahyoid neck. In addition to soft tissue algorithm reconstruction, bone algorithm reconstruction is required to assess better any widening or compromise of skull base foramina and facial bone involvement. Thin sections (0.3–1.5 mm), high-resolution images, and 2D reconstructions in the axial and coronal plane are mandatory. As with MR imaging, if CT is used alone, imaging of the entire course of the trigeminal nerve is essential, because clinical examination cannot always precisely locate a lesion along the course of the nerve.

At the authors' institution, patients who have trigeminal neuropathy are imaged using a combination of MR imaging and CT. First, an MR imaging examination of the brain and face is performed and if pathology involves the skull base or bony structures of the face, a thin-slice CT with bone window algorithm and without administration of contrast material is added. Interpretation of findings will then be made from the combined information from both examinations.

The role of ultrasound and angiography in imaging trigeminal neuropathy is minor, because the former is used only to guide fine-needle aspiration biopsies, and the latter may be performed either to assess precisely arteriovenous malformations (AVMs) and dural fistulae or before interventional procedures.

CLINICAL SYMPTOMS

Symptoms arising from pathologic conditions involving the trigeminal nerve (trigeminal neuropathy) depend on the segment and division of the nerve that is affected.[2–6] Because V1 (ophthalmic), V2 (maxillary), and V3 (mandibular) divisions have sensory fibers, patients typically complain of pain, burning, or anesthesia and analgesia in the regions innervated by any of the three divisions. In addition, when V1 is affected, the corneal reflex may be absent (nasociliary nerve), with an increased risk of corneal injury and ulceration (neurokeratitis). When V3 is affected, patients may complain of weakness in chewing and deviation of the jaw on mouth opening (muscles of mastication), or they may present with serous otitis media (eustachian tube dysfunction from malfunction of the tensor veli palatini muscle).

Pathologic processes affecting the cavernous sinus may present clinically with ophthalmoplegia (cranial nerves III, IV, and VI), anisocoria or mydriasis (III), V1 and V2 deficits, chemosis, and proptosis.

Pathologic processes affecting the cisternal portion of the trigeminal nerve may result in trigeminal neuralgia (TN). TN, or tic douloureux, is the most frequently occurring condition of all nerve pain disorders.[10–13] The pain, which comes and goes, feels like bursts of sharp, stabbing, electric shocks in the V1 or V2 distribution of the trigeminal nerve, and can last from a few seconds to a few minutes. Although the onset of TN is most often seen in middle or old age, young adults and children can also be affected.[10] People with "classic" or "idiopathic" TN become plagued by intermittent severe sharp or stabbing pain that interferes with common daily activity. They live in fear of unpredictable painful attacks, which may lead to sleep deprivation, irritability, severe anticipatory anxiety and depression, dehydration, and malnutrition. A characteristic feature of TN is the trigger zone, a small area in the central part of the face, usually on a cheek, nose, or lip, that, when stimulated, triggers a typical burst of pain. A light touch or vibration is the most effective trigger.[10–17] Because of this, common daily activities, such as brushing the teeth, shaving, eating, drinking, or talking, trigger the attacks. Typically, attacks are similar in individual patients and no neurologic deficits are clinically evident. Between paroxysmal attacks, most patients usually become relatively pain free. However, in time, the pain usually becomes more intense and the attacks more frequent. In some cases, the pain does not exactly fit these criteria; patients may experience a persistent ache between paroxysms (steady component) or mild sensory loss. Such disease has been labeled "atypical" TN.[10] Less commonly, autonomic symptoms, such as conjunctival injection, lacrimation, eyelid edema, and nasal congestion as features of trigeminal autonomic cephalgias may be seen in association with TN.[12,13] Although the clinical diagnosis of TN is straightforward in most cases, other causes of facial pain, such as dental pain, temporomandibular joint pain, migraine, temporal arteritis, trigeminal deafferentation pain, and atypical facial pain should be eliminated in patients in whom a paroxysmal and a steady pain component are noted. As opposed to TN, trigeminal deafferentation pain is pain that results from intentional injury to the trigeminal nerve system in an attempt to treat TN, particularly after destructive neurosurgical intervention. Numbness of the face and excruciating facial pain, sometimes accompanied by trophic wounds in the areas innervated by the trigeminal nerve, are a constant part of this syndrome, which has also been referred to as anesthesia dolorosa.[14] Atypical facial pain, also called persistent idiopathic facial pain, is characterized by steady aching or throbbing pain, described as pressure and a sensation of swelling in the face. It has a strong female predominance, with typically no trigger zone on the face.[15]

Diseases affecting the brainstem and the upper spinal cord nuclei may result not only in trigeminal neuropathy but also in other cranial nerve deficits (III, IV, VI, VII–XII) and brainstem syndromes, such as the lateral medullary syndrome (Wallenberg syndrome) and the medial medullary syndrome, and less common syndromes, such as Parinaud syndrome or Foville's syndrome. A detailed discussion of these syndromes is, however, beyond the scope of this article.

Last but not least, some patients who have pathologic conditions of the trigeminal nerve may not have TN, facial pain, or numbness at all,[3,15–17] and trigeminal pathology is discovered incidentally at imaging.

PATHOLOGIC CONDITIONS OF THE TRIGEMINAL NERVE

For the purpose of this article, the clinical, radiologic, and pathologic features of the most common conditions affecting the trigeminal nerve are reviewed at each specific anatomic level: brainstem, cisternal, Meckel's cave, cavernous sinus, and peripheral divisions. Various vascular, infectious and inflammatory, neoplastic, traumatic, and congenital conditions are discussed for each specific anatomic site.

Brainstem

Vascular lesions

The brainstem is the site of approximately 25% of acute strokes. Infarction at this site may cause diverse and complex patterns of dysfunction, depending on the site of the lesion and its relationship to the cranial nerve nuclei, long tracts, and brainstem connections. Most brainstem strokes are seen in patients over 60 years of age. At MR imaging, most patients have solitary acute ischemic brainstem lesions. However, as many as 15% have additional cerebellar lesions and 10% have acute supratentorial ischemic stroke lesions.[18] The most common brainstem infarcts are seen in the dorsolateral medulla (occlusion of the ipsilateral posterior inferior cerebellar artery (PICA)) and in the paramedian pons (occlusion of pontine branches of the basilar artery). Spinal cord infarction, which may present with trigeminal neuropathy by affecting the dorsally located trigeminal tracts, is less common than brainstem infarction. Since the introduction of diffusion-weighted imaging, which is particularly sensitive to ischemic changes, diagnosis of ischemic strokes in the brainstem and upper spinal cord has become standard in most institutions (**Fig. 1**).

Hemorrhage involving the trigeminal nuclei and other cranial nerve nuclei may be caused by

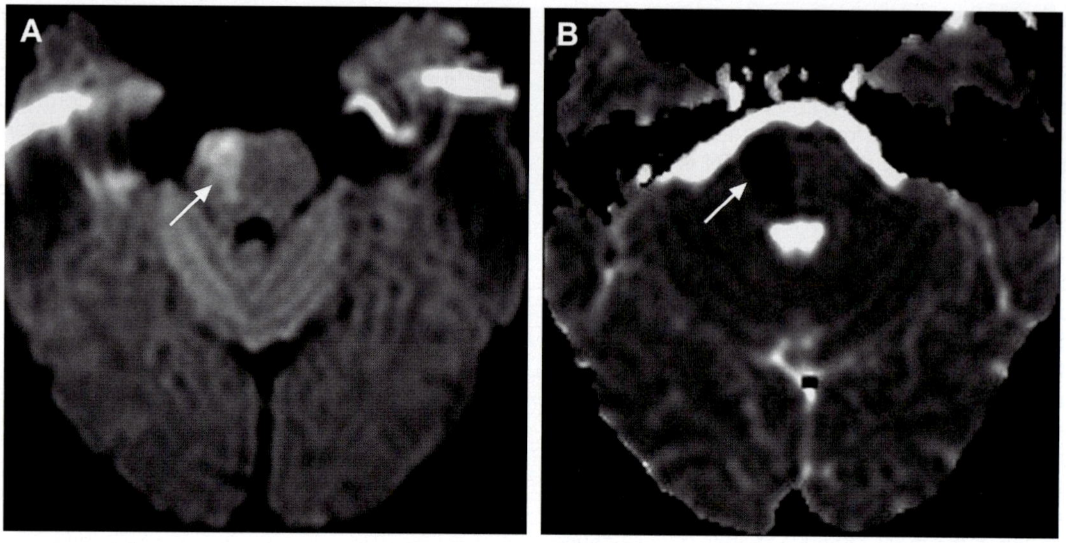

Fig. 1. Acute ischemic infarct in a 40-year-old man with hypoesthesia of the right face and a burning sensation in the territory of V2. (*A*) Axial diffusion-weighted image (b = 1000 s/mm^2) shows a hyperintense lesion in the right brainstem (*arrow*) involving the trigeminal fibers located between the brainstem nuclei and the trigeminal roots. (*B*) Axial apparent diffusion coefficient map shows that the lesion is hypointense (*arrow*), compatible with an acute stroke.

hypertension, cavernous angiomas, AVMs, or trauma (Duret's hemorrhage).[19–21] As a cause of hemorrhage, cavernous angiomas are far less common than hypertension; nevertheless, they must be excluded as a cause of hemorrhage, especially in young patients. Cavernous angiomas are considered to be congenital vascular hamartomas composed of endothelial-lined sinusoidal collections without significant amounts of interspersed neural tissue. A sporadic form and a familial form of disease with a genetic component have been observed.[20] Cavernous angiomas are frequently located in the brainstem and have a characteristic MR imaging appearance caused by the presence of blood degradation products (**Fig. 2**).

Brainstem AVMs are less common than cavernous angiomas and can be divided into pial lesions and parenchymal lesions. Pial AVMs typically receive arterial input from dilated branches of the superior cerebellar artery or the anterior inferior cerebellar artery and drain into the prepontine or petrosal sinuses. Because they are restricted to the pial surface, they can sometimes be completely resected. In contrast, parenchymal brainstem AVMs receive arterial inflow from brainstem perforating vessels, show a deep insinuation pattern within vital neural tissue, and drain through venous channels of the brainstem substance, which then empty into the petrosal sinus and galenic system. Therefore, safe microsurgical extirpation is not possible in most cases. The characteristic radiologic aspect of a brainstem AVM is seen in **Fig. 3**.

Duret's hemorrhages are delayed, secondary brainstem hemorrhages. They occur in craniocerebral trauma victims with rapidly evolving descending transtentorial herniation.[21] In most cases, the outcome is fatal. On the basis of recent observations, it is believed that arterial hypertension and advanced age are risk factors for the development of Duret's hemorrhage.[21] The diagnosis is made on CT or MR imaging of the brain.

Inflammatory and infectious lesions

Demyelinating diseases of the white matter may affect one or more cranial nerve nuclei located in the brainstem. Multiple sclerosis (MS) is the single most common pathologic entity leading to trigeminal neuropathy, which may be the first presenting symptom or may be found in association with other cranial nerve deficits. The diagnosis of MS is based on clinical presentation (optic neuritis, transverse myelitis, internuclear ophthalmoplegia, paresthesias, and other neurologic abnormalities), cerebral spinal fluid analysis, and typical findings on MR imaging. MS plaques are hyperintense on T2-w and FLAIR images and hypointense on T1-w sequences. Specific signal intensities of MS lesions vary, depending on the magnetic field strength, the pulse sequence parameters, and partial volume effects. Occasionally, acute plaques may have a thin rim of relative T2 hypointensity or T1 hyperintensity. The T1

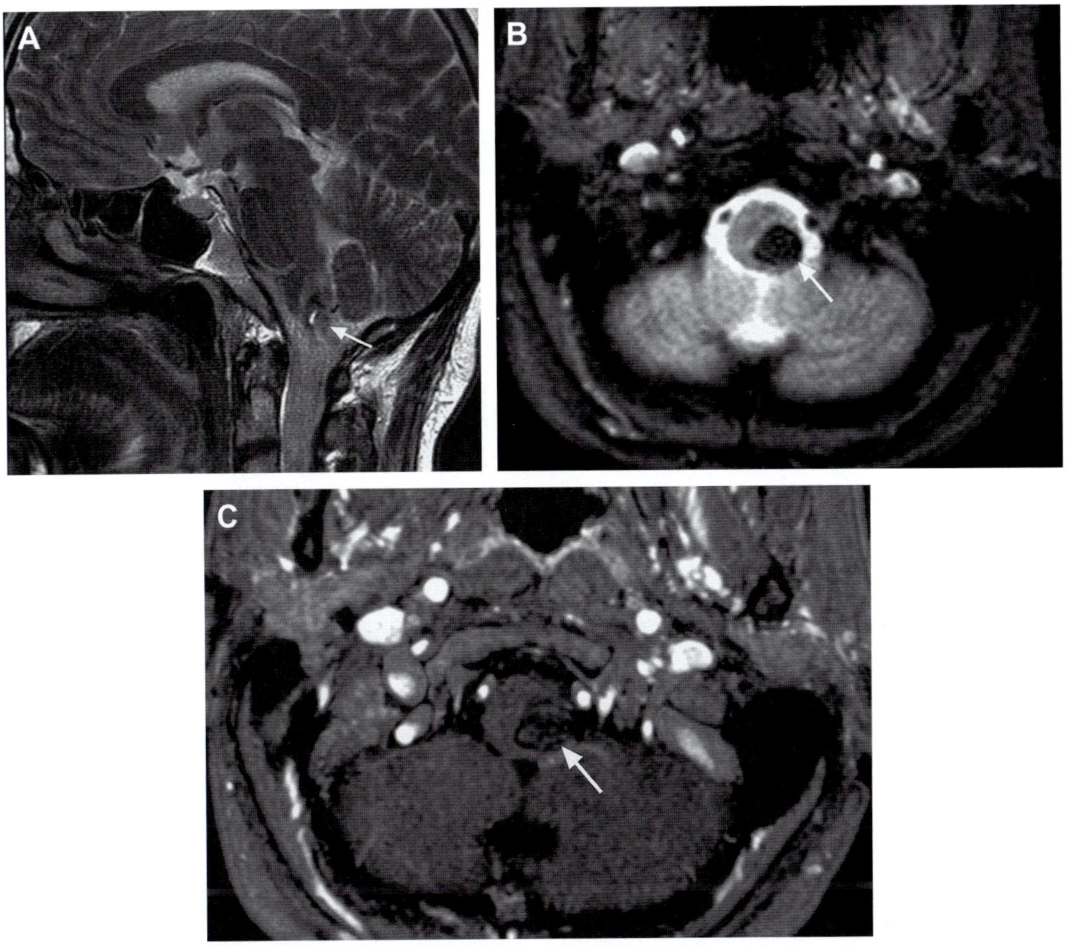

Fig. 2. Cavernous angioma in a 38-year-old man with facial pain, hypoesthesia in the distribution of V2 and V3, headache, and vertigo. (*A*) Sagittal T2-w image shows a popcorn-like, smoothly circumscribed, well-delineated complex lesion in the posterolateral medulla (*arrow*) with a heterogeneous core that is surrounded by a low-signal-intensity hemosiderin rim. (*B*) Axial gradient-refocused T2-w image shows that the hypointensity of this rim becomes more prominent because of magnetic susceptibility effects (*arrow*). No associated mass effect or edema. (*C*) Contrast-enhanced 3D time-of-flight image shows no enhancement of the lesion (*arrow*), no feeding artery, and no draining vein.

hyperintensity is attributed to free radicals, lipid-laden macrophages, and protein accumulations. Most MS plaques are small and irregular, but larger lesions can coalesce to form a confluent, tumefactive pattern. Active plaques may enhance after intravenous administration of contrast material because of transient breakdown of the blood–brain barrier 8 to 12 weeks after acute demyelination, whereas old plaques typically do not enhance (**Fig. 4**).[22] Isolated tumefactive MS plaques may mimic mass lesions and should be differentiated from other inflammatory or neoplastic lesions.

Various other inflammatory and infectious diseases may produce lesions similar to those of MS in the brainstem, such as acute disseminated encephalomyelitis, progressive multifocal leukoencephalopathy, HIV encephalitis, Behcet's disease, Lyme disease, progressive neurosarcoidosis, Whipple's disease, Bickerstaff's brainstem encephalitis, vasculitis due to systemic lupus erythematosus, and listeria rhombencephalitis. Listeria rhombencephalitis–causing TN may occur in otherwise healthy subjects, and should be looked for in a specific endemic context (**Fig. 5**). On MR imaging, transient enhancement of brainstem nuclei is observed.

Neoplasms

The trigeminal nuclei may be affected by gliomas, lymphomas, and hematogenous metastases to the brainstem. Brainstem gliomas account for 10% to 20% of all childhood brain tumors.[23,24]

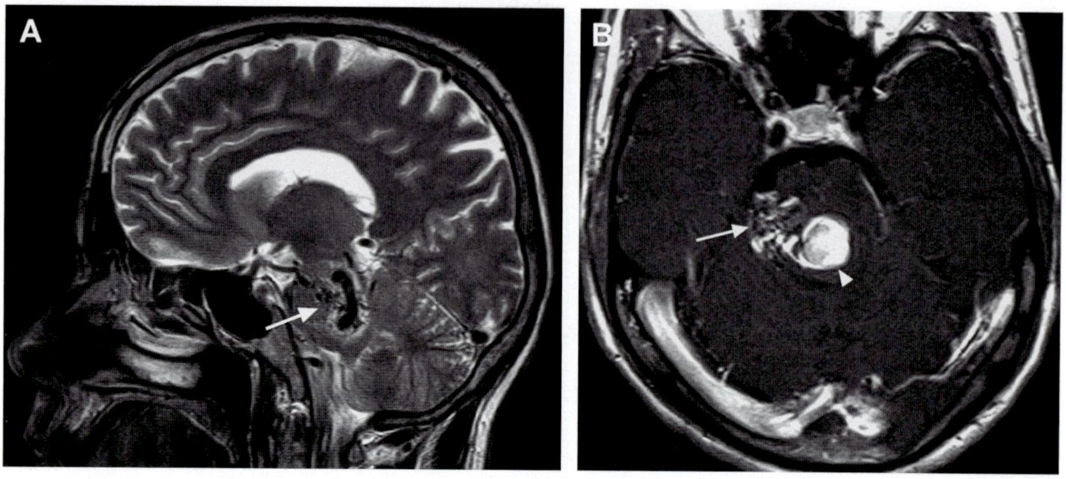

Fig. 3. Arteriovenous malformation in a 44-year-old man with right-sided V2 and V3 hypoesthesia. (*A*) Sagittal T2-w image shows the arteriovenous malformation with enlarged and tortuous vessels (*arrow*) involving the posterolateral pons. (*B*) Axial contrast-enhanced T1-w image better shows the nidus of the malformation (*arrow*) involving the right pons and an enlarged venous component (*arrowhead*).

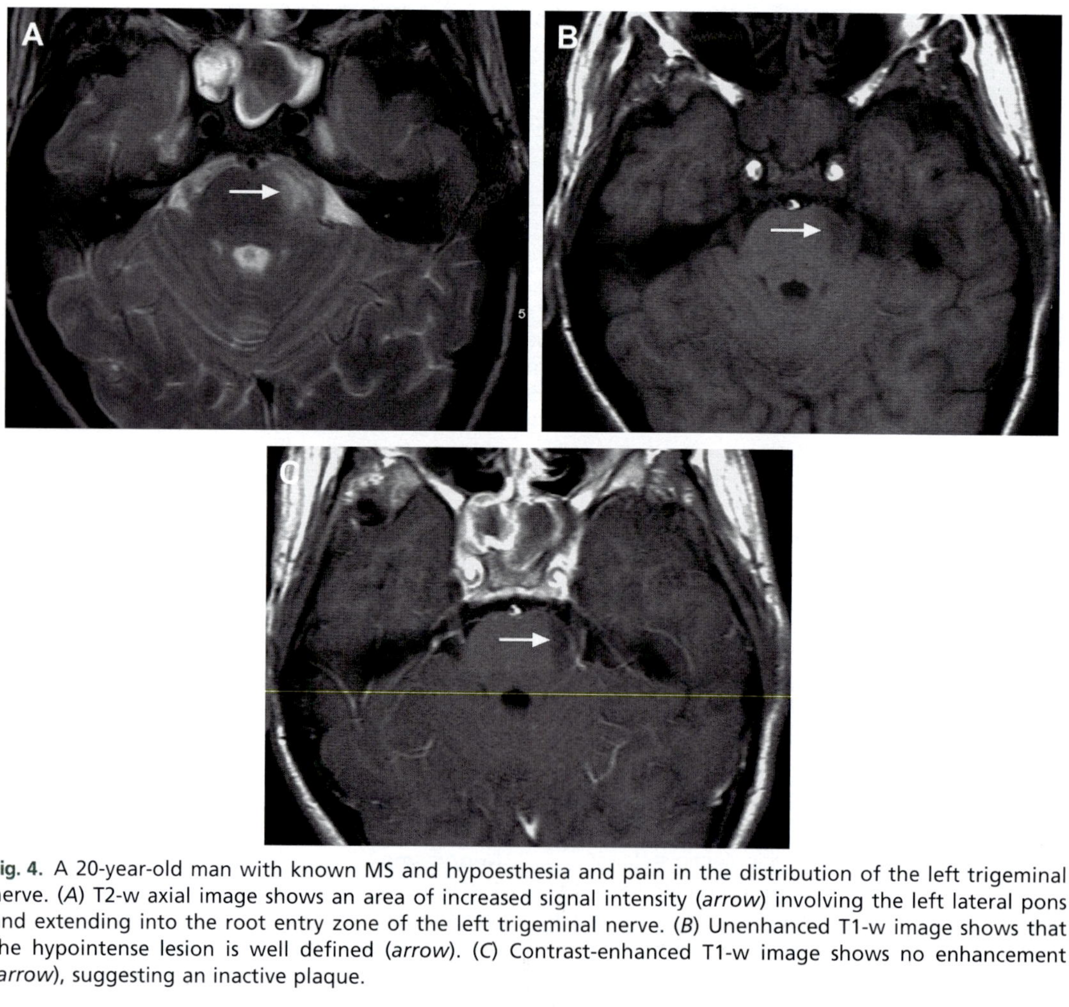

Fig. 4. A 20-year-old man with known MS and hypoesthesia and pain in the distribution of the left trigeminal nerve. (*A*) T2-w axial image shows an area of increased signal intensity (*arrow*) involving the left lateral pons and extending into the root entry zone of the left trigeminal nerve. (*B*) Unenhanced T1-w image shows that the hypointense lesion is well defined (*arrow*). (*C*) Contrast-enhanced T1-w image shows no enhancement (*arrow*), suggesting an inactive plaque.

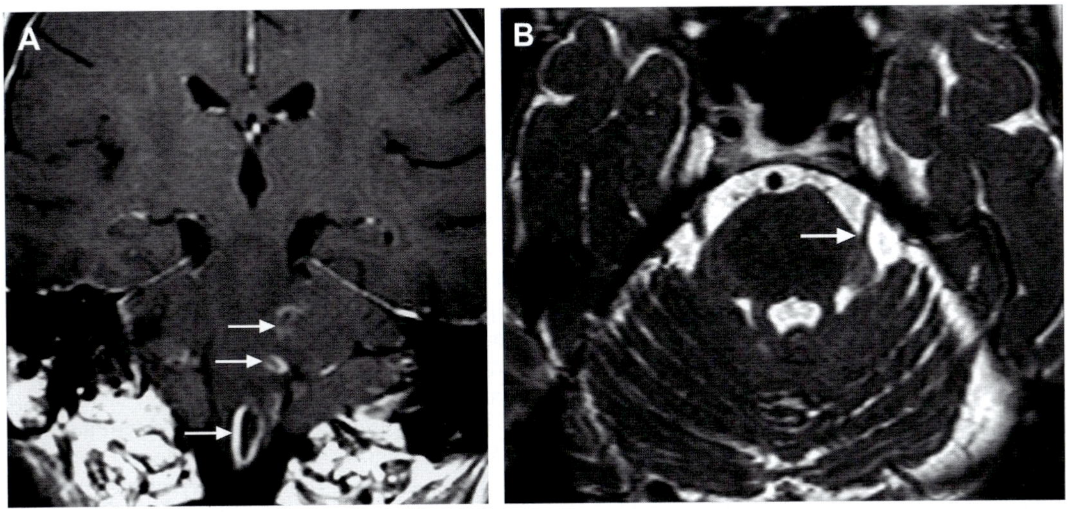

Fig. 5. Listeria rhombencephalitis in a 45-year-old man with decreased pain and thermal sense of the left face. (*A*) Contrast-enhanced coronal T1-w image shows multiple left pontomedullary lesions (*arrows*) involving the left-sided trigeminal nerve nuclei, including the spinal nucleus (*lowest arrow*). The patient was treated successfully with antibiotics. (*B*) Five years later, he developed left-sided TN, hyperesthesia in the distribution of the left V2 and V3, and hypoesthesia of the left tongue. T2-w axial image shows atrophy of the preganglionic segment of the left trigeminal nerve (*arrow*) as a sequela of brainstem rhombencephalitis.

The incidence in adults is lower than that in children younger than 16. In adults, brainstem gliomas follow a more indolent course than in children and are more likely to remain localized. Diffuse glioma is the most common form of brainstem glioma. It leads to progressive cranial nerve deficits, often asymmetric, and trigeminal symptoms are only rarely striking clinical features. Long tract signs and ataxia of trunk and limbs are common, whereas hydrocephalus is uncommon, even with large tumors. The histology of brainstem glioma is variable, although most of these tumors are of low-grade malignancy. Almost all occur in the pons but they may spread in any direction into the mesencephalon or medulla (**Fig. 6**) or may show exophytic growth that may encase and elevate the basilar artery. The typical MR imaging appearance of a brainstem glioma is an expansive, infiltrative process with low-to-normal signal intensity on T1-w images and heterogeneous

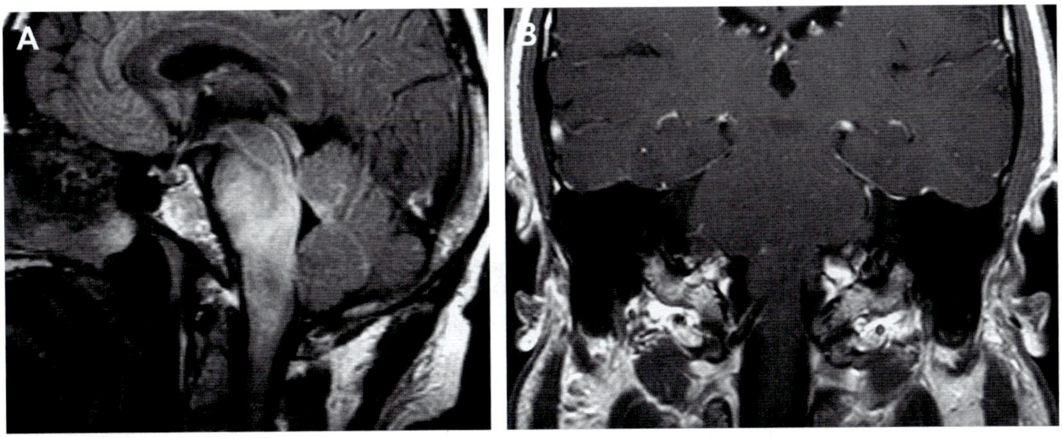

Fig. 6. Diffuse pontine glioma in a 38-year-old man with ophthalmoplegia, vertigo, left trigeminal paresthesia, and V3 motor atrophy. (*A*) Sagittal FLAIR image shows diffuse pontine and medullary enlargement with ill-defined, confluent hyperintense areas involving the anterior and posterior brainstem. (*B*) Coronal contrast-enhanced T1-w image shows absent enhancement of the tumor mass. Spectroscopy and biopsy revealed glioma grade II.

high-signal intensity on T2-w and FLAIR images, with or without contrast enhancement.

The most frequent metastatic tumors to the brain are bronchogenic carcinoma and breast carcinoma. Most commonly, hematogenous metastases are seen as multiple lesions located at the gray-white corticomedullary junction. Less frequently, metastases may be found in the brainstem, leading to cranial nerve deficits. Enhancement is characteristic for most lesions.

Congenital lesions

Congenital lesions involving the trigeminal nerve are rare and include aplasia and hypoplasia of the nerve and brainstem nuclei. Aplasia and hypoplasia of the trigeminal nerve have been described in association with Goldenhar-Gorlin syndrome, also called oculo-auriculo-vertebral syndrome, or as an isolated lesion.[3–5,25]

Cisternal (Preganglionic) Segment

Vascular lesions

Increasing evidence suggests that the most frequent cause (80%–90%) of classic TN is compression of the trigeminal nerve root close to its point of entry into the pons (root entry zone) by aberrant loops of arteries or veins, large or small, that may simply contact or indent the trigeminal nerve. The axons of the root entry zone of the trigeminal nerve are coated with central nervous system myelin, which extends up to 5 mm along the root into the prepontine cistern.[10,26,27] In consequence, the junction between central nervous system myelin and peripheral nervous system myelin, which is approximately 2 mm in length, is located some distance away from the pons. Examination of trigeminal nerve roots from patients with compression of the nerve root by an overlying blood vessel has revealed focal demyelination in the region of compression,[10,27,28] which results in the abnormal generation of ectopic sensory impulses with subsequent spread to adjacent fibers, so that spontaneous nerve activity increases. Over time, this nerve activity is thought to cause hyperactivity of the trigeminal brainstem nucleus, resulting in the generation of TN pain. Decompression of the nerve root by surgery produces rapid and long-term relief of symptoms in most patients who have vessel-associated TN, and intraoperative assessments report immediate improvement in trigeminal conduction on decompression. This phenomenon is thought to reflect the reversal of compression-induced conduction block in larger myelinated fibers outside the region of demyelination.[10] Similarly, vascular compression of the facial and glossopharyngeal nerves is thought to be responsible for most cases of hemifacial spasm and glossopharyngeal neuralgia, respectively.[2,5,10]

In classic TN, the superior cerebellar artery or one of its branches, the anterior inferior cerebellar artery, the PICA, or the basilar artery, usually compresses the root entry zone.[6,29,30] Rarely, the conflicting vessel is a petrous vein, a saccular aneurysm, a persistent trigeminal artery, or an AVM.[31,32] Recently, it has been shown that the size of the cerebellopontine cistern, as measured with MR imaging, may play a role in favoring a neurovascular conflict, because a significantly smaller volume of the cistern was found in patients who had TN on the affected side.[33]

Because contact between the cisternal portion of the trigeminal nerve and a blood vessel may also be seen in asymptomatic patients, the diagnosis of a neurovascular conflict should only be made at MR imaging with caution. Only in the presence of an appropriate clinical setting, if the site of contact is the root entry zone, the offending vessel crosses the nerve perpendicularly, the nerve itself is deviated or indented by the respective vessel, or it is encased by two or more vessels[27,34] should the diagnosis of neurovascular compression be made on MR imaging (**Fig. 7**). Using high-resolution MR angiography and 3D gradient echo SSFP sequences, the areas of compression and the conflicting vessels can be identified preoperatively.[6,8] Recently, it has been shown that neurovascular conflicts can be identified at MR imaging in 88% of the typical TN cases and in 56% of the atypical TN cases. Although arterial compression is much more common than venous compression (90% of cases with typical TN and 52% of cases with atypical TN), pure venous compression is seen more often in patients who have atypical TN (24%) than in patients who have typical TN (1%).[6] At many institutions, MR imaging is involved nowadays in the decision making when considering microvascular decompression[6] because it can differentiate between the types of compression; in MR imaging–negative cases for atypical TN, treatment modalities other than microvascular decompression can be considered.

Recently, two additional features of trigeminal nerves affected by TN have been observed at MR imaging, namely atrophy in cases with severe TN, and loss of anisotropy revealed by diffusion tensor imaging.[9,35] Based on observations performed on a small number of patients with TN, it appears that a significant reduction of FA may be observed in the affected nerves, with accompanying nerve–vessel conflict (see **Fig. 7**), and that reversibility of an abnormally low FA may be seen after successful microvascular decompression.[9] Results of a reduced FA are explained by tissue

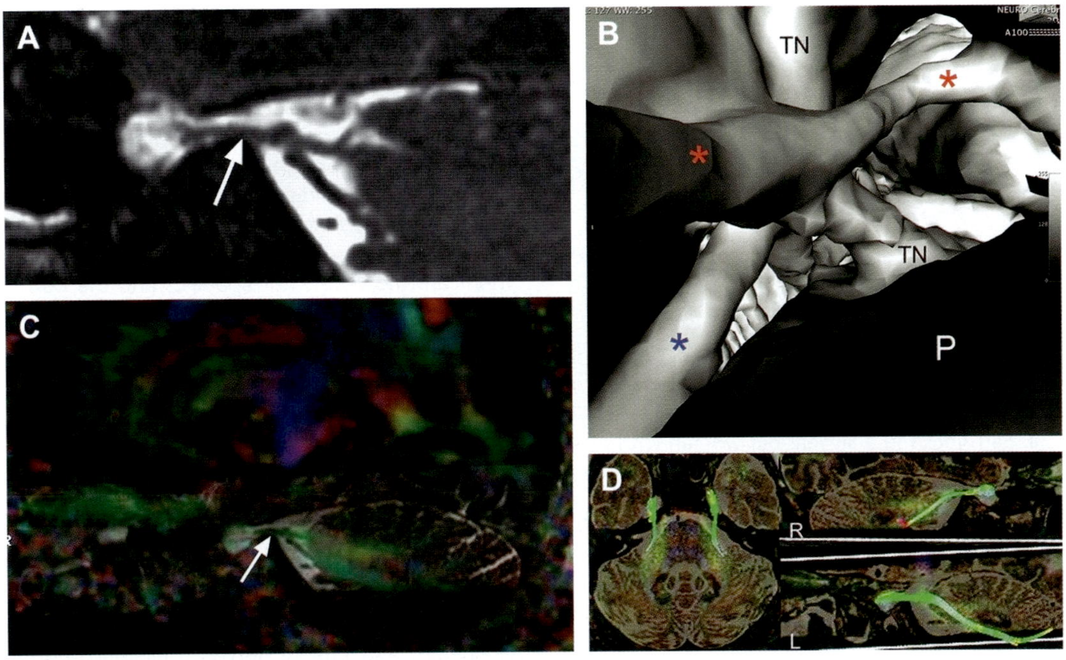

Fig. 7. Neurovascular conflict in a 45-year-old woman with right-sided TN. (*A*) Sagittal oblique 2D reconstruction from a CISS sequence shows the preganglionic segment of the right trigeminal nerve (*arrow*) as it is encased by the PICA from below and a petrosal vein from above. (*B*) Tridimensional navigation reconstruction view from below based on a CISS sequence shows the pons (P) and the cisternal portion of the trigeminal nerve (TN), which is encased by the PICA (*red asterisks*) and a petrosal vein (*blue asterisk*). (*C*) Fusion of CISS sequence and color-coded diffusion tensor image (the color-coding scheme is anterior-posterior/green; left-right/red; cranio-caudal/blue) showing the right trigeminal nerve in green (*arrow*). The calculated FA value of the right trigeminal nerve was lower than the FA value on the left (0.32 and 0.44, respectively). The root entry zone (*arrow*) is fully covered by the slice. (*D*) Fiber tracts superimposed on 3D CISS and FA color-coded map images show diminished fibers on the right (R), as opposed to the left (L).

damage associated with demyelination. However, these interesting observations have to be confirmed by larger series.

Inflammatory and infectious lesions

The symptoms of MS-related TN are identical to those of typical TN. Approximately 1.9% of patients who have MS develop TN and 4% of patients who have TN have MS.[10,22] In general, patients who have MS-related TN tend to be younger, and bilateral involvement is seen more often than in patients without MS. In MS-related TN, a plaque of demyelination involves the root entry zone, which results in gadolinium enhancement at MR imaging in the active phase.

Chronic inflammatory demyelinating polyneuropathy is a rare, immunologically mediated and acquired, sensory-motor neuropathy, considered to be the chronic variety of the Guillain-Barré syndrome. It may have a remitting relapsing, chronic progressive, or monophasic course. On MR imaging, enlargement and enhancement of multiple cranial nerves may be seen, including the cisternal and peripheral extracranial segments of the trigeminal nerve. This finding may persist for several years.

Enhancement of the preganglionic segment of the trigeminal nerve is also seen in various granulomatous diseases such as sarcoidosis (**Fig. 8**), tuberculosis, and syphilis and is the result of granulomatous neuritis. Transient enhancement of the cisternal preganglionic segment with or without enlargement may be seen in fungal and bacterial infections (**Fig. 9**), in viral neuritis secondary to herpes simplex or varicella zoster, and in idiopathic trigeminal sensory neuropathy with no underlying disease.[36] In these conditions, MR imaging typically reveals complete resolution of abnormalities on follow-up examinations 3 to 6 months later.

Neoplasms

A wide range of neoplastic lesions can cause trigeminal nerve dysfunction (including TN) by compressing or distorting the cisternal portion of the trigeminal nerve. Compression of the trigeminal nerve root may be mediated by the tumor itself or by displacement of the nerve root against

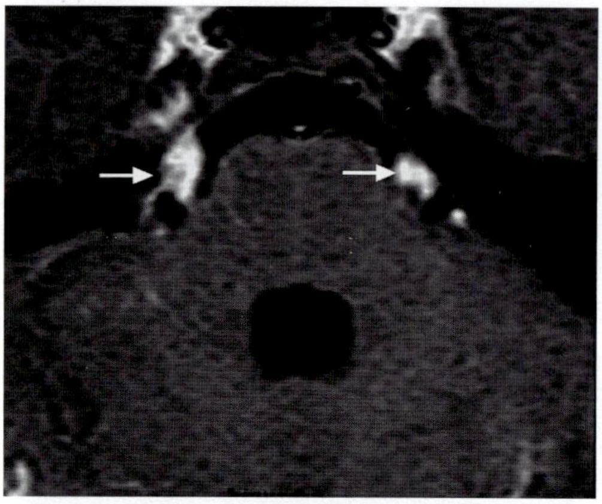

Fig. 8. Sarcoidosis in a 56-year-old woman with bilateral atypical TN. Axial contrast-enhanced T1-w image shows thickening and bilateral enhancement of the cisternal portion of both trigeminal nerves (*arrows*).

a vessel of the skull base. The most common benign tumors compressing the cisternal segment of the trigeminal nerve include vestibular schwannoma (**Fig. 10**), meningioma, cerebellopontine angle epidermoid cyst (**Fig. 11**), lipoma, and posterior fossa meningioma. Less commonly, benign tumors may originate directly from the nerve itself (trigeminal schwannoma) and may involve the preganglionic segment. Trigeminal schwannomas represent less than 0.3% of all intracranial neoplasms, and account for about 6% of all intracranial schwannomas.[37] Peak incidence is in the fourth to fifth decade. Three different types of trigeminal schwannomas are distinguished: schwannomas of the roots located exclusively in the posterior fossa; schwannomas of the gasserian ganglion; and schwannomas of the trigeminal distal branches. Multiple cranial nerve schwannomas are characteristic for neurofibromatosis type 2 (NF2) (**Fig. 12**).

The most common malignant lesions affecting the preganglionic segment of the trigeminal nerve are meningeal carcinomatosis and perineural spread from an extracranial malignant tumor. Involvement of the cisternal segment in both benign and malignant tumors results in gadolinium enhancement. In addition, the preganglionic segment may be enlarged and may show irregular or smooth margins. Both enhancement and enlargement are, however, not specific, and the correct diagnosis can only be suggested if the clinical background is known.

Congenital/developmental lesions

Congenital/developmental lesions involving the preganglionic segment of the trigeminal nerve include aplasia (**Fig. 13**), hypoplasia, and arachnoid cysts.[3–6,25,38] Arachnoid cysts may be found in the parasellar area, interpeduncular cistern, prepontine cistern, and cerebellopontine angle cisterns. Arachnoid cysts are usually developmental lesions and may exert mild to severe mass effect on the brainstem and cranial nerves traversing the cisterns. Typically, these lesions have the attenuation value and signal intensity characteristics of cerebrospinal fluid at CT and MR imaging, respectively, and they do not enhance after administration of contrast material.

Meckel's Cave and Cavernous Sinus

Vascular lesions

Giant aneurysms of the cavernous portion of the internal carotid artery may present with cavernous sinus syndrome caused by compression of cranial nerves III, IV, VI, V1, and V2,[39] or they may present with subarachnoid hemorrhage or subdural hematoma caused by aneurysm rupture. In unruptured aneurysms, trigeminal nerve involvement has been reported in up to 37% of cases.[39] Carotid cavernous fistulas have a low incidence in closed

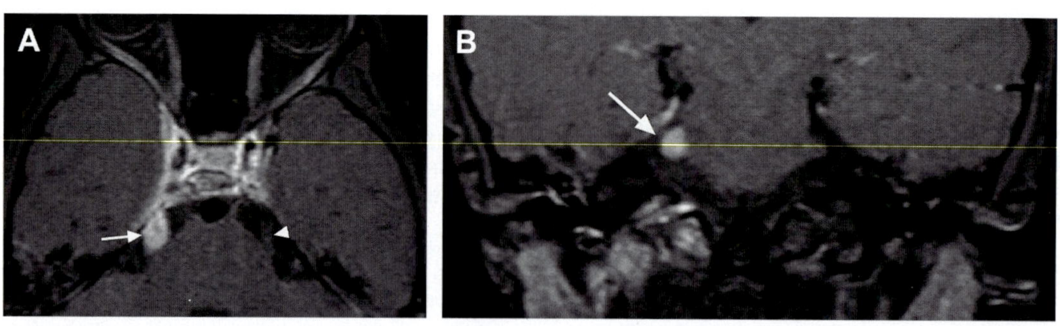

Fig. 9. Complicated otomastoiditis with neuritis of the trigeminal nerve in a 7-year-old boy with hypoesthesia of the right face. Axial (*A*) and coronal (*B*) contrast-enhanced fat-saturated T1-w images show thickening and enhancement of the cisternal portion of the right trigeminal nerve and of the adjacent dura (*arrows*). Note for comparison the normal appearance of the left preganglionic trigeminal nerve (*arrowhead*).

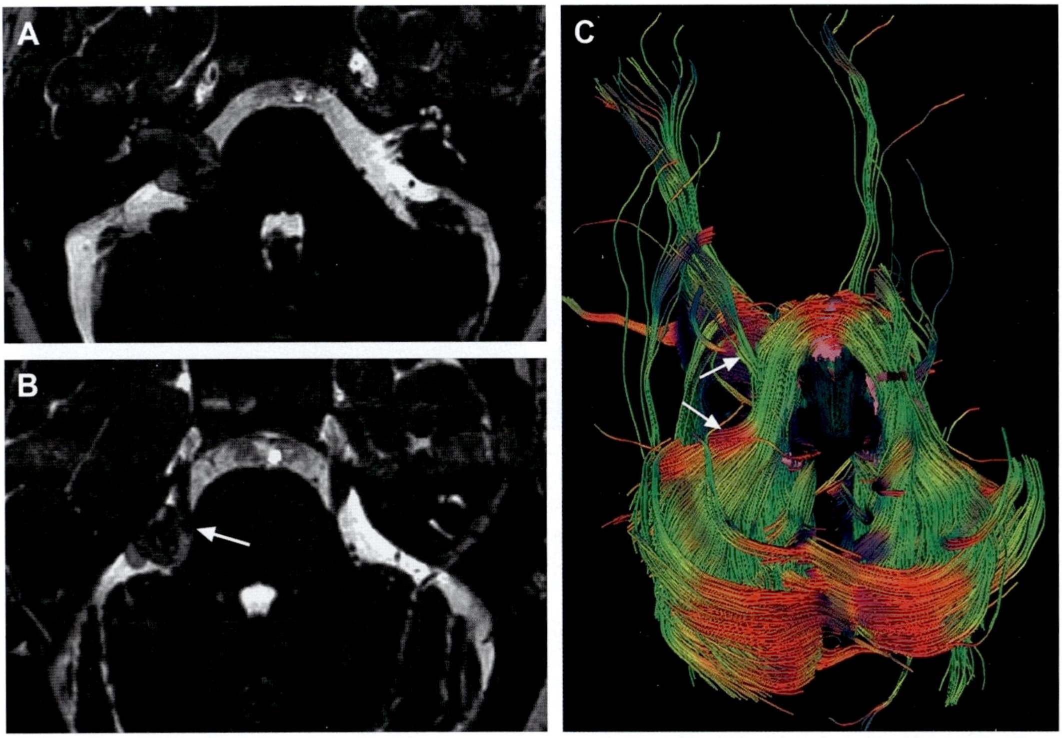

Fig. 10. A 59-year-old woman with right-sided sensorineural hearing loss and hypoesthesia in the distribution of V2 and V3. (*A*) and (*B*) Axial CISS images demonstrate a large vestibulocochlear schwannoma extending into the cerebellopontine angle cistern that has a mass effect on the lateral pons and indents the root entry zone of the right trigeminal nerve (*arrow*). (*C*) Fiber tract map reconstructed from diffusion tensor imaging sequence. Fiber tracts in the lateral pons and of the root entry zone are displaced (*arrows*) by the vestibulocochlear schwannoma.

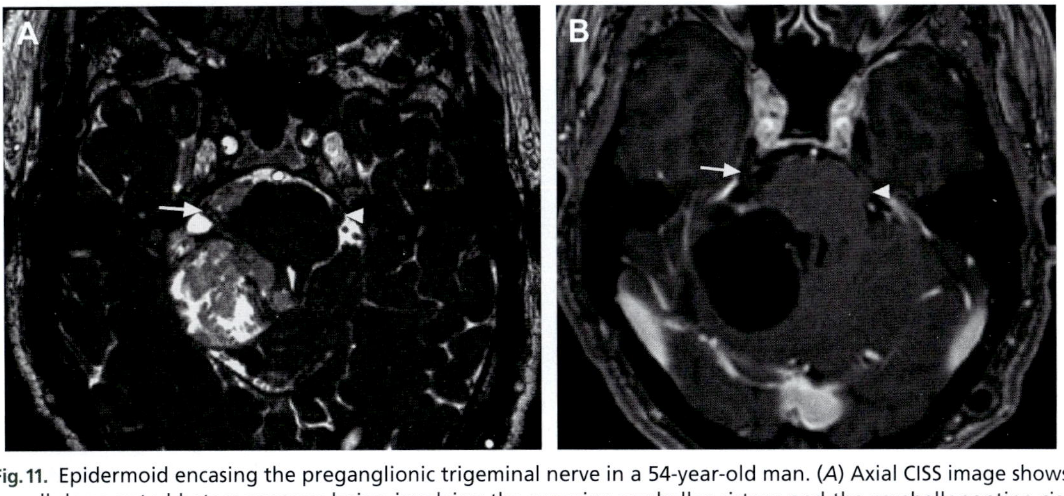

Fig. 11. Epidermoid encasing the preganglionic trigeminal nerve in a 54-year-old man. (*A*) Axial CISS image shows a well-demarcated heterogeneous lesion involving the superior cerebellar cistern and the cerebellopontine cistern extending above the tentorium. It has a mass effect on the pons and fourth ventricle. The lesion encases and displaces the right preganglionic trigeminal nerve, which is slightly atrophic (*arrow*). Note the normal appearance of the left preganglionic trigeminal nerve (*arrowhead*). (*B*) Axial contrast-enhanced T1-w image shows no enhancement of the lesion compressing the root entry zone of the right trigeminal nerve. Note the marked hypointensity of the right trigeminal nerve (*arrow*), as opposed to the left (*arrowhead*).

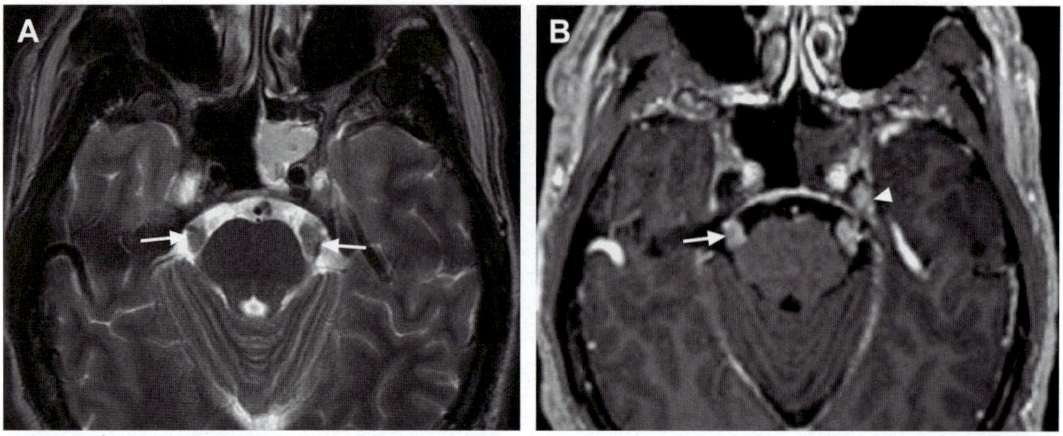

Fig. 12. Asymptomatic bilateral schwannoma in a 40-year-old man with NF2. (*A*) T2-w image shows enlargement and hyperintensity of the cisternal segment of the right and left trigeminal nerves (*arrows*). Note that on the left, the high signal intensity normally found within Meckel's cave is partially obliterated. (*B*) Contrast-enhanced T1-w image obtained at the same level shows marked enlargement and enhancement of the preganglionic trigeminal nerve on the right (*arrow*) and similar findings on the left but extending more anteriorly into Meckel's cave (*arrowhead*).

head trauma but are the most common posttraumatic intracranial vascular anomaly.[40] Acceleration–deceleration injury usually results in a direct fistula by causing a tear in the muscular wall of the internal carotid artery, or by completely transecting the internal carotid artery by shearing forces. Indirect fistulas may occur spontaneously or as a result of minor trauma, and can be associated with abnormalities in collagen deposition such as those seen in Ehlers-Danlos syndrome and osteogenesis imperfecta.

Inflammatory and infectious lesions

Aggressive bacterial and fungal sinusitis, typically seen in immunocompromised or diabetic patients, may spread to the cavernous sinus along nerves and vessels, causing thrombophlebitis or thrombosis. Inflammatory lesions affecting the

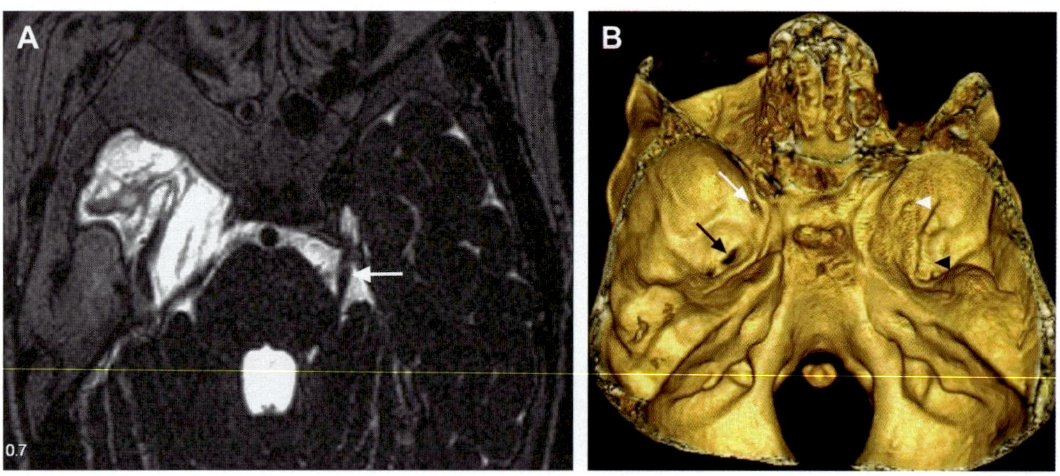

Fig. 13. Congenital absence of the preganglionic segment of the right trigeminal nerve seen in a 9-year-old boy with anesthesia in the distribution of the right trigeminal nerve, impaired mastication, and left-sided hemiparesis. (*A*) Axial CISS sequence shows atrophy of the right temporal lobe associated with absence of the right preganglionic trigeminal nerve. Note the normal left preganglionic trigeminal nerve (*arrow*). (*B*) 3D reconstruction of the skull base from CT data set (view from above [intracranial skull base surface]) shows absence of the right foramen ovale (*black arrowhead*) and right foramen rotundum (*white arrowhead*). Note normal foramen ovale (*black arrow*) and normal foramen rotundum on the left (*white arrow*).

cavernous sinus and Meckel's cave are infrequent, and include granulomatous diseases, such as sarcoidosis and Wegener's granulomatosis and idiopathic lesions, such asTolosa-Hunt syndrome (**Fig. 14**).[41] Nonspecific inflammation within the cavernous sinus or superior orbital fissure is the cause of constant retro-orbital pain in Tolosa-Hunt syndrome. Classic symptoms include ophthalmoparesis, pupillary dysfunction, and paresthesia of the forehead. Tolosa-Hunt syndrome is related to the histopathologic entity of orbital pseudotumor, and has the same imaging features and a similar clinical presentation.[3,41] MR imaging and CT may show an enhancing soft tissue mass with enlargement of the affected cavernous sinus, with lateral bulging of the outer dura (see **Fig. 14**). The cavernous portion of the internal carotid artery is often narrowed. After corticosteroid therapy, MR imaging typically shows complete resolution of the lesions within 8 weeks.

Neoplasms

Tumors of Meckel's cave comprise less than 0.5% of all intracranial tumors. The most common lesions at this site are schwannomas, meningiomas, and malignant nerve sheath tumors (malignant schwannoma). Malignant nerve sheath tumors arising from the trigeminal nerve are rare. They typically present with burning facial pain, sensory paresthesia, or diminished corneal reflex. They originate in the gasserian ganglion and may extend in an antegrade and retrograde fashion into the trigeminal distal branches and the preganglionic segment. Differentiation of malignant nerve sheath tumors from benign schwannoma is not always possible with MR imaging because both lesions may show similar spreading and enhancing patterns, therefore necessitating biopsy (**Fig. 15**). However, the rapid growth pattern and earlier and disproportionate erosion of skull base foramina may suggest the malignant nature.[42] Involvement of the gasserian ganglion in Meckel's cave is easily recognized on MR imaging because of replacement of high signal intensity fluid on T2-w images by low signal intensity tissue and because of abnormal enhancement after injection of contrast material (see **Fig. 15**).

Based on the surgical approach, primary tumors of the cavernous sinus have been subdivided into interdural and intracavernous tumors.[43] Interdural tumors include nerve sheath tumors (schwannomas and malignant nerve sheath tumors), melanocytomas, and epidermoid cysts. Interdural nerve sheath tumors displace the internal carotid artery medially without encasement or narrowing. Intracavernous tumors include meningiomas and hemangiopericytomas. They typically encase the internal carotid artery with or without bone erosion or hyperostosis, and show dural extension along the tentorium (**Fig. 16**). Aggressive pituitary adenomas have a tendency to encase the cavernous portion of the internal carotid artery and to invade the skull base. Hemorrhagic infarction in these tumors may result in V1 and V2 palsy, which may be the first presenting symptom in some patients. Primary tumors of the central skull base (chordoma and chondrosarcoma), hematogenous metastases, and lymphoma may invade the cavernous

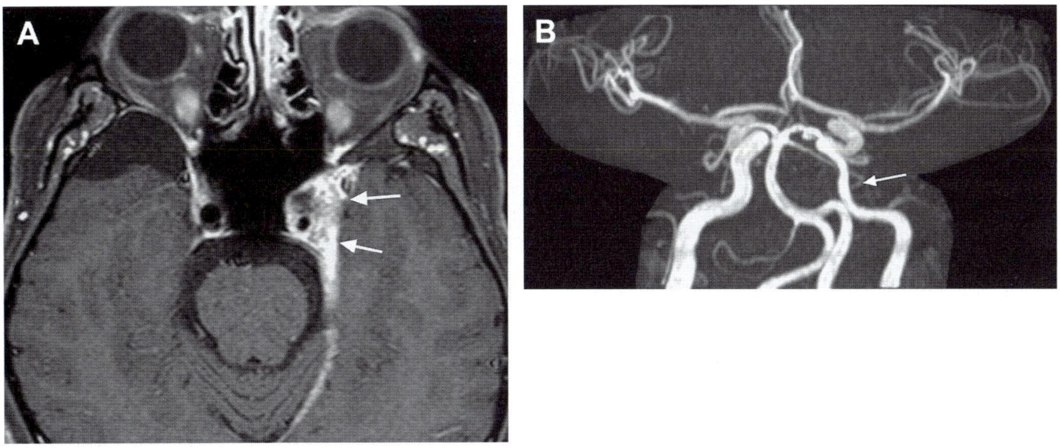

Fig. 14. Tolosa-Hunt syndrome in a 30-year-old man with left retro-orbital pain, ophthalmoplegia, and left V2 and V3 paresthesia. (*A*) Axial contrast-enhanced T1-w image shows enlargement and heterogeneous enhancement of the left cavernous sinus, and thickening and enhancement of the adjacent dura (*arrows*). (*B*) Maximum intensity projection reconstruction of a time-of-flight angiography sequence shows narrowing of the cavernous portion of the internal carotid artery on the left (*arrow*) caused by infiltration of the cavernous sinus by the inflammatory pseudotumor. The patient responded rapidly to steroids.

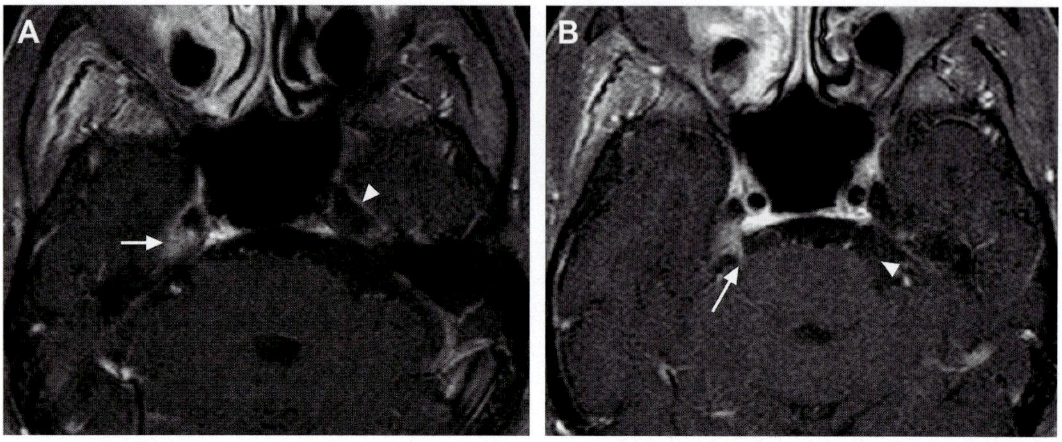

Fig. 15. Gasserian malignant peripheral nerve sheath tumor in a 64-year-old man with right V1-V3 paresthesia. (*A*) Axial contrast-enhanced fat-suppressed T1-w image shows a well-defined enhancing lesion within the posterior portion of Meckel's cave (*arrow*) bulging the lateral dura. Note the normal aspect of the left Meckel's cave (*arrowhead*). (*B*) Axial contrast-enhanced fat-suppressed T1-w image obtained at a higher level shows involvement of the preganglionic segment (*arrow*). Note the normal appearance of the left preganglionic trigeminal nerve (*arrowhead*). The MR imaging appearance is nonspecific and differentiation between a benign and a malignant nerve sheath tumor is not possible. Neurosurgical biopsy revealed malignant peripheral nerve sheath tumor. The patient underwent radiation therapy.

sinus and result in V1 and V2 palsy. Chordomas originate from notochord remnants, and are typically located in the clivus, whereas chondrosarcomas can be located on the midline and off midline arising from the spheno-occipital and petro-occipital synchondrosis, respectively. Lymphoma invading the cavernous sinus may present clinically with the same symptoms as the Tolosa-Hunt syndrome. As in most lymphomas, involvement of the cavernous sinus occurs simultaneously with lymphoma manifestations elsewhere in the body, and the diagnosis is often suggested by the clinical history (**Fig. 17**). However, in rare cases of primary cavernous sinus lymphomas, diagnosis has to be confirmed by biopsy.

Skull Base and Extracranial V1

Inflammatory and infectious lesions

Aggressive bacterial or fungal sinusitis may traverse the bony sinus wall and involve the orbit, sometimes affecting V1 within the supraorbital fissure. Involvement of V1 may also be seen in invasive forms of mucormycosis and aspergillosis. Fungal mycelia and hypha have a characteristic aspect on MR imaging because of the presence of manganese, which has paramagnetic properties. On T1-w and T2-w images, low signal intensity areas are seen, which show major enhancement after administration of contrast material.

Neoplasms

The most common primary tumors of the ophthalmic nerve are neural sheath tumors, such as schwannoma and plexiform neurofibroma. Only 5% of all trigeminal schwannomas arise in the distal intracranial branches and extend extracranially. Most distal trigeminal branch schwannomas originate from the ophthalmic division (**Fig. 18**). Plexiform neurofibromas are associated with neurofibromatosis type 1 (NF1). They arise as a result of diffuse proliferation of Schwann cells of the peripheral nerve, and involve fibroblastic elements of

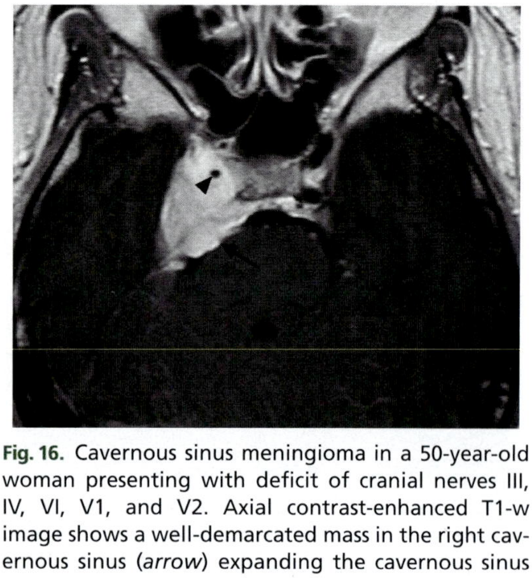

Fig. 16. Cavernous sinus meningioma in a 50-year-old woman presenting with deficit of cranial nerves III, IV, VI, V1, and V2. Axial contrast-enhanced T1-w image shows a well-demarcated mass in the right cavernous sinus (*arrow*) expanding the cavernous sinus and narrowing the internal carotid artery (*arrowhead*). Note the associated dural tail sign characteristic of a cavernous sinus meningioma.

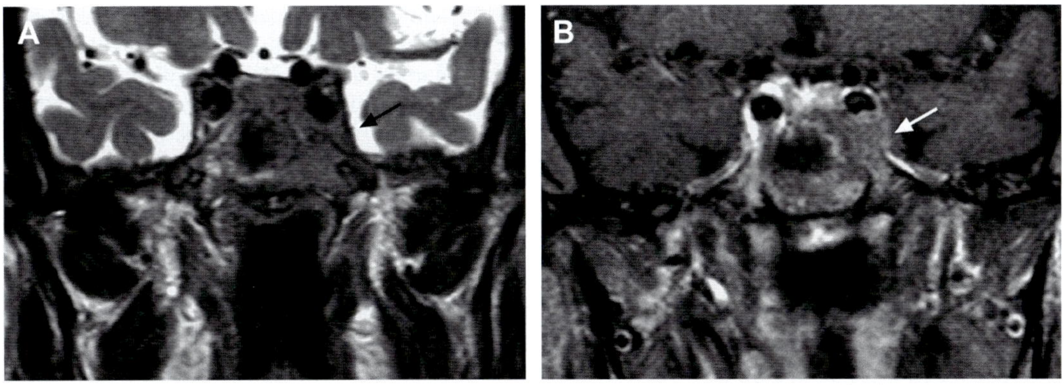

Fig. 17. An 81-year-old man with generalized lymphoma and deficit of cranial nerves III, V1, and V2. (*A*) Coronal T2-w image shows replacement of the normal fatty marrow of the sphenoid bone by hypointense, poorly defined tissue that extends into the left cavernous sinus (*arrow*). (*B*) Coronal contrast-enhanced T1-w image obtained at the same level demonstrates enhancement of the poorly defined tissue (*arrow*), suggesting leukemic infiltration.

the endoneurium and perineurium. Later, some proliferations occur within the sheath, leading to enlargement and tortuosity of the nerve. The distribution of V1 is frequently involved, and the tumor can often be seen extending into the orbital fat and around the orbital muscles, causing proptosis, ptosis, and visual impairment. Plexiform neurofibromas are often associated with bony spheno-orbital deformity (egg-shaped enlargement of the anterior orbital rim, bony defects in the posterior orbit, and anteroposterior enlargement of the middle cranial fossa). Although these changes had been understood to take place without tumoral involvement of the orbit and skull, recent observations support the concept of secondary dysplasia, in which interaction of plexiform neurofibromas with the developing skull is a major component of the craniofacial changes in NF1.[44]

Perineural tumor spread along V1 may occur in lacrimal gland tumors or skin tumors, which may use this route of spread through the superior orbital fissure to the gasserian ganglion.[5,17] Hematogenous metastases to the orbit may be seen in breast, kidney, and lung tumors, and may occasionally compress V1.

Trauma

The supraorbital nerve may be injured in orbital roof fractures and superior orbital rim fractures, whereas fractures involving the superior orbital

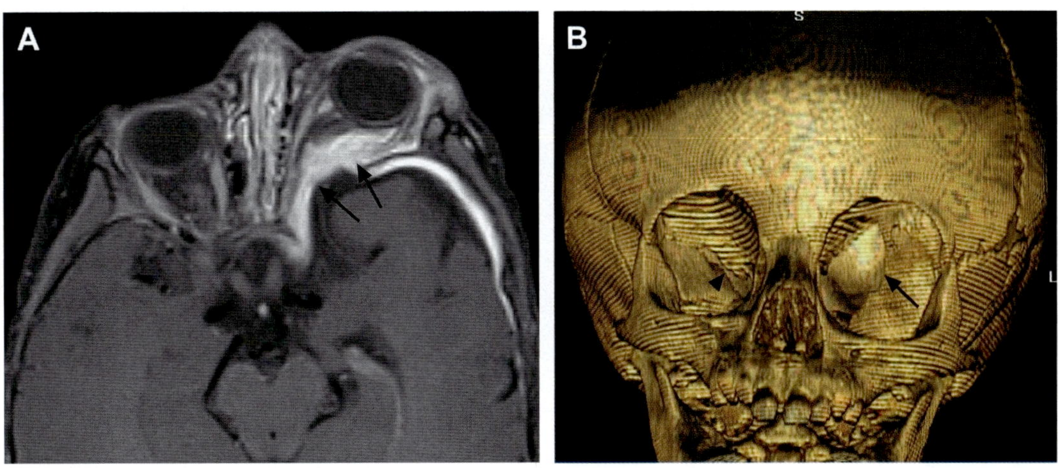

Fig. 18. Plexiform neurofibroma of the V1 nerve in a 7-year-old girl with NF1. The plexiform neurofibroma started to develop soon after birth. (*A*) Axial contrast-enhanced T1-w image shows an enlarged and strongly enhancing tortuous plexiform neurofibroma arising from the left ophthalmic nerve (*arrows*). (*B*) 3D reconstruction of the face from CT data set shows the associated deformity of the left orbit with sphenoid wing defect, and enlargement of the superior orbital fissure (*arrow*). Normal superior orbital fissure is on the right (*arrowhead*).

fissure may damage the entire trunk of V1. Superior orbital fissure syndrome is a rare complication of facial trauma, characterized by ophthalmoplegia, ptosis, proptosis, and hypoesthesia due to palsies of the cranial nerves III, IV, VI, and V1. It can occur in midface fractures, including Le Fort II and III, zygomaticomaxillary, and orbital fractures, and in complex skull base fractures. Nerve injury can be caused by displaced bony fragments or by hemorrhage. CT is the modality of choice for identifying these fractures.

Skull Base and Extracranial V2

Inflammatory and infectious lesions

Patients who have certain predisposing conditions (diabetes, corticosteroids, HIV) may develop aggressive bacterial or fungal infections of the paranasal sinuses, maxilla, temporal bone or, less commonly, central skull base (skull base osteomyelitis). V2 may be involved within the infraorbital canal, palatine foramina, pterygopalatine fossa, or foramen rotundum. Involvement of V2 within the pterygopalatine fossa and foramen rotundum is characterized by loss of normal fatty signal on T1-w images, enhancement of the nerve after intravenous injection of contrast material, and, occasionally, enlargement of the nerve. Because differentiation between inflammatory and neoplastic involvement of V2 is not always possible on the basis of radiologic findings alone, the diagnosis of infectious involvement of V2 should be made only in the appropriate clinical context. In skull base osteomyelitis, MR imaging may depict early involvement of the bony marrow caused by the inflammatory marrow edema, which precedes massive destruction. Abnormal, diffusely infiltrating, enhancing soft tissues around the sphenoid and clivus and along the extracranial V2 are typically seen in this clinical context (**Fig. 19**).[45] Wegener's granulomatosis may affect the maxillary sinus and the orbit and may cause V2 involvement. Imaging findings are, however, nondistinguishable from other infectious and inflammatory entities.

Neoplasms

The maxillary nerve and its branches may be affected by primary (nerve sheath) tumors (**Fig. 20**); by tumors that may destroy bony structures and secondarily invade the pterygopalatine fossa and neurovascular foramina, causing V2 neuropathy; and by metastases. Tumors of the paranasal sinuses produce few, if any, signs while the tumor is in its early stage. Therefore, when patients seek medical advice, the tumors are already advanced and destruction of bony structures with extension into the orbit, pterygopalatine fossa, pterygopalatine canal, or anterior skull base may already be present. Malignant tumors arising from the paranasal sinuses include squamous cell carcinoma, adenocarcinoma, esthesioneuroblastoma, melanoma, lymphoma, and sarcoma. One half of all hard palate cancers are squamous cell carcinoma, whereas nonsquamous cell

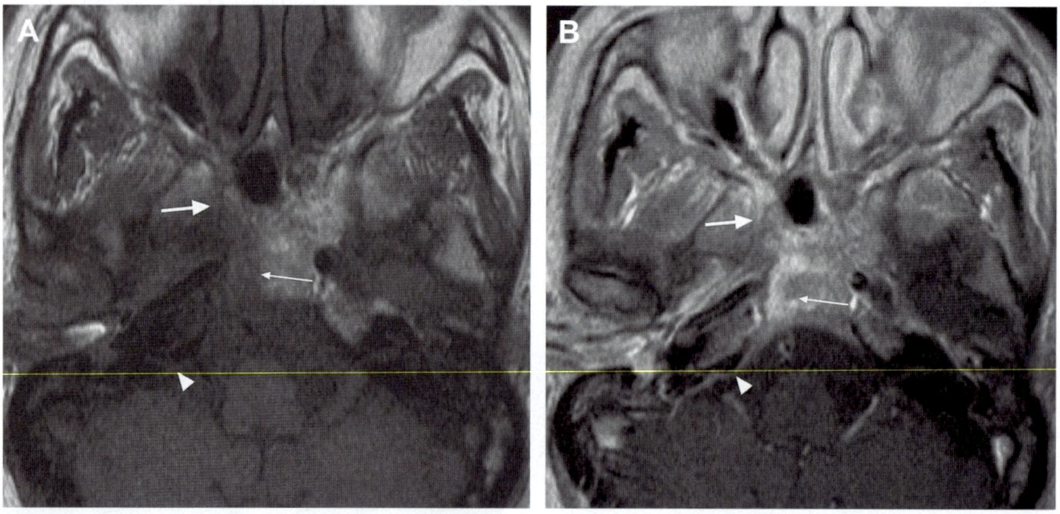

Fig. 19. Skull base osteomyelitis caused by actinomycosis in a 71-year-old diabetic woman presenting with sepsis, and multiple cranial nerve deficits on the right. (*A*) T1-w image shows hypointense bony marrow of the right clivus (*long arrow*) and of the apex of the right temporal bone (*arrowhead*). Note hypointensity around the vidian canal and fat in the pterygopalatine fossa on the right (*thick arrow*). (*B*) Contrast-enhanced T1-w image obtained at the same level shows enhancement of the clivus (*arrow*), of the apex of the right temporal bone (*arrowhead*), around the vidian canal, and of the fat in the pterygopalatine fossa (*thick arrow*).

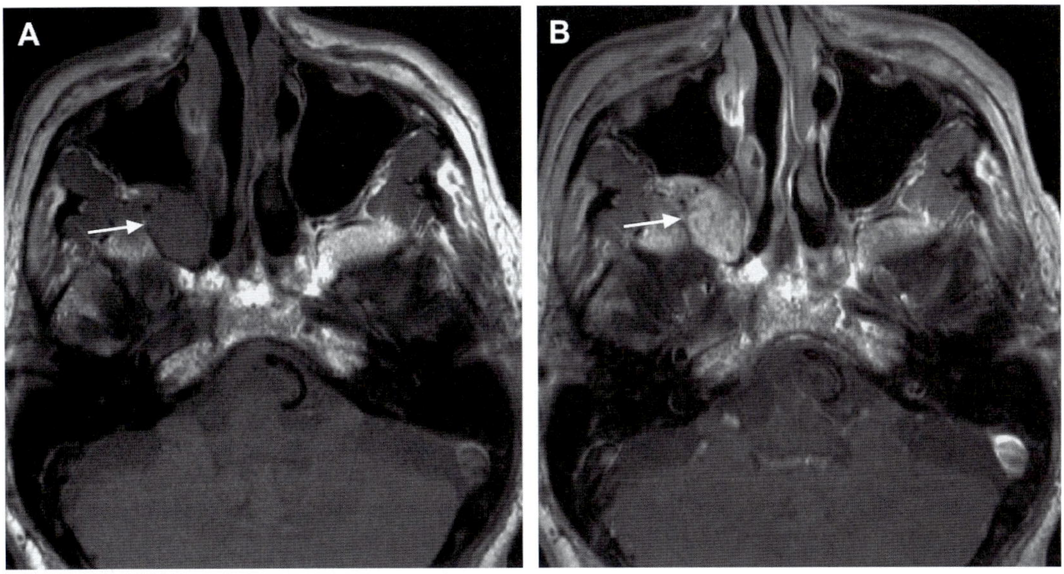

Fig. 20. Biopsy-proven schwannoma of the pterygopalatine fossa in an asymptomatic 70-year-old woman. (*A*) Axial T1-w image shows a well-defined hypointense mass that enlarges the right pterygopalatine fossa (*arrow*) and displaces the maxillary artery laterally. Note scalloping of the posterior wall of the maxillary sinus due to the slow growth. (*B*) Contrast-enhanced T1-w image at the same level shows slightly inhomogeneous enhancement of the mass (*arrow*).

cancers (adenoid cystic carcinoma, mucoepidermoid carcinoma, melanoma, and sarcoma) account for the other half. Although cancers of the hard palate are often confined to the site of origin at the time of diagnosis, advanced tumors with invasion of the maxilla, palatine foramina, nasal cavity, or retromolar trigone are seen occasionally. From the palatine foramina and pterygopalatine fossa, tumors may spread along V2 to the foramen rotundum, which constitutes one of the most common pathways of perineural spread to and through the central skull base. A detailed review of patterns of perineural spread and their radiologic aspect is provided elsewhere in this issue.

Juvenile angiofibroma is a benign, nonencapsulated fibrovascular tumor that usually originates from the superolateral aspect of the choana, but may also arise more medially, near the vomer, from the pharyngeal roof or adjacent pterygoid plates. It extends submucosally into the adjacent open spaces and passages. The location and routes of extension are characteristic and can be seen with either CT or MR imaging. MR imaging is superior to CT, allowing differentiation of tumor from mucosal inflammation and sinus fluid. In almost every case, the tumor extends into the sphenopalatine foramen and pterygopalatine fossa, occasionally causing sensory deficits in the distribution of V2. As the tumor grows, the posterior wall of the maxillary sinus and the pterygoid plates are remodeled, and the tumor then grows into the sphenoid sinus, the cavernous sinus, and middle cranial fossa.

Hematogenous metastases can reach V2 from primary tumors in the lung, kidney, breast, and prostate (**Fig. 21**). The imaging findings are usually those of lytic destruction of bony structures or

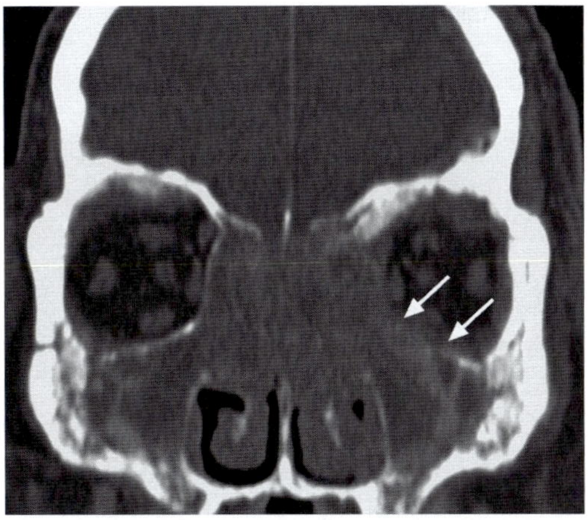

Fig. 21. Hematogenous metastasis from prostate cancer in a 73-year-old patient presenting with left V2 paresthesia. Contrast-enhanced coronal 2D reformatted CT image shows massive involvement of the nose and paranasal sinuses with permeative type destruction of the cribriform plate, left lamina papyracea, and left infraorbital rim (*arrows*). The left infraorbital nerve is compressed within the infraorbital canal.

sclerotic changes around neurovascular foramina at CT associated with enlargement and enhancement of V2 at CT or MR imaging. Nevertheless, in patients in whom a primary tumor is not known, biopsy is required to make the correct diagnosis of a metastatic lesion involving V2.

Trauma

Fractures of the central skull base may extend through the foramen rotundum, contusing, crushing, or disrupting the maxillary nerve. In addition, V2 may be injured with orbital floor blow-out fractures, zygomaticomaxillary (tripod) fractures, or LeFort II and LeFort III fractures (**Fig. 22**).

Skull Base and Extracranial V3

Infectious and inflammatory lesions

Odontogenic infection is most often caused by periapical or periodontal disease or by extraction of a carious tooth. Dental infections may result in cellulitis, abscess formation, myositis, fasciitis, and osteomyelitis. Depending on their origin, dental abscesses may spread in a variable fashion. Odontogenic infection of the maxillary molars and lower second and third molars may produce abscesses in the masticator space, whereas infection of the lower first molar and premolar teeth tends to involve the sublingual space. Myositis and abscess formation within the pterygoid muscles may involve the proximal part of V3 just as V3 enters the masticator space, resulting in V3 neuropathy. Acute osteomyelitis of the mandible is the result of tooth infection and less often of dental manipulation, whereas chronic osteomyelitis results from either inadequately treated acute osteomyelitis or by a long-term reaction to a subclinical infection. Acute and chronic osteomyelitis may progress to involve the mandibular canal and, therefore, the inferior alveolar nerve, causing intense pain and numbness of the chin and lips. CT may show multiple, ill-defined radiolucent areas, cortical disruption, sequestrae, areas of sclerosis, and periosteal reactions (**Fig. 23**). On MR imaging, inflammatory changes involving the marrow and soft tissues demonstrate an increased signal intensity on T2-w and short tau inversion recovery (STIR) images, hypointensity on T1-w images, and enhancement after injection of contrast material (see **Fig. 23**). Enlargement and enhancement of the nerve within the mandibular canal and up to the foramen ovale may be seen in this context and correspond to V3 neuritis.

Osteoradionecrosis of the mandible typically occurs months or years after high-dose irradiation of oral cavity or oropharyngeal tumors. Because of compromise of the inferior alveolar nerve, patients may present with paresthesia or pain. The CT and MR imaging aspect is similar to that of osteomyelitis, but the clinical context is different (**Fig. 24**). A particular feature is the presence of prominent, mass-like soft tissue thickening and enhancement in the adjacent musculature or soft tissues, which is, however, not related to recurrent tumor or metastatic disease.[46]

Neoplasms

The most common primary tumors of the mandibular nerve are benign neural sheath tumors,

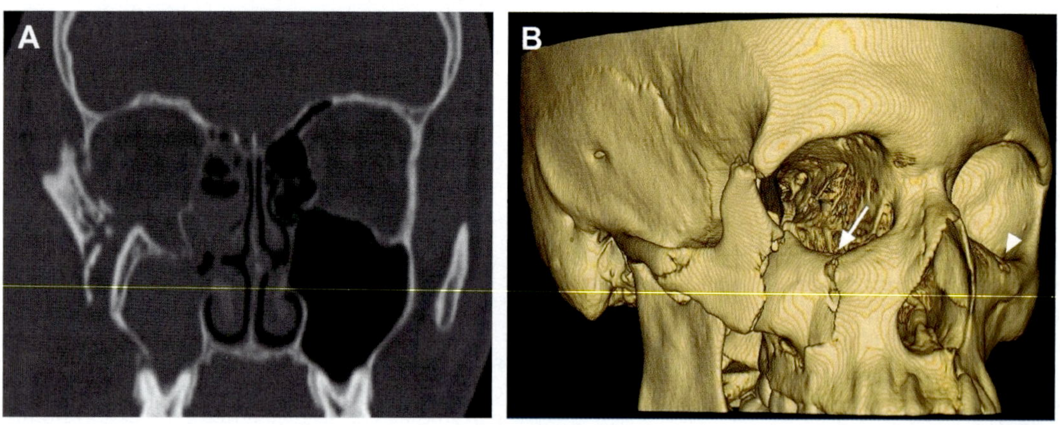

Fig. 22. Tripod fracture in a 21-year-old man presenting with right V2 paresthesia after a motor vehicle accident. (*A*) Coronal 2D reformatted image shows inferior displacement of orbital floor fragments with entrapped fat. No muscle herniation. (*B*) A 3D reformatted image better shows the multiple fracture lines involving the zygoma, lateral orbital rim, and orbital floor. The most anterior fracture line passes through the anterior wall of the maxillary sinus and right infraorbital foramen (*arrow*), causing V2 paresthesia. Note the normal aspect of the infraorbital foramen on the left (*arrowhead*).

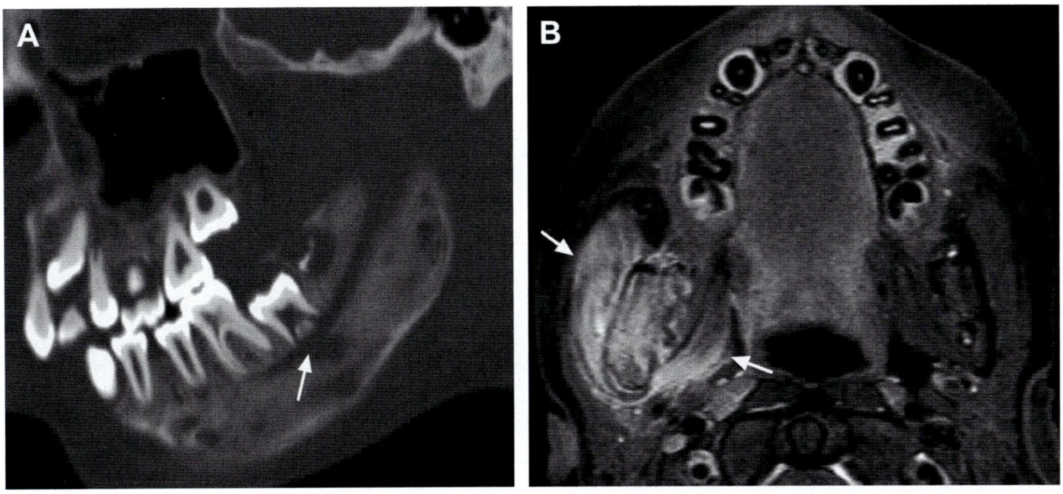

Fig. 23. Chronic osteomyelitis of the mandible in a 10-year-old girl presenting with swelling of the right cheek, pain, and V3 numbness. (*A*) Sagittal oblique 2D reconstruction from a CT data set (bone window setting) shows multiple areas of lysis corresponding to intraosseous abscesses, which are surrounded by extensive sclerosis of the mandible. One area of lysis extends into the canal of the inferior alveolar nerve (*arrow*). (*B*) Axial contrast-enhanced fat-suppressed T1-w image shows major enlargement of the ascending ramus of the mandible and enhancement of the marrow and of the muscles of mastication (*arrows*), suggesting osteomyelitis and myositis. Biopsy confirmed the radiologic findings. The patient was treated with intravenous antibiotics.

followed by meningioma and malignant schwannoma (**Fig. 25**).[3,5,47] Multiple cranial nerve schwannomas are common with NF2. However, involvement of the mandibular nerve is rare.

Invasion of the mandible and masticator space is usually a late manifestation of carcinoma of the oral cavity, oropharynx, paranasal sinuses, and nasopharynx, and it appears to correlate with survival after treatment. Patients typically present with trismus, V3 numbness, or denervation atrophy of the muscles of mastication. Squamous cell carcinoma and adenoid cystic carcinoma may enter the masticator space by direct extension from the faucial tonsil or retromolar trigone, or by way of direct mandibular invasion from the floor of the mouth. Subtle cortical erosion of the mandible is best assessed by thin-slice CT with bone algorithm, and evaluation of the inferior alveolar nerve may require additional DentaScan (GE Healthcare, Princeton, New Jersey) software with 2D curved reconstructions along the mandibular canal. On MR imaging, the diagnosis of neoplastic invasion of the mandibular marrow and inferior alveolar nerve is made in the presence of hypointensity on T1-w images, hyperintensity on T2-w and STIR images, and contrast material enhancement (**Fig. 26**). As shown recently, these findings are highly sensitive and specific for the assessment of mandibular invasion.[48–50]

Because the masticator space is mainly composed of muscle tissue and bone tissue, only few lesions are seen to originate in this location. These include rhabdomyosarcoma, lymphoma, and tumor or tumor-like lesions originating from the mandible, such as ameloblastoma, osteosarcoma, chondrosarcoma, and fibrous dysplasia. Rhabdomyosarcoma is one of the most common soft tissue sarcomas, not only in children under 15 years of age but also in adolescents and young adults. The head and neck are one of the main locations, and these tumors are typically found in the orbit, paranasal sinuses, and masticator space (**Fig. 27**). Ameloblastoma is a benign epithelial odontogenic tumor thought to arise from ameloblasts. More than 80% of all ameloblastomas arise in the mandible and show characteristic uni- or multilocular lesions filled with fluid of variable protein content. Osteogenic sarcomas of the mandible are rare and have a peak incidence in the third decade. The main symptoms are swelling, pain, and paresthesia caused by compression of the inferior alveolar nerve. Fibrous dysplasia is an idiopathic benign bone disease that may affect the peripheral branches of the trigeminal nerve by causing narrowing of skull base foramina with subsequent cranial nerve deficits. Three types of fibrous dysplasia are observed: the monostotic form, the multiostotic form, and the McCune-Albright syndrome (with associated endocrine anomalies). The skull and the face, including the maxilla and mandible, are frequently involved, often with obvious asymmetry

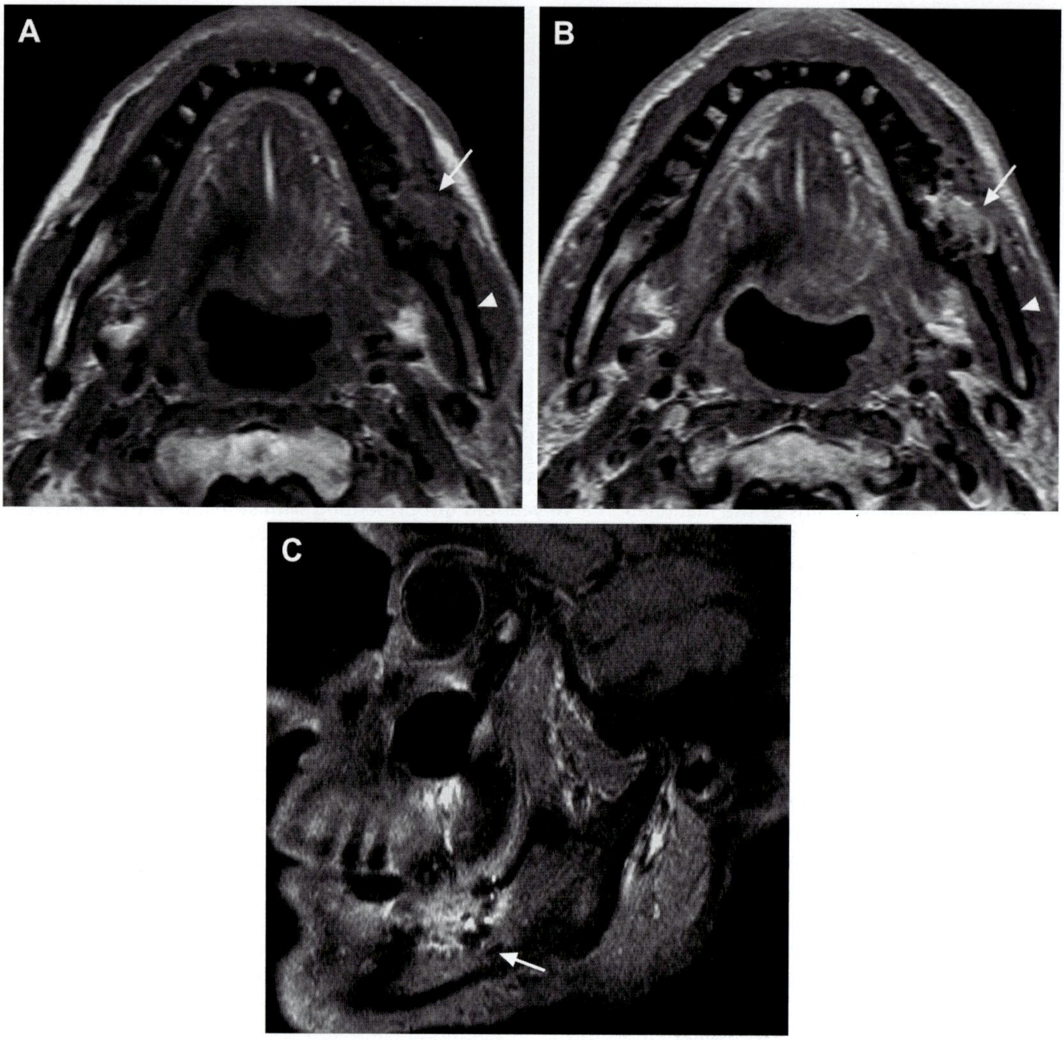

Fig. 24. Osteoradionecrosis of the mandible in a 50-year-old man presenting with intense pain and numbness in the distribution of the left inferior alveolar nerve. The patient was irradiated 4 years previously for squamous cell carcinoma of the floor of the mouth. (*A*) Axial T1-w image shows abnormally low signal intensity of the left mandibular bone marrow (*arrowhead*), and an area of lysis and hypointense soft tissue mass (*arrow*) in the region of teeth 36 to 38. (*B*) Contrast-enhanced T1-w image obtained at the same level shows enhancement of the area of lysis around teeth 36 to 38 and of the soft tissues around the mandible (*arrow*). The rest of the abnormal mandibular marrow (*arrowhead*) shows no obvious enhancement due to reduced vascularization and fibrosis. (*C*) Sagittal oblique contrast-enhanced fat saturated T1-w image shows that the area of lysis extends into the inferior alveolar canal (*arrow*). Note bone sequestrae seen as scattered hypointense structures around the area of lysis. The patient underwent surgical resection of the mandible, with subsequent reconstruction. Histology confirmed osteoradionecrosis of the mandible and no tumor. The enhancing soft tissue mass seen on MR imaging corresponded histologically to granulation tissue.

secondary to bony expansion. Radiologically, the bony lesions are either dense or radiolucent (**Fig. 28**).

Metastases to the mandible are uncommon. They may be asymptomatic or may cause pain and V3 numbness. The most common primary tumors are in the breast, lung, kidney, and thyroid.

Trauma

Fractures of the central skull base may extend through the foramen ovale, contusing, crushing, or disrupting the mandibular nerve. V3 injury may also occur from displaced mandibular neck fractures within the masticator space. Fractures of the mandibular canal between the mandibular

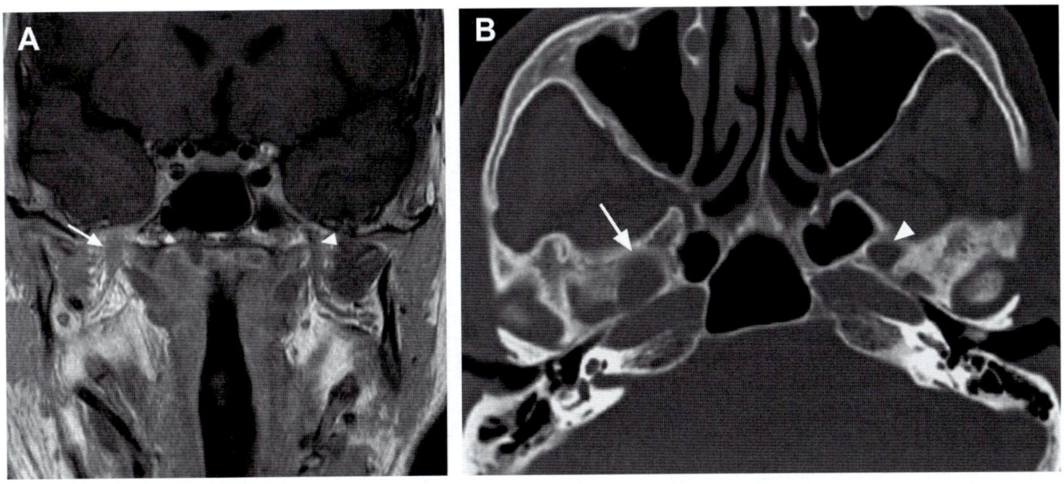

Fig. 25. Biopsy-proven V3 recurrent malignant peripheral nerve sheath tumor seen 1 year after radiation therapy and chemotherapy of the patient shown in Fig. 15. (*A*) Coronal contrast-enhanced T1-w image demonstrates a right-sided tumor mass involving V3 (*arrow*) within the masticator space. Note the normal appearance of the left V3 (*arrowhead*). (*B*) Axial CT image through the base of the skull shows major enlargement of the right foramen ovale (*arrow*) as opposed to the left (*arrowhead*). The tumor that initially originated from Meckel's cave has recurred along the V3 division of the trigeminal nerve.

foramen and the mental foramen may cause numbness and paresthesia caused by involvement of the inferior alveolar nerve (**Fig. 29**).

SUMMARY

Imaging of the trigeminal nerve requires a thorough understanding of its anatomy and function, clinical symptoms related to malfunction, and key pathologies. Although MR imaging has almost completely replaced CT as the diagnostic modality of choice for investigating trigeminal neuropathy, CT still plays a role in the assessment of skull base foramina and facial skeleton. High-resolution MR imaging studies with tailored dedicated protocols allow recognition of a multitude

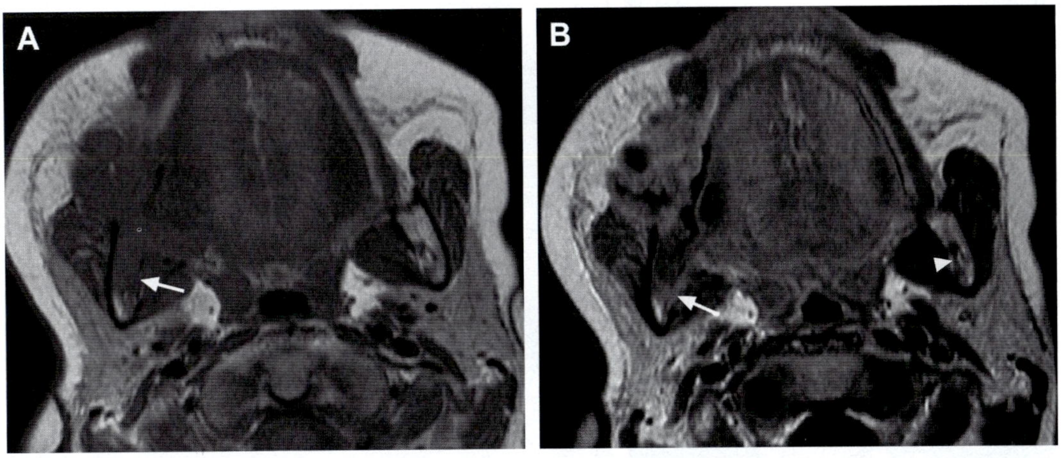

Fig. 26. Squamous cell carcinoma in a 43-year-old woman presenting with V3 paresthesia. (*A*) Axial T1-w image shows a tumor originating from the cheek mucosa extending into the buccal space and masticator space. Invasion of the masseter muscle and of the mandibular marrow (*arrow*). (*B*) Axial contrast-enhanced T1-w image obtained at the same level shows inhomogeneous enhancement of the tumor mass and of the mandibular marrow. The mandibular canal with the inferior alveolar nerve is invaded (*arrow*). Note for comparison the normal mandibular canal on the left (*arrowhead*).

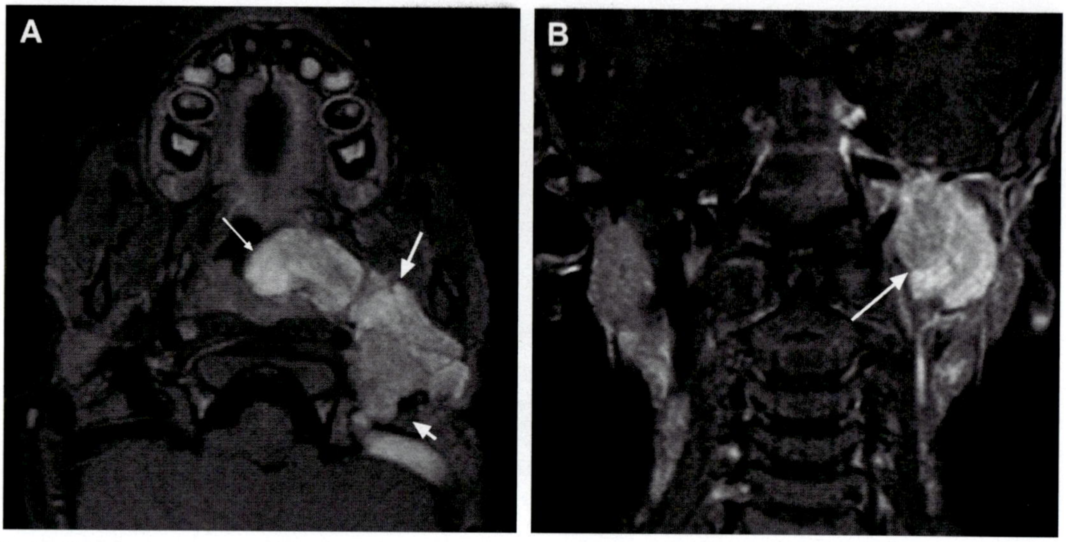

Fig. 27. Rhabdomyosarcoma with V3 involvement within the masticator space in a 5-year-old boy presenting with pain, burning sensation in the left cheek, and facial nerve palsy. (*A*) Axial contrast-enhanced fat-saturated T1-w image demonstrates a large tumor mass that invades the left parapharyngeal space and masticator space (*long arrow*); extends laterally into the parotid gland and posteriorly into the jugular foramen, eroding the inferior part of the temporal bone (*short arrow*); and spreads anteriorly into the nasopharynx (*thin arrow*). (*B*) Coronal contrast-enhanced fat-saturated T1-w image shows the craniocaudal extent of the lesion (*arrow*).

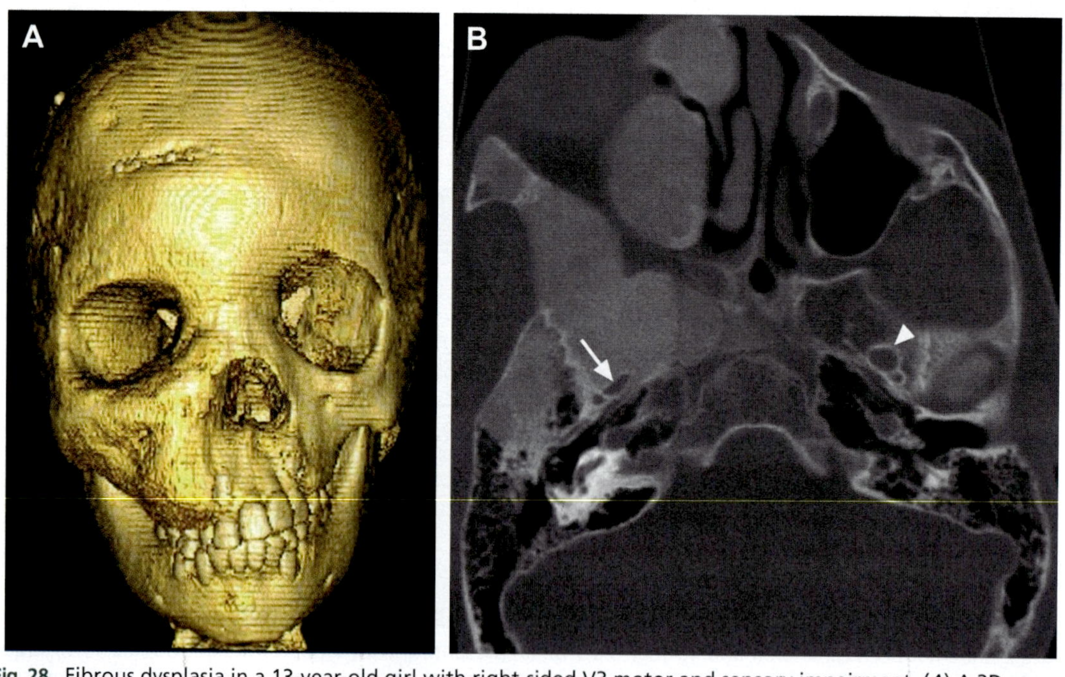

Fig. 28. Fibrous dysplasia in a 13-year-old girl with right-sided V3 motor and sensory impairment. (*A*) A 3D reconstruction from CT data set shows the marked facial deformity. (*B*) Axial unenhanced CT with bone window settings shows major narrowing of the foramen ovale on the right (*arrow*) caused by the fibro-osseous lesion that involves the right sphenoid, frontal bone, and temporal bone. Note the normal aspect of the left foramen ovale (*arrowhead*).

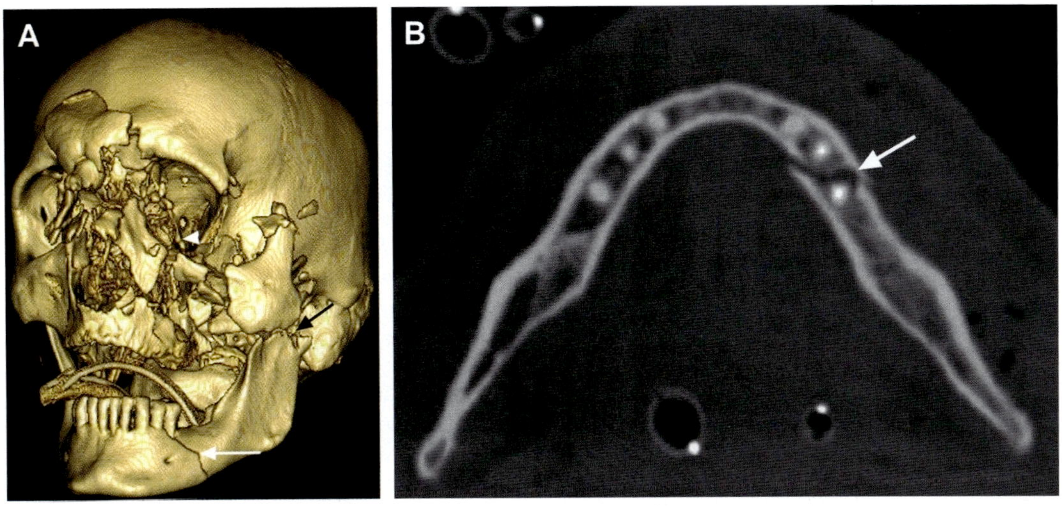

Fig. 29. Mandibular fracture with involvement of the mandibular canal and inferior alveolar nerve in a 52-year-old male patient who sustained multiple facial injuries following an attack with an axe. A 3D reconstruction from CT data set (*A*) and axial CT image through the mandibular body (*B*) show panfacial fractures involving the frontal bone, orbit, maxilla, and mandible. Displaced fracture involving the infraorbital foramen and canal (*arrowhead*), fracture of the ascending ramus of the mandible (*black arrow*) and fracture through the body of the mandible (*white arrow*) posterior to the mental foramen.

of pathologic conditions and diffusion tensor MR imaging techniques also offer insights into the underlying pathophysiologic mechanisms of dysfunction.

REFERENCES

1. Hutchins LG, Harnsberger HR, Jacobs JM, et al. Trigeminal neuralgia (tic douloureux): MR imaging assessment. Radiology 1990;175:837–41.
2. Borges A. Trigeminal neuralgia and facial nerve paralysis. Eur Radiol 2005;15:511–33.
3. Borges A, Casselman J. Imaging the cranial nerves: part I: methodology, infectious and inflammatory, traumatic and congenital lesions. Eur Radiol 2007; 175(8):2112–25.
4. Borges A, Casselman J. Imaging the cranial nerves: part II: primary and secondary neoplastic conditions and neurovascular conflicts. Eur Radiol 2007;17(9): 2332–44.
5. Delavelle J, Becker M, Megret, et al. Diagnostic features of intracranial and extracranial pathologic conditions of the trigeminal nerve. International Journal of Neuroradiology 1998;4(6):445–65.
6. Kuncz A, Vörös E, Barzo P, et al. Comparison of clinical symptoms and magnetic resonance angiographic (MRA) results in patients with trigeminal neuralgia and persistent idiopathic facial pain. Medium-term outcome after microvascular decompression of cases with positive MRA findings. Cephalalgia 2006;26:266–76.
7. Casselman JW. The skull base: tumoral lesions. Eur Radiol 2005;15:534–42.
8. Ishimori T, Nakano S, Kagawa M, et al. Virtual endoscopic images by 3D FASE cisternography for neurovascular compression. Magn Reson Med Sci 2003;2(3):145–9.
9. Herweh C, Kress B, Rasche D, et al. Loss of anisotropy in trigeminal neuralgia revealed by diffusion tensor imaging. Neurology 2007;68:776–8.
10. Love S, Coakham HB. Trigeminal neuralgia. Pathology and pathogenesis. Brain 2001;124:2347–60.
11. Mac Donald BK, Cockerell OC, Sander JW, et al. The incidence and lifetime prevalence of neurological disorders in a prospective community-based study in the UK. Brain 2000;123:665.
12. Al-Din AS, Mir R, Davey R, et al. Trigeminal cephalgias and facial pain syndromes associated with autonomic dysfunction. Cephalgia 2005;25: 605–11.
13. Leone M, Mea E, Genco S, et al. Coexistence of TACS and trigeminal neuralgia: pathophysiological conjectures. Headache 2006;46:1565–70.
14. Tatli M, Keklikci U, Aluclu U, et al. Anesthesia dolorosa caused by penetrating cranial injury. Eur Neurol 2005;56:162–5.
15. Eskandar E, Barker FG 2nd, Rabinov JD. Case 21-2006: a 61-year-old man with left sided facial pain. Case records of the Massachusetts General Hospital. N Engl J Med 2006;355(2):183–8.
16. Laine FJ, Braun IF, Jensen ME, et al. Perineural tumor extension through the foramen ovale: evaluation with MR imaging. Radiology 1990;174:65–71.

17. Maroldi R, Battaglia G, Farina D, et al. Tumours of the oropharynx and oral cavity: perineural spread and bone invasion. JBR-BTR 1999;82(6):294–300.
18. Fitzek S, Fitzek C, Marx J, et al. Lesion pattern of brain stem infarctions. Clinical Neuroradiology 2003;203–7.
19. Mendelowitsch A, Radu EW, Gratzl O. Aneurysm, arteriovenous malformation and arteriovenous fistula in posterior fossa compression syndrome. Eur Neurol 1990;30:338–42.
20. Liquori CL, Berg MJ, Siegel AM, et al. Mutations in a gene encoding a novel protein containing a phosphotyrosine-binding domain cause type 2 cerebral cavernous malformations. Am J Hum Genet 2003;73(6):1459–64.
21. Parizel PM, Makkat S, Jorens PG, et al. Brainstem hemorrhage in descending transtentorial herniation (Duret hemorrhage). Intensive Care Med 2002;28(1):85–8.
22. Gass A, Kitchen N, MacManus DG, et al. Trigeminal neuralgia in patients with multiple sclerosis: lesion localization with magnetic resonance imaging. Neurology 1997;49:1142–4.
23. Fischbein NJ, Prados MD, Wara W, et al. Radiologic evaluation of brain stem tumors. Correlation of MRI appearance with clinical outcome. Pediatr Neurosurg 1996;24:9–23.
24. Milstein JM, Geyer JR, Berger MS, et al. Favorable prognosis for brainstem gliomas in neurofibromatosis. J Neurooncol 1989;7(4):367–71.
25. Villanueva O, Atkinson DS, Lambert SR. Trigeminal nerve hypoplasia and aplasia in children with Goldenhar syndrome and corneal hypoesthesia. J AAPOS 2005;9(2):202–4.
26. Peker S, Kurtkaya O, Uzun I, et al. Microanatomy of the central myelin peripheral myelin transition zone of the trigeminal nerve. Neurosurgery 2006;59(2):354–9.
27. Brisman R, Kandji AG, Mooji RB. Trigeminal nerve-blood vessel relationship as revealed by high resolution magnetic resonance imaging and its effect on pain relief after gamma knife radiosurgery for trigeminal neuralgia. Neurosurgery 2002;50:1261–6.
28. Devor M, Govrin-Lippmann R, Rappaport ZH. Mechanism of trigeminal neuralgia: an ultrastructural analysis of trigeminal root specimens obtained during microvascular decompression surgery. J Neurosurg 2002;96:532–43.
29. Umehara F, Kamishima K, Kashio N, et al. Magnetic resonance tomographic angiography: diagnostic value in trigeminal neuralgia. Neuroradiology 1995;37:353–5.
30. Majoie CB, Hulsmans FJ, Verbeeten B Jr, et al. Trigeminal neuralgia: comparison of two MR imaging techniques in the demonstration of neurovascular contact. Radiology 1997;204:455–60.
31. de Bondt BJ, Stokroos R, Casselman J. Persistent trigeminal artery associated with trigeminal neuralgia: hypothesis of neurovascular compression. Neuroradiology 2007;49(1):23–6.
32. Garcia-Pastor C, Lopez-Gonzalez F, Revuelta R, et al. Trigeminal neuralgia secondary to arteriovenous malformations of the posterior fossa. Surg Neurol 2006;66(2):207–11.
33. Kress B, Schindler M, Rasche D, et al. MRI volumetry for the preoperative diagnosis of trigeminal neuralgia. Eur Radiol 2005;15:1344–8.
34. Patel NK, Aquilina K, Clarke Y, et al. How accurate is magnetic resonance angiography in predicting neurovascular compression in patients with trigeminal neuralgia? A prospective, single-blinded comparative study. Br J Neurosurg 2003;17:60–4.
35. Erbay SH, Bradelia RA, O'Callaghan M, et al. Nerve atrophy in severe trigeminal neuralgia: noninvasive confirmation at MR imaging - initial experience. Radiology 2006;298:689–92.
36. Seidel E, Hansen C, Urban PP, et al. Idiopathic trigeminal sensory neuropathy with gadolinium enhancement in the cisternal segment. Neurology 2000;54:1191–2.
37. Tancioni F, Gaetani P, Villani L, et al. Neurinoma of the trigeminal root and atypical trigeminal neuralgia. Surg Neurol 1995;44:36–42.
38. Ramaesh K, Stokes J, Henry E, et al. Congenital corneal anesthesia. Surv Ophthalmol 2007;52(1):50–60.
39. Hahn CD, Nicolle DA, Lownie SP, et al. Giant cavernous carotid aneurysms: clinical presentation in fifty-seven cases. J Neuroophthalmol 2000;20(4):253–8.
40. Biffl WL, Moore EE, Ryu RK, et al. The unrecognized epidemic of blunt carotid arterial injuries: early diagnosis improves neurologic outcome. Ann Surg 1998;228:462–70.
41. Yousem DM, Atlas SN, Grossman RI, et al. MR imaging of Tolosa-Hunt syndrome. AJR Am J Roentgenol 1990;154:167–70.
42. Stone JA, Cooper H, Castillo M, et al. Malignant schwannoma of the trigeminal nerve. AJNR Am J Neuroradiol 2001;22:505–7.
43. Larson JJ, van Loeveren HR, Balko G, et al. Evidence of meningioma infiltration into cranial nerves: clinical implications for cavernous sinus meningiomas. J Neurosurg 1995;83:596–9.
44. El- Kalliny M, Van Loeveren H, Keller JT, et al. Tumors of the lateral wall of the cavernous sinus. J Neurosurg 1992;17:508–14.
45. Jacquemin C, Bosley TM, Svedberg H. Orbit deformities in craniofacial neurofibromatosis type 1. AJNR Am J Neuroradiol 2003;24:1678–82.
46. Chang PC, Fischbein NJ, Holliday RA. Central skull base osteomyelitis in patients without otitis

externa: imaging findings. AJNR Am J Neuroradiol 2003;24:1310–6.

47. Chong J, Hinckley LK, Ginsberg LE. Masticator space abnormalities associated with mandibular osteoradionecrosis: MR and CT findings in five patients. AJNR Am J Neuroradiol 2000;21(1):175–8.
48. Marsot-Dupuch K, Matozza F, Firat MM, et al. Mandibular nerve: MR versus CT in 10 proved unusual tumors. Neuroradiology 1990;23(3):482–6.
49. Bolzoni A, Cappiello J, Piazza C, et al. Diagnostic accuracy of magnetic resonance imaging in the assessment of mandibular involvement in oral-oropharyngeal squamous cell carcinoma: a prospective study. Arch Otolaryngol Head Neck Surg 2004; 130(7):837–43.
50. Lee JH, Lee MS, Lee BH, et al. Rhabdomyosarcoma of the head and neck in adults: MR and CT findings. AJNR Am J Neuroradiol 1996;17:1923–8.

Pathology of the Facial Nerve

F. Veillon, MD[a,*], L. Ramos Taboada, MD[a], M. Abu Eid, MD[a], S. Riehm, MD[a], C. Debry, MD[b], P. Schultz, MD[b], A. Charpiot, MD[b]

KEYWORDS

- Facial nerve • Fallopian canal • Temporal bone
- Computer Tomography • MR imaging

The facial nerve is responsible for the motion of the face and for lacrimal, nasal, and salivary secretions. The main clinical sign that leads a clinician to ask for imaging is peripheral facial nerve palsy, which has different causes but is most frequently caused by inflammation. Both MR and computer tomography (CT) of the temporal bone are used when the facial nerve must be examined.

The following anatomic areas must be imaged when the facial nerve is studied:

- The brain and pons (precentral-, postcentral-, central gyrus, posterior limb of the internal capsule)
- The cerebellopontine angle (CPA)
- The internal auditory canal (IAC)
- The labyrinthine part of the facial nerve canal (VII-1) and geniculate ganglion (GG)
- The tympanic part of the facial nerve canal (VII-2)
- The mastoid part of the facial nerve canal (VII-3)
- The stylomastoid foramen (SF) and the parotid gland (PG)

TECHNIQUE: 1 TO 1.5 TESLA

Sequences

T2 weighted, fluid attenuated inversion recovery

These images are acquired in the axial plane, perpendicular to the brainstem using a head coil. To study the brain and pons, a slice thickness of 4 mm to 5 mm and a 256 matrix is used.

T1 weighted, spin echo

T1 images are achieved parallel to the roof of the orbit using a head coil; additional surface coils centered on the ears can also be used (at 1.5 Tesla). The CPA, IAC, VII-1, GG, VII-2, VII-3 are studied on gadolinium-enhanced images, with or without fat saturation, and with a slice thickness ranging from 1 mm to 2 mm. Additional contrast enhanced T1-weighted images in the coronal plane can provide valuable information of the VII-1, VII-2, VII-3 segments of the facial nerve, and contrast enhanced sagittal T1-weighted images can be helpful in the study of VII-3.

High resolution 3-dimensional heavily T2-weighted images

Images are made in the axial plane, parallel to the roof of the orbit. Gradient echo (GE) or spin echo (SE) or fast spin-echo (FSE) sequences are used depending on the MR-unit used. These axial images have a thickness of 0.35 mm to 0.7 mm, and provide detail visualization of the nerve in the CPA, internal auditory meatus (IAM), or of the VII-1, VII-2, and VII-3 segments. Images reformatted in the coronal (VII-1, VII-2, VII-3) and para-sagittal (VII-2, VII-3) plane are very helpful in the evaluation of the different nerve segments.

T1-weighted SE images through the stylomastoid foramen and parotid gland

Axial 2-mm to 3-mm thick images parallel to the soft palate make evaluation of the facial nerve at the level of the SF and PG possible. This can be achieved using a head coil or surface coils.

[a] Service de Radiologie I, Hôpital de Hautepierre, 67098 Strasbourg Cedex, France
[b] Service d'O.R.L., Hôpital de Hautepierre, 67098 Strasbourg Cedex, France
* Corresponding author.
E-mail address: francis.veillon@chru-strasbourg.fr (F. Veillon).

Neuroimag Clin N Am 18 (2008) 309–320
doi:10.1016/j.nic.2008.01.002
1052-5149/08/$ – see front matter

Brain and Pons

Sequences: T2 and fluid attenuated inversion recovery (FLAIR)
Coils: head coil
Imaging plane: Axial, perpendicular to the brainstem
Slice thickness: 4 mm
Matrix: 256

CPA, IAM, VII-1, VII-2, VII-3: at 1.5 Tesla

T1-weighted images

Sequence: T1-weighted SE, with and without intravenous (IV) contrast administration, with or without fat saturation pulse
Coils: head coil or surface coils centered on the ears, or a combination of both
Imaging plane: axial plane, parallel to the roof of the orbit
Slice thickness: 1 mm to 2 mm, depending on the quality of the MR system

T2-weighted images

Sequence: high resolution T2-weighted GE or turbo spin-echo or FSE three-dimensional (3D) images, with IV contrast administration
Coils: head coil or surface coils centered on the ears, or a combination of both
Imaging plane:

- Parallel to the roof of the orbit
- Axial reformatted images parallel to the lateral semicircular canal for visualization of VII-2
- Sagittal reformatted images for visualization of the nerve in the IAC and VII-1, VII-2, and VII-3 segments of the nerve. These sagittal images, in combination with IV gadolinium administration, are very useful to identify a tumor or enhancement inside the facial canal.

Slice thickness: 0.4 mm to 0.7 mm

In case a tumor is detected

Sequence: SE T1-weighted images
Imaging plane: coronal plane with IV gadolinium administration from the GG to the VII-3 segment and in the sagittal plane for evaluation of the VII-3 segment.
Slice thickness: 1 mm to 2 mm

Stylomastoid Foramen and Parotid Gland

Sequence: SE T1-weighted image with IV gadolinium administration without fat suppression
Imaging plane: axial
Slice thickness: 2 mm to 3 mm

In summary, T2 and FLAIR sequences are used for imaging of the brain and pons (especially the motor nucleus). T1 and T2 gadolinium-enhanced high-resolution images are used to study the cerebellopontine angle and the facial nerve inside its canal in the petrous bone. For both sequences, better image quality is achieved when surface coils are used, alone or in combination with the head coil. Routine 2-mm to 3-mm thick T1-weighted SE images are used to evaluate the stylomastoid foramen and the parotid gland.

IMAGING OF THE PATHOLOGIC NERVE

The most common indications for imaging of the facial nerve are as follows:

Peripheral facial nerve palsy. This is the most frequent indication. It can be caused by infectious diseases, Bell's palsy, tumors (schwannomas or other tumors), pseudotumoral lesions, brainstem lesions, trauma, and malformations.
Tinnitus, conductive or sensorineural hearing loss, or vertigo related to a schwannoma of the facial nerve without any facial nerve palsy.
Evaluation of the facial nerve position before surgery. This is indicated before surgery in patients with otosclerosis, ossicular malformations, CPA, and IAC pathology.
Hemifacial spasm.

Evaluation of a Peripheral Facial Nerve Palsy

Nontumoral lesions of the pons with facial nerve palsy

The most frequent nontumoral lesions of the brain and pons are ischemia, multiple sclerosis, hemorrhagic cavernous hemangioma, and arteriovenous malformations. They can all cause peripheral facial nerve palsy. On T2 or FLAIR images they appear as areas of hypersignal in the region of the facial nerve motor nucleus or facial nerve fibers, close to the fourth ventricle (**Figs. 1 and 2**). Acute ischemic lesions in this region can be distinguished on diffusion weighted images (DWI) as a diffusion restriction (high signal on b-1000 images, low signal on apparent diffusion coefficient images) and, therefore, the DWI sequence should be added as a routine sequence in these patients.

Inflammation of the facial nerve

In these patients, the radiologist is asked to confirm inflammation and to eliminate a tumor. Patients most often present with Bell's palsy[1] without any other cranial neuropathy. The unilateral paralysis is most frequently acute and there can be associated trouble of taste or pain around the ear. The herpes simplex virus is most often

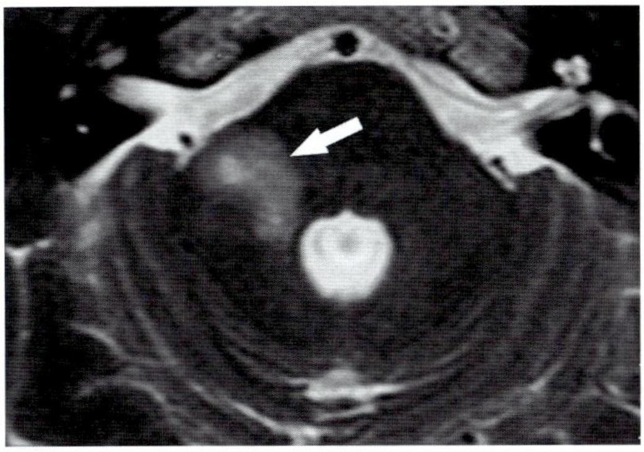

Fig. 1. Multiple sclerosis. Axial T2-weighted SE image through the pons in a patient with peripheral facial nerve palsy on the right. A hyperintense lesion (*white arrow*) is seen in the course the motor fibers of the facial nerve.

causing the symptoms but cannot always be traced by laboratory tests.

In other cases, the viral origin is evident, as in the case of patients presenting with a Ramsay Hunt syndrome. Varicella-like cutaneous lesions of the external ear in association with a peripheral facial nerve palsy confirm the viral origin. Nerves V, VIII, IX, and X are then also commonly affected. There is no need for imaging in typical Bell's palsy or Ramsay Hunt syndrome when the inflammation is clinically obvious. Imaging should be reserved for atypical Bell's palsies, with a persistent peripheral facial nerve paralysis lasting for more than 2 months, and for recurrent or slowly progressive palsies. Imaging can also be used to confirm inflammation in anxious patients with slow or bad recovery of the facial nerve palsy.

The diagnosis of neuritis can be made in the petrous facial nerve canal (VII-1, GG, VII-2). The most interesting sequences (see above) to detect inflammation are the gadolinium enhanced T1-weighted SE and the high resolution T2-weighted sequences, such as GE constructive interference in steady state (CISS) after intravenous gadolinium injection. Viral infection can cause rupture of the blood-nerve barrier, causing edema and diffusion of gadolinium along the labyrinthine segment (VII-1) of the facial nerve (**Fig. 3**). On axial T1-weighted SE images, this contrast material diffusion appears as a more or less important enhancement following the curvature of the labyrinthine segment of the facial nerve.[2]

The enhancement of the tympanic and mastoid segment of the facial nerve is more difficult to delineate and evaluate. The normal veins that surround the tympanic and mastoid segment of the facial nerve in its canal[3] take up gadolinium after IV administration as well. This results in a more or less high physiologic signal on contrast-enhanced images,[4,5] which is not so easily differentiated from an abnormal condition (eg, neuritis) (**Fig. 4**). The diffusion of gadolinium along the labyrinthine segment of the facial nerve and in the fundus of the IAC is always pathologic. High resolution SE or GE (eg, CISS) images can be used to exclude a mass or nodule in the course of the facial nerve or in the facial nerve canal. This is especially helpful in the superior upper quadrant of the IAC, where mass lesions are best excluded, or demonstrated on para-sagittal reformatted images. The facial nerve can easily be delineated in the fundus of the IAC when there is

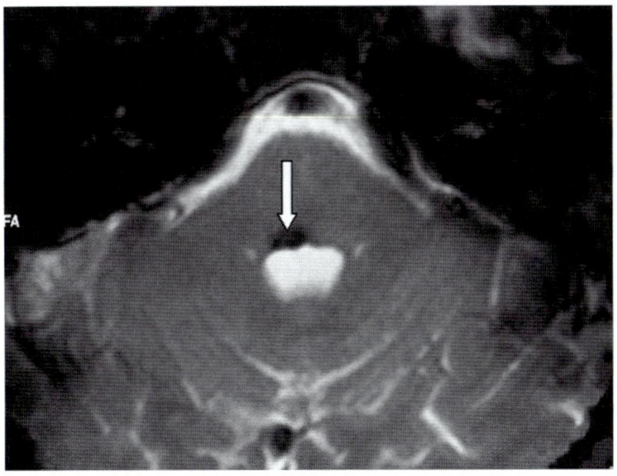

Fig. 2. Cavernous hemangioma. Axial T2-weighted SE image at the level of the pons. The malformation is localized at the level of the facial colliculus, close the floor of the fourth ventricle, where the facial nerve fibers course around the nucleus of the sixth nerve (*white arrow*).

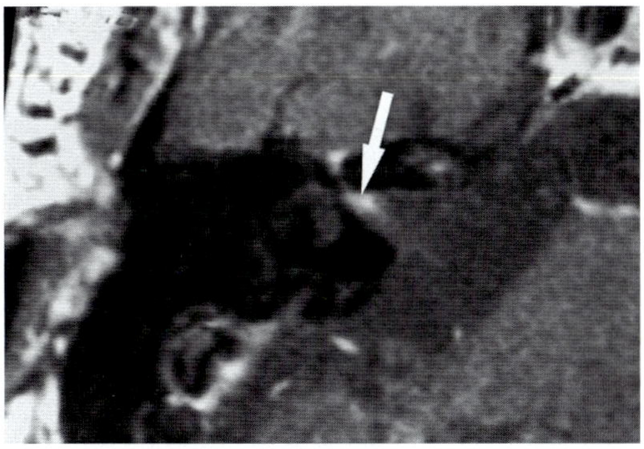

Fig. 3. Neuritis of the right facial nerve (right peripheral facial palsy). Gadolinium enhanced axial T1-weighted SE image in a patient presenting with peripheral facial palsy on the right side. Abnormal enhancement of the facial nerve in the anterior and superior part of the IAC (*white arrow*).

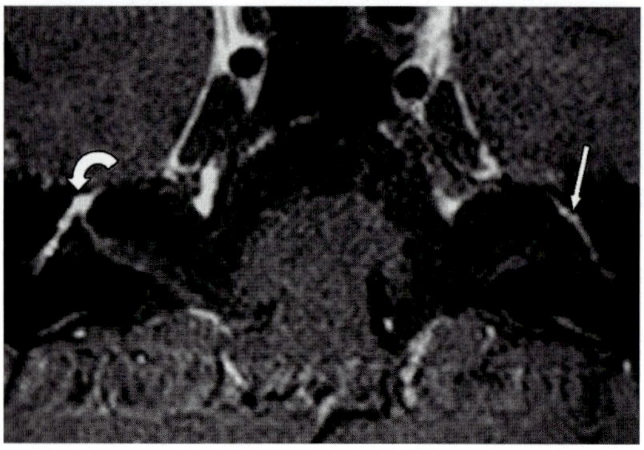

Fig. 4. Neuritis of the right facial nerve. Gadolinium-enhanced axial T1-weighted SE image in a patient presenting with peripheral facial nerve palsy on the right side. On the right side the enhancement in the GG and VII-2 segment is caused by inflammation and normal veins (*curved arrow*); there is no enhancement in the IAC or along the VII-1 segment. The enhancement inside the left facial nerve canal is caused by vessels, and more particularly by the veins that are surrounding the facial nerve (*straight arrow*).

sufficient cerebrospinal fluid surrounding the nerve (**Fig. 5**). On the other hand, if the IAC is narrow, the different nerves (facial nerve, vestibular nerves, cochlear nerve) may be squeezed together, and then it can becomes impossible to exclude a mass. Hence, it is important to analyze the IAC in detail on contrast-enhanced T1-weighted images.

Inflammation of the tympanic and mastoid segment of the facial nerve canal can be nicely demonstrated on contrast-enhanced high resolution T2-weighted images (eg, CISS GE sequence). The T1 effect of gadolinium makes it possible to depict inflammation of the tympanic and mastoid segment of the facial nerve because of the high signal intensity on these 3D high resolution T2-weighted images (**Fig. 6**).[6] Such a high signal is never seen inside the facial nerve canal on these images (eg, CISS) in noninflammatory cases. Therefore, there are two ways to demonstrate inflammation within the facial nerve canal: rupture of the blood-nerve barrier with abnormal gadolinium diffusion along the labyrinthine segment of the facial nerve, and high signal of the second and third segment of the facial nerve inside the facial nerve canal on the high resolution T2-weighted CISS sequence. In several cases, and especially in case of herpes simplex infection, labyrinthitis can also be present. Contrast enhancement along the superior or inferior branch of the vestibular nerve and inside the cochlea, vestibule, and semicircular canals can be seen in these patients.[7,8] The perilymphatic fluid can even have a spontaneous high-signal intensity on the precontrast T1 SE images.

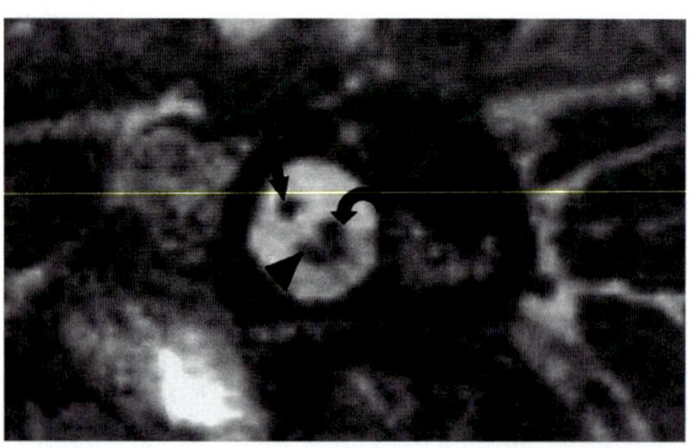

Fig. 5. Normal facial nerve inside the internal auditory canal. Sagittal high resolution T2-weighted GE CISS image. Facial nerve (*arrow*), common vestibular nerve (*curved arrow*), cochlear nerve (*arrowhead*).

In summary, in most of the cases it is possible to localize the inflammation with a combination of contrast-enhanced SE T1-weighted images and high-resolution 3D T2-weighted images (CISS). However, there is no clear relation between the prognosis and the contrast enhancement. Other viruses—in case of borellia and HIV, for exmple—can also affect the facial nerve inside the facial nerve canal.

Peripheral facial nerve palsy can also occur in cases of malignant external otitis (MEO). MEO is caused by *Pseudomonas aeroginosa* and usually results in a localized tympanic bone infection, with a more or less important osteitis. It preferentially occurs in elderly diabetic patients. CT may nicely demonstrate the destruction of the anterior or posterior walls of the tympanic bone. Usually the inflammation spreads along the soft tissues superficial to the temporal bone and around the external auditory canal, with potential extension to the temporo-mandibular joint, the middle ear cavity, the upper part of the carotid space in the neck, the lateropharyngeal space, and more rarely the posterior or middle cranial fossa. Surgical and medical treatment may be required in patients with an associated peripheral facial nerve palsy and in whom a tumor is excluded.

Facial nerve schwannoma with facial palsy

Facial nerve schwannomas occur less frequent than eighth nerve schwannomas. Usually the lesion originates in the schwann cells with a frequent clinical sign: peripheral facial nerve palsy.[9] However, one has to know that the peripheral facial nerve palsy is absent in 30% of the cases. Multiple schwannomas occur in patients with neurofibromatosis type II. Neurofibromas are found in type I neurofibromatosis. In these patients, additional schwannomas or neurofibromas can also be detected along the major side branches of the facial

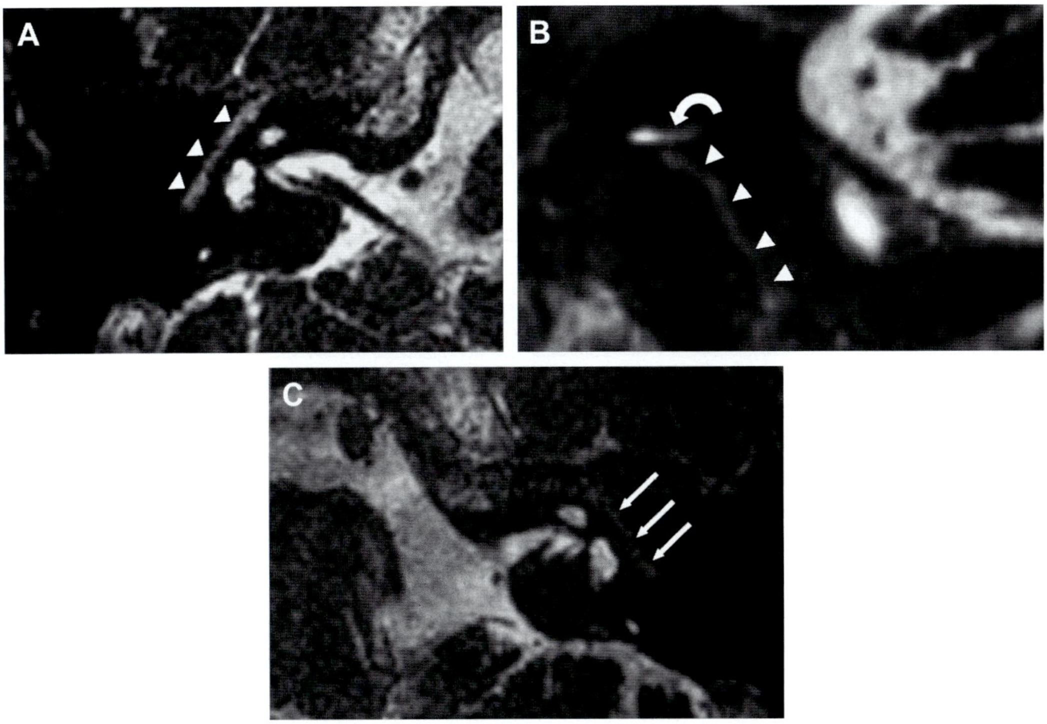

Fig. 6. Neuritis of the right facial nerve. Axial (*A*) and para-sagittal reformatted (*B*) gadolinium-enhanced high resolution T2-weighted CISS image of the right facial nerve, and axial (*C*) similar image of the left facial nerve in a patient with facial nerve palsy on the right side. (*A*) A hyperintense signal caused by inflammation is seen in the course of the tympanic segment of the right facial nerve (*white arrowheads*). (*B*) The para-sagittal reformatted image also shows abnormal high-signal intensity along the second and third segment of the facial nerve (*white arrowheads*). Fluid inside the lateral semicircular canal (*curved arrow*). (*C*) Normal enhancement inside the tympanic segment of the left facial nerve canal following intravenous gadolinium injection (*white arrows*). The patient had no facial nerve palsy on the left side.

nerve, such as the greater superficial petrosal nerve and the chorda tympani. Local or more extensive enlargement of the facial nerve canal can be seen on CT. The diagnosis is easy when a mass is seen along one or several segments of the facial nerve inside the facial nerve canal.[10] Schwannomas appear as round, well-delineated masses in the CPA, IAC, or facial nerve canal (**Fig. 7**A). They can extend to the middle ear, the stylomastoid foramen, or parotid gland. Schwannomas can also cause enlargement of the chorda tympani canal, situated between the mastoid segment of the facial nerve canal and the middle ear cavity, and this is often more subtle and more difficult to depict. The lesions can also present as a small mass in the external auditory meatus or the tympanic cavity. This "double nodule or mass" sign (tumoral lesions both in the mastoid segment of the facial nerve canal and along the chorda tympani) is typical for a nervous tumor of the facial nerve. In the middle ear, schwannomas or neurofibromas can also destroy the long process of the incus or can compress the stapes.

MR imaging is useful in the demonstration of the mass itself, from the CPA to the facial nerve canal and the parotid gland. On T1-weighted images, schwannoma have a slightly high signal intensity that can be found along the course of the facial nerve. On contrast-enhanced SE T1-weighted images, schwannomas are well delineated and strongly enhancing masses (**Fig. 7**B), with sizes ranging from several millimeters to 3 to 5 centimeters. A dumbbell appearance is classical along the facial nerve canal.[11]

On the high-resolution T2-weighted images it is also possible to distinguish nodular masses in the CPA, the fundus of the internal auditory canal, or in the facial nerve canal (**Fig. 7**C).

Small IAC schwannomas of the facial nerve should be studied on para-sagittal reformatted images. On these images one can check if the schwannoma is localized in the anterior upper quadrant of the IAC, while the normal cochlear nerve is located in the inferior anterior quadrant and the normal vestibular nerves are located in the superior and inferior posterior quadrants.

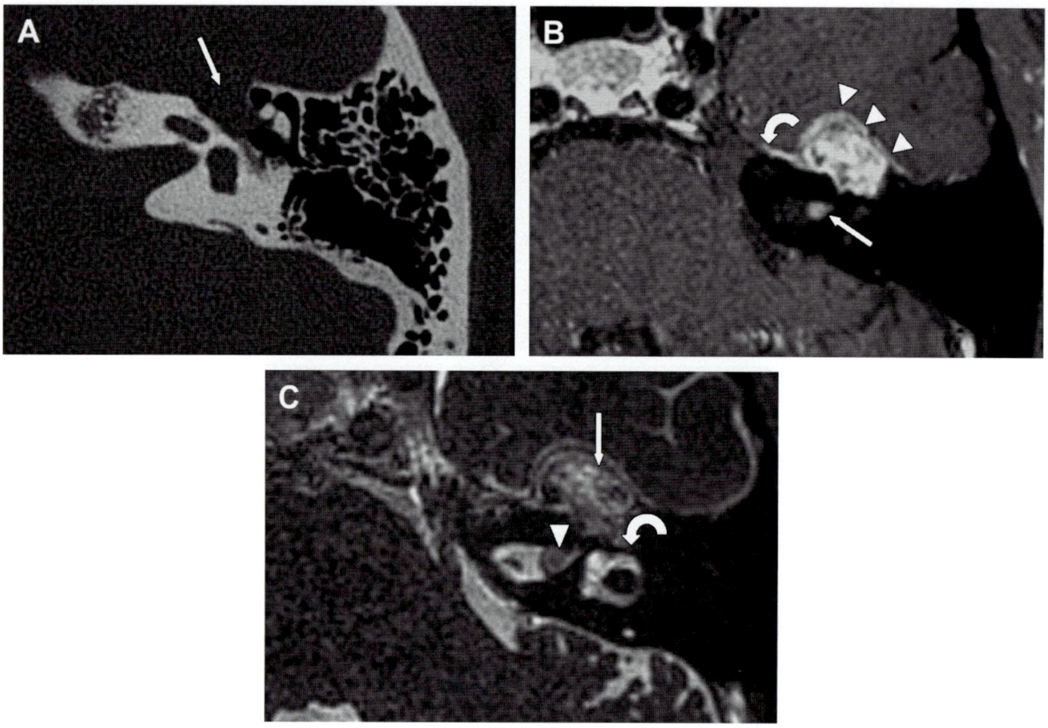

Fig. 7. Schwannoma of the left seventh facial nerve. Axial CT image (*A*), contrast-enhanced T1-weighted images (*B*) and CISS image (*C*) of the left geniculate ganglion area in a patient presenting with a left peripheral facial nerve palsy. CT axial section. (*A*) A mass in the region of the geniculate ganglion is destroying the cortical bone of the anterior tympanic recess (*white arrow*). (*B*) The schwannoma in the region of the geniculate ganglion (*white arrowheads*) has smooth margins. The dura anterior to the petrous apex is thickened and is enhancing (*curved arrow*). Note the extension of the schwannoma in the fundus of the internal auditory canal (*arrow*). (*C*) The solid tumor in the region of the geniculate ganglion (*arrow*) with an extension along the proximal tympanic segment of the facial nerve (*curved arrow*) and in the internal auditory canal (*white arrowhead*) can again be recognized.

Finally, large schwannomas (several centimeters) can be very heterogeneous on MR and can have large cystic areas.

Other tumors and pseudotumors of the facial nerve

The pons Pontine malignancies, metastatic tumors, and lymphomas may all cause peripheral facial nerve palsy. On MR, and especially on the FLAIR images, it is easier to recognize and delineate these tumors.

The CPA and IAC Lesions occurring in these regions and which are causing peripheral facial nerve palsy are usually malignant: metastasis or lymphoma. These lesions enhance strongly on contrast-enhanced SE T1-weighted images (**Fig. 8**). The margins are hazy and the meninges are usually thickened in case of metastasis. In lymphoma, the diagnosis can be more difficult, especially when the margins of the masses, for example in the IAC, are sharp and are therefore mimicking a neurofibroma or schwannoma. Special attention must be paid when clinical signs evolve quickly. In some cases, arachnoiditis can have the appearance of a pseudotumor; however, the thickened meninges will decreased in size under medical treatment and will heal without any scars.

The facial nerve canal Several benign and malignant tumors or pseudotumors involve the facial nerve canal and compress the facial nerve.

Hemangioma: Based on the vascular caliber, hemangiomas are classified as capillary, cavernous or a combination of both. They are usually located in the geniculate ganglion fossa and have a short extension along the labyrinthine segment of the facial nerve canal into the IAC or along the tympanic facial nerve segment. On CT these lesions have poorly defined margins. The diagnosis is made easy if bone spiculae are present. On MR, a hemangioma can be seen as a mass in the geniculate ganglion, with intermediate signal

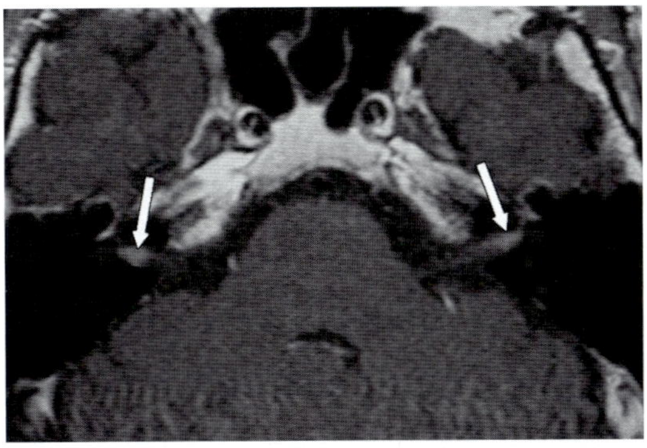

Fig. 8. Lymphoma. Gadolinium-enhanced axial T1-weighted SE image in a patient presenting with peripheral facial palsy on the right side. An enhancing mass is seen in the fundus of both the right and left IAC (*arrows*).

intensity on unenhanced T1-weighted MR images. Following IV contrast administration, they enhance strongly[12] but also become somewhat heterogeneous because of the presence of the calcified spiculae (**Fig. 9**). Special attention must be paid to subtle extension and associated enhancement along the labyrinthine segment of the facial nerve canal. Hemangiomas are usually small, the facial nerve fibers are disorganized, and patients frequently present with facial nerve palsy. In contrast, schwannomas compress the facial nerve fibers, and in these patients often no neurologic abnormalities or clinical signs are present.

Meningioma: A meningioma may compress the facial nerve in any part of the facial nerve canal and does this most often in the geniculate ganglion fossa, causing a peripheral facial nerve palsy.

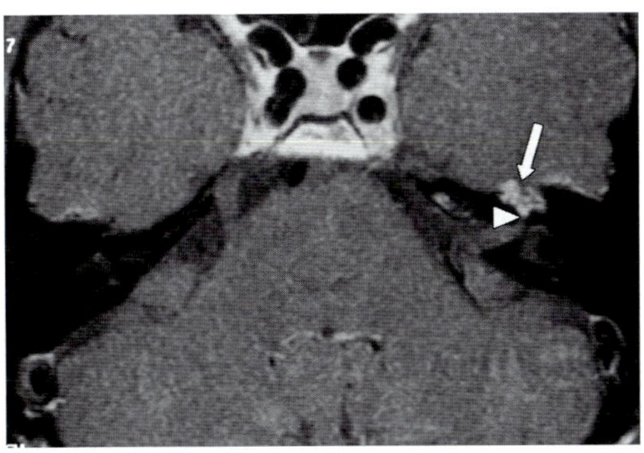

Fig. 9. Hemangioma of the left geniculate ganglion fossa. Gadolinium-enhanced axial T1-weighted SE image. An enhancing lesion is seen in the left geniculate ganglion fossa. The margins are irregular, the enhancement is strong, and the signal is heterogenous because of the presence of small bone spiculae (*arrow*). Subtle extension in the labyrinthine segment of the facial nerve canal can be seen (*arrowhead*).

Strong enhancement of the thickened meninges can be seen on axial and coronal gadolinium-enhanced T1-weighted images. The surrounding bone is heterogeneous and has irregular margins. Meningiomas can also originate in the middle cranial fossa and can then invade the Eustachian tube, the middle ear, the greater superficial petrosal nerve canal, and the geniculate ganglion fossa.[13] Facial nerve palsy is rarely found in association with such an extension.

Secondary cholesteatoma: Secondary cholesteatoma with peripheral facial nerve palsy is rare and usually occurs after a long history of chronic otitis media. Cholesteatoma usually invades the attic superiorly, may fistule toward the labyrinth, and can compress the facial nerve in the region of the geniculate ganglion. CT can demonstrate the sequelae of chronic otitis media and is able to visualize the extension of the lesion (**Fig. 10**A). Cholesteatoma presents as a nonenhancing mass on gadolinium enhanced T1-weighted images, has an intermediate to low signal intensity on T2-weighted images (**Fig. 10**B), and has a high signal intensity on diffusion images (**Fig. 10**C). The region of the geniculate ganglion is most often involved, but the lesion can attack any part of the facial nerve canal. The cholesteatoma can also erode or invade the labyrinth and can eventually grow into the IAC.

Congenital cholesteatoma: Congenital cholesteatoma develops from some remnants of cutaneous epithelium, which at birth are usually situated in the bony interface between the labyrinthine capsule and the tympanic cavity. Facial nerve palsy occurs when the geniculate ganglion (or more rarely the tympanic segment) is compressed. CT demonstrates a sharply marginated mass, sometimes multiloculated, with a more or less important destruction of the bone. On MR imaging, the signal is intermediate on T1-weighted images and there is no enhancement following IV gadolinium administration. The mucosa close to the cholesteatoma can be congestive, resulting in a peripheral rim enhancement. The lesion has a high signal intensity on diffusion-weighted images, especially when the lesion is superior to 5 mm in size. On high-resolution T2-weighted images, the signal is low or intermediate, depending on the amount of water within the keratoma.

Paragangliomas: Jugular paragangliomas may compress the facial nerve because the jugular foramen is very close to the mastoid segment of the facial nerve. They have a heterogeneous appearance on T2-weighted images, with signal voids corresponding to arteries within the mass. Strong enhancement is seen on gadolinium-enhanced T1-weighted images.

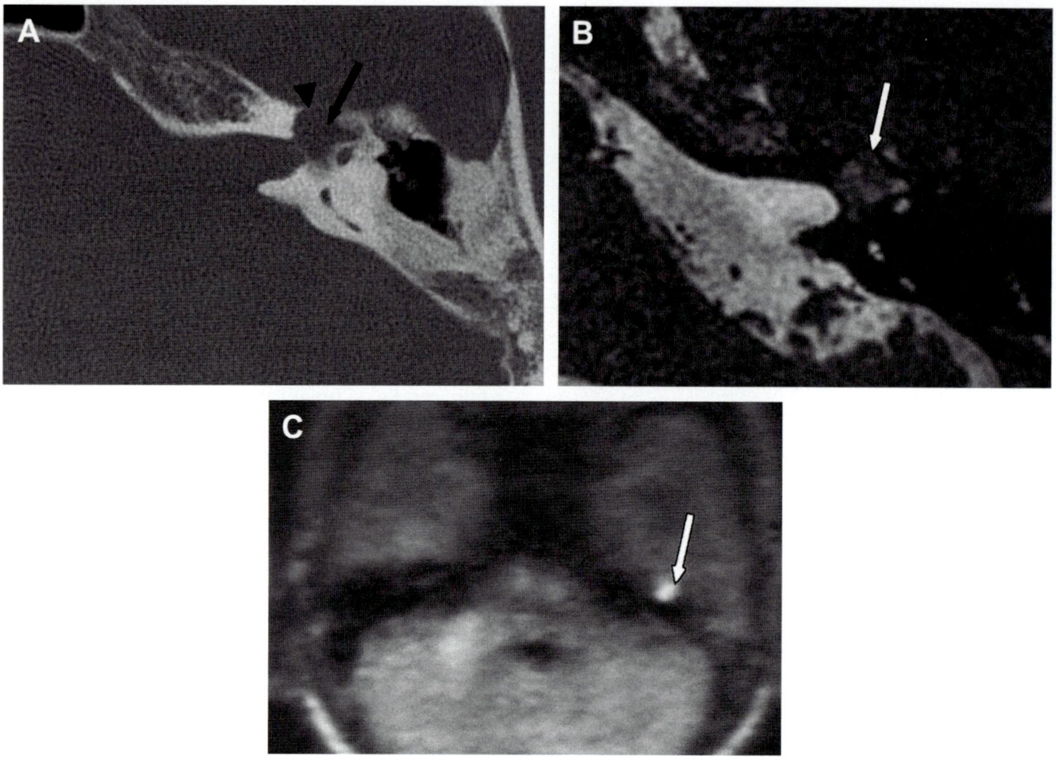

Fig. 10. Secondary cholesteatoma in the left geniculate ganglion fossa with left facial palsy. Axial CT image (*A*) and high-resolution T2-weighted CISS image (*B*) and diffusion half-Fourier acquisition single-shot turbo image (*C*) through the left geniculate ganglion in a patient presenting with left facial nerve palsy. (*A*) Lesion with regular margins is enlarging the left geniculate ganglion fossa (*arrow*) and an erosion of the anterior wall of the petrous bone is seen (*arrowhead*). (*B*) The lesion has an intermediate signal intensity on the T2-weighted GE image (*arrow*). (*C*) A high signal intensity can be seen in the left geniculate ganglion area, compatible with cholesteatoma (*arrow*).

Histiocytosis: Histiocytosis is a macrophage localized in the skin and traveling in the lymphatic system. The development of these cells may lead to an aggressive lesion in the temporal bone (eosinophilic granuloma), causing destruction in the squamous and petrosal parts of the temporal bone. The facial nerve canal may be compressed, with peripheral facial nerve palsy dominating the clinical signs. CT can demonstrate the destruction of the middle and inner ear, with potential fistula formation toward the cochlea and all the semicircular canals. The soft tissue component in the middle and inner ear can be recognized on MR, and these soft tissues enhance strongly following IV contrast administration. The radiologist should always consider the diagnosis when such a mass is found in young children. A biopsy, showing multiple granulomas with Langerhans (LH) cells, is needed before surgery to prove the diagnosis. The immunohistochemical technics show specific cyclin-dependent kinase inhibitor 1A (LH specific cytoplasmic membranous tracer). There is no need for a large surgical approach. When the result of the biopsy is known and is positive, then chemotherapy is the treatment of choice.

Malignant tumors involving the petrous bone: Sarcoma, lymphoma, and metastasis of a neuroblastoma can lead to peripheral facial nerve palsy in children, with possible destruction of the petrous bone. There are no specific signs; usually the enhancement on gadolinium-enhanced T1-weighted images is strong and heterogeneous. The diagnosis is made by biopsy. In adults, chondrosarcoma is a frequent primary tumor that appears as a multilobulated mass with a high signal intensity on T2, heterogeneous enhancement on after contrast T1-weighted images, and destruction of bone with bone spiculae visible on CT. In adults metastases of the temporal bone have their origin in the lung, breast, prostate, kidney, pharynx, stomach, and liver. The petrous apex, the geniculate ganglion fossa, and the internal auditory canal are the most commonly involved sites.

The parotid gland A malignant tumor of the parotid gland may be responsible for a peripheral facial nerve palsy: carcinomas originating in the parotid gland itself (mucoepidermoid, cystadenocarcinoma)[14], metastasis (especially from the lung), or lymphoma. Extension along the facial nerve is possible in the region of the stylomastoid foramen, where the lesion can enter the facial nerve canal with further extension toward the geniculate ganglion and even to the internal auditory canal. CT shows a partial or total enlargement of the facial nerve canal in these cases. On MR, the tumor in the parotid gland can be seen as a low or intermediate signal intensity lesion on T1- and T2-weighted images. Gadolinium-enhanced SE T1-weighted images are very useful in the evaluation of tumor extension in the facial nerve canal, with possible further involvement of the fundus of the IAC where the tumor extension can then be seen as a nodular-enhancing mass (**Fig. 11**).

Trauma

Peripheral facial nerve palsy may be secondary to a head trauma. Most of the fractures run in the direction of the middle ear (extralabyrinthine longitudinal fractures, 88%), while other fractures run perpendicular to the petrous bone (translabyrinthine fractures, 7%). In 5% of cases, the trauma involves the middle ear and the labyrinth, with involvement of the oval and round window. The weakest point of the facial nerve canal is the geniculate ganglion fossa. Most longitudinal fractures will eventually end or run through this fossa (**Fig. 12**). Moreover, the facial nerve may be injured by bony spiculae or can be directly contused by the shock wave.

On MR imaging, the gadolinium-enhanced T1-weighted images demonstrate the swollen injured area of the nerve (geniculate ganglion, tympanic segment), with strong enhancement that can be compared with the normal opposite side. Other parts of the facial nerve, like the mastoid segment, especially in the area close to the pyramid eminence, can also be affected. Postoperative facial nerve injuries causing peripheral facial nerve palsy are most often located laterally or posterior to the stapes.

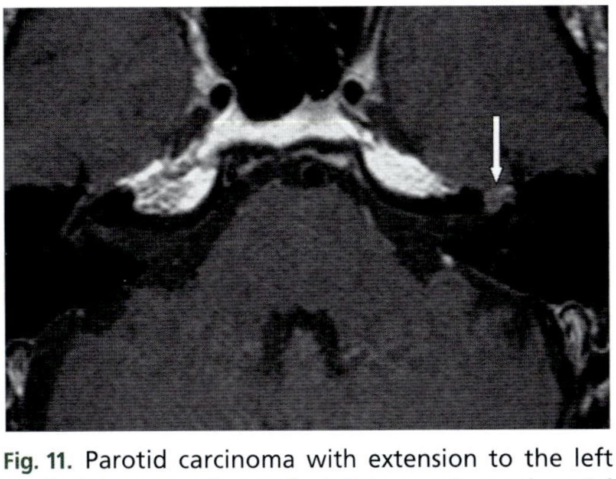

Fig. 11. Parotid carcinoma with extension to the left geniculate ganglion. Gadolinium-enhanced axial T1-weighted SE image. An enhancing tumor (*arrow*) is seen in the geniculate ganglion. The parotid lesion grew along the facial nerve in the stylomastoid foramen and nerve inside the facial nerve canal to reach the geniculate ganglion.

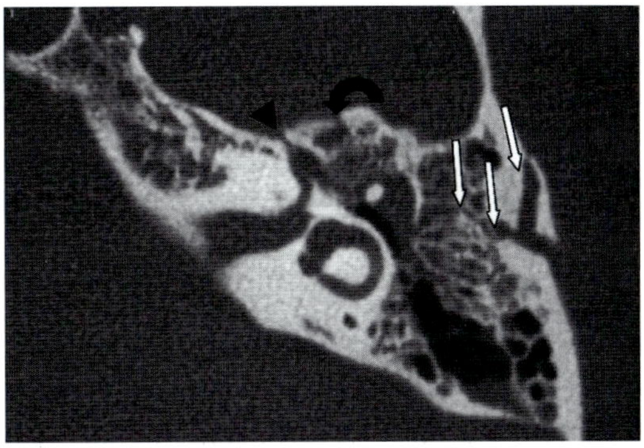

Fig. 12. Trauma of the left temporal bone with peripheral facial palsy. Axial CT image of the left temporal bone in a patient with posttraumatic facial nerve palsy. Fractures of the vertical and horizontal parts of the squamous temporal bone (*white arrows*), with a fracture involving the geniculate ganglion fossa (*black arrowhead*) and the anterior wall of the tympanic cavity (*black curved arrow*).

Congenital absence of the facial nerve

The facial nerve can be absent. This is best demonstrated on para-sagittal reformatted MR images. Thin slices through the IAC are used to show the absence of the facial nerve, while the other three nerves, the two vestibular branches and the cochlear branch, can still be visualized (**Fig. 13**). CT can be used to demonstrate the absence of the labyrinthine, tympanic, and mastoid segments of the facial nerve canal in case of congential absence of the facial nerve.

Schwannoma of the Facial Nerve without Facial Nerve Palsy

Tinnitus, conductive or sensorineural hearing loss, and vertigo may be the only clinical signs in patients with a facial nerve schwannoma[15]. CT and MR are then initially performed to find more frequent causes of the above-mentioned clinical signs, but will depict the facial nerve schwannoma. Any part of the facial nerve may be involved. The most difficult area to distinguish a facial nerve schwannoma from an eighth nerve schwannoma is the CPA (**Fig. 14**). When facial nerve schwannomas are situated deep in the IAC, then special

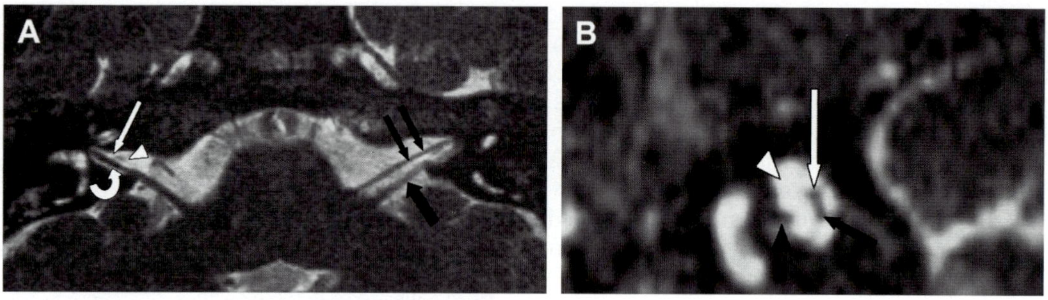

Fig. 13. Congenital absence of the right facial nerve. High resolution T2-weighted CISS image through both IACs in the axial plane (*A*) and sagittal reformatted through the right IAC (*B*) in a 3-year-old child with congenital facial nerve palsy on the right side. (*A*) Absence of the right facial nerve (*white arrow*), upper part of the cochlear branch (*arrowhead*), superior vestibular nerve (*curved arrow*), normal left facial nerve (*black arrows*), and left superior vestibular nerve (*thick black arrow*). (*B*) Absence of the right facial nerve (*white arrowhead*), superior vestibular nerve (*white arrow*), inferior vestibular nerve (*black arrow*), and cochlear branch (*black arrowhead*).

attention must be paid to detect extension in and enlargement of the labyrinthine segment of the facial nerve canal. In 30% of the facial nerve schwannomas, there is no facial nerve palsy. Therefore, the detection of a mass inside the facial nerve canal on MR or CT, sometimes in combination with an extension along the greater superficial petrosal nerve or chorda tympani, must be considered as a schwannoma in the absence of helpful clinical signs. Similarly, a nodule in the parotid gland in a patient with neurofibromatosis type I must be suspected to be a facial nerve neurofibroma.

Evaluation of the Position of the Facial Nerve in Malformations of the Middle Ear or Before Surgery

The position of the facial nerve must always be analyzed by the radiologist, especially in malformations of the middle ear or before surgery in patients with otosclerosis, CPA tumors, or congenital malformed ossicles. In patients with congenital malformations, the facial nerve can follow its own canal in the inner ear, separate from the IAC, and will join the mastoid segment of the nerve in the roof of the middle ear. The tympanic portion of the facial nerve canal may be absent, leading to a vertical course of the facial nerve in the middle ear cavity, where the nerve will be running on the surface of the promontory. The tympanic segment of the facial nerve can also be found in a lower position, running close to or even over the oval window. This is the most frequently found congenital abnormal position of the facial nerve, especially in patients with an absent or closed oval window or small tympanic cavity, and the nerve may be found very close to the footplate in these cases. Sometimes the facial nerve is passing through the middle ear without any surrounding bony canal, and can even run through the round window recess. The mastoid segment of the nerve can also be displaced anterior or medially in the middle ear, and can run close to the jugular foramen. In these cases, CT is the method of choice to precisely delineate the abnormal course of the nerve (**Fig. 15**). Special attention must be paid to the position of the facial nerve canal when surgery of abnormal ossicles—and more particularly the stapes—is planned. The radiologist should also evaluate the exact position of the facial nerve on every single MR study of CPA and IAC eighth nerve schwannomas. In otosclerosis cases, the position of the facial nerve above the oval window recess and its exact distance to the footplate must be known before surgery.

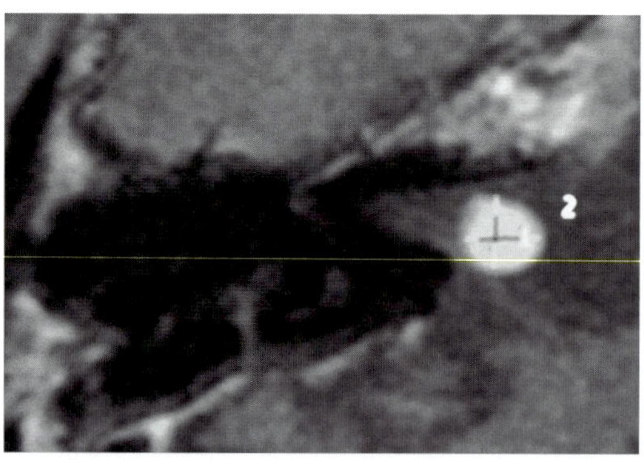

Fig. 14. Schwannoma of the right facial nerve without facial palsy. Gadolinium-enhanced axial T1-weighted SE image. A small tumor with smooth margins and strong enhancement can be seen in the right IAC but also has a component extending in the CPA.

Hemifacial Spasm

Hemifacial spasm, or facial nerve vascular loop syndrome, is an isolated involuntary sudden contraction of the facial muscles caused by a vascular

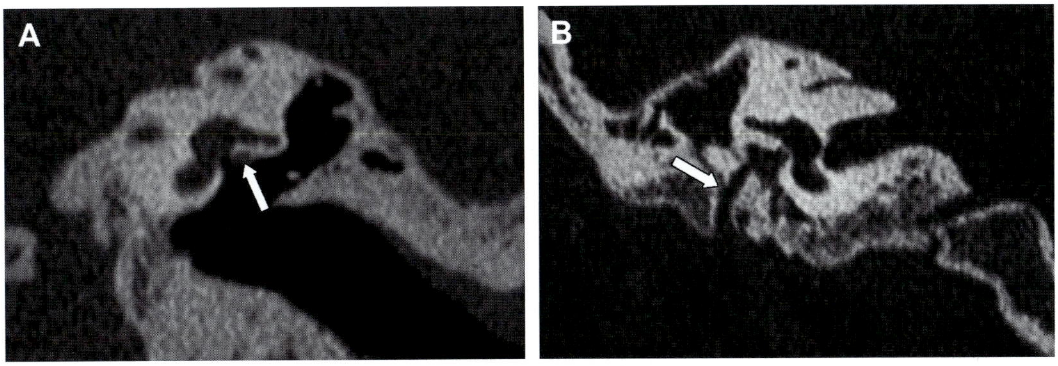

Fig. 15. Congenital abnormal course of the left facial nerve. Coronal CT image of a left (*A*) and right (*B*) temporal bone of two different patients. (*A*) The tympanic segment of the facial nerve is running too far medially and too low, close to oval window and in contact with the stapes (*arrow*). (*B*) Anteriorly shifted mastoid segment of the facial nerve canal (*arrow*).

loop of the anterior cerebellar artery (AICA), posterior inferior cerebellar artery (PICA), or vertebral artery (VA). The location is the root exit zone, situated at the site where the nerve exits the brainstem. MR is the method of choice to demonstrate the neurovascular conflict. High-resolution T2-weighted images or MR-angiography images are particularly suited to detect the contact between the AICA, PICA, VA, and the facial nerve. Displacement of the nerve by an artery and perpendicular crossing of the nerve at the root exit zone are the MR findings that can explain a hemifacial spasm.[16,17]

SUMMARY

The exact anatomy of the facial nerve must be known and all segments of the facial nerve must be evaluated in detail on every CT or MR examination of the temporal bone. This will lead to the right diagnosis not only in lesions of the nerve itself, but also when an abnormal position of the nerve is present or when the nerve has an abnormal course. This will avoid dangerous surprises during surgery.

REFERENCES

1. Lustig J, Niparko J. Disorders of the facial nerve. In: Lalwani A, editor. Current diagnosis and treatment in otolaryngology—head and neck surgery. New York: Lange Medical Books/Mc Graw-Hill; 2004. p. 903–29.
2. Sartoretti-Schefer S, Brändle P, Wichmann W, et al. Intensity of MR contrast enhancement does not correspond to clinical and electroneurographic findings in acute inflammatory facial nerve palsy. AJNR Am J Neuroradiol 1996;17:1229–36.
3. May M. Anatomy for the clinician. In: May M, Schaitkin B, editors. The facial nerve. 2nd edition. New York: Thieme Medical Publishers; 2000. p. 19–56.
4. Gebarski SS, Telian SA, Niparko JK. Enhancement along the normal facial nerve in the facial canal: MR imaging and anatomic correlation. Radiology 1992;183:391–4.
5. Martin-Duverneuil N, Sola Martinez MT, Miaux Y, et al. Contrast enhancement of the facial nerve in MRI normal or pathological? Neuroradiology 1997; 39:207–12.
6. Shigematsu Y, Yukunori K, Toshinori H, et al. Contrast enhancement CISS MRI of vestibular schwannomas: phantom and clinical studies. J Comput Assist Tomogr 1999;23:224–31.
7. Swartz J, Harnsberger H. The facial nerve (cranial nerve VII). In: Swartz J, Harnsberger H, editors. Imaging of the temporal bone. 3rd edition. New York: Thieme Medical Publishers; 1998. p. 345–93.
8. Stokroos RJ, Albers FW, Krikke AP, et al. Magnetic resonance imaging of the inner ear in patients with idiopathic sudden sensorineural hearing loss. Eur Arch Otorhinolaryngol 1998;9:433–6.
9. Sterkers O, Chobaut JC, Martin C, et al. Paralysies faciales tumorales. In: Charachon R, Bebear JP, Sterkers O, editors. La paralysie faciale, le spasme hémifacial. Société Française d'Oto-Rhino-Laryngologie et de Pathologie Cervico-Faciale; 1997. p. 188–98 [In French].
10. Jager L, Reiser M. CT and MR imaging of the normal and pathologic conditions of the facial nerve. Eur J Radiol 2001;40:133–46.
11. Wiggins RH, Harnsberger H, Salzman KL, et al. The many faces of facial nerve schwannoma. AJNR Am J Neuroradiol 2006;27:694–9.
12. Lo WW, Shelton C, Waluch V, et al. Intratemporal vascular tumors: detection with CT and MR imaging. Radiology 1989;171:443–8.

13. Nager GT. Hemangiomas and vascular malformations. In: Nager GT, editor. Pathology of the ear and temporal bone. Baltimore: William and Wilkins; 1993. p. 858–78.
14. Mukherji S, Chong V. Mucoepidermoid carcinoma. Adenoid cystic carcinoma. In: Mukherji S, Chong V, editors. Atlas of head and neck imaging. New York: Thieme Medical Publishers; 2004. p. 91–104.
15. Kubota Y, Kawamata T, Kubo O, et al. Large facial nerve schwannomas without facial palsy: case reports and review of the literature. Neurosurg Rev 2005;28:234–8.
16. Magnan S, Caces F, Girard N, et al. Spasme hémifacial idiopathique. In: Charachon R, Bebear JP, Sterkers O, editors. La paralysie faciale, le spasme hémifacial. Société Française d'Oto-Rhino-Laryngologie et de Pathologie cervico-faciale; 1997. p. 391–408 [In French].
17. Harnsberger H. Diagnostic imaging, head and neck. Manitoba (Canada): Amirsys, Elsevier Saunders; 2004.

Pathology of the Vestibulocochlear Nerve

Joel D. Swartz, MD

KEYWORDS

- Internal auditory canal • Vestibulocochlear nerve
- Hearing loss

This article covers congenital deformity of the internal auditory canal (IAC), neoplastic and pseudoneoplastic lesions with special detailed emphasis on schwannoma of the eight cranial nerve (acoustic neuroma), non-neoplastic IAC/cerebellopontine angle mass (CPA) pathology, including vascular loops and numerous additional differential diagnostic entities with particular emphasis on nonneoplastic meningeal disease.

CONGENITAL DEFORMITY OF THE INTERNAL AUDITORY CANAL

The caliber of the internal auditory canal (IAC) depends upon the development of the vestibulocochlear nerve.[1] This is consistent with findings noted in the evaluation of the other skull base foramina, virtually all of which develop in response to the presence of the regional nerve or artery. As such, congenital vestibulocochlear nerve deficiency commonly is associated with a hypoplastic IAC containing only the facial nerve (**Fig. 1**). Although measurements are somewhat arbitrary, the IAC is considered hypoplastic when less than 2 mm in diameter. This usually is appreciated best upon examination in the axial and coronal plane; however, high-resolution thin-section oblique sagittal T2W MR imaging not only allows demonstration of this small canal but also depicts to best advantage absence/hypoplasia of the vestibulocochlear nerve (**Fig. 2**).[2] The cochlear nerve is defined as hypoplastic when similar in size or smaller than either of the vestibular nerves.

Cochlear nerve deficiency in the presence of a normal-sized internal auditory canal implies that it is acquired after formation of the IAC. This has been observed most commonly in patients who have labyrinthitis ossificans (**Fig. 3**).

Abnormality of vestibulocochlear nerve caliber has crucial implications for patients requiring cochlear implantation.[3] Absence of the cochlear nerve is the only complete contraindication to this procedure. In addition to the IAC caliber, the imaging specialist must evaluate the status of the cochlear nerve aperture at the fundus of the IAC. Stenosis of this aperture consistently is associated with cochlear nerve deficiency also (**Fig. 1**B).[4] Additional considerations regarding cochlear implantation are discussed later in this article.

Narrowing of the IAC may occur secondary to exostoses or osteomas. These bony lesions are rare, but they may clinically mimic vestibular schwannomas by compression of the vestibulocochlear nerve. Hearing loss and vestibular symptoms including dizziness and vertigo may improve after surgical removal of the bony lesion. Compromise of the IAC also may occur as a complication of several of the otodystrophies, including Paget's disease and fibrous dysplasia.

A large IAC (greater than 9mm) may be incidental. Bilateral IAC enlargement is seen with neurofibromatosis (NF)-2 secondary to bilateral acoustic tumors. NF also may result in IAC widening because of dural ectasia without neoplasm.

The large IAC also has other important implications. Special attention to the fundus (lateralmost aspect) of the canal may reveal an unusually wide neural aperture leading to the cochlea or vestibule. This implies increased pressure within the perilymphatic space and predisposes to abnormal flow of perilymph (gusher) upon stapes manipulation. This can occur with various congenital inner ear malformations but is a classic manifestation of x-linked progressive mixed deafness (XLPMD) (**Fig. 4**).[5] These male patients present with mixed hearing loss possibly masquerading

Germantown Imaging Associates, Gladwyne, PA 19085, USA
E-mail address: swartzjd@aol.com

Neuroimag Clin N Am 18 (2008) 321–346
doi:10.1016/j.nic.2008.02.001

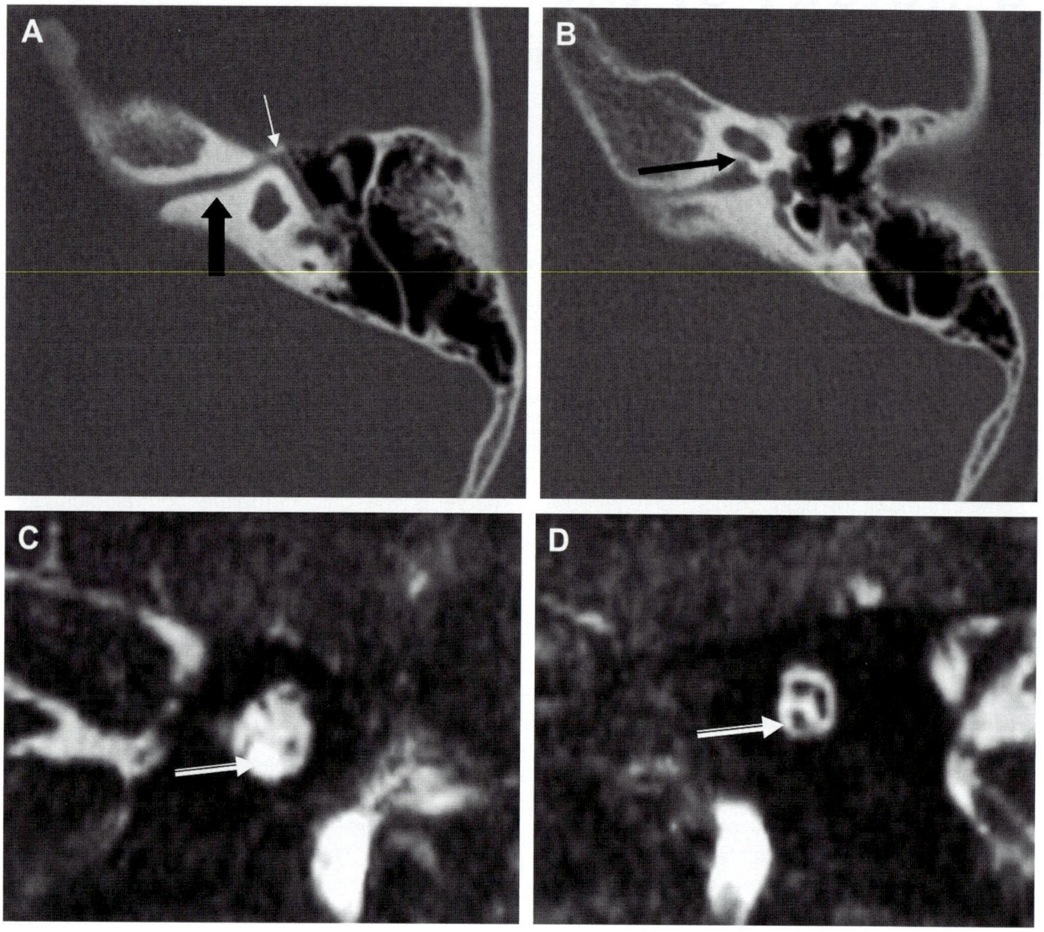

Fig. 1. Hypoplastic internal auditory canal (IAC), occluded cochlear neural foramen. (*A,B*) Axial CT images of the left ear reveal an extremely narrow internal auditory canal (*thick black arrow*) contiguous with the anterior genu of the facial nerve canal (*white arrow*) with a bony plate occluding the cochlear neural foramen (*long black arrow*). (*C*) Sagittal T2WI of the left ear reveals a vacant anteroinferior fundal IAC quadrant (*white arrow*) indicating that the cochlear nerve is absent. (*D*) Sagittal T2WI of the right ear reveals a normal cochlear nerve (*white arrow*). (*Courtesy of* C.D. Phillips, MD, Charlottesville, VA.)

as otosclerosis clinically. If the deformity is recognized before middle ear exploration, the imaging specialist can provide a potentially life-saving service.

NEOPLASTIC AND PSEUDONEOPLASTIC

The differential diagnosis of the IAC/cerebellopontine angle mass (CPA) is fairly clear-cut in that there is universal agreement regarding the four most common entities. Schwannoma of the eighth cranial nerve (acoustic neuroma) is the most common, followed by meningioma, arachnoid cyst, and epidermoid (in that order). The next several paragraphs summarize the most important clinical and imaging findings of these entities. Subsequent paragraphs will focus on the less common diagnostic entities.

Schwannoma of the Eighth Cranial Nerve (Acoustic Neuroma)

Overview

Schwannoma of the eighth cranial nerve (acoustic neuroma) is by far the most common CPA neoplasm.[6–9] They are noncalcifying, slow-growing, well-encapsulated lesions of midlife that account for 6% to 10% of all intracranial tumors and 60% to 90% of CPA tumors. They are somewhat more common and tend to be larger in women. There are strong indications that pregnancy may accelerate the growth of this tumor. Schwannomas most commonly present as a combined IAC/CPA lesion; however, they may be entirely intracanalicular in nature. Interestingly, this latter subgroup of lesions is more common in men. Schwannomas arising from the extracanalicular portion of

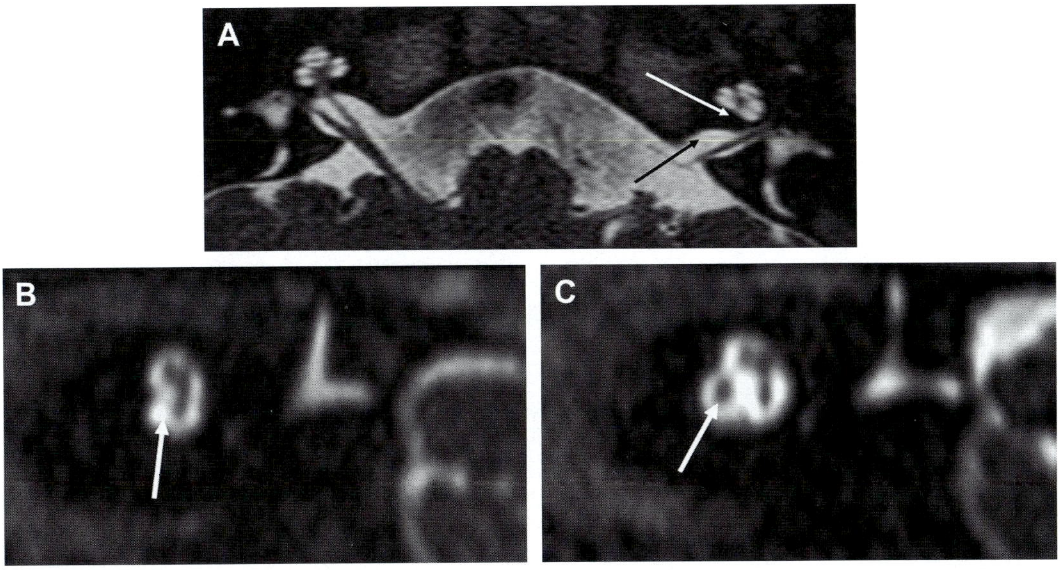

Fig. 2. Cochlear nerve aplasia. (*A*) Axial T2W drive image reveals that the cochlear nerve is absent (*black arrow*) from the anteroinferior quadrant of the internal auditory canal. The cochlear neural foramen is developmentally occluded (*white arrow*). (*B*) Sagittal T2W drive image of the left ear confirms the vacant anteroinferior quadrant (*white arrow*). (*C*) Sagittal T2W drive image of the right ear for comparison reveals a normal cochlear nerve (*white arrow*). (*Courtesy of* Jan W. Casselman, MD, PhD, Bruges, Belgium.)

the nerve may involve only the CPA cistern, sparing the IAC and masquerade as meningioma, metastasis, or exophytic brainstem tumor. Intralabyrinthine schwannomas are rare and will be discussed in detail later.

Clinical issues

Eighth nerve schwannomas typically present with progressive unilateral high-frequency retrocochlear sensorineural hearing loss, presumably resulting from compression/infiltration of auditory (cochlear) nerve fibers. This hearing loss is often manifested clinically by disproportionately deficient speech discrimination (compared with pure tone loss) as measured by brainstem electric response audiometry.[8] Sudden worsening of hearing deficit occurs commonly (26%) and presumably is associated with occlusion of the internal auditory branch of the anterior inferior cerebellar artery (AICA). A small number of patients have normal hearing (or symmetric loss). The clinician must maintain suspicion when nonauditory symptoms predominate such as tinnitus or vertigo. Tinnitus in this context is typically high-pitched and unilateral (tumor side). Vertigo, an episodic illusion of motion, and horizontal nystagmus, are manifestations of peripheral vestibular dysfunctions that typically occur early in the course of tumor development, possibly because of disruption of vascular supply. Disequilibrium, a continuous sense of instability, occurs with larger lesions, possibly because of deafferentation (compromise of sensory nerve impulses caused by injury of sensory nerve fibers). The presence of vertical nystagmus often implies a large tumor with brainstem compression. The facial nerve may undergo substantial torsion without losing its functional integrity; therefore associated facial palsy is unusual. Recall that although the facial nerve is predominately motor, there is a sensory component that supplies a portion of the external auditory canal and pinna. Diminished sensation in this distribution is referred to as Hitselberger's sign. Large lesions are more likely to cause fifth nerve symptoms (facial numbness, diminished corneal reflex). Facial pain, presumably caused by vascular impingement on the trigeminal root entry zone, is uncommon but not rare. Intention tremor and ataxia result from cerebellar compression.

Despite the progressive nature of the hearing deficit, eighth nerve schwannomas arise from the vestibular rather than the cochlear portion of the nerve in approximately 85% of these patients. The superior and inferior vestibular nerves are equally likely to be the site of origin.

Imaging issues

The internal auditory canals have a strong tendency for symmetry, similar to the optic canals. This was the historical basis for schwannoma diagnosis with plain film and polytomography, modalities that required precise comparative

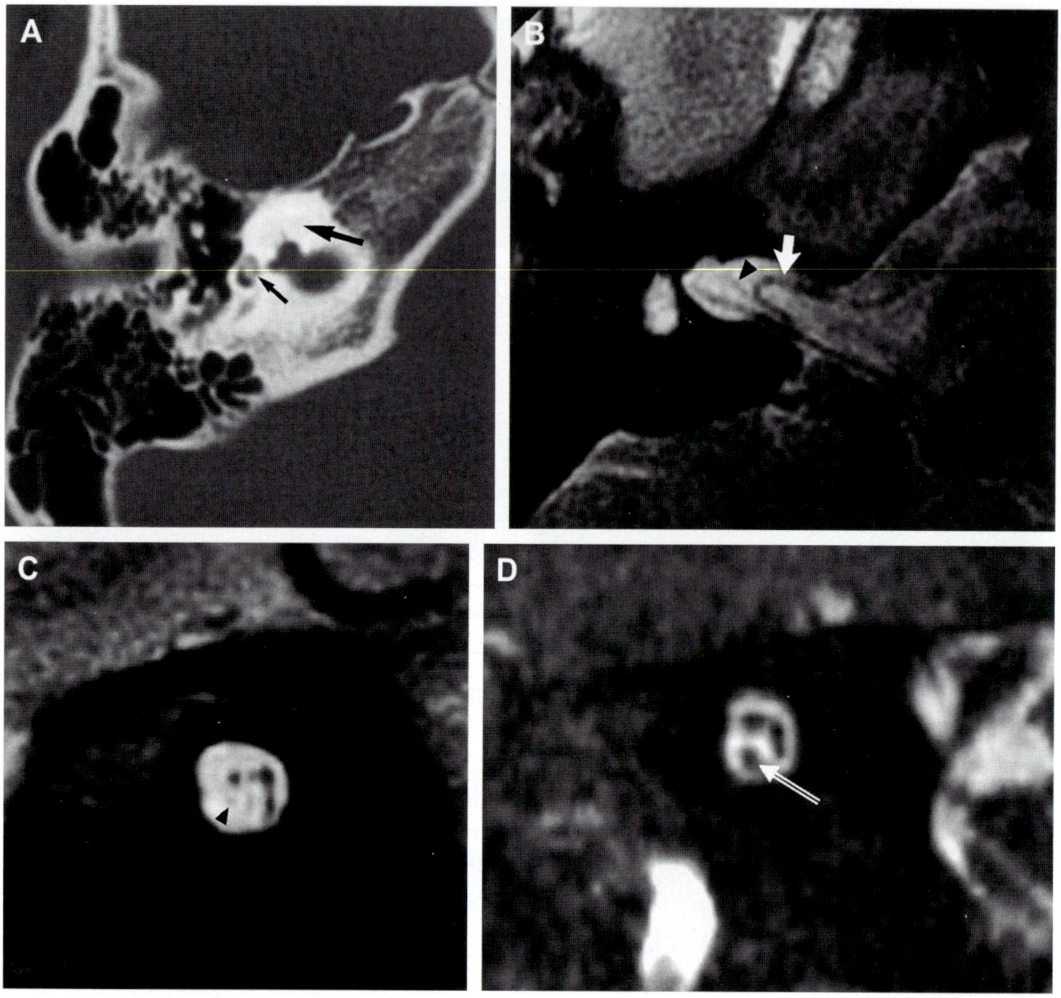

Fig. 3. Acquired cochlear nerve atrophy. (*A*) Axial CT. The cochlea (*large black arrow*) and to a lesser degree, the vestibule (*small black arrow*) are ossified. Axial (*B*) and sagittal (*C*) T2W fast-spin-echo (FSE) images. A small caliber cochlear nerve (*black arrowhead*) is identified within the anteroinferior IAC quadrant. Incidental note is made of a vascular loop (*white arrow*). (*D*) Normal axial T2W FSE image for comparison reveals a normal cochlear nerve (*white outlined arrow*). (*From* Swartz JD, Harnsberger HR. Imaging of the temporal bone. New York: Thieme, Incorporated; 1998; with permission.)

measurements and identification of subtle erosive change. With the development of CT, direct visualization of the CPA component of the tumor could be accomplished, and it simultaneously was discovered that a significant percentage of normal individuals have asymmetric IACs. Despite advancements in CT, the direct diagnosis of intracanalicular lesions remained difficult until the development of gas CT cisternography. This technique required the placement of a small amount (2 to 3 mL) of intrathecal air or CO_2 by means of lumbar puncture.[9] The patient was imaged in the decubitus position with the affected ear up. Using this technique, very small lesions first were diagnosed, and an appreciation of CPA/IAC neurovascular anatomy was mandated. The emergence of thin-section gadolinium-enhanced T1 weighted MR imaging sequences revolutionized diagnosis, as very small lesions easily could be diagnosed less invasively, and larger lesions were characterized more readily (**Figs. 5 and 6**). More recently, thin-section T2 weighted fast-spin-echo (FSE) and gradient-echo techniques have been developed that provide highly sensitive screening for these lesions without the use of gadolinium. FSE images have the advantage of far less tendency for magnetic susceptibility artifact, and resolution is increased further by the use of phased array receiver coils. Cerebrospinal fluid (CSF) provides an excellent contrast in this context, as virtually all schwannomas are of lower T2 signal intensity. This contrast is more apparent with longer TR

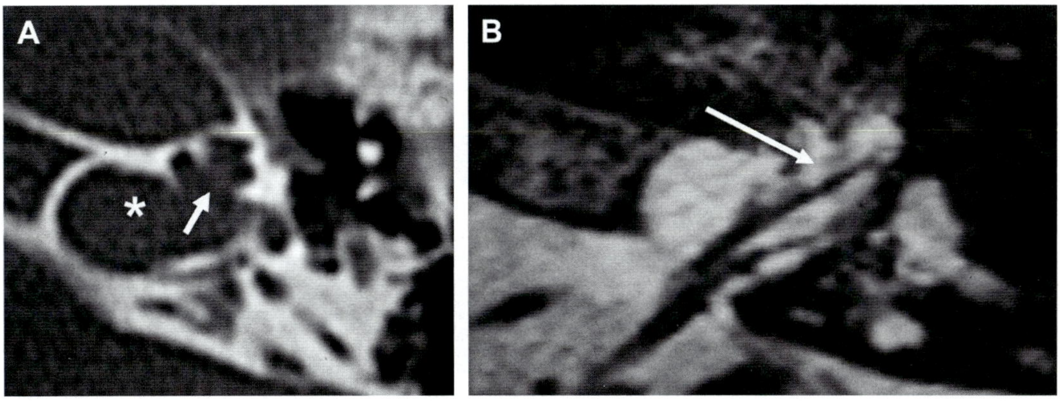

Fig. 4. X-linked deafness. (*A*) Axial CT reveals patulous internal auditory canal (IAC) (*) and large defect at IAC fundus resulting in direct communication with the cochlear apex (*white short arrow*). (*B*) Axial T2WI reveals normal caliber neural structures and confirms wide communication (*white long arrow*). (*Courtesy of* Jan W. Casselman, MD, PhD, Bruges, Belgium.)

(4000 to 5000 ms). Such long repetition times (TR) are practical because of the decreased acquisition time resulting from the long echo trains inherent to this technique.[10]

There is some disagreement regarding the precise site of origination of eighth nerve schwannomas. It has been postulated that they arise in most cases at the transition zone between the myelin produced by the oligodendroglia (central myelin) and that produced by Schwann's cells (peripheral myelin). This neuroglial/neurilemmal junction, referred to as the Obersteiner-Redlich zone, occurs most commonly at the Scarpa's (vestibular) ganglion typically (but not invariably) located at or in close proximity to the meatus (porus) of the IAC. Others have suggested that these tumors originate from Scarpa's ganglion because this is the area of the highest concentration of Schwann cells.[11] Extracanalicular lesions invariably arise in close proximity to the meatus. No vestibular Schwannoma ever has been diagnosed at the brainstem root entry zone or even within the medial half of the cisternal segment of the nerve. Schwannomas only uncommonly arise within the lateral IAC (fundus), and therefore, imaging diagnosis of intracanalicular lesions in this specific location must be viewed with suspicion (**Fig. 7**). False-positive examinations are associated with the presence of relatively faint fundal enhancement. Nonneoplastic conditions encountered during surgical exploration of these lesions has lead to speculation that perhaps a wait-and-see approach should be advocated in this circumstance, with reimaging in 6 months. Disappearance of this faint enhancement has been documented in several patients.

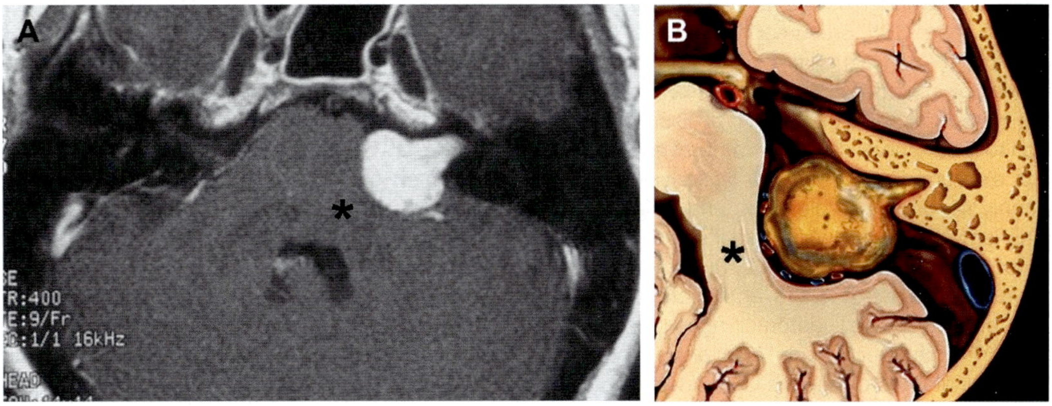

Fig. 5. 8th nerve schwanoma with corresponding drawing. (*A*) Axial T1W postcontrast image reveals an intensely enhancing cerebellopontine angle mass (CPA) mass. (*B*) Corresponding drawing depicts a mass emanating from the internal auditory canal, bulging into CPA and impinging upon the middle cerebellar peduncle. (*Courtesy of* Amirsys, Inc., Salt Lake City, UT; with permission.)

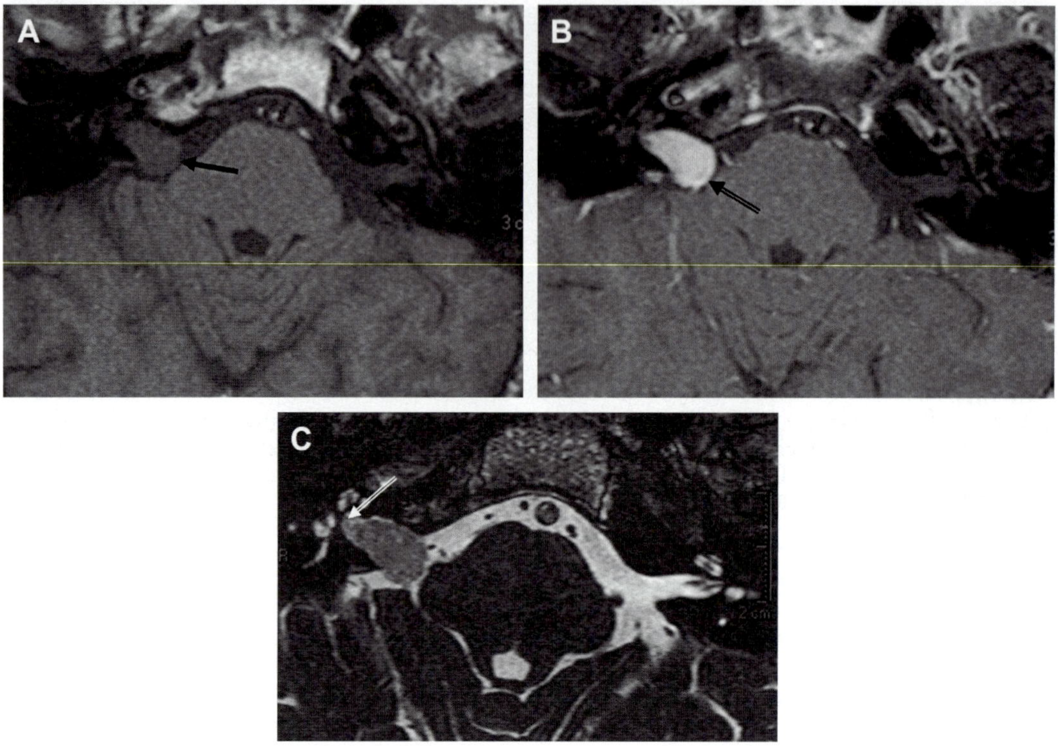

Fig. 6. 8th nerve schwannoma. (*A*) Axial T1W image. There is an isointense intracanalicular expansion (*black arrow*) bulging into the cerebellopontine angle mass. (*B*) Axial T1W image after contrast reveals intense homogeneous enhancement (*outlined black arrow*). (*C*) Axial T2W fast-spin-echo image reveals that the lesion extends throughout the fundus (*outlined white arrow*). (*Courtesy of* C.D. Phillips, MD, Charlottesville, VA.)

Histologic examination of schwannomas reveal compact Antoni type A tissue and loose textured, often cystic, Antoni type B tissue. The predominance of the Antoni type A variety helps explain this tendency toward T2 hyposignal relative to CSF. As schwannomas enlarge, regions of internal necrosis/cyst formation may result in a heterogeneous appearance. These are of higher signal intensity than CSF presumably because of the presence of hemorrhagic byproducts, necrotic material, or colloid-rich fluid. These larger lesions have a predominance of Antoni type B cells. In addition to intratumoral cysts, extramural (arachnoid) cysts also are associated with large lesions presumably secondary to elevation and deformation of the leptomeninges, which results in the formation of peritumoral adhesions, thereby creating a pseudoduplication of the arachnoid, trapping fluid between the leptomeninges and the mass.[12,13] Extramural cysts also are associated with meningiomas by means of a similar mechanism. Intratumoral hemorrhage is rare and associated with head injury or vigorous physical exertion. Both intratumoral hemorrhage and cystic expansion may result in a rapid increase in tumor volume. These patients often develop a sudden severe worsening of symptomatology (**Fig. 8**).

The reader should be aware that diminished signal intensity in the vestibule on T2-weighted images has been demonstrated in patients who have cerebellopontine angle/IAC schwannoma (acoustic neurinoma), but not in patients who have CPA meningioma. This decreased signal intensity may result from increased protein concentration in the perilymph associated with acoustic tumors.[14] Some patients who have vestibular schwannoma larger than 2 cm in diameter demonstrate a tiny area of hyperintensity in the dorsal brain stem on T2 weighted images at the lateral angle of the fourth ventricle floor. This may represent degeneration of the vestibular nucleus. This should not be confused with infarction.[15]

Eighth nerve schwannomas are typically benign and slow growing. Malignant degeneration is rare and usually associated with NF 1. These patients have an increased incidence of schwannomas; however, fewer than 5% have eighth nerve schwannoma. By contrast, the identification of bilateral eighth nerve schwannomas is the cornerstone of imaging diagnosis of the far less common

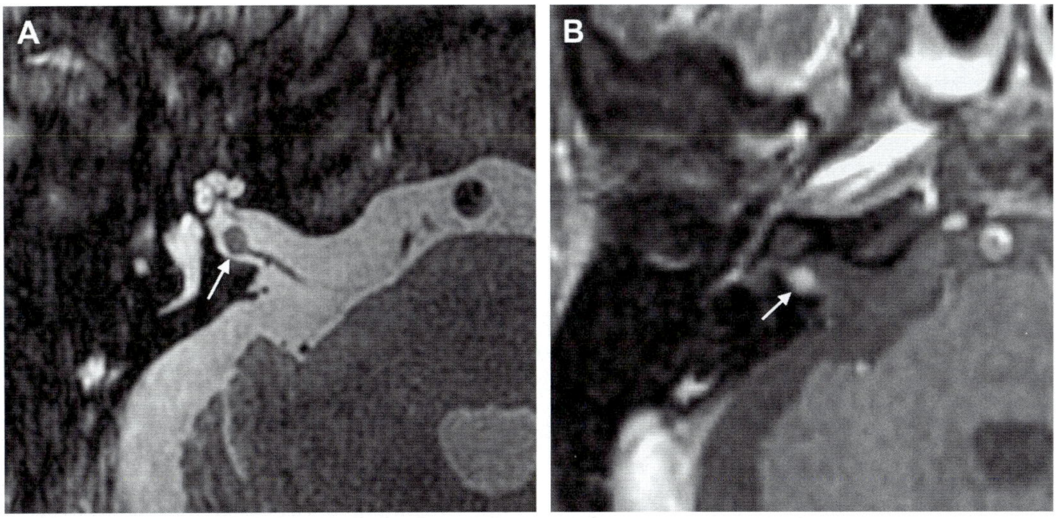

Fig. 7. 8th schwannoma of the inferior vestibular nerve. Axial T2W image (*A*) and axial postcontrast T1W image (*B*) reveals a lesion (*white arrows*) within the posteroinferior internal auditory canal quadrant at the level of the fundus. (*Courtesy of* Amirsys, Inc., Salt Lake City, UT; with permission.)

NF 2, so-called central NF (**Fig. 9**). These patients typically also have multiple meningiomas, neurofibromas, and glial tumors. Eighth nerve lesions may develop at a young age and MR imaging screening is recommended.[9] The gene responsible for this neoplasm has been isolated to the long arm of chromosome 22.

Surgical issues

The collaboration of the imaging specialist and the surgical team is required in the choice of a definitive surgical procedure when an eighth nerve tumor is diagnosed. Three major approaches are employed: translabyrinthine (TL), retrosigmoid (RS), and middle fossa (MF). Factors influencing the decision include the depth of tumor extension into the lateralmost IAC (fundal involvement), the size of a CPA component, and the prognosis for hearing conservation.[9,16]

If there is no serviceable hearing, or the prognosis for acceptable hearing is dim, the TL approach is most desirable, as surgical morbidity is reduced greatly. The TL approach is the most direct and allows for identification of the facial nerve and easy access to the fundus; it is required when an intralabyrinthine component is present. Despite

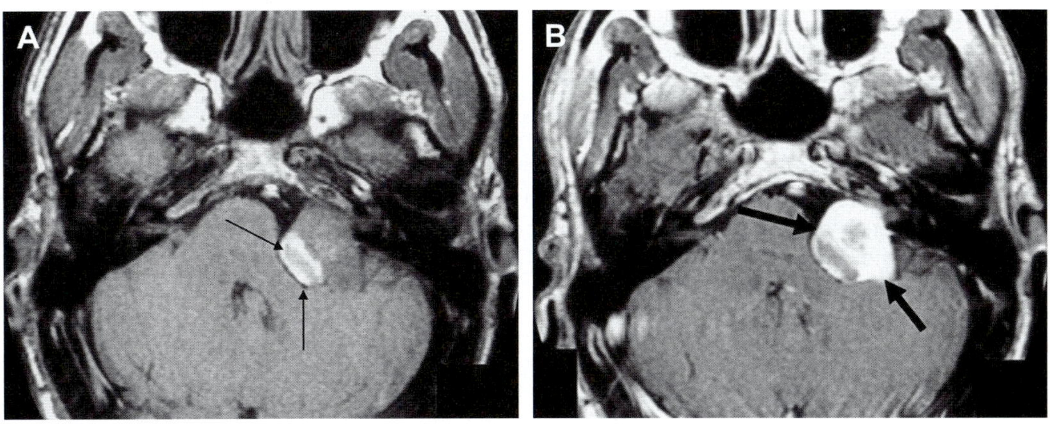

Fig. 8. 8th nerve schwannoma, hemorrhagic. (*A*) Axial T1W image, noncontrast: cerebellopontine angle mass mass with an area of hypersignal indicating the presence of methemoglobin (*thin black arrows*). (*B*) Axial T1W image, postcontrast reveals extent of lesion (*thick black arrows*). (*Courtesy of* Amirsys, Inc., Salt Lake City, UT; with permission.)

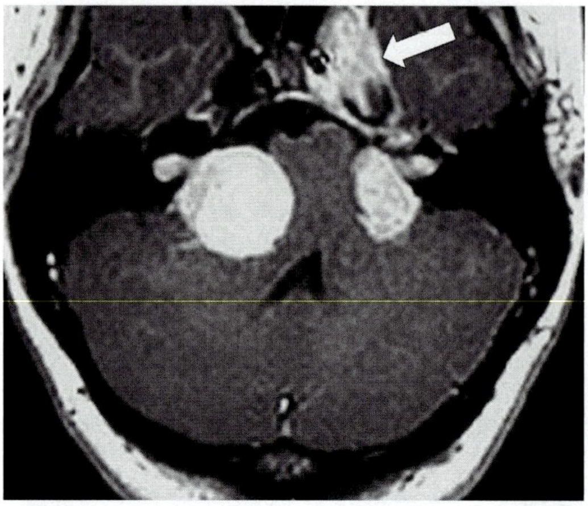

Fig. 9. Neurofibromatosis 2, bilateral vestibular schwannomas. Enhanced axial T1W image reveals bilateral intensely enhancing cerebellopontine angle mass/ internal auditory canal lesions. The right-sided lesion is larger, and there is shift of the fourth ventricle to the left. The left cavernous sinus is also abnormal (*white arrow*). (*Courtesy of* C.D. Phillips, MD, Charlottesville, VA.)

common misconception, the surgical exposure necessary for removal of large CPA components can be accomplished in experienced hands.

Hearing conservation requires either an MF or RS approach. In this context, the imaging findings become especially crucial. The presence of a significant CPA component (greater than 1.5 cm) precludes the MF technique because of inadequate surgical exposure. The presence of a fundal component precludes the RS technique, because a portion of the labyrinth would have to be removed to expose the lateral third of the IAC (see **Fig. 6**). There are strong indications that FSE magnetic resonance sequences using T2 weighting are more sensitive to the presence of fundal tumor, because bright CSF provides better contrast than the dark CSF visualized on gadolinium MR imaging (T1 weighting).

The MF approach is ideal for fundus lesions. The MF technique affords the greatest likelihood of hearing conservation but does so at the expense of the need for greater facial nerve manipulation, as the anterosuperior location of the nerve within the IAC places the nerve between the surgeon and the tumor. This is especially true when the neoplasm arises from the inferior (IVN) instead of the superior vestibular nerve (SVN).

The RS approach is another example of potential hearing preservation surgery and affords the exposure to remove lesions with large CPA components. A suboccipital craniotomy medial to the sigmoid sinus is followed by cerebellar retraction and removal of the posterior lip of the IAC.

CSF leak can occur with any of the three surgical approaches, although this complication is more common with the retrosigmoid approach and with larger tumors. Translabyrinthine surgery can result in a middle ear CSF fistula that drains through the nose through the eustachian tube, resulting in rhinorrhea.

Loss of inner ear signal on T2WI correlates with loss of hearing in patients who have undergone surgery for CPA and IAC vestibular schwannoma, perhaps reflecting developing inner ear fibrous changes or ossification.[17] Normal cochlear T2 signal is associated with hearing preservation in this circumstance.

Radiosurgery (gamma knife treatment [GKT]) may be recommended, and the imaging specialist should be familiar with this procedure and the post-treatment appearance.[18] This method has been helpful for patients who for other health reasons might be considered poor operative candidates. Often, there is paradoxically more heterogeneous enhancement in the first 6 to 12 months after GKT, as the center of the lesion undergoes cell death and fibrosis. Temporary enlargement has been reported within 2 years following treatment; therefore lesions larger than 3 cm and those with significant brainstem compression are excluded from radiosurgery.

Postoperative imaging

The imaging diagnosis of recurrent schwannoma may be challenging. Postoperative intracanalicular enhancement with gadolinium is very common. Such enhancement may be caused by recurrent tumor, adhesions, or meningeal irritation. Temporalis muscle and fascia, commonly used to seal the bony IAC defect created with the MF approach, results in a globular enhancement pattern. A linear enhancement pattern within the postoperative IAC is another predictable postoperative appearance.[19–22] Other postoperative features include T1 shortening in the labyrinth, possibly representing methemoglobin or elevated protein concentration, and the presence of new labyrinthine enhancement, which may be caused by labyrinthitis or granulation tissue. Intracanalicular enhancement also may occur within the facial nerve as the result of surgical manipulation of this structure and must not be confused with tumor recurrence.

Postoperative MR imaging study performed within 3 days after surgery may be the most helpful asset for determining the presence of residual disease and serves as a baseline study for subsequent evaluation for recurrence. Follow-up studies that demonstrate a change in the enhancement pattern should be viewed with suspicion, especially when this enhancement becomes nodular.[23] The retrosigmoid approach has the greatest risk of unintentional residual tumor in the lateral (fundal) aspect of the IAC, and this area should be searched carefully with postoperative scans.[24]

Intralabyrinthine schwannoma

Intralabyrinthine schwannomas (ILS) arise from distal branches of the cochlear, superior vestibular, or inferior vestibular nerves. They may originate from vestibular nerve fibers of any of the cristae or maculae within the vestibule or nerve fibers of the cochlear nerve within the cochlea **Box 1**.

ILS is rare, although recently a larger series and a more frequent occurrence has been reported.[25] They are somewhat more common in patients who have NF-2, but most cases are sporadic.[26] Lesions that are limited to the labyrinth are classified as intracochlear, intravestibular, and intravestibulocochlear. Lesions that also involve the IAC are described as transmodiolar (cochlea and IAC) or transmacular (vestibule and IAC) (**Figs. 10 and 11**). Lesions that also involve the middle ear are described as transotic (ME, labyrinth, and IAC) or tympanolabyrinthine (ME and labyrinth). All patients report sensorineural hearing loss that is of sudden onset in perhaps one third of cases. ILS is histologically identical to IAC counterparts and occasionally presents with Meniere-type symptoms, although recent data indicate that presentation is typically indistinguishable from that which occurs with typical eighth nerve schwannoma. A loss of conductive hearing is not uncommon and results from blockage of sound wave movement through inner ear fluid.

Box 1
Intralabyrinthine schwannoma

Localized to labyrinth

Intracochlear

Intravestibular

Intravestibulocochlear

Internal auditory canal involvement

Transmodiolar (cochlea and IAC)

Transmacular (vestibule and IAC)

Middle ear involvement

Transotic (ME, labyrinth and IAC)

Tympanolabyrinthine (ME and labyrinth)

Data from Tieleman A, Casselman JW, Somers TH, et al. Imaging of intralabyrinthine schwannomas: a retrospective study of 52 cases with emphasis on lesion growth. AJNR Am J Neuroradiol 2008 [Epub ahead of print].

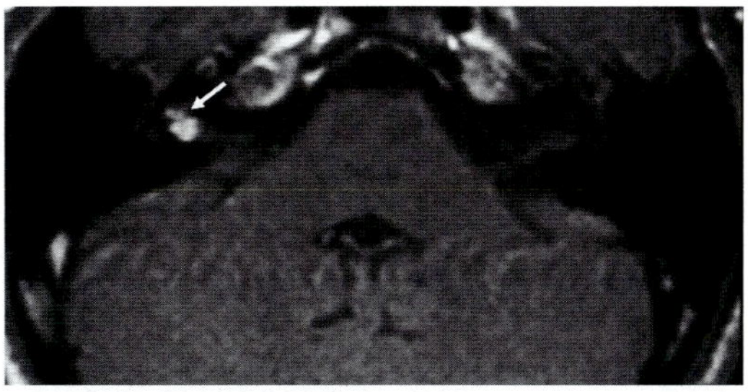

Fig. 10. Transmodiolar schwannoma. Axial enhanced T1W image reveals an enhancing lesion within the fundus of the internal auditory canal extending into the cochlea (*white arrow*). (*From* Swartz JD. Lesions of the cerebellopontine angle and internal auditory canal: diagnosis and differential diagnosis. Semin Ultrasound CT MR 2004;25(4):332–52; with permission.)

Prior to the development of modern imaging methods, diagnosis usually was made during surgical labyrinthine ablation. Currently, the mainstays of diagnosis are thin-section Gadolinium-enhanced T1 weighted images that demonstrate a focal area of intense localized enhancement within the labyrinth (**Fig. 12**).[27] This appearance is usually quite different from the faint, diffuse enhancement seen with labyrinthitis. Most cases will be discovered during routine evaluation of the "rule out acoustic" patient. The observer is encouraged to avoid IAC tunnel vision and meticulously examine the fluid-filled spaces of the labyrinth also. ILS also can be visualized with carefully preformed thin-section FSE T2WI as regions of hyposignal within the normally fluid intensity (bright) labyrinth (see **Figs. 11 and 12**).

The reader should be aware that nontumorous labyrinthine enhancement may occur secondary to a fundal IAC lesion likely caused by venous engorgement and inflammation. This is referred to as IAC block.[26]

Intralabyrinthine neoplasms other than schwannoma are even more rare. Intralabyrinthine meningiomas are also intensely enhancing lesions.[28,29] IAC meningioma likely arises from arachnoid granulations located along the dural lining of the neural foramina.[30] They may spread to the labyrinth, resulting in intense enhancement, often with ossification and demineralization reminiscent of otospongiosis. The presence of associated ossification may be the key to diagnosis, although an atypically positioned ossified hemangioma also must be considered as a differential diagnostic possibility under this circumstance.

Intravestibular lipomas have been reported manifest by precontrast T1 hypersignal, which disappears with fat suppression techniques. Neural

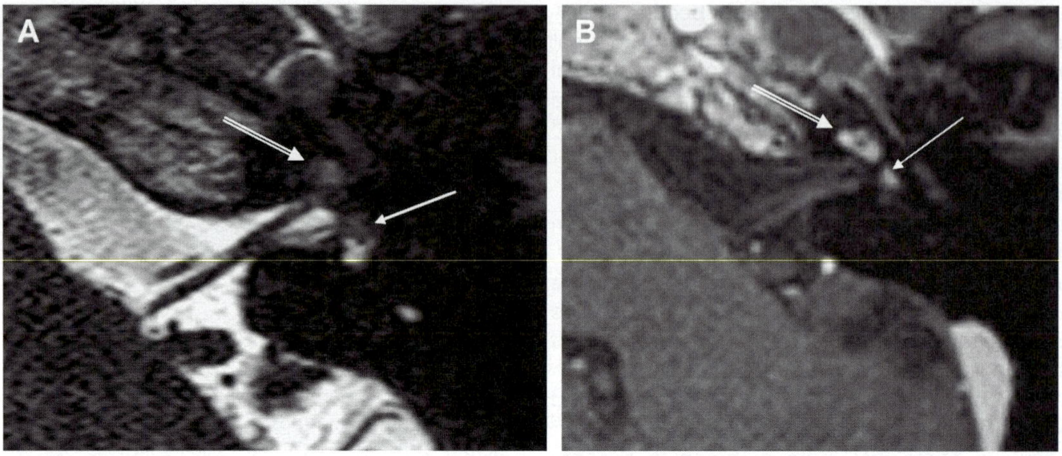

Fig. 11. Cochleovestibular schwannoma. (*A*) Axial T2W image reveals abnormal hyposignal throughout the cochlear apex (*outlined white arrow*) and a portion of the vestibule (*white arrow*). (*B*) Axial contrast-enhanced T1W image reveals abnormal enhancement throughout the cochlear apex (*outlined white arrow*) and a portion of the vestibule (*white arrow*). (*Courtesy of* Jan W. Casselman, MD, PhD, Bruges, Belgium.)

transport of the meninx primitiva along the developing eighth nerve has been proposed as an etiology.[31]

Other Cerebellopontine Angle Mass Schwannomas

Vestibular schwannoma is clearly the most common intracranial nerve sheath tumor; however, schwannomas arising from CN5 to CN12 may result in a CPA mass. The nerve of origin of most CPA schwannomas often can be determined by the clinical symptomatology and specific imaging epicenter. The facial nerve schwannoma (FS) arising in the IAC or CPA may cause the most difficulty with differentiation from vestibular schwannoma.[32] The key differentiating feature is the presence of an enhancing component extending along the labyrinthine segment of the facial nerve to the geniculate ganglion.[33] At CT, bone windows may reveal enlargement of the facial nerve canal.

Meningiomas

Meningiomas are extra-axial neoplastic lesions arising from arachnoidal cap cells.[7] Approximately 10% of all intracranial meningiomas arise in the posterior fossa. They are the second most common CPA tumor, constituting approximately 10% of masses in this location. CPA meningiomas usually arise from the posterior petrous surface or the underside of the tentorium. Intense enhancement

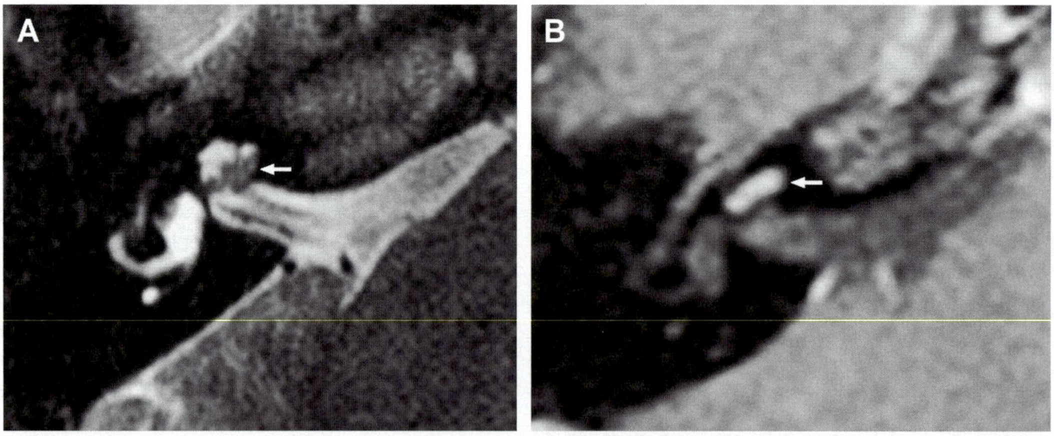

Fig. 12. Intralabyrinthine schwannoma in the cochlear apex. Axial T2W fast-spin-echo image (*A*) and axial postcontrast T1W image (*B*) reveal a mass (*white arrow*) at the cochlear apex that enhances on the contrast enhanced image. (*Courtesy of* Amirsys, Inc., Salt Lake City, UT; with permission.)

is the rule. Relative T2 hyposignal is characteristic of many of these lesions, especially the transitional and fibroblastic varieties (**Fig. 13**).[9]

Differentiation from acoustic tumor is based primarily on remoteness of the epicenter from the porus of the IAC and the presence of a broad base. Occasionally, meningiomas will masquerade as acoustic tumors when the epicenter is indeed at the meatus. Extension of tumor into the IAC is not rare in this context. The presence of a dural tail once was thought to be pathognomonic of meningioma and represent tumor extending along the adjacent dura; however, not only have histologic studies proven that the tail is often merely an inflammatory response, but numerous neoplasms and even non-neoplastic entities have been discovered to exhibit this nonspecific imaging characteristic.[34–37] Nonetheless, in some circumstances, this remains a somewhat useful imaging finding.

Up to 75% of CPA meningiomas present with hearing loss similar to acoustic tumors.[36] These tumors tend to present in middle-aged to elderly patients, especially women, and they are rare in young patients in the absence of NF2. As with meningiomas elsewhere, there is a tendency toward multiplicity, and the current and follow-up scans should be evaluated carefully for additional lesions.

As with meningiomas found elsewhere, they tend to be hyperdense to brain at noncontrast CT imaging with homogeneous contrast enhancement. Focal areas of calcification are appreciated best before contrast and evident in up to 25% of cases.

In contradistinction to schwannoma, necrosis and cystic degeneration are uncommon with meningiomas. Rarely, meningiomas may originate within the internal auditory canal, or even within the labyrinth. In these latter circumstances, differentiation from schwannoma is even more

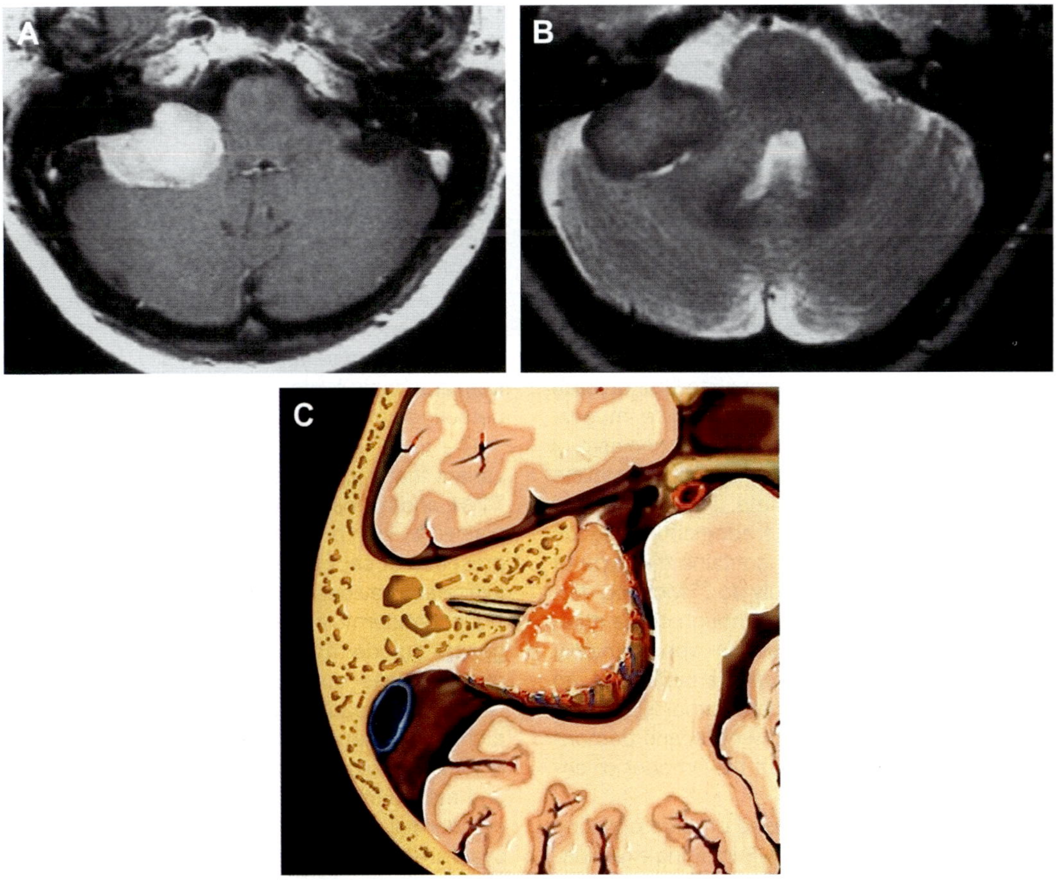

Fig. 13. Meningioma. (*A*) Axial enhanced T1W image. (*B*) Axial T2W image. (*C*) Artist rendering. There is a homogeneously enhancing cerebellopontine angle mass mass (*A*) with a broad base and epicenter along the posterior petrous surface. The lesion is hypointense on the T2W image (*B*), characteristic of meniningioma (see text). There is fourth ventricle displacement confirming mass effect. Artist rendering (*C*) indicates a broad-base lesion that does not emanate from the IAC. (*Courtesy of* Amirsys, Inc., Salt Lake City, UT; with permission.)

difficult. IAC meningiomas may spread to the labyrinth, often with ossification and demineralization reminiscent of otospongiosis. Relative T2 hypointensity is a helpful imaging finding, suggesting dense cellularity, and supports a diagnosis of tumor rather than reactive enhancement.[38–40]

Epidermoid

An epidermoid is an ectodermal inclusion that develops during neural tube closure in the third to fifth week of embryogenesis and comprises .2% to 1.8% of primary intracranial masses. Histologically identical to congenital cholesteatoma, they consist of a sac of exfoliated keratin lined by stratified squamous epithelium. They grow very slowly by means of desquamation and therefore often do not present until adulthood despite their congenital etiology. Epidermoids may become quite large before becoming symptomatic, because they have a strong tendency to grow along paths of least resistance, and, as such, conform to the surface of the brain tending to surround (encase) normal neural and vascular structures rather than displace or invade them. This tendency also often makes complete surgical resection difficult.[41,42]

The CPA is the most common location for the intracranial epidermoid (40% to 50%). They are the third most common overall CPA/IAC mass (3% to 7%) (after acoustic schwannoma and meningioma).

At CT, most epidermoids are CSF density and do not enhance. Calcification is present in 10% to 25% of cases. An occasional lesion will have a faintly enhancing border or flecks of calcification.

Most epidermoids are isointense to CSF on both T1 and T2 weighted magnetic resonance images. They exhibit this signal, because the cholesterol in epidermoid tumors is in the solid/crystalline state rather than the liquid state. The latter would result in bright T1 signal. The adamantinomatous craniopharyngioma typically contains this type of cholesterol; epidermoids rarely do.[41] Most epidermoid cysts do not enhance, although some minimal rim enhancement occurs in approximately 25% of cases. Malignant transformation of an epidermoid (squamous cell carcinoma) is rare but should be considered if follow-up scans demonstrate a significant increase in the amount of enhancement (**Box 2**).

Often, MR imaging is focused on differentiation from arachnoid cyst. Careful MR imaging examination commonly will reveal multiple internal septations within the epidermoid that are not present with arachnoid cyst. Furthermore, many epidermoids often have a lamellated appearance because of surface desquamation. This lamellation

Box 2
Imaging epidermoid and arachnoid cyst

Epidermoid

Internal septations

Lamellated appearance

Encase

Insinuate

Higher signal than csf on flair

Diffusion weighted imaging (DWI): restricted diffusion-marked hyperintensity

Arachnoid cyst

Homogeneous

Smooth contour

Displace

Expand

Identical to CSF on flair

DWI: unrestricted diffusion—identical to CSF

as well as the tendency to have internal septations and to insinuate rather than displace are far more characteristic of epidermoid. They do not suppress completely on fluid-attenuated inversion recovery imaging and therefore are higher in signal intensity than CSF.[43] State-of-the-art differentiation of epidermoids from arachnoid cysts requires DWI (**Fig. 14**). Epidermoids are bright on diffusion imaging because of low water diffusability (low apparent diffusion coefficient, or ADC). This restricted diffusion results in marked hyperintensity, quite different from arachnoid cysts.[44] DWI signal also is useful for detecting postoperative residual epidermoid.[45]

The rare "white epidermoid" is an interesting variant that is hyperdense at CT, hyperintense on T1WI, and hypointense on T2W.[46] This may be explained by high protein content, hemorrhage or the presence of saponified keratinized debris, and as indicated previously, cholesterol in the liquid state.

Like epidermoid cysts, dermoid *cysts* are congenital ectodermal inclusions but are extremely rare, far less common than epidermoid cysts. Growth can lead to rupture of the cyst, causing a chemical meningitis. A common misconception is that dermoid cysts arise from both ectodermal and mesodermal elements. Their origin is entirely ectodermal. Imaging findings vary. Unruptured cysts are hyperintense, similar to fat on T1 weighted images. The masses have heterogeneous signal intensity on T2-weighted magnetic resonance images and vary from hypo- to hyperintense. Fat-like leptomeningeal and intraventricular deposits are diagnostic of a ruptured dermoid cyst.[47]

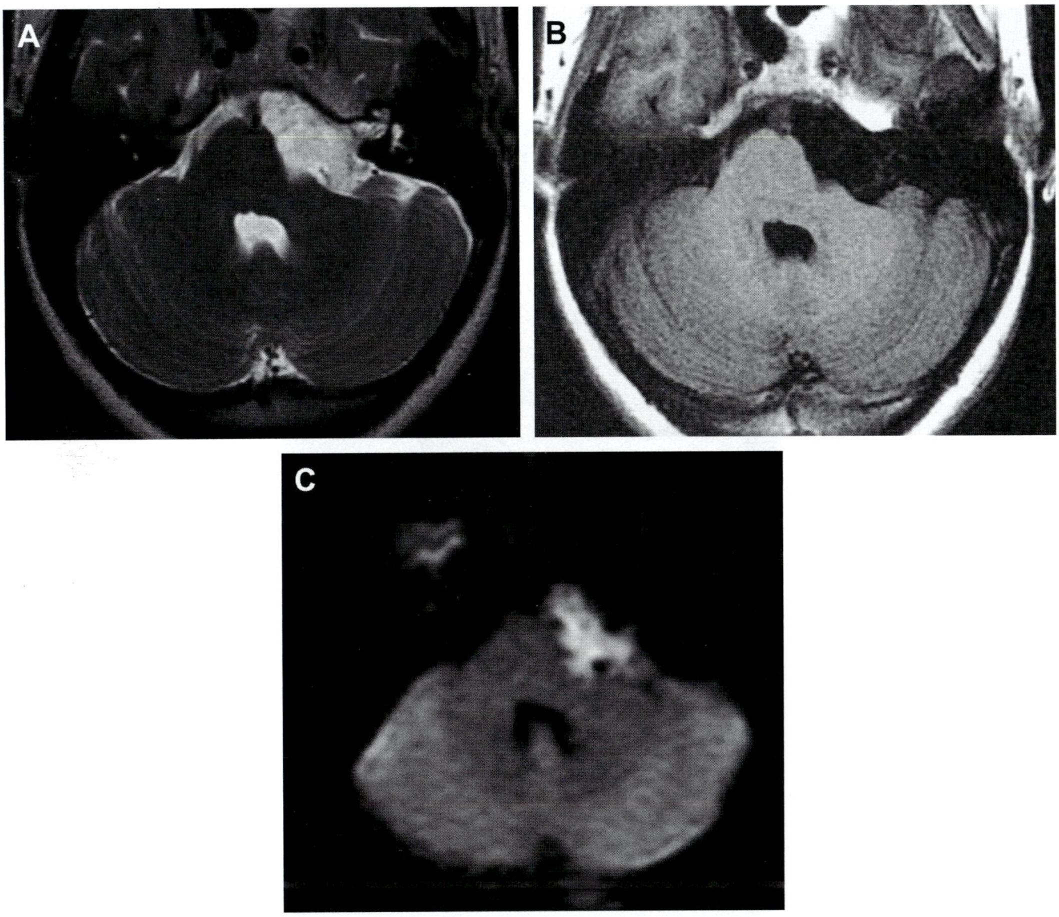

Fig. 14. Epidermoid. (*A*) Axial T2W image. (*B*) Axial T1W image. (*C*) Axial diffusion image. (*D*) Artist rendering. There is a homogeneous mass in the left cerebellopontine angle mass, isointense with cerebrospinal fluid (*A,B*) and with fourth ventricle displacement. There is restricted diffusion (*C*). (*Courtesy of* C.D. Phillips, MD, Charlottesville, VA.)

Arachnoid Cysts

Arachnoid cysts are benign space-occupying lesions containing CSF. They reside entirely within the subarachnoid space but are surrounded by a thin membrane. They are typically unilocular, smoothly marginated, and expansile; they do not communicate with the ventricular system.

The precise mechanism for arachnoid cyst development is unknown. These lesions may develop through failure of embryonic meninges to merge or they may occur secondary to "splitting" of the developing arachnoid. Arachnoid cysts are generally stable over time.[48] The cyst wall is lined by flattened arachnoid cells rather than epithelium.

Most arachnoid cysts are supratentorial. Fifty percent to 60% are found in the middle cranial fossa, anterior to the temporal lobes. Approximately 10% occur in the posterior fossa, most commonly in the CPA.

Arachnoid cysts are well demarcated extra-axial lesions that can displace adjacent structures. There is no identifiable internal architecture. They are isodense to CSF at CT and isointense to CSF on all magnetic resonance sequences. They do not enhance with either modality (**Fig. 15**). Occasionally, hemorrhage, high protein content, or lack of flow within the cyst may complicate the magnetic resonance appearance. As discussed previously, the most difficult lesion to distinguish from the arachnoid cyst is epidermoid.

Meningeal Metastases

Cerebellopontine angle metastatic disease can present as a distinct extra-axial mass mimicking schwannoma/meningioma or as meningeal metastases associated with diffuse seeding of the CSF (**Fig. 16**). Meningeal metastases is referred to by several ambiguous terms including

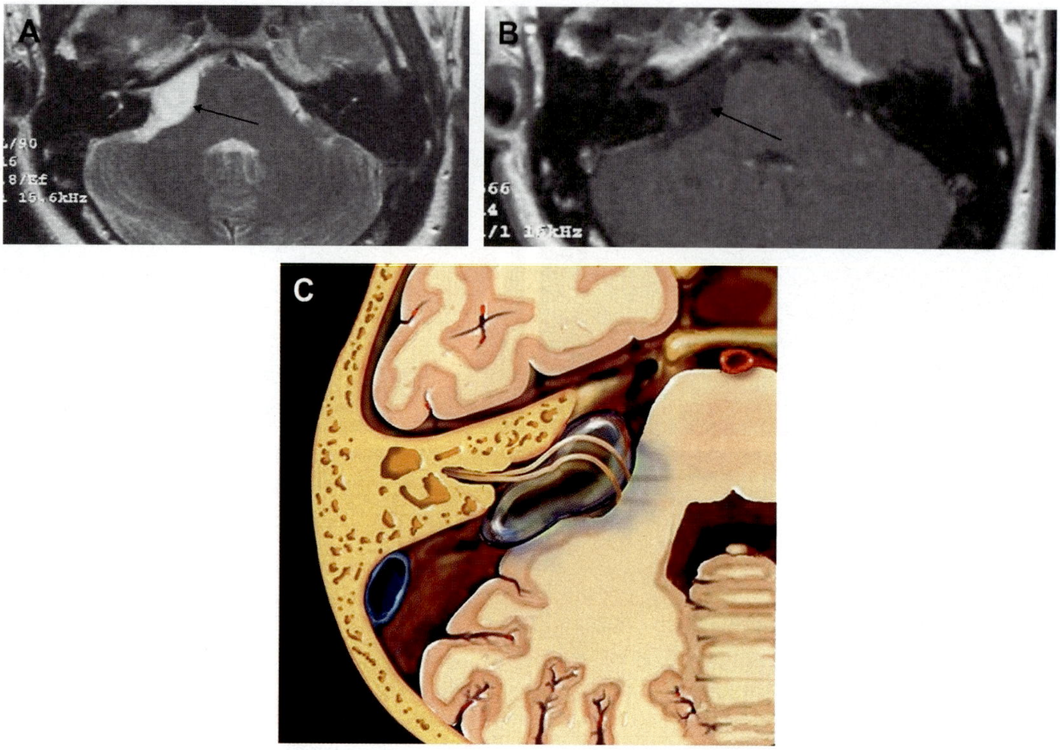

Fig. 15. Arachnoid cyst. (*A*) Axial T2W image. (*B*) Axial enhanced T1W image. (*C*) Artist's rendering. There is a homogeneous fluid intensity nonenhancing right cerebellopontine angle mass mass (*black arrow*), compatible with an arachnoid cyst. The diffusion images were negative (*unrestricted diffusion*). Drawing illustrates that these lesions displace rather than encase the neural structures. (*Courtesy of* Amirsys, Inc., Salt Lake City, UT; with permission.)

leptomeningeal carcinomatosis, meningeal carcinomatosis, and carcinomatous meningitis.[9] These terms are inexact, as these neoplasms are not always carcinomas. Additionally, they often involve the pachymeninges and the leptomeninges and may not contain an inflammatory (-itis) component.[49] Meningeal metastases from solid tumors (ie, breast) and lymphoproliferative malignancy

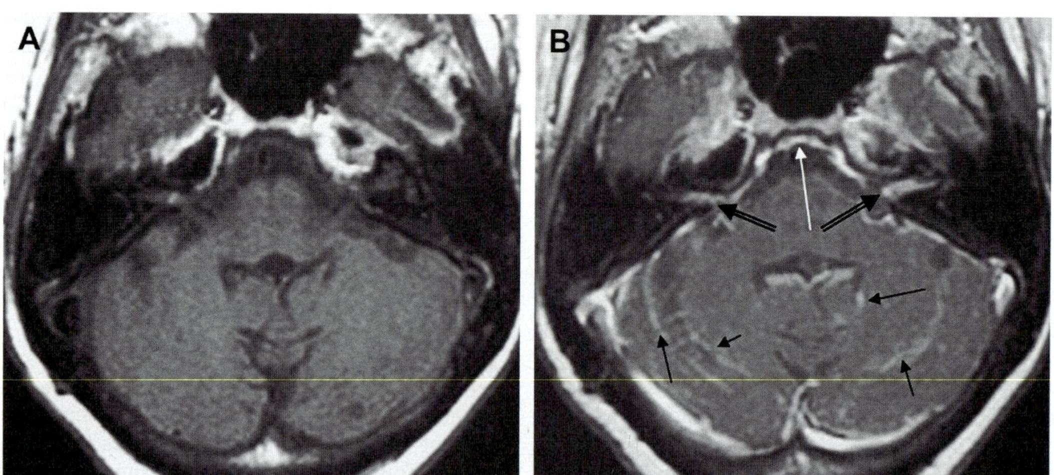

Fig. 16. Meningeal metastases. (*A*) Axial unenhanced T1W image. (*B*) Axial enhanced T1W image. There is diffuse enhancement within the internal auditory canal bilaterally (*black outlined arrows*). In addition, there is diffuse thickening and enhancement of the leptomeninges (*black arrows*) and pachymeninges (*white arrow*).

(ie, lymphoma) involve both the pachymeninges and the leptomeninges. Seeding from primary central nervous system (CNS) tumors involve only the leptomeninges. Leptomeningeal neoplasm may be diffuse or discrete and nodular. Nodular disease may masquerade as a primary neoplasm such as schwannoma or meningioma. Involvement of multiple cranial nerves is common. In this context, both facial nerve dysfunction and vertigo/hearing loss may result from CPA/IAC dissemination. A new diagnosis of NF2 in an adult patient should be considered suspect even when bilateral CPA/IAC lesions are diagnosed, and a thorough search should be performed for other intracranial metastases and the CSF sampled for malignant cells. Metastatic melanoma has a predilection for the leptomeninges and as such distinctively involve the IAC/CPA.[50] Amelanotic lesions appear identical to schwannoma; however, melanotic lesions are hyperintense on precontrast T1WI, resulting in a confusing imaging picture suggestive of lipomatous infiltratration. There is no fat suppression, which aids in diagnosis.

Lipoma and Mimics

Lipomas are composed of mature adipose tissue, which is thought to arise from aberrant differentiation of the meninx primitiva. They are mesodermal inclusions, distinguishing them from epidermoid and dermoid, which are ectodermal in nature. They may be found in the CPA, IAC, or even more rarely, within the vestibule. Intracanalicular lipomas, despite their rarity, mandate routine precontrast thin-section T1 weighted images as part of a complete IAC examination.[51]

At CT, lipomas are of fatty density and do not enhance. At MR imaging, they follow the signal intensity of fat, with suppression of signal on fat saturation images (**Fig. 17**).

CPA lipomas may present with symptoms related to cranial nerve irritation such as trigeminal neuralgia (CN5) or hemifacial spasm (CN7). Most commonly, they present with vertigo and hearing loss (CN8). Conservative management usually is preferred unless the symptoms are disabling, as neurovascular structures often pass through or are adherent to the lesion.

Noncontrast T1 hypersignal also could result from a dermoid; in particular, ruptured dermoid must be considered in the differential diagnosis if CPA/IAC hypersignal is accompanied by numerous other subarachnoid hyperintense deposits.

Retained pantopaque (iophendylate) also has signal characteristics identical to fat. T1 hypersignal within the IAC masquerading as lipoma has been described. Clinical history of previous myelogram is needed to suggest this diagnosis.[9]

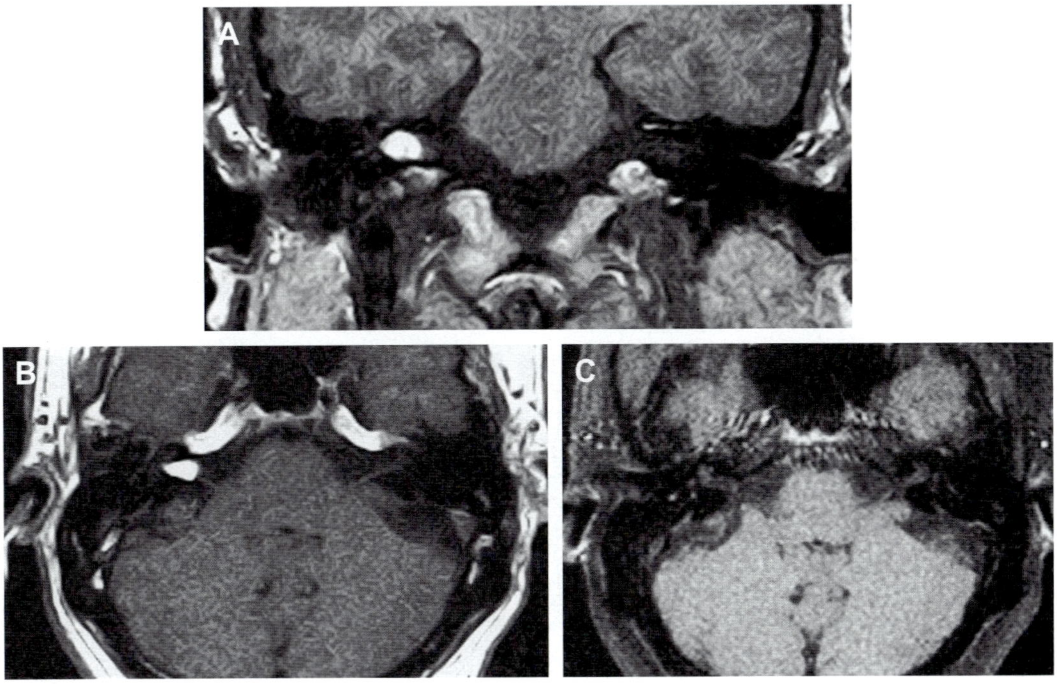

Fig. 17. Lipoma, intracanalicular. Axial (*A*) and coronal T1W image (*B*) reveal a hyperintense intracanalicular expansion. (*C*) Axial T1W fat-suppressed image confirms the diagnosis of lipoma. (*Courtesy of* C.D. Phillips, MD, Charlottesville, VA.)

Hamartomas of the IAC also have a tendency for adherence to neurovascular structures, making resection technically difficult.[52] Lipochoristomas are rare tumors of the acoustic nerve containing mature adipose tissue mixed with varied amounts of fibrous tissue, vessels, and muscle fibers.[53]

Primary Parenchymal Neoplasms

Lesions of the brainstem or cerebellum rarely may have an exophytic component resulting in a CPA mass. Careful attention to all magnetic resonance pulse sequences usually will reveal an infiltrative intra-axial component that clarifies the diagnosis. Childhood neoplasms such as medulloblastoma, astrocytoma, and ependymoma may present in this fashion. Astrocytoma is the most common lesion to result in this phenomenon in the adult patient.

Choroid Plexus Papilloma

The choroid plexus courses into the lateral recess of the fourth ventricle by means of the foramen of Luschka and extends as far laterally as the CPA; therefore, choroid plexus papilloma must be kept in mind when a CPA mass is identified. Intense homogeneous enhancement with iodinated contrast (CT) and gadolinium (MR imaging) is the rule.[54]

ADDITIONAL DIFFERENTIAL DIAGNOSTIC ENTITIES

Vascular

Vascular loops

Surgical decompression of a vascular loop is often useful in the treatment of unremitting facial pain (fifth nerve) and hemifacial spasm (seventh nerve). There is, however, considerable debate as to whether vascular loops can produce auditory or vestibular symptoms.[55–57] A recent study attempted to correlate hearing loss with AICA loops.[55] The study's authors used the following definitions: type 1 loops (within the CPA), type 2 loops (at the porus extending up to 50% of IAC), and type 3 loops (extending beyond 50% of IAC). These authors found a statistically significant association with unilateral hearing loss and type 2 and 3 AICA loops. Other studies, however, have been less supportive of surgical intervention. These have indicated that radiologic demonstration of contact between a vascular loop formed by the AICA and the eighth cranial nerve on MR imaging scans should be considered a normal anatomic finding and should not, on its own, be used to support the diagnosis of a vascular compression syndrome. Clinical correlation is needed, and a cause and effect may be difficult to establish (**Fig. 18**). I would certainly advise that all vascular structures within the CPA/IAC be reported to the referring physician.

Aneurysms

Aneurysms localized to the CPA/IAC may arise from the AICA.[58,59] They are rare and may be misinterpreted as vestibular schwannoma (**Fig. 19**). They may present with headache (subarachnoid hemorrhage); however, symptoms related to facial and vestibulocochlear nerve dysfunction frequently are described. At CT, AICA aneurysms are usually slightly hyperdense with strong uniform enhancement. Multidetector CT angiography depicts these lesions to excellent advantage, even when they are intracanalicular in nature. At MR imaging, a flow void is expected on T1 and T2 weighted images unless thrombus is present, which may result in variable signal intensities.

Cavernous hemangiomas

Cavernous hemangiomas of the IAC are rare.[60,61] They manifest increased T1 signal and focal regions of decreased T2 signal. There is typically a heterogeneous enhancement pattern and regions of increased magnetic susceptibility.

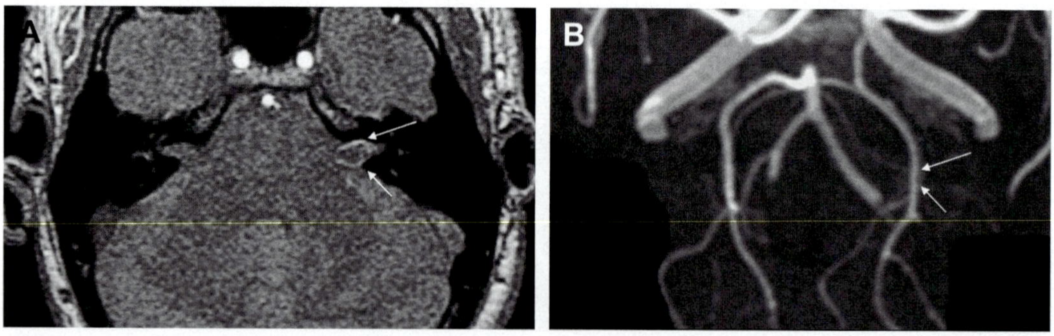

Fig. 18. Vascular loop, hearing loss, and vertigo. (*A*) Magnetic resonance angiography source image reveals that the loop (*white arrows*) extends into the canal as far as the fundus. (*B*) Conventional angiogram confirms an anterior inferior cerebellar artery loop (*white arrows*). (*Courtesy of* C.D. Phillips, MD, Charlottesville, VA.)

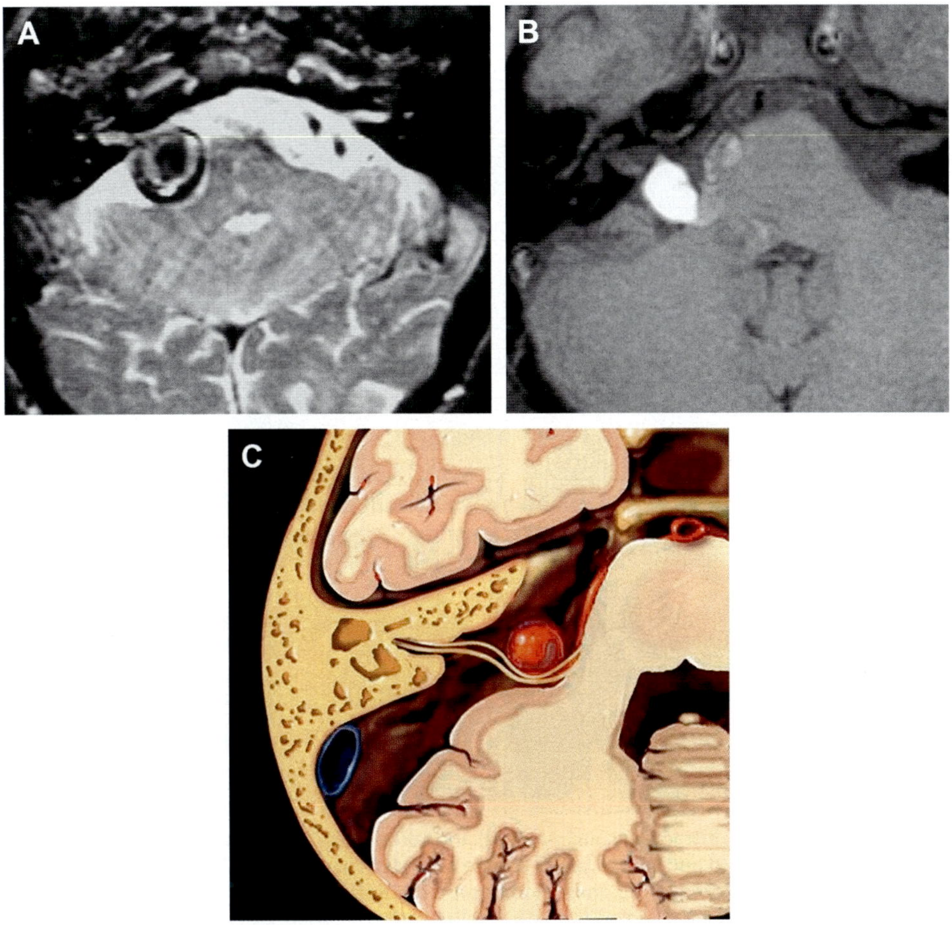

Fig. 19. Aneurysm in the cerebellopontine angle. (*A*) Axial T2W fast-spin-echo image reveals a cerebellopontine angle mass containing regions of heterogeneous T2 hyposignal, indicating the presence of hemorrhage in this partially thrombotic aneurysm. (*B*) The axial source image reveals T1 hypersignal. (*C*) Corresponding drawing depicts an aneurysm displacing the neural structures. (*Courtesy of* Amirsys, Inc., Salt Lake City, UT; with permission.)

Multiple cavernoma syndrome is a familial process that can present in an autosomal dominant fashion.

Vascular malformations

Areteriovenous malformations characterized by enlarged intensely enhancing vessels are rare in the CPA. As with other cerebral AVMs, angiography will demonstrate the feeding and draining vessels best and determine the best therapeutic management. An important differential is the acquired dural arteriovenous fistula with venous varix.

Ossifying hemangioma

Ossifying hemangioma is an uncommon but well-known temporal bone lesion, typically originating along the facial nerve canal, particularly at the first genu.[62] This lesion is characterized by intense contrast enhancement and bony spiculations similar to hemangiomas noted elsewhere. Hemangiomas of the IAC tend to be more symptomatic than an acoustic schwannoma of equal size (**Fig. 20**). Differentiation from meningioma may be difficult.

Non-Neoplastic Meningeal Disease

Overview

The meninges are the dura, dense connective tissue attached to the calvarium, the pia, a membrane firmly attached to the surface of the brain, and the arachnoid, which is a complex network of reticular fibers interposed between the pia and the dura.[50] Importantly, the pia and arachnoid collectively are referred to as the leptomeninges; the dura is referred to as the pachymeninges.

The leptomeninges is contiguous with the vestibulocochlear nerve. Any leptomeningeal disease process may manifest within the IAC and cause

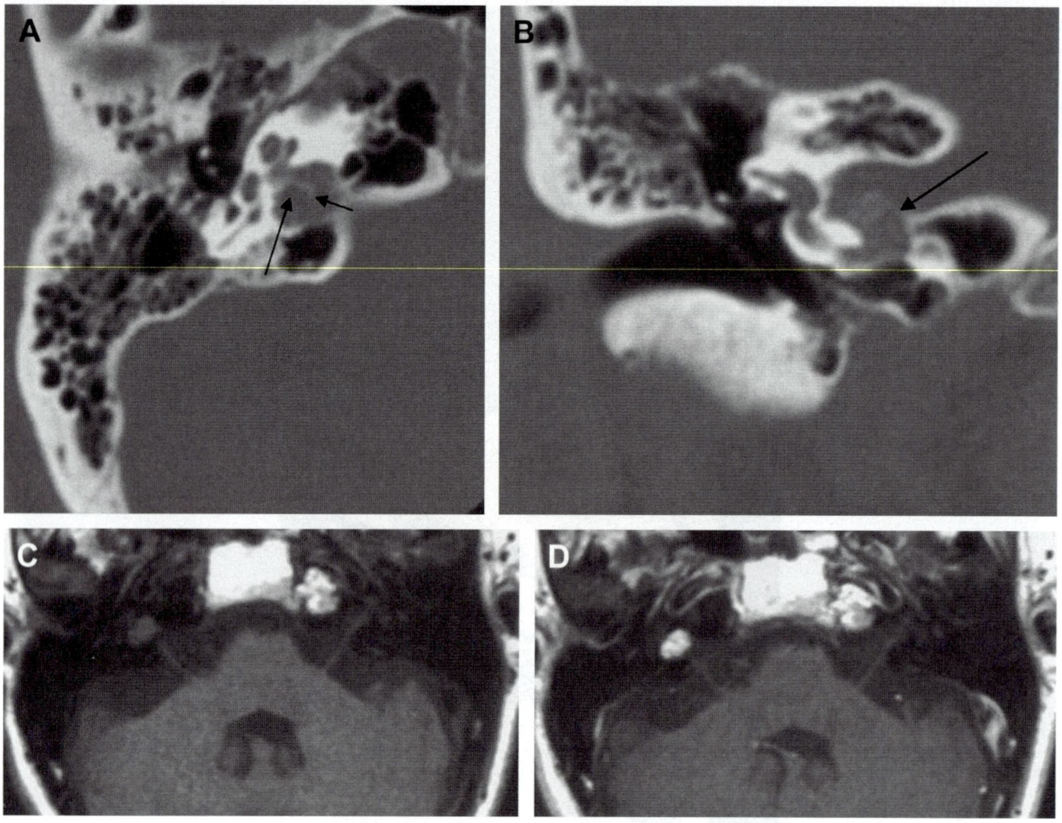

Fig. 20. Ossifying hemangioma, intracanalicular. Axial (*A*) and coronal (*B*) CT images reveal an eccentric expansion within the fundus of the internal auditory canal. There are calcifications within the lesion (*black arrows in A*), and a generalized hyperdensity is noted in (*B*). These findings are highly suggestive of an ossifying hemangioma. Axial precontrast (*C*) and postcontrast (*D*) images reveal intense contrast enhancement. (*From* Swartz JD. Lesions of the cerebellopontine angle and internal auditory canal: diagnosis and differential diagnosis. Semin Ultrasound CT MR 2004;25(4):332–52; with permission.)

vertigo or retrocochlear hearing loss. Pathologic enhancement within the CPA and IAC may occur as a consequence of the entire gamut of meningeal disease. There is extensive overlap in the imaging appearance of benign and malignant disease.

Meningitis

Meningitis may result in pathologic leptomeningeal enhancement identical to that caused by neoplasm and commonly involves the IAC/CPA. Bacterial and fungal diseases are more predisposed to this manifestation than viral disease.[63]

Neurosarcoidosis

Neurosarcoidosis occurs in up to 25% of patients who have systemic sarcoidosis and typically manifests as leptomeningeal thickening and enhancement (**Fig. 21**). The leptomeninges are involved somewhat more commonly than the pachymeninges. This granulomatous process may result in both diffuse and nodular enhancement patterns. IAC/CPA involvement is not uncommon and is often bilateral, perhaps masquerading as NF-2. This often results in retrocochlear sensorineural hearing loss.[9] Involvement of other cranial nerves is also very common.

Additional conditions

Pathologic enhancement of the meninges may result from various additional conditions. Pachymeningeal enhancement routinely is seen in postcraniotomy patients. On occasion, such enhancement is extensive and quite thick and may persist for several years. Intracranial hypotension may be spontaneous or result from lumbar puncture or head trauma.[64] The spontaneous variety (SIHH) is associated with a distinctive postural headache. Occult CSF leak is the presumed cause. The meningeal enhancement associated with this condition is often quite extensive and is most commonly pachymeningeal but may involve the leptomeninges including the IAC (**Fig. 22**).

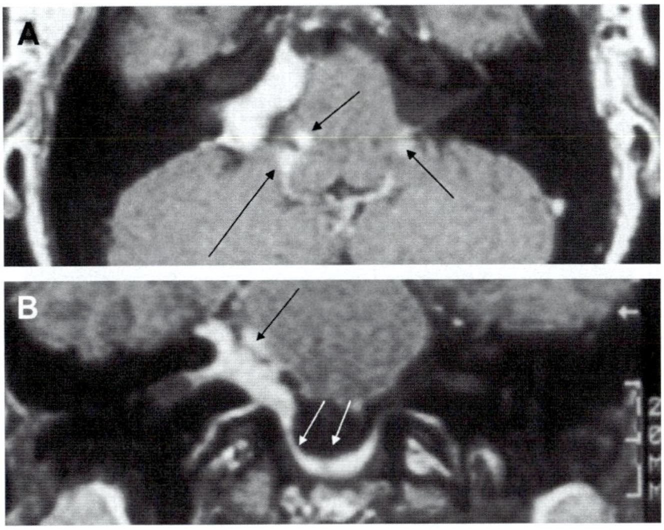

Fig. 21. Neurosarcoidosis. Axial (*A*) and coronal (*B*) enhanced T1W image reveals a cerebellopontine angle mass and nodules of enhancement in the adjacent leptomeninges (*black arrows*) and pachymeninges (*white arrows*). (*From* Swartz JD. Lesions of the cerebellopontine angle and internal auditory canal: diagnosis and differential diagnosis. Semin Ultrasound CT MR 2004;25(4):332–52; with permission.)

Miscellaneous Conditions

Siderosis

Superficial siderosis is characterized by deposition of hemosiderin in the leptomeninges resulting from subarachnoid hemorrhage that overwhelms the ability of the blood stream to remove the hemosiderin-laden macrophages.[65,66] Hearing impairment is an important feature, and its absence is exceptional.[66]

The vestibulocochlear nerve (VCN) is vulnerable to hemosiderin for several reasons. The VCN is lined extensively with central myelin, which is supported by microglia. These microglia are uniquely sensitive to iron-mediated cell damage. Furthermore, the VCN has a long and tortuous course and as such is exposed to substantial CSF flow. The olfactory tract and bulb are also vulnerable because of their similar anatomy.[66]

MR imaging findings of siderosis are pathognomonic. T2 weighted and, in particular, gradient echo susceptibility imaging reveals characteristic hypointensity most easily appreciated along the surface of the brain stem and cerebellar vermis (**Fig. 23**). The multiple refocusing 180° pulses of FSE imaging may make the hemosiderin less apparent as they reduce the T2* effect, and low field magnets are also less susceptible to the paramagnetic effects of hemosiderin. Gradient echo imaging is the ideal sequence as it results in blooming of the T2* effect.

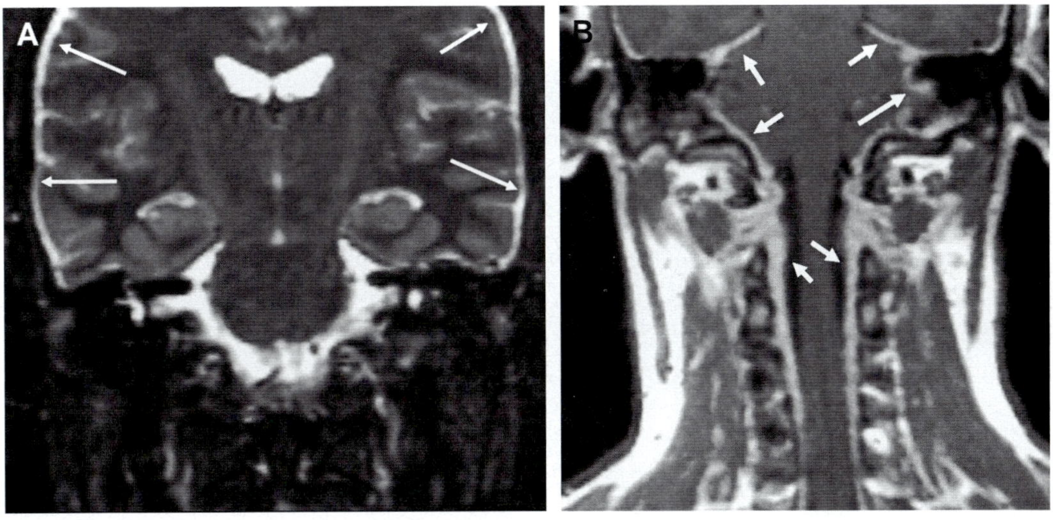

Fig. 22. Intracranial hypotension in a 34-year-old patient with postural headaches. (*A*) Coronal T2W image reveals T2 hypersignal reflecting thickening of the pachymeninges (*white arrows*). (*B*) Enhanced coronal T1W image confirms pathologic thickening and enhancement along the tentorium, cerebellopontine angles, and the cervical epidural space (*white arrows*).

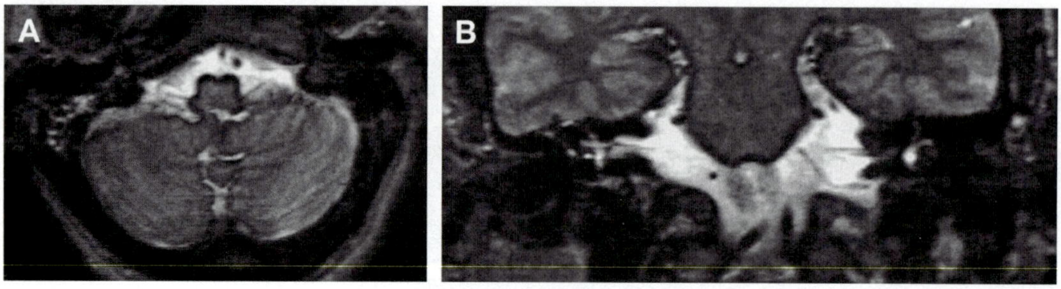

Fig. 23. Siderosis. Axial (*A*) and coronal (*B*) T2W images reveal extensive T2 hyposignal along the surface of the brainstem and temporal lobes, reflecting increased magnetic susceptibility caused by hemosiderin deposition.

The extent of siderosis does not necessarily correlate with the severity of clinical disease.[65,66] Some patients who have extensive imaging evidence have minimal symptoms, whereas others with less severe findings may be debilitated significantly.

Labyrinthitis

Labyrinthitis refers to inflammatory disease of the perilymphatic spaces of the inner ear, which results in secondary changes within the endolymphatic spaces (membranous labyrinth).[67] The most common symptoms are sensorineural hearing loss and vertigo, which may be recurrent or debilitating.

Tympanogenic labyrinthitis is typically unilateral and secondary to middle ear disease. Meningogenic labyrinthitis is usually bilateral and occurs secondary to meningitis. The latter probably results from spread by means of the fundus of the IAC into the vestibule or by means of the cochlear nerve foramen into the cochlear apex with internal dissemination via the modiolus.[68] Propagation by means of the cochlear aqueduct is probably less common. Meningogenic labyrinthitis typically occurs in children and is the most common cause of acquired childhood deafness.[69]

Labyrinthitis may be viral (most common) as well as autoimmune, bacterial or luetic. Otosyphilis also may manifest as an osteitis, resulting in otic capsule demineralization or a meningitis involving the IAC.[70]

The classic imaging finding in acute/subacute labyrinthitis is enhancement of the normally nonenhancing fluid-filled spaces of the labyrinth as seen on contrast-enhanced T1 weighted images (**Fig. 24**).[71] The reader should be aware that most patients diagnosed with viral labyrinthitis will not have labyrinthine enhancement (or any other imaging finding).

If acute labyrinthitis does not resolve, a progression to chronic disease initially results in fibrous changes followed by ossification. The fibrous stage of this disorder manifests as T2 hyposignal on MR

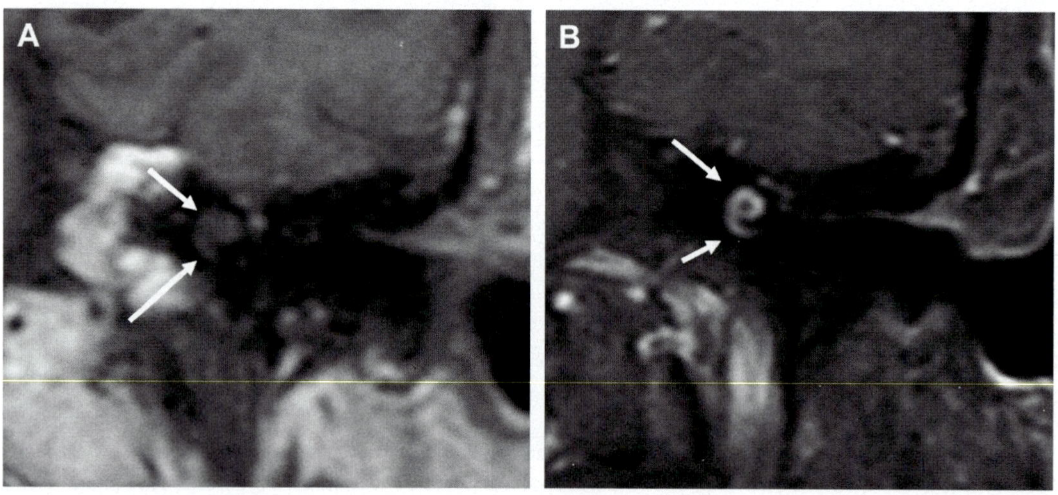

Fig. 24. Viral labyrinthitis. Recent onset of hearing loss and vertigo in a 47-year-old man. (*A*) Precontrast coronal T1W image of the left ear. (*B*) Postcontrast coronal T1W image of the left ear. The normally fluid-filled spaces of the anterior cochlear turns enhance intensely after contrast administration (*white arrows*).

imaging and a normal CT. The ossific stage is characterized by labyrinthine ossification at CT that often is profound (see **Fig. 3**). MR imaging is also abnormal at this stage. Intermediate stages also exist.

Trauma

Hearing loss is a common sequela of temporal bone injury. SNHL may of course result from fracture through the IAC or bony labyrinth; however, it may also develop because of a severe concussive force (labyrinthine concussion) in the absence of demonstrable fracture.[67] There are no CT findings, and MR imaging is negative unless intralabyrinthine hemorrhage is present. SNHL also could result from brain stem contusion at the level of the upper medulla. Shearing force at the root entry zone is an additional cause. Rarely, contusions of the inferior colliculi may be diagnosed consequent to the traumatic event. Impaction of tentorium against the dorsal midbrain secondary to acceleration–deceleration forces is the presumed cause. Delayed or fluctuating SNHL associated with persistent vertigo may result from a perilymphatic fistula, an aberrant perilymphatic leakage into the middle ear.

Intralabyrinthine hemorrhage

Imaging documentation of intralabyrinthine hemorrhage (ILH) is rare.[67,72,73] Noncontrast thin-section T1 weighted images easily demonstrate the bright signal from the methemoglobin in distinct contrast to the low signal/signal void of surrounding bone. The ability to make this diagnosis mandates the need for precontrast thin-section T1 weighted images (**Fig. 25**).

There are numerous potential causes of ILH, and there have been numerous individual case reports documenting this process in various disease states. ILH can be secondary to coagulopathy, tumor, trauma, and sickle cell disease.

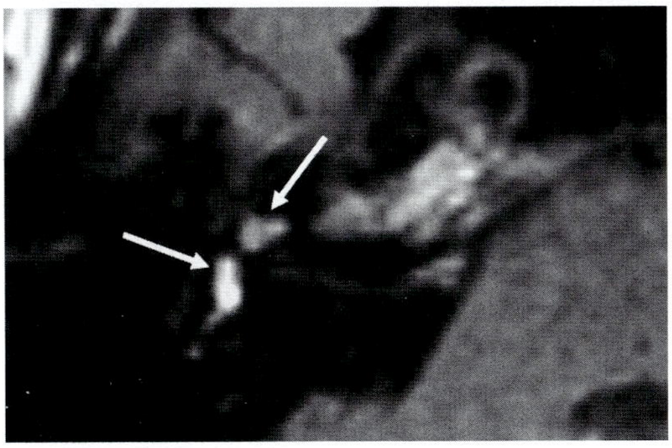

Fig. 25. Intralabyrinthine hemmorhage. Noncontrast T1W image reveals pathologic hypersignal throughout the cochlea and vestibule (*white arrows*) in a trauma patient. (*Courtesy of* Jan W. Casselman, MD, PhD, Bruges, Belgium.)

AUDITORY PATHWAY

The hair cells of the organ of Corti subtend the neurons of the spiral (cochlear) ganglion, which reside within the modiolus and give origin to the cochlear nerve. The cochlear nerve travels through the cochlear nerve aperture at the apex of the cochlea and subsequently along the anteroinferior quadrant of the internal auditory canal and through the cerebellopontine angle cistern to the dorsal and ventral cochlear nuclei that lie along the lateral surface of the inferior cerebellar peduncle at the rostral pole of the upper medulla.[69,74] Fibers from the cochlear nuclei course superiorly to the lateral lemniscus and subsequently to the inferior colliculus in the midbrain where they synapse. The auditory pathway continues to the medial geniculate body of the thalamus and subsequently to the auditory cortex in the temporal lobe. There are a few collaterals from the cochlear nuclei that course to the superior olive and then cross in the pons through the trapezoid body.

Lesions involving the cochlear nuclei in the medulla result in unilateral retrocochlear hearing loss identical to that caused by compression of the cochlear nerve (**Figs. 26 and 27**). Avoidance of internal auditory canal tunnel vision is paramount when evaluating these patients. Lesions involving the more peripheral auditory pathway result in less severe and bilateral deficits or perhaps even an auditory agnosia.[74] This is defined as

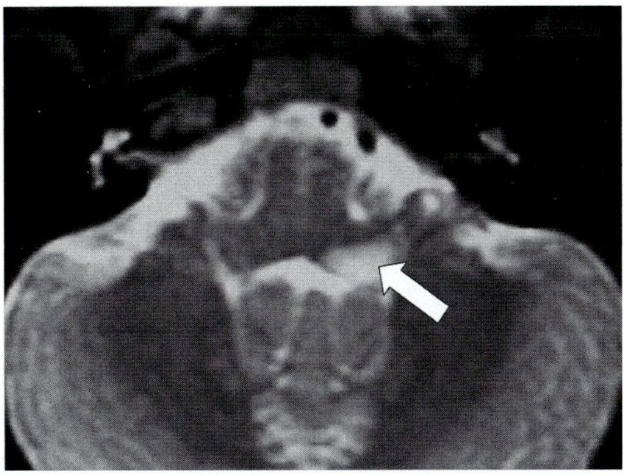

Fig. 26. Acute disseminated encephalomyelitis (ADEM). This patient suffered hearing loss following a vaccination. There is a hyperintense lesion within the posterolateral aspect of the upper medulla on the left (*white arrow*) in the vicinity of the cochlear and vestibular nuclei. Differential diagnosis includes demyelinating disease (in this case monophasic) and ischemic disease. (*Courtesy of* C.D. Phillips, MD, Charlottesville, VA.)

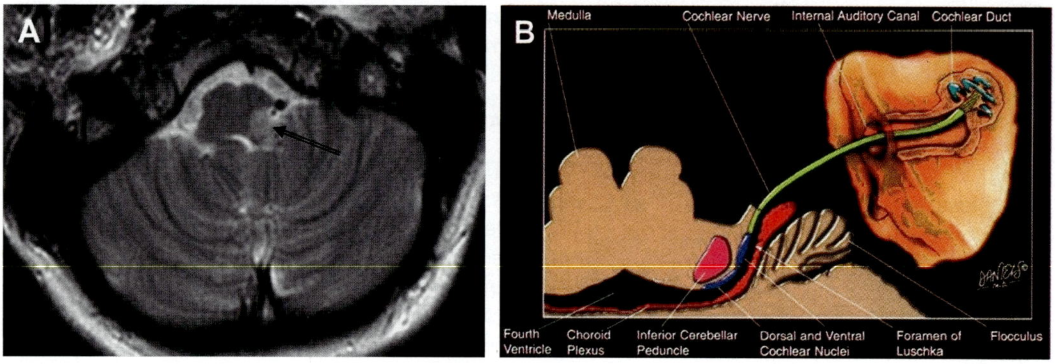

Fig. 27. Multiple sclerosis, retrocochlear hearing loss. (*A*) Axial T2W images; there is a focus of hypersignal within the posterolateral part of the upper medulla (*outlined black arrow*) in a patient with demyelinating disease. (*B*) Artist's rendering; note corresponding location of cochlear nuclei. (*From* Swartz JD, Daniels DL, Harnsberger HR, et al. Hearing, II: the retrocochlear auditory pathway. AJNR Am J Neuroradiol 1996;17:1479–81; with permission.)

preservation of the sensation of hearing but impaired recognition of sound and words.[75]

Intra-axial lesions responsible for SNHL can be ischemic, demyelinating, traumatic, vascular, and neoplastic. The most common are infarcts and demyelinating disease (multiple sclerosis).

COCHLEAR IMPLANT SURGERY

Components of the Cochlear implant include a speech processor, a headset and microphone, a receiver and stimulator, and an intracochlear electrode array responsible for stimulating the

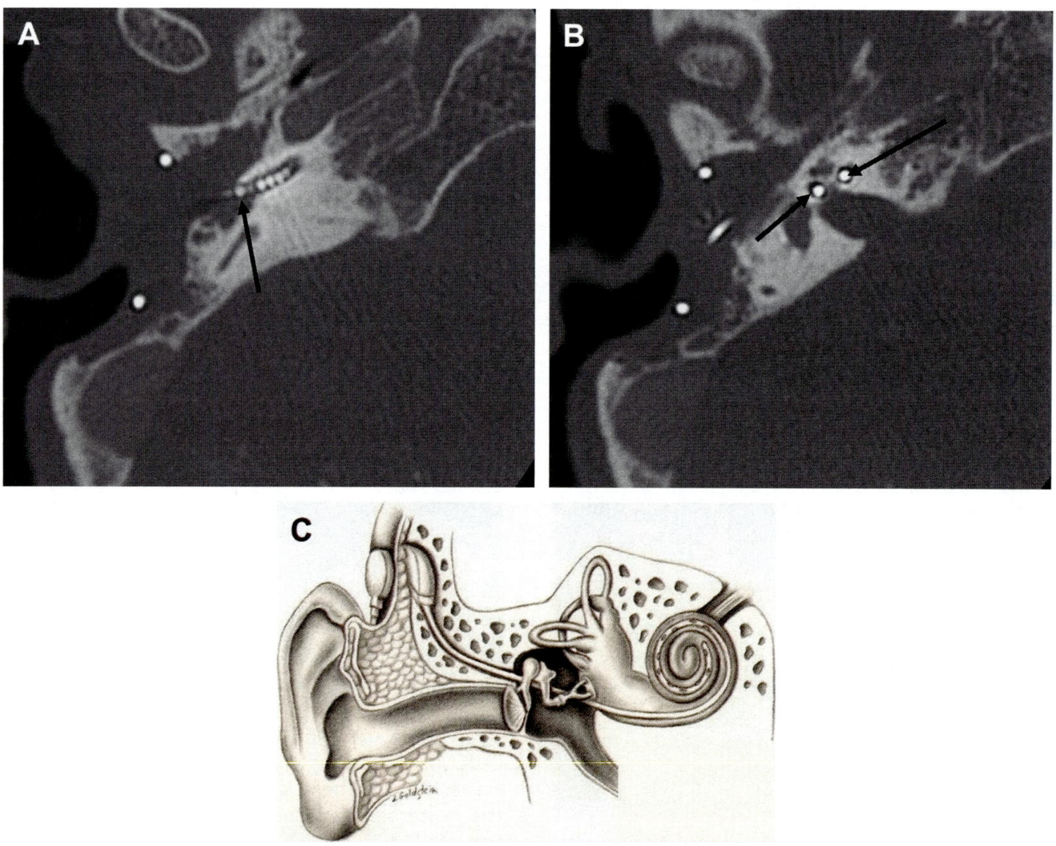

Fig. 28. Cochlear implant. (*A*) Axial CT image demonstrates an electrode array at the site of introduction by means of a cochleostomy (*black arrow*) in the vicinity of the round window. (*B*) Axial CT image through the cochlear apex indicates that the device (*black arrows*) is well-positioned in the middle and basal cochlear turn. (*C*) Artist's rendering of the device.

cochlear nerve.[76] The receiver/stimulator is placed beneath the postauricular soft tissues within the calvarium. The electrode array is inserted for a variable distance by means of the round window (or anteroinferior basilar turn fenestration–cochleostomy) into the scala tympani of the basilar turn (**Fig. 28**). The interscalar septum and the basilar membrane provide protection for the scala media (cochlear duct). Scala vestibuli insertions are much more likely to cause damage to Reissner's membrane and residual hair cells. An attempt is made to replicate the tonotopic organization of the cochlea by orienting the electrode to specific electrode contacts along the electrode array. The electrical stimulation that corresponds with the highest pitches is delivered within the basilar region of the cochlea, and the lowest pitches are delivered toward the apical region of the cochlea consistent with normal physiology.

Auditory brainstem implants (ABI) are used at some institutions. They are placed in the lateral recess of the fourth ventricle and allow for direct stimulation of the cochlear nuclei in the medulla in individuals with nonfunctioning or absent cochlear nerves. The flat rectangular shape of the stimulating array facilitates placement in the foramen of Luschka. An ABI is similar to a cochlear implant in the way it receives and processes sound.[77,78]

Preoperative CT without contrast is recommended for all cochlear implant candidates[79] MR imaging may be of significant value also. Analysis of these images not only aids in determining the likelihood of success of the procedure, but also influences the choice of implant and allows the surgeon to choose the best side for implantation.

Ossification obliterates the membranous labyrinth and potentially limits cochlear patency. When extensive, such ossification may effectively preclude implantation in many patients. Preoperative imaging in individuals who have diffuse inner ear malformation also must focus on the potential for perilymph gusher following insertion of the electrode.[80] Specifically the images must evaluate the anatomy of the fundus of the IAC and the base of the cochlea.

The number of contraindications to cochlear implant is diminishing rapidly as the technology and surgical skill increase.[81,82] The lone complete contraindication is an absent cochlear nerve, which may be congenital or acquired.[1]

Plain film (radiograph) provides an excellent overview and assessment of insertion depth of the device.[83] A modified Stenver's view has been suggested for this purpose. In difficult cases, postoperative CT has been advanced to provide an assessment of the intracochlear position of the electrode array.[84] The precise location of each electrode contact can be assessed in this manner. Successful CI requires that the electrodes be restricted to the scala tympani, and CT is useful in this regard.

The presence of a functioning cochlear implant was a contraindication to MR imaging examination. This is unfortunate, as many of these patients may develop conditions for which MR imaging may be a useful diagnostic procedure. Recently one cochlear implant manufacturer officially announced that their implant is compatible with MR imaging at or below 1.5 Tesla. Some precautions have to be made, and a tape has to be tightened around to head to keep the magnet in place. Unfortunately many other companies did not announce magnetic resonance compatibility yet. Hence magnetic resonance compatibility has to be checked in every case before MR imaging.

REFERENCES

1. Glastonbury CM, Davidson HC, Harnsberger HR, et al. Imaging findings of cochlear nerve deficiency. AJNR Am J Neuroradiol 2002;23:635–43.
2. Loevner L, Glastonbury C. The vestibulocochlear nerve. In: Swartz JD, Loevner L. Imaging the temporal bone, 4th edition, in press.
3. Govaerts PJ, Casselman J, Daemers K, et al. Cochlear implants in aplasia and hypoplasia of the cochleovestibular nerve. Otol Neurotol 2003;24:887–91.
4. Fatterpekar GM, Mukherji SK, Alley J, et al. Hypoplasia of the bony canal for the cochlear nerve in patients with congenital sensorineural hearing loss: initial observations. Radiology 2000;215:243–6.
5. Tang A, Parnes LS. X-linked progressive mixed hearing loss: computed tomography findings. Ann Otol Rhinol Laryngol 1994;103:655–7.
6. Smirniotopolous JG, Yue NC, Rushing EJ. Cerebellopontine angle masses: radiologic–pathologic correlation. Radiographics 1993;13:1131–47.
7. Maya MM, Lo WWM, Kovanlikaya I. Temporal bone tumors and cerebellopontine angle lesions. In: Som PM, Curtin HD, editors. Head and neck imaging. 4th edition. St. Louis (MO): Mosby-Yearbook; 2003. p. 1275–360.
8. Jackler RK. Acoustic neuroma (vestibulocochlear schwannoma). In: Jackler RK, Brackman DE, editors. Neurotology. St. Louis (MO): Mosby-Yearbook; 1994. p. 729–85 Chapter 41.
9. Swartz JD. Lesions of the cerebellopontine angle and internal auditory canal: diagnosis and differential diagnosis. Semin Ultrasound CT MR 2004;25: 332–52.
10. Allen RW, Harnsberger HR, Shelton C, et al. Low-cost high-resolution fast spin-echo MR of acoustic schwannoma: an alternative to enhanced

conventional spin-echo MR? AJNR Am J Neuroradiol 1996;17:1205–10.
11. Xenellis JE, Linthicum FH. On the myth of the glial/schwann junction (Obersteiner-Redlich zone): origin of vestibular nerve schwannomas. Otol Neurotol 2003;24:1.
12. Tali ET, Yuh WTC, Nguyen HD, et al. Cystic acoustic schwannomas: MR characteristics. AJNR Am J Neuroradiol 1993;14:1241–7.
13. Spickler EM, Govila L. The vestibulocochlear nerve. Semin Ultrasound CT MR 2002;23:218–37.
14. Ishikawa K, Okamoto K, Furusawa T, et al. Inner ear signals on mr cisternography: clues to differentiate between acoustic neurinomas and cerebellopontine angle meningiomas. Presented at the Radiological Society of North America. Chicago (IL), 2006.
15. Okamoto K, Furusawa T, Ishikawa K, et al. Focal T2 hyperintensity in the dorsal brain stem in patients with vestibular schwannoma. AJNR Am J Neuroradiol 2006;27:1307–11.
16. Copelan BB, Sarver CE, Zee C, et al. Imaging of the postoperative temporal bone: an educational review. Presented at the Radiological Society of North America. Chicago (IL), 2006.
17. Warren FM, Kaylie DM, Aulino JM, et al. Magnetic resonance appearance of the inner ear after hearing-preservation surgery. Otol Neurotol 2006;27:393–7.
18. Pollock BE. Management of vestibular schwannomas that enlarge after stereotactic radiosurgery: treatment recommendations based on a 15-year experience. Neurosurgery 2006;58:241–8.
19. Weissman JL, Hirsch BE, Fukui MB, et al. The evolving MR appearance of structures in the internal auditory canal after removal of an acoustic neuroma. AJNR Am J Neuroradiol. 1997;18:313–23.
20. Smith M, Castillo M, Campbell J, et al. Baseline and follow-up MRI of the internal auditory canal after suboccipital resection of acoustic schwannoma: appearances and clinical correlations. Neuroradiology 1995;37:317–20.
21. Kremer P, Forsting M, Hamer J, et al. MR enhancement of the internal auditory canal induced by tissue implant after resection of acoustic neurinoma. AJNR Am J Neuroradiol 1998;19:115–8.
22. Thedinger BA, Glasscock ME, Cueva RA, et al. Postoperative radiographic evaluation after acoustic neuroma and glomus jugulare removal. Laryngoscope 1992;102:261–6.
23. Larson TL. Understanding the post-treatment appearance of the internal auditory canal and cerebellopontine angle. Semin Ultrasound CT MR 2003;24:133–46.
24. Brors D, Schafers M, Bodmer D, et al. Postoperative magnetic resonance imaging findings after transtemporal and translabyrinthine vestibular schwannoma resection. Laryngoscope 2003;113:420–6.
25. Tieleman A, Casselman JW, Somers T, et al. Imaging of intralabyrinthine schwannomas: a retrospective study of 52 cases with emphasis on lesion growth. AJNR Am J Neuroradiol, in press.
26. Kennedy RJ, Shelton C, Salzman KL, et al. Intralabyrinthine schwannomas: diagnosis, management, and a new classification system. Otol Neurotol 2004;25:160–7.
27. Hegarty JL, Patel S, Fischbein N, et al. The value of enhanced magnetic resonance imaging in the evaluation of endocochlear disease. Laryngoscope 2002;112:8–17.
28. Aho TR, Daspit CP, Dean BL, et al. Intralabyrinthine meningioma. AJNR Am J Neuroradiol 2003;24:1642–5.
29. Hamilton BE, Salzman KL, Patel N, et al. Imaging and clinical characteristics of temporal bone meningioma. AJNR Am J Neuroradiol 2006;27:2204–9.
30. Bacciu A, Piazza P, Di Lella F, et al. Intracanalicular meningioma: clinical features, radiologic findings, and surgical management. Otol Neurotol 2007;28:391–9.
31. Dahlen RT, Johnson CE, Harnsberger HR, et al. MR imaging characteristics of intravestibular lipoma. AJNR Am J Neuroradiol 2002;23:1413–7.
32. Bonneville F, Sarrazin J, Marsot-Dupuch K, et al. Unusual lesions of the cerebellopontine angle: a segmental approach. Radiographics 2001;21:419–38.
33. Kertesz TR, Shelton C, Wiggins RH, et al. Intratemporal facial nerve neuroma: anatomical location and radiological features. Laryngoscope 2001;111:1250–6.
34. Stasolla A, Bellussi A, Bibbolino C. Dural tail: another face of facial nerve schwannoma? AJNR Am J Neuroradiol 2006;27:1804–7.
35. Rokni-Yazdi H, Sotoudeh H. Prevalence of dural tail sign in patients with different intracranial pathologies. Eur J Radiol 2006;60:42–5.
36. Oner AY, Tokgoz N, Tali ET, et al. Imaging meningiomas: is there a need for postcontrast FLAIR? Clin Radiol 2005;60:1300–5.
37. Martinez R, Vaquero J, Areitio E, et al. Meningiomas of the posterior fossa. Surg Neurol 1983;19:237–43.
38. Asaoka K, Barrs DM, Sampson JH, et al. Intracanalicular meningioma mimicking vestibular schwannoma. AJNR Am J Neuroradiol 2002;23:1493–6.
39. Magliulo G, Zardo F, Bertin S, et al. Meningiomas of the internal auditory canal: two case reports. Skull Base 2002;12:19–26.
40. Roche PH, Regis J. Cerebellopontine angle meningiomas. J Neurosurg 2005;103:935–7, author reply 937–8.
41. Ben Hamouda M, Drissi C, Sebai R, et al. Atypical CT and MRI aspects of an epidermoid cyst. J Neuroradiol 2007;34:129–32.
42. Eldevik OP, Blaivas M, Gabrielsen TO, et al. Craniopharyngioma: radiologic and histologic findings and recurrence. AJNR Am J Neuroradiol 1996;17:1427–39.

43. Ikushima I, Korogi Y, Hirai T, et al. MR of epidermoids with a variety of pulse sequences. AJNR Am J Neuroradiol 1997;18:1359–63.
44. Annet L, Duprez T, Grandin C, et al. Apparent diffusion coefficient measurements within intracranial epidermoid cysts in six patients. Neuroradiology 2002;44:326–8.
45. Dechambre S, Duprez T, Lecouvet F, et al. Diffusion-weighted MRI postoperative assessment of an epidermoid tumour in the cerebellopontine angle. Neuroradiology 1999;41:829–31.
46. Osborn AG. Miscellaneous tumors, cysts, and metastases. In: Osborn AG, editor. Diagnostic neuroradiology. St Louis (MO): Mosby; 1994. p. 631–49.
47. Osborn AG, Preece MT. Intracranial cysts: radiologic-pathologic correlation and imaging approach. Radiology 2006;239:650–64.
48. Choi JU, Kim DS. Pathogenesis of arachnoid cyst: congenital or traumatic. Pediatr Neurosurg 1998; 29:260–6.
49. Cinnamon J, Sharma M, Gray D, et al. Neuroimaging of meningeal disease. Semin Ultrasound CT MR 1994;15:466–98.
50. Brackmann DE, Doherty JK. CPA Melanoma: diagnosis and management. Otol Neurotol 2007;28: 529–37.
51. Tankere F, Vitte E, Martin-Duverneuil N, et al. Cerebellopontine angle lipomas: report of four cases and review of the literature. Neurosurgery 2002;50: 626–32.
52. Carvalho GA, Matthies C, Osorio E, et al. Hamartomas of the internal auditory canal: report of two cases. Neurosurgery 2003;52:944–9.
53. Wu SS, Lo WW, Tschirhart DL, et al. Lipochoristomas (lipomatous tumors) of the acoustic nerve. Arch Pathol Lab Med 2003;127:1475–9.
54. Kieserman S, Linstrom C, McCormick S, et al. Choroid plexus papilloma of the cerebellopontine angle. Am J Otol 1996;17:119–22.
55. McDermott AL, Dutt SN, Irving RM, et al. Anterior inferior cerebellar artery syndrome: fact or fiction. Clin Otolaryngol Allied Sci 2003;28:75–80.
56. Makins AE, Nikolopoulos TP, Ludman C, et al. Is there a correlation between vascular loops and unilateral auditory symptoms? Laryngoscope 1998; 108:1739–42.
57. De Carpentier J, Lynch N, Fisher A, et al. MR imaged neurovascular relationships at the cerebellopontine angle. Clin Otolaryngol Allied Sci 1996;21: 312–6.
58. Yamakawa H, Hattori T, Tanigawara T, et al. Intracanalicular aneurysm at the meatal loop of the distal anterior inferior cerebellar artery: a case report and review of the literature. Surg Neurol 2004;61:82–8.
59. Jayaraman MV, Mayo-Smith WW, Doberstein CE. Intracanalicular aneurysm of the anterior inferior cerebellar artery revealed by multidetector CT angiography. AJNR Am J Neuroradiol 2003;24: 1338–40.
60. Aquilina K, Nanra JS, Brett F, et al. Cavernous angioma of the internal auditory canal. J Laryngol Otol 2004;118:368–71.
61. Cotton CA, Beall DP, Winter BJ, et al. Cavernous angioma of the cerebellopontine angle. Curr Probl Diagn Radiol 2006;35:120–3.
62. Brackmann DE, Weisskopf PA, Lo WWM. Ossifying hemangioma of the internal auditory canal. Otol Neurotol 2005;26:1239–40.
63. Smith JK, Matheus MG, Castillo M. Imaging manifestations of neurosarcoidosis. AJR Am J Roentgenol 2004;182:289–95.
64. Albayram S, Wasserman BA, Yousem DM, et al. Intracranial hypotension as a cause of radiculopathy from cervical epidural venous engorgement: case report. AJNR Am J Neuroradiol 2002;23:618–21.
65. Kale S, Donaldson I, West RJ, et al. A superficial siderosis of the meninges and its otolaryngologic connection: a series of five patients. Otol Neurotol 2003;24:90–5.
66. Hsu WC, Loevner LA, Forman MS, et al. Superficial siderosis of the CNS associated with multiple cavernous malformations. AJNR Am J Neuroradiol 1999;20:1245–8.
67. Swartz JD, Loevner LA. Imaging the temporal bone. 4th edition. New York: Thieme Inc., in press.
68. Merchant SN, Gopen QA. Human temporal bone study of acute bacterial meningogenic labyrinthitis. Am J Otol 1996;17:375–85.
69. Fortnum H, Davis A. Hearing impairment in children after bacterial meningitis: incidence and resource implications. Br J Audiol 1993;27:43–52.
70. Smith MM, Anderson JC. Neurosyphilis as a cause of facial and vestibulocochlear nerve dysfunction: MR imaging features. AJNR Am J Neuroradiol 2000;21:1673–5.
71. Stokroos RJ, Albers FW, Krikke AP, et al. Magnetic resonance imaging of the inner ear in patients with idiopathic sudden sensorineural hearing loss. Eur Arch Otorhinolaryngol 1998;255:433–6.
72. Weissman JL, Weber PC, Bluestone CD. The CT appearance of the middle ear and inner ear in patients with congenital perilymphatic fistula. Otolaryngol Head Neck Surg 1994;111:243–9.
73. Weissman JL, Curtin HD, Hirsch BE, et al. High signal from the otic labyrinth on unenhanced magnetic resonance imaging. AJNR Am J Neuroradiol 1992; 13:1183–7.
74. Armington WG, Harnsberger HR, Smoker WR, et al. Normal and diseased acoustic pathway: evaluation with MR imaging. Radiology 1988;167: 509–15.
75. Demanez JP, Demanez L. Anatomophysiology of the central auditory nervous system: basic concepts. Acta Otorhinolaryngol Belg 2003;57:227–36.

76. Witte RJ, Lane JI, Driscoll CL, et al. Pediatric and adult cochlear implantation. Radiographics 2003; 23:1185–200.
77. Niparko J. Cochlear implants, auditory brainstem implants, and surgically implantable hearing aids. In: Cummings CW, Fredickson JM, Harker LA, et al, editors. Otolaryngology head and neck surgery. 3rd edition. St. Louis (MO): Mosby. p. 2934–62.
78. Lo WW. Imaging of cochlear and auditory brain stem implantation. AJNR Am J Neuroradiol. 1998;19: 1147–54.
79. Lane JI, Driscoll CL, Witte RJ, et al. Scalar Localization of the electrode array after cochlear implantation: a cadaveric validation study comparing 64-slice multidetector computed tomography with microcomputed tomography. Otol Neurotol 2007;28:191–4.
80. Kusuma S, Liou S, Haynes DS. Disequilibrium after cochlear implantation caused by a perilymph fistula. Laryngoscope 2005;115:25–6.
81. Sennaroglu L, Sarac S, Ergin T. Surgical results of cochlear implantation in malformed cochlea. Otol Neurotol 2006;27:615–23.
82. Mecca MA, Wagle W, Lupinetti A, et al. Complication of cochlear implantation surgery. AJNR Am J Neuroradiol 2003;24:2089–91.
83. Shpizner BA, Holliday RA, Roland JT, et al. Postoperative imaging of the multichannel cochlear implant. AJNR Am J Neuroradiol 1995;16:1517–24.
84. Verbist BM, Frijns JH, Geleijns J, et al. Multisection CT as a valuable tool in the postoperative assessment of cochlear implant patients. AJNR Am J Neuroradiol 2005;26:424–9.

Pathologic Conditions of the Lower Cranial Nerves IX, X, XI, and XII

Bruno A. Policeni, MD*, Wendy R.K. Smoker, MS, MD, FACR

KEYWORDS

• Lower cranial nerves • Imaging • Pathology
• Differential diagnosis • Palsy

Radiologic evaluation of the patient who has isolated or combined deficits of the lower four cranial nerves requires knowledge of the course of each nerve and the muscles innervated by these nerves. Because glossopharyngeal (CN IX), vagus (CN X), and spinal accessory (CN XI) nerves share some functions and nuclei, they are most often discussed as a group. There are some unique characteristics of each nerve that are also described, however. Although the hypoglossal nerve has a different skull base pathway, it is located in close proximity to the other lower cranial nerves. The severity of symptoms that result from insults to these nerves depends on the chronicity of the insult. If the cause is a slow-growing tumor or a chronic insult, the patient may adapt well, with only a partial palsy.[1] If the event is acute, however, such as traumatic or postsurgical, the patient usually has severe complete paralysis.[2]

In this article, a brief overview of the anatomy of the lower four cranial nerves is presented, because this topic has been discussed in detail elsewhere in this issue. The clinical manifestations associated with impairment of the lower four cranial nerves are also discussed, and the commonly associated pathologic conditions and their classic imaging findings are reviewed.

ANATOMY AND CLINICAL MANIFESTATIONS

Glossopharyngeal Nerve—Cranial Nerve IX

CN IX is composed of motor and sensory fibers. By itself, the glossopharyngeal nerve provides motor innervation to a single muscle, the stylopharyngeus muscle. The sensory segment of CN IX forms the first synapse in the superior ganglion and enters the medulla to synapse further in the nucleus spinalis of the trigeminal nerve—CN V. Parasympathetic fibers of CN IX, originating in the inferior salivary nucleus, go to the parotid glands, stimulating gland secretion. There are also special sensory fibers, part of the nucleus solitarius, for taste from the posterior one third of the tongue.[3]

After exiting the brain stem in the retro-olivary sulcus, CN IX crosses the cistern and exits the skull base through the pars nervosa of the jugular foramen. In the suprahyoid neck, CN IX runs in the high carotid space, medial to the styloid process and anterior to the internal carotid artery (ICA) and internal jugular vein.

As previous noted, given the close proximity of the glossopharyngeal nerve to the vagus and spinal accessory nerves, pathologic conditions commonly affect all three nerves simultaneously, often related to the so-called "jugular foramen (Vernet's) syndrome".[4] Pathologic conditions affecting CN IX in isolation are rare.[3] Patients usually present with external otalgia, slight dysphagia, and changes in taste from the posterior one third of the tongue. Physical examination demonstrates loss of the gag reflex on the affected side, deviation of the uvula to the opposite side, and differences in sensation between sides of the soft palate and pharynx. Because there are also parasympathetic fibers to the parotid gland and carotid body, secretions of saliva from the parotid gland are decreased and the heart rate may be accelerated (**Box 1**). This last finding has only been described in patients immediately after surgical sectioning of the nerve.[3]

Department of Radiology, University of Iowa Hospitals and Clinics, 200 Hawkins Drive, Iowa City, IA 52242, USA
* Corresponding author.
E-mail address: bruno-policeni@uiowa.edu (B.A. Policeni).

Neuroimag Clin N Am 18 (2008) 347–368
doi:10.1016/j.nic.2007.12.012
1052-5149/08/$ – see front matter

Box 1
Clinical findings of lower cranial nerve palsies

Glossopharyngeal nerve (CN IX)
- External otalgia
- Slight dysphagia
- Loss of taste from the posterior one third of the tongue
- Loss of gag reflex on the affected side
- Decreased saliva secretion from the parotid gland
- Accelerated heart rate (only after surgical sectioning)

Vagus nerve (CN X)
- Soft palate droops on the affected side
- Deviation of the posterior pharyngeal wall on the affected side
- Hoarseness attributable to vocal cord paralysis
- Bilateral palsy results in a dilated and atonic esophagus, stomach, and intestine

Accessory nerve (CN XI)
- Shoulder droop secondary to trapezius muscle denervation
- Diminished strength on turning the head toward the paralyzed side
- Weakness elevating the shoulder above the horizontal plane

Hypoglossal nerve (CN XII)
- Compromised motor function of the tongue

Vagus Nerve—Cranial Nerve X

The vagus nerve is a long nerve extending from the brain stem to the splenic flexure of the colon, with branchial motor, visceral motor, general sensory, and visceral sensory functions. The branchial motor segment carries fibers to the laryngeal musculature, extralaryngeal neck muscles, and pharyngeal muscles. The vagus nerve originates from the nucleus ambiguus that continues cranially with the motor nuclei of the facial and trigeminal nerves. General sensory fibers come from the dura mater, external ear canal, tympanic membrane, and pharyngeal and laryngeal mucosa. Visceral sensory fibers originate from the intrathoracic and intra-abdominal structures, related to cardiovascular, respiratory, and gastrointestinal reflexes. The visceral motor (parasympathetic) fibers of the nerve go to glands of the pharynx and larynx, thoracic and abdominal viscera, and cardiac muscle.[5]

The vagus nerve has three major branches: pharyngeal, superior laryngeal, and recurrent laryngeal.[6] The pharyngeal branch is the principal motor nerve to the pharynx, supplying all muscles of the pharynx and soft palate, with the exception of the stylopharyngeus and tensor veli palatini muscles, which are supplied by CN IX and CN V3 (mandibular nerve), respectively. The superior laryngeal nerve divides into internal (mainly a sensory nerve from the hypopharynx and larynx above the vocal cords) and external (a motor nerve to the inferior constrictor and cricopharyngeus muscles) branches. The distal branch is the recurrent laryngeal nerve (RLN), which has different right and left pathways that are described subsequently.

The vagus nerve exits the brain stem in the retro-olivary sulcus of the medulla. Eight to 10 rootlets emerge, caudal to those of CN IX. After crossing the perimedullary cistern, the nerve exits the skull base through the pars vascularis of the jugular foramen, sharing the same dural sheath as the accessory nerve. In the high carotid space, the vagus nerve lies posterior to, and in a groove between, the internal jugular vein and the ICA.[7] Descending within the carotid sheath, the vagus nerve gives branches to the pharynx, larynx, and constrictor muscles, as described previously. In the mediastinum, each vagus nerve takes a different pathway to reach the esophageal, cardiac, and pulmonary plexuses.

The right and left RLNs exit the vagus at different levels, which is extremely important to remember when evaluating patients who have vocal cord paralysis. The right RLN nerve exits higher, looping under the right subclavian artery before ascending in the right tracheoesophageal groove. The left RLN branches from the vagus in the thorax and loops under the aortic arch to ascend in the left tracheoesophageal groove. Because of these differing origins, it is essential to continue scanning caudally to the level of the aortopulmonary window when evaluating patients who have left vocal cord paralysis or the entire course of the left vagus nerve or RLN is not included on cross-sectional imaging examinations.

Patients who have unilateral vagal paralysis present with multiple findings. The soft palate droops and does not rise on phonation, and the palatal reflex is absent. Examination of the oropharynx demonstrates deviation of the posterior pharyngeal wall, known as the "side scenes phenomenon".[1] Hoarseness is present because of ipsilateral vocal cord paralysis. Pooling of secretions on the side of paralysis is usually identified during laryngoscopy. Dysphasia may be present because of swallowed food being pushed toward the paralyzed side of the hypopharynx by muscles of the intact side. Blood pressure and heart rate increase for approximately 2 months because of loss of parasympathetic innervation. Bilateral vagus nerve paralysis results in bilateral vocal cord paralysis and more severe dysphasia. Bilateral loss of visceromotor innervation results in dilatation and atony of the esophagus, stomach, and intestine (see **Box 1**).[1]

When clinical findings implicate involvement of CN IX and CN X, the offending pathologic findings can be localized to the brain stem, subarachnoid cisterns, skull base, or suprahyoid carotid space. Isolated distal vagal neuropathy, manifested by isolated vocal cord dysfunction, places the pathologic findings below the level of the hyoid.

Spinal Accessory Nerve—Cranial Nerve XI

The spinal accessory nerve is purely motor, providing innervation to the sternocleidomastoid and trapezius muscles. The nerve has two separates components: cranial and spinal. The cranial component originates in the nucleus ambiguus, along with CN IX and CN X. The spinal component arises as multiple roots in the anterior horn of the spinal cord from C1 to C6. These fibers ascend within the spinal canal, passing posterior to the vertebral artery (VA), to enter the posterior cranial fossa. The two components course through the perimedullary cistern and exit the skull base through the pars vascularis of the jugular foramen along with nerve X. Within the high carotid space, the spinal accessory nerve courses lateral to the vagus nerve.[8]

Because of the proximity of CN IX, CN X, and CN XI at the skull base, at the subarachnoid cisterns, and within the high carotid space, it is not surprising that patients who have CN XI palsy typically have involvement of other lower cranial nerves. Paralysis of the spinal accessory nerve is diagnosed clinically by ipsilateral shoulder droop, as a result of trapezius muscle denervation, and decreased strength on turning the head toward the paralyzed side, as a result of sternocleidomastoid denervation. There may also be weakness of shoulder elevation because of insufficient fixation of the scapula to the thorax wall (see **Box 1**).[1]

An important finding of which the radiologist should be aware when interpreting studies of patients who have trapezius and sternocleidomastoid muscle atrophy or resection (ie, after radical neck dissection) is that there is often compensatory hypertrophy of the ipsilateral levator scapula muscle. This occurs as the muscle attempts to assume some of the functions of the denervated muscles and should not be confused with a mass (**Fig. 1**).[4]

Hypoglossal Nerve—Cranial Nerve XII

The hypoglossal nerve supplies motor innervation to the tongue and also contributes to innervation of the infrahyoid strap muscles through the ansa hypoglossi. The nucleus is located in the paramedian floor of the fourth ventricle, bulging into the ventricle, producing the hypoglossal trigone.[9] The nerve courses anteriorly though the medulla, between the olive (laterally) and the medial longitudinal fasciculus, medial lemniscus, accessory olivary nucleus, and pyramidal tract (medially). Rootlets exit the brain stem in the preolivary sulcus and course posterolateral to the VA within the perimedullary cistern to exit the skull base through the hypoglossal (anterior condylar) canal. In the high nasopharyngeal carotid space, the nerve lies in

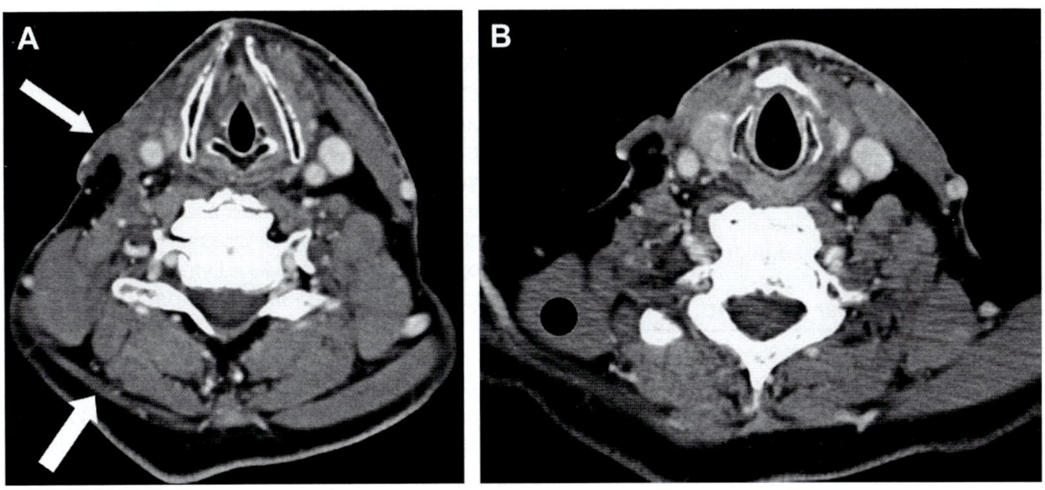

Fig. 1. Right levator scapula hypertrophy in a 64-year-old man after a right neck dissection. Axial CT images of the neck demonstrate chronic long-standing denervation atrophy of the sternocleidomastoid and trapezius muscles (*A; arrows*) and compensatory levator scapula hypertrophy (*B; dot*).

the carotid sheath in close proximity to the other lower four cranial nerves. At the level of the mandible, the hypoglossal nerve loops anteriorly around the occipital artery, lying inferior to the posterior belly of the digastric muscle. It then runs along the surface of the hyoglossus muscle in the sublingual space, above the mylohyoid sling, to reach the tongue musculature.[7]

Patients who have hypoglossal paresis present clinically with ipsilateral tongue paralysis and fasciculation (see Box 1). Approximately 4 to 6 weeks after injury, the intrinsic and extrinsic muscles of the tongue undergo atrophy and fatty replacement (see the article by Smoker and Reede elsewhere in this issue).[4]

PATHOLOGIC FINDINGS OF THE LOWER CRANIAL NERVES

When paralysis of one or more of the lower four cranial nerves is identified, complete evaluation of the nerves from their brain stem nuclei to their "end organs" must be performed. For purposes of organization and discussion, this can best be accomplished by considering the nerves in five segments: (1) brain stem or nuclear segment; (2) cisternal segment, affecting the nerves as they transverse the cisterns; (3) skull base segment: jugular foramen and hypoglossal canal; (4) suprahyoid neck segment, compromising the nerves as they course through the nasopharyngeal and oropharyngeal carotid spaces; and (5) infrahyoid neck or mediastinal segment, only affecting the vagus nerve. With this organization, a reasonable differential diagnosis can be constructed for pathologic findings in each segment (ie, inflammatory or infectious, traumatic, miscellaneous) (**Box 2**). It should be noted, however, that many lesions may affect the nerves in more than one segment (ie, nerve sheath tumors may involve any segment other than the nuclear segment, paragangliomas can be located in the suprahyoid and cisternal segments in addition to the skull base, aneurysms can also be located in more than one segment). In the following discussion, lesions are presented as they occur in their major segments.

Brain Stem or Nuclear Segment

Vascular, neoplastic, and inflammatory lesions are the most common pathologic findings to involve the brain stem segment. The brain stem receives its arterial supply from the posterior circulation. The medulla is supplied anteromedially and anterolaterally by the VA and anterior spinal arteries. Laterally and posteriorly, the medulla is supplied by the posterior inferior cerebellar artery (PICA).[10] Occlusion of the VA or PICA can cause a lateral medullary infarct, clinically described as the Wallenberg syndrome (**Fig. 2**).[11] This syndrome is composed of the following clinical signs: difficulty in swallowing, hoarseness, dizziness, nausea, vomiting, nystagmus, and balance or gait incoordination. Because the infarct also affects the descending sympathetic pathway, Horner's syndrome is usually present. Involvement of the nucleus of CN V and lateral spinothalamic tract produces loss of pain and temperature to the ipsilateral face and contralateral limbs and trunk.[11]

Diffusion-weighted imaging (DWI) is recommended for evaluation of brain stem infarcts. False-negative diffusion of lateral medullary strokes has been described within the first 24 hours, however.[12] This is probably attributable to the low resolution of DWI echo planar imaging for detection of small lesions.[13] If symptoms persist, the study should be repeated.

Primary hemorrhage of the medulla is rare. Brain stem hemorrhage is often restricted to the pons. Hypertension and vascular malformations are the most common causes. Anticoagulation has also been described as a cause of primary brain stem hemorrhage.[14] Vascular malformations, such as cavernomas and arteriovenous malformations, can cause lower cranial nerve palsies, commonly associated with other neurologic symptoms, especially when they bleed and produce mass effect.[15]

Metastases, gliomas, and lymphoma are the principal neoplasms to affect the brain stem and lower cranial nerve nuclei. The nerve palsy can be bilateral if the tumor is midline, affecting both nuclei, or unilateral when the lesion is eccentric or exophytic. Syringobulbia associated with ependymoma has also been reported to cause lower cranial nerve paralysis.[16]

MS can involve the brain stem and is reported to affect 30% of patients at the onset of disease.[17] The pons is the most commonly affected site, followed by the midbrain and, less commonly, the medulla.[18] In patients who have lower cranial nerve involvement, the vagus nerve is the most commonly affected cranial nerve at the onset of disease.[17] An infectious etiology that may mimic MS is Lyme disease, and it can rarely cause lower cranial nerve palsy.[19]

Cisternal Segment

Major pathologic findings that affect the lower cranial nerves in their cisternal segments include vascular, infectious, neoplastic, and congenital lesions. VBD refers to elongation and dilatation of the vertebrobasilar vessels typically associated with hypertension. Although the pathogenesis of

Box 2
Segmental approach "to assess" lower cranial nerve pathologic findings

Brain stem or nuclear segment
- Vascular
  - Wallenberg's syndrome (stroke)
  - Hemorrhage
  - Vascular malformations
- Inflammatory
  - Multiple sclerosis (MS)
  - Lyme disease
- Neoplastic
  - Gliomas
  - Lymphoma
  - Metastases
  - Ependymoma

Cisternal segment
- Inflammatory
  - Tuberculosis
  - Sarcoidosis
- Vascular
  - Vascular malformations
  - Vertebrobasilar dolichoectasia (VBD)
  - Posterior inferior cerebellar and VA aneurysm
  - VA dissection
- Neoplastic
  - Leptomeningeal metastases
  - Leptomeningeal lymphoma
  - Nerve sheath tumors
  - Meningioma
- Congenital
  - Chiari I

Skull base segment
- Inflammatory
  - Osteomyelitis
- Trauma
  - Skull base fractures
- Neoplastic
  - Paragangliomas
  - Meningiomas
  - Nerve sheath tumors
  - Chordomas
  - Metastases
  - Nasopharyngeal carcinoma
  - Lymphoma

Suprahyoid segment
- Inflammatory
  - Carotid space abscess
- Neoplastic
  - Paragangliomas
  - Meningiomas
  - Nerve sheath tumors
  - Nasopharyngeal carcinoma
- Vascular
  - ICA dissection and aneurysm
- Miscellaneous
  - Second branchial cleft cyst

Infrahyoid or mediastinum segment
- Inflammatory
  - Mediastinitis
  - Inflammatory adenopathy
- Neoplastic
  - Bronchogenic carcinoma
  - Metastases
  - Lymphoma
- Vascular
  - Aortic aneurysm
  - Cardiomegaly
- Miscellaneous
  - Bronchogenic cyst

VBD is unclear, a vessel wall abnormality has been implicated.[20] VBD can be asymptomatic or can produce cranial nerve symptoms attributable to compression. Facial and trigeminal nerves are most commonly affected, resulting in hemifacial spasm or trigeminal neuralgia, but isolated lower cranial nerve palsies have also been reported.[21] Aneurysms of the VA and PICA, especially fusiform aneurysms, and vascular malformations within the cisterns[22] can also cause lower cranial nerve symptoms produced by the mass effect (**Fig. 3**). Isolated hypoglossal palsy has been reported in association with VA dissection.[23]

Various infectious and inflammatory processes that have a predisposition to affect the cisterns around the brain stem may also cause lower cranial nerve impairment, particularly granulomatous diseases. Tuberculous meningitis preferentially

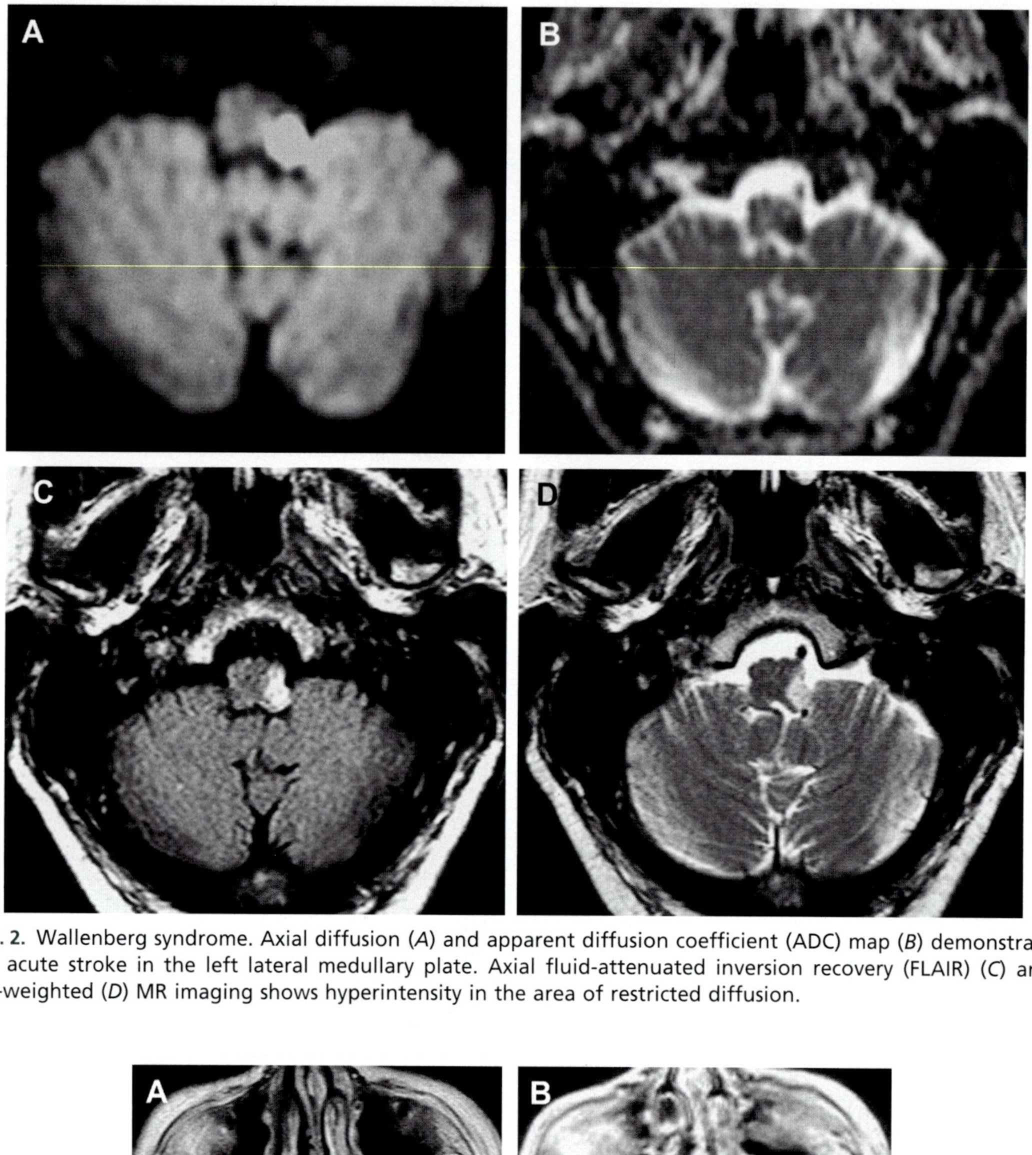

Fig. 2. Wallenberg syndrome. Axial diffusion (*A*) and apparent diffusion coefficient (ADC) map (*B*) demonstrate an acute stroke in the left lateral medullary plate. Axial fluid-attenuated inversion recovery (FLAIR) (*C*) and T2-weighted (*D*) MR imaging shows hyperintensity in the area of restricted diffusion.

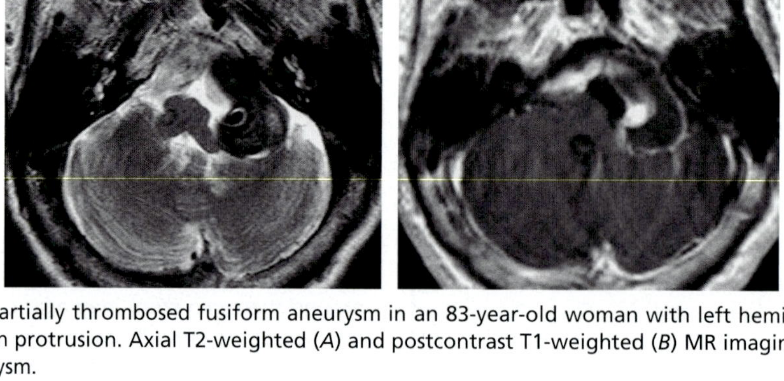

Fig. 3. Left VA partially thrombosed fusiform aneurysm in an 83-year-old woman with left hemitongue atrophy and deviation on protrusion. Axial T2-weighted (*A*) and postcontrast T1-weighted (*B*) MR imaging demonstrates the large aneurysm.

involves the basal cisterns and sylvian fissures and coats the cerebellum and brain stem with a thick gelatinous exudate.[24] Cranial nerve palsies occur in 20% to 30% of patients and may be the presenting manifestation.[24] Sarcoidosis frequently affects the central nervous system, with symptoms from leptomeningeal involvement being the most common manifestation, present in 40% of patients.[25] Leptomeningeal sarcoidosis has a similar appearance to leptomeningeal tuberculosis. There is poor correlation between the imaging findings and the clinical symptoms in sarcoidosis, because some patients have symptoms without imaging findings and some asymptomatic patients have prominent imaging findings of cisternal involvement.[25,26] As described with tuberculosis, any cranial nerve can be involved. MR imaging is more sensitive than CT for demonstration of the abnormal findings, with thickening and enhancement of the leptomeninges seen on postcontrast T1-weighted images (**Fig. 4**). Idiopathic hypertrophic pachymeningitis is a rare entity, essentially a diagnosis of exclusion, that can also cause lower cranial nerve palsies.[27] In summary, any inflammation or infection affecting the subarachnoid cisterns around the medulla may produce lower cranial nerve symptoms.

Central nervous system lymphoma can affect the cranial nerves when leptomeningeal spread of disease is present. The radiologic appearance is similar to that of leptomeningeal sarcoidosis or tuberculosis.[28] Meningiomas (**Fig. 5**) and nerve sheath tumors (**Fig. 6**) can originate or extend to involve the cisternal segment. These are further discussed in the segment on the skull base in this article.

Lower cranial nerve dysfunction, such as vocal cord paralysis and tongue hemiatrophy, has been reported to be present in 20% of patients who have the Chiari I malformation.[29] Controversy exists regarding the exact mechanism related to this phenomenon. One proposed mechanism is that traction and compression of the lower cranial nerves is attributable to herniation of the cerebellar tonsils through the foramen magnum (**Fig. 7**).[30]

Skull Base Segment

Neoplasms (benign and malignant), infections, or trauma injuries may damage the lower cranial nerves as they traverse the skull base. Three main neoplasms are located in the vicinity of the jugular foramen: paragangliomas, nerve sheath tumors, and meningiomas.

Paragangliomas are highly vascular lesions arising from nonchromaffin cells of neural crest origin. There are four common locations for these neoplasms within the head and neck: carotid artery bifurcation (carotid body paraganglioma), along the vagus nerve (vagal paraganglioma), at the jugular foramen (jugular paraganglioma), and in the middle ear (tympanicum paraganglioma). These neoplasms may occur sporadically or in an inherited familial pattern.[31] Paragangliomas are hypervascular and show dense tumor staining on conventional angiography.

Jugular paragangliomas commonly affect the lower cranial nerves at the level of the skull base.

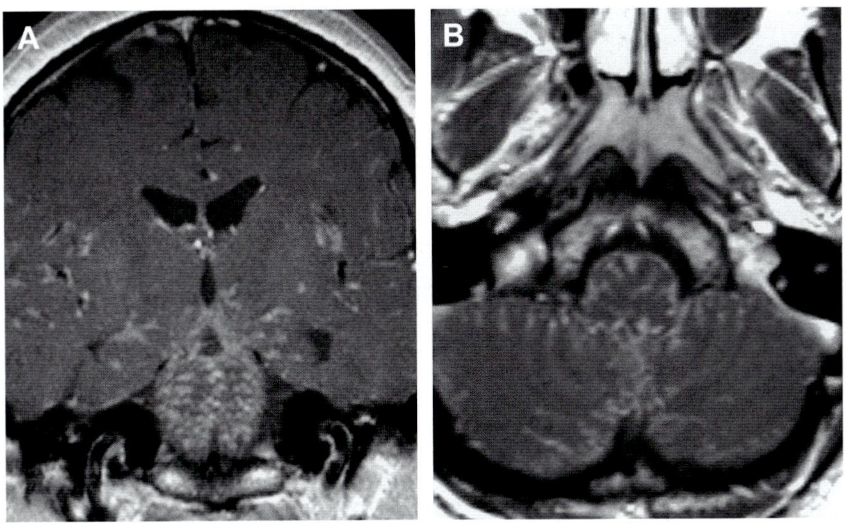

Fig. 4. Leptomeningeal sarcoidosis. Axial (*A*) and coronal (*B*) postcontrast T1-weighted MR imaging demonstrates leptomeningeal enhancement around the medulla, pons, cerebellar folia, and Sylvian fissures.

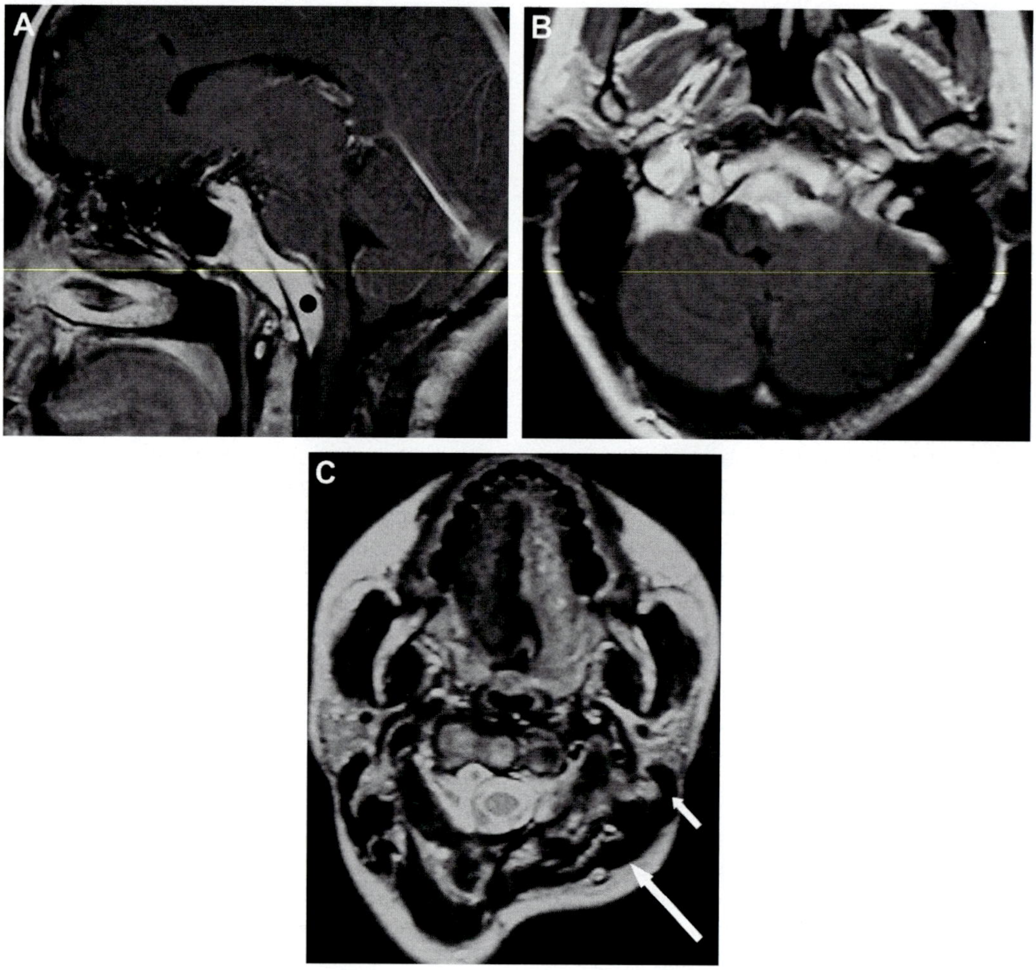

Fig. 5. Foramen magnum meningioma in a 42-year-old woman with palsies of CN XI and CN XII. Sagittal (*A*) and axial (*B*) postcontrast T1-weighted MR imaging demonstrates a dural-based enhancing lesion along the lower clivus at the level of the foramen magnum (*A; dot*). (*C*) Axial T2-weighted MR imaging at the level of the oral cavity reveals changes of late chronic denervation atrophy of the left hemitongue and atrophy of the left trapezius (*long arrow*) and sternocleidomastoid (*short arrow*) muscles.

They arise within the jugular foramen, from paraganglia surrounding the jugular bulb, Arnold's nerve (branch of CN X), or Jacobsen's nerve (branch of CN IX).[32] MR imaging demonstrates a soft tissue mass; if the lesion is large enough, a salt and pepper appearance may be identified on standard spin echo imaging.[31] The "salt" represents slow flow versus hemorrhage, and "pepper" represents flow voids within the mass. Jugular paragangliomas may extend to involve the middle ear cavity (jugulotympanicum paraganglioma).[32] CT may be helpful in demonstrating a "moth-eaten" pattern of jugular foramen or spine erosion attributable to progressive growth of the tumor (**Fig. 8**).[33]

This destructive pattern is not associated with schwannomas, which remodel and expand the jugular foramen, or meningiomas, which are frequently associated with sclerosis.

Schwannomas and neurofibromas are benign primary neoplasms that can affect the cranial nerves.[34] Approximately 40% of these tumors occur in the head and neck, and they can originate from any cranial nerve, including the lower four cranial nerves.[35] Schwannomas and neurofibromas cannot be differentiated by their imaging characteristics;[36] however, cranial nerve neurofibromas are extremely rare.[37] Calcification and hemorrhage are uncommon, but cystic or fatty degeneration is frequently associated with schwannomas.[31] As opposed to paragangliomas, which occur exclusively in the jugular canal, schwannomas can also arise within the hypoglossal canal. The clinical manifestations of these tumors, when

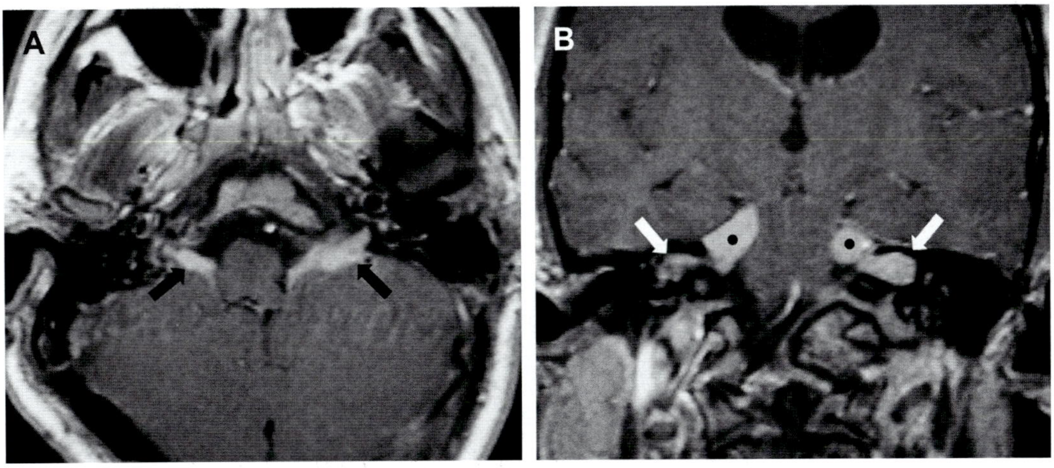

Fig. 6. Multiple cranial nerve schwannomas (presumed) in a patient who has neurofibromatosis type II. Axial (*A*) and coronal (*B*) postcontrast T1-weighted MR imaging reveals bilateral tumors of glossopharyngeal or vagus (*A; black arrows*), trigeminal (*B; dots*), and vestibulocochlear (*B; white arrows*) nerves.

located in the jugular foramen or hypoglossal canal, are variable, depending on tumor growth patterns.[38] These neoplasms cause expansion and remodeling of the jugular foramen (**Fig. 9**) or hypoglossal canal (**Fig. 10**) without osseous destruction.[37] As opposed to paragangliomas, extension to involve the middle ear is not a feature of these tumors. MR imaging signal characteristics of nerve sheath tumors are similar in all locations: isointense to hypointense signal on T1-weighted images; heterogeneous to homogeneous hyperintense signal on T2-weighted images; and variable enhancement, depending on the proportion of Antoni A and Antoni B cells and the amount of cystic degeneration.[31]

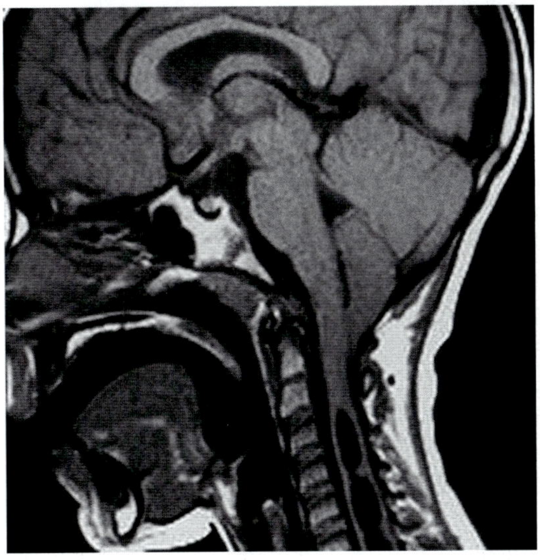

Fig. 7. Chiari I malformation in a 17-year-old girl with CN X paresis. Midsagittal T1-weighted MR imaging demonstrates caudal displacement of the cerebellar tonsils, well below the plane of the foramen magnum. There is no cerebrospinal fluid (CSF) surrounding the brain stem at this level. There is also an associated syringohydromyelic cavity visible in the cervical cord.

Posterior fossa meningiomas account for 10% of intracranial meningiomas. They are described as occurring in six major locations: (1) cerebellar convexity, (2) cerebellopontine angle, (3) jugular foramen, (4) petroclival, (5) foramen magnum, and (6) unclassified.[39] A review of 161 cases by Roberti and colleagues[40] reported that 2 of 14 patients who had cerebellar convexity meningiomas, 1 of 9 patients who had cerebellopontine angle meningiomas, 2 of 7 patients who had jugular foramen meningiomas, 8 of 110 patients who had petroclival meningiomas, and 6 of 21 patients who had foramen magnum meningiomas had CN IX, CN X, and CN XI deficits. Additionally, 1 patient who had a cerebellar convexity meningioma, 1 patient who had a jugular foramen meningioma, 4 patients who had petroclival meningiomas, and 4 patients who had foramen magnum meningiomas had CN XII deficits. Meningiomas that originate in the posterior fossa can extend to involve the internal auditory canal, hypoglossal canal, or middle ear.[41] They usually manifest isointense to hypointense signal on T1-weighted images, isointense signal on T2-weighted images, and enhancement on postcontrast T1-weighted images. Flow voids are not associated with these lesions. CT of meningiomas located around the jugular foramen often demonstrates sclerosis, which, together with

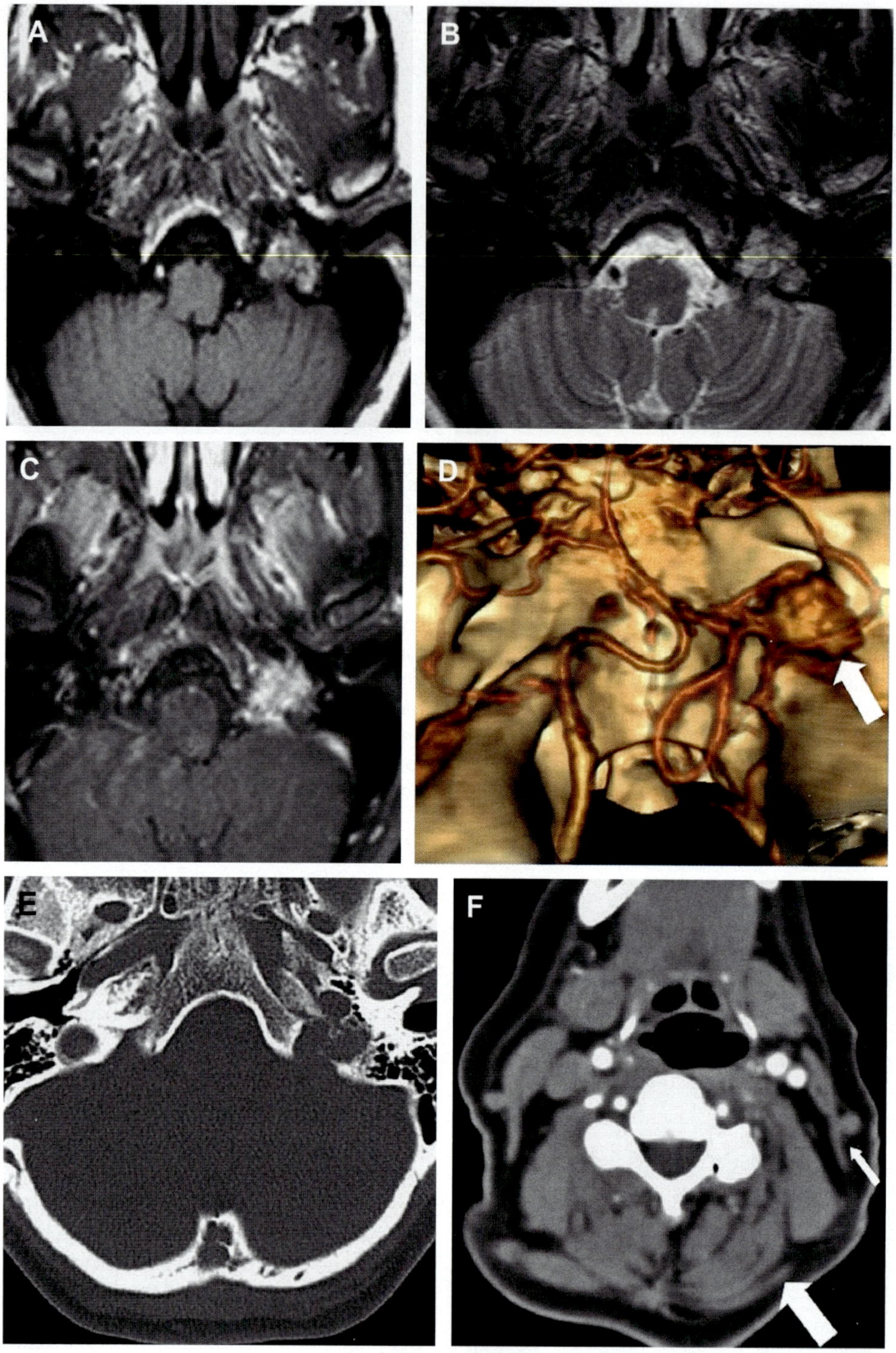

Fig. 8. Jugular paraganglioma in a 65-year-old woman with hoarseness and dysphagia. (*A*) T1-weighted MR imaging demonstrates a mass, centered in the region of the left jugular foramen, that is isointense with foci of hyperintensity probably representing hemorrhage or slow-flow within vessels. (*B*) T2-weighted MR imaging reveals lesion isointensity with small flow voids. (*C*) Fat-suppressed, postcontrast, T1-weighted MR imaging shows intense enhancement. (*D*) CT angiogram (three-dimensional reconstruction) demonstrates lesion hypervascularity, with a density similar to blood (*arrow*). (*E*) CT image at the level of the skull base reveals destruction of the left jugular foramen with a "moth-eaten" appearance. (*F*) CT at the level of the hyoid bone shows atrophy of the left sternocleidomastoid (*small arrow*) and trapezius (*large arrow*) muscles.

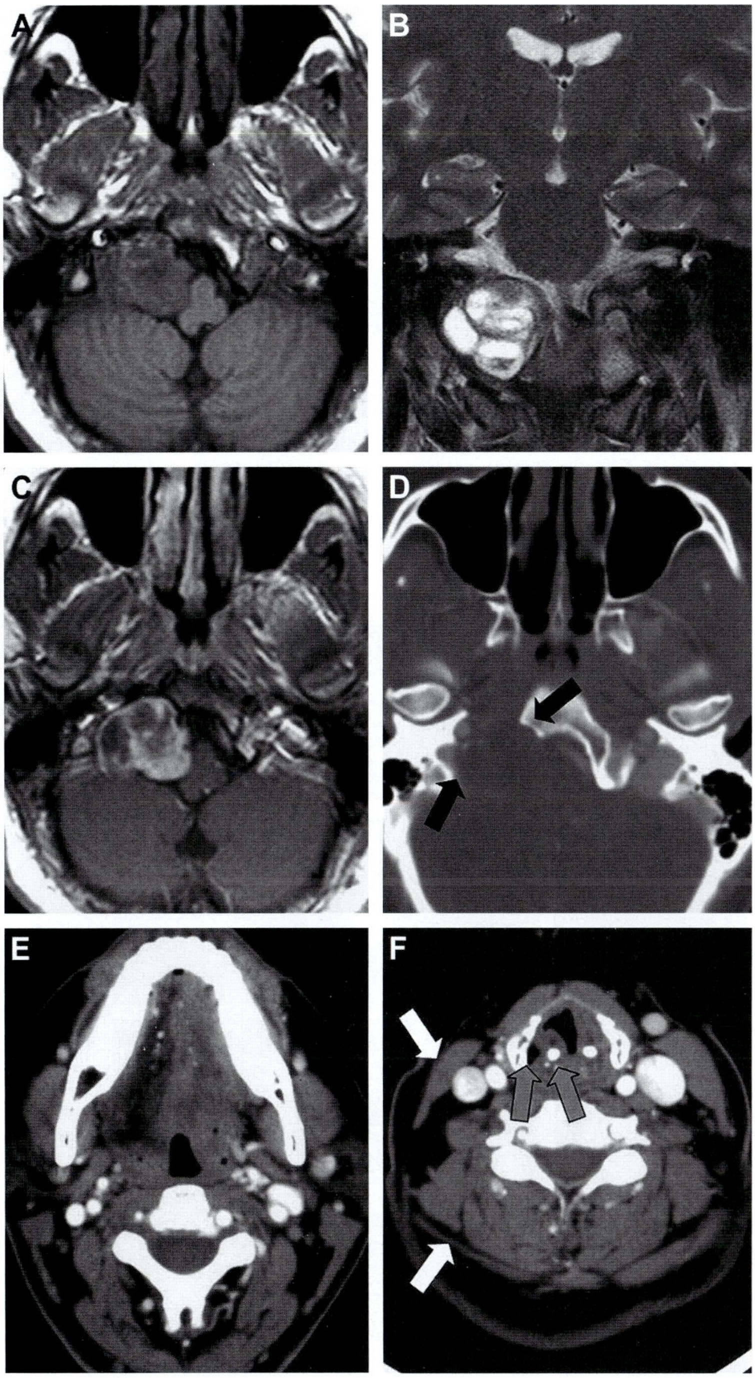

Fig. 9. Jugular foramen schwannoma in a 52-year-old woman presenting with hoarseness, right hemitongue atrophy, and decreased right shoulder shrug. (*A*) Axial T1-weighted MR imaging shows an isointense mass in the right jugular foramen. (*B*) Coronal T2-weighted MR imaging reveals multiloculation and heterogenous signal within the lesion. (*C*) Axial postcontrast, fat-suppressed, T1-weighted MR imaging demonstrates heterogenous enhancement. (*D–F*) Contrast-enhanced axial CT images demonstrate expansion and remodeling of the jugular foramen (*D; black arrows*), long-standing chronic right hemitongue denervation atrophy with fatty infiltration (*E*), and atrophy of the sternocleidomastoid and trapezius muscles (*F; white arrows*), in addition to enlargement of the right piriform sinus and rotation and medial positioning of the right arytenoid cartilage attributable to vocal cord paralysis (*F; gray arrows*).

the lack of vascular flow voids, is helpful in differentiating these tumors from paragangliomas (**Fig. 11**).[41]

Another tumor that can extend to involve the lower cranial nerves is the clivus chordoma. Although chordomas are histologically benign neoplasms, they are locally aggressive.[42] They originate from embryonic notochordal remnants, most commonly encountered in the sacrum and clivus.[43] Clivus chordomas can produce lower cranial nerve palsies as they extend to involve the skull base or, if they have an eccentric component, by abutting the nerves in their cisternal segments. CT typically shows an expansile, destructive, lytic

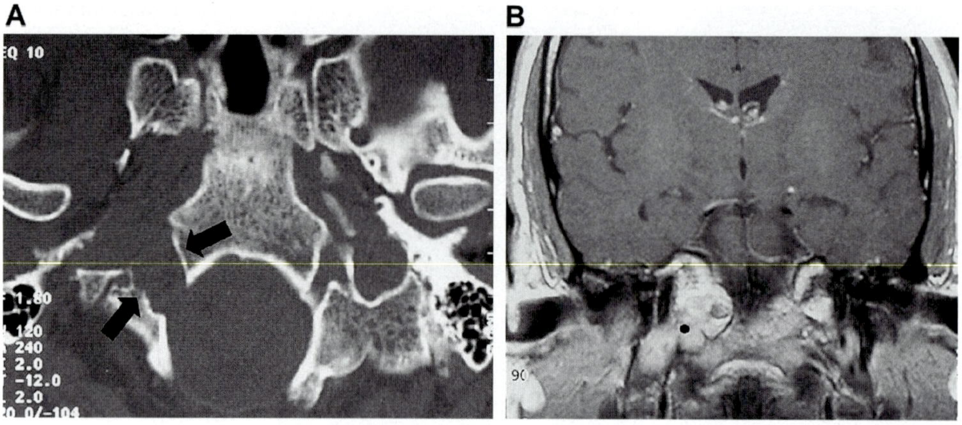

Fig. 10. Hypoglossal schwannoma. (*A*) Unenhanced axial CT image at the level of the hypoglossal canal reveals right hypoglossal canal expansion and remodeling without destruction (*black arrows*). (*B*) Coronal postcontrast T1-weighted MR imaging demonstrates marked lesion in the right hypoglossal canal (*dot*).

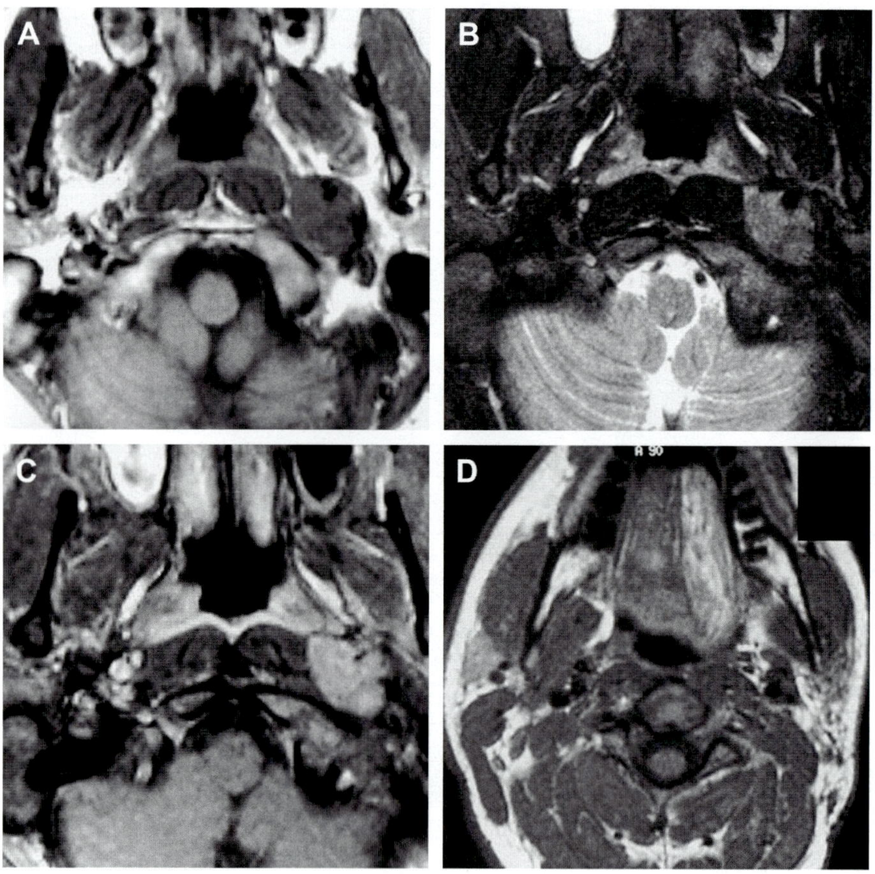

Fig. 11. Jugular foramen meningioma in a 17-year-old boy who was trying to "bulk up" before his prom but noted that his left neck was getting smaller while the right neck was getting larger. Axial T1-weighted (*A*) and T2-weighted (*B*) MR imaging shows an isointense mass in the left jugular foramen. (*C*) Axial postcontrast T1-weighted MR imaging demonstrates avid homogeneous enhancement of the mass. (*D*) Axial T1-weighted imaging at the level of the oral cavity shows left hemitongue fatty infiltration attributable to denervation atrophy. (*E*) Axial T1-weighted imaging through the lower neck demonstrates left sternocleidomastoid and trapezius muscle atrophy (*white arrows*). (*F, G*) Axial CT images at the level of the jugular foramen show high left carotid space soft tissue calcifications (*F; gray arrow*) and left jugular foramen sclerosis (*G; black arrows*).

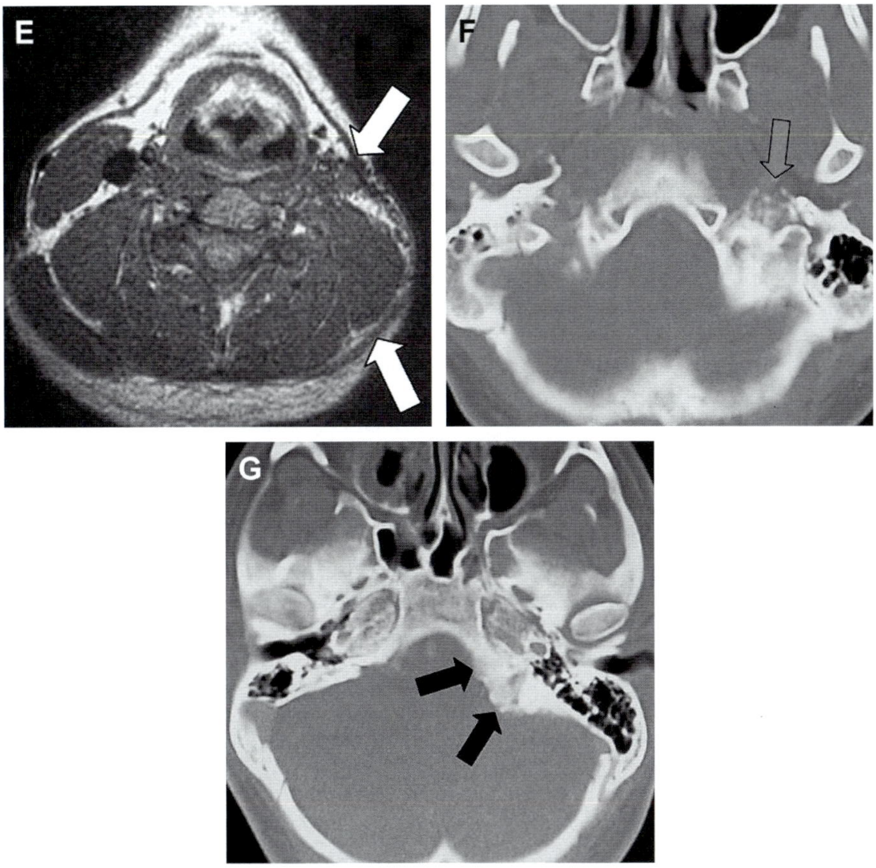

Fig. 11. (*continued*)

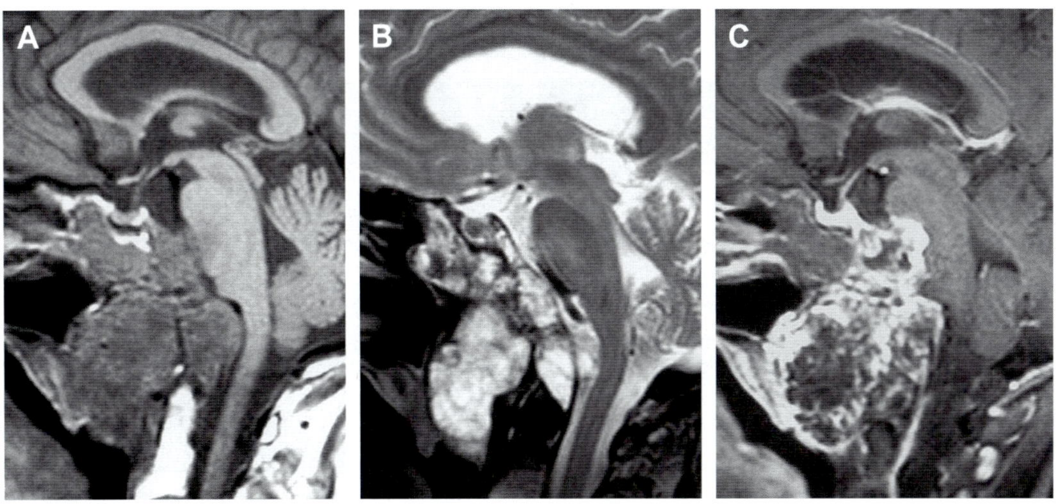

Fig. 12. Clivus chordoma in a 70-year-old man with right hemitongue atrophy. (*A*) Sagittal T1-weighted MR imaging demonstrates an isointense clivus mass with anterior extension into the nasopharynx and posterior extension into the premedullary and prepontine cisterns. (*B*) Sagittal T2-weighted MR imaging reveals marked inhomogeneous lesion hyperintensity, typical of chordomas. (*C*) Sagittal postcontrast T1-weighted MR imaging demonstrates heterogeneous enhancement in a "honeycomb" pattern.

lesion with an associated soft tissue mass centered within the clivus.[42] Bone windows are helpful to define the osseous destruction. MR imaging is the best modality for the evaluation of chordomas because it provides excellent soft tissue contrast.[42] T1-weighted MR imaging demonstrates a low signal intensity mass; however, some areas of high T1 signal may be identified as a result of intratumoral hemorrhage or mucous pools. The typical chordoma has characteristic high T2 signal intensity with low signal septations that represent the multilobulated feature of these lesions. Marked enhancement is present in most chordomas, described as a "honeycomb" appearance (**Fig. 12**).[42]

Metastatic disease can affect cranial nerves by perineural spread or skull base involvement. Skull base metastases from distant tumors occur in 4% of patients who have cancer.[44] In a review of 43 skull base metastasis by Greenberg and colleagues,[45] lung, prostate, and breast neoplasms were reported to be the most common primary neoplasms. Laigle-Donadey and colleagues[44] reported cranial nerve palsies associated with skull base metastases as the presenting symptom in 28% of patients. MR imaging is the best modality to demonstrate marrow replacement and an enhancing skull base mass (**Fig. 13**). CT is a complementary modality that better demonstrates the osseous destruction and is particularly helpful in differentiating fibrous dysplasia (FD) from metastases, a distinction that is often quite challenging on MR imaging.[46]

Nasopharyngeal squamous cell carcinoma (NPSCCa) is another malignancy that can extend to involve the skull base, producing lower cranial nerve symptoms.[47] This tumor originates in the high posterolateral nasopharynx, just below the skull base.[48] Based on the fifth American Joint Committee on Cancer (AJCC) staging system, NPSCCa

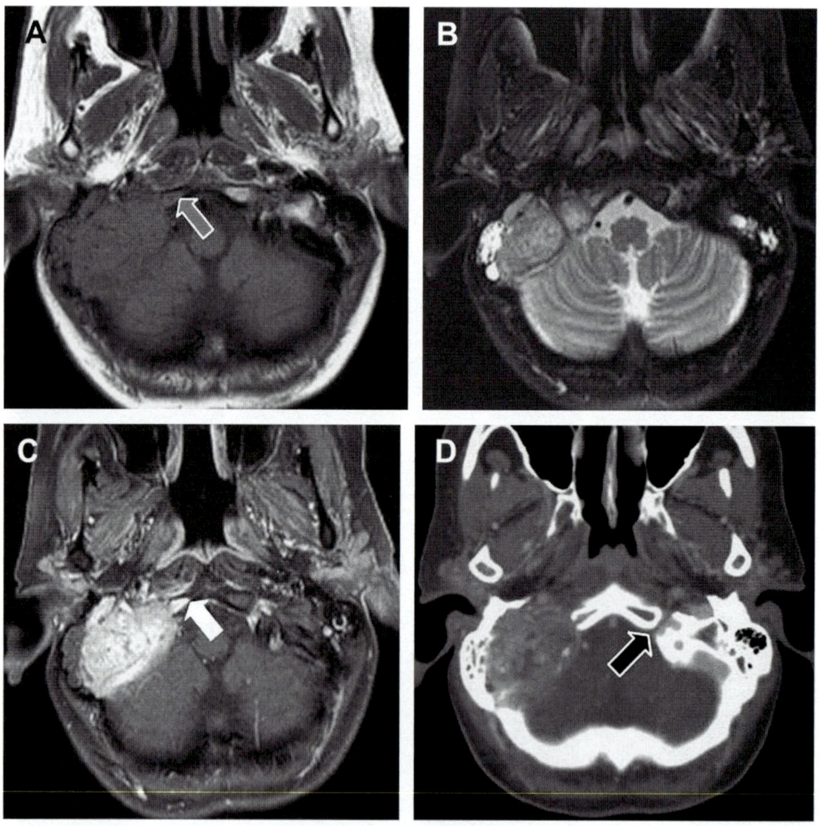

Fig. 13. Skull base metastasis in a 42-year-old woman with breast carcinoma and right CN XII palsy. Axial T1-weighted (*A*), T2-weighted (*B*), and postcontrast T1-weighted (*C*) MR imaging demonstrates a T1 isointense soft tissue mass with osseous destruction involving the right skull base with marrow replacement of the right half of the clivus (A; *gray arrow*), hypointensity on T2, and pathologic enhancement of the lesion and the infiltrated portion of the clivus (*C; white arrow*). (*D*) Axial postcontrast CT image shows the large destructive lesion involving the right hypoglossal canal. The hypoglossal canal on the left (*black arrow*) is normal.

with associated skull base involvement but without cranial nerve involvement is considered a T3 lesion. If, however, there is intracranial extension or cranial nerve involvement, it is considered a T4 lesion.[49] After radiation therapy, recovery of cranial nerve function can occur.[47] MR imaging is significantly more sensitive than CT in demonstrating skull base involvement and intracranial extension.[50] CT reveals the osseous erosion, but replacement of fatty marrow is best demonstrated on T1-weighted MR imaging on which the high signal of fat is replaced by the intermediate signal intensity of tumor (**Fig. 14**).[51]

Skull base osteomyelitis may occur as a complication of paranasal sinus or ear infections, typically encountered in the immunocompromised patient.[52] Patients can present with an isolated lower cranial palsy without obvious signs of infection.[53] CT optimally demonstrates the osseous skull base destruction, but MR imaging better demonstrates the associated soft tissue inflammatory changes.[52] CT is unreliable in the early stages of disease, however, and in the appropriate clinical setting, a bone scan should be obtained.[53]

Head trauma with skull base fractures can be associated with lower cranial nerve palsies.

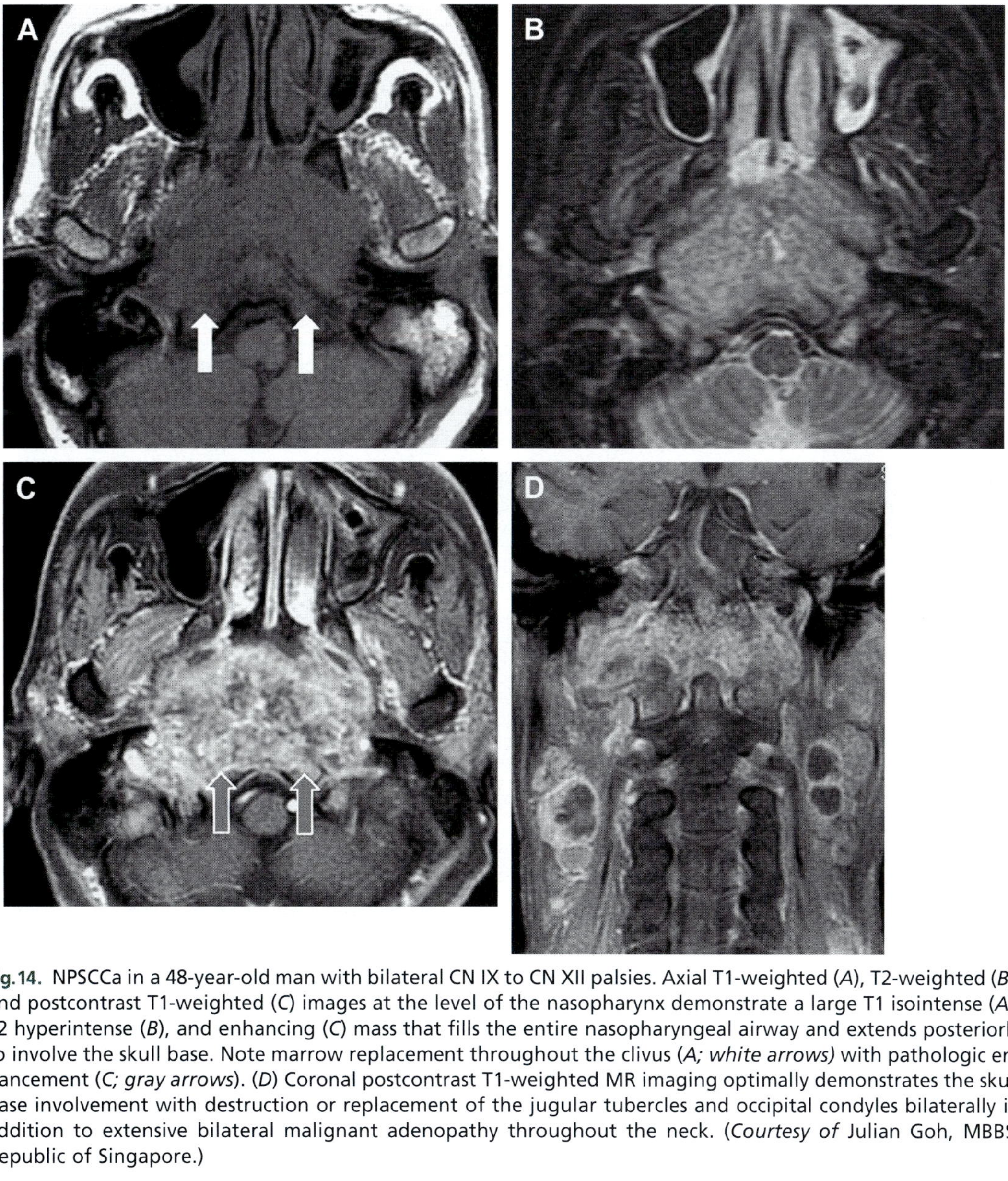

Fig. 14. NPSCCa in a 48-year-old man with bilateral CN IX to CN XII palsies. Axial T1-weighted (*A*), T2-weighted (*B*), and postcontrast T1-weighted (*C*) images at the level of the nasopharynx demonstrate a large T1 isointense (*A*), T2 hyperintense (*B*), and enhancing (*C*) mass that fills the entire nasopharyngeal airway and extends posteriorly to involve the skull base. Note marrow replacement throughout the clivus (*A; white arrows*) with pathologic enhancement (*C; gray arrows*). (*D*) Coronal postcontrast T1-weighted MR imaging optimally demonstrates the skull base involvement with destruction or replacement of the jugular tubercles and occipital condyles bilaterally in addition to extensive bilateral malignant adenopathy throughout the neck. (*Courtesy of* Julian Goh, MBBS, Republic of Singapore.)

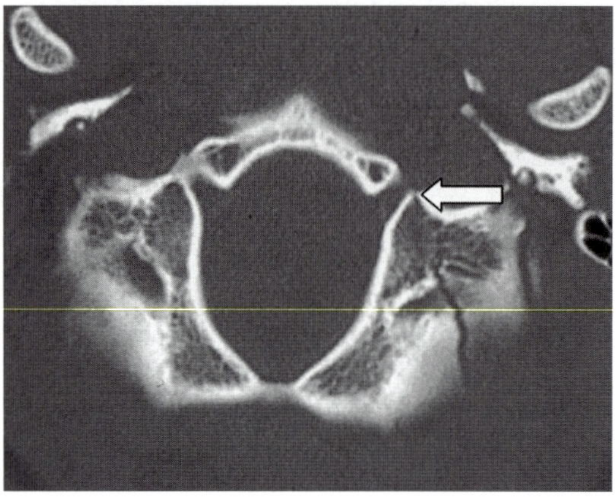

Fig. 15. Type II occipital condyle fracture in a patient who fell from a truck 2 weeks previously and presented with left CN XII paresis. Axial CT images of the skull base demonstrate a left occipital bone fracture that extends to involve the left occipital condyle and hypoglossal canal (*arrow*).

Because of the close proximity of the occipital condyle, hypoglossal canal, and jugular foramen, mixed neuropathies are common.[54,55] Fractures are better evaluated by high-resolution CT of the skull base than by MR imaging. The cranial nerve palsy may not be present immediately but may manifest in a delayed fashion because of callus formation or fragment displacement (**Fig. 15**).[56]

Suprahyoid Neck

Lower cranial nerve involvement in the suprahyoid neck can result from a wide range of pathologic findings. These include benign and malignant tumors, inflammatory processes, and vascular lesions.

As previously described, vagal and carotid body paragangliomas are located in the carotid space. Carotid body paragangliomas arise from nonchromaffin cells in the carotid body and characteristically splay the common carotid artery bifurcation (**Fig. 16**).[32] Vagal paragangliomas typically arise from tissue rests within the nodose (inferior) ganglion and typically displace the carotid vessels anteromedially and the lateral pharyngeal wall medially.[32] Because these lesions are usually not in close proximity to the skull base, bone destruction is absent. Vagal paragangliomas can, however, arise from the superior ganglion and assume a dumbbell shape consisting of intracranial and extracranial components.[33] These lesions are usually asymptomatic slow-growing masses. Some of these lesions may be associated with lower cranial nerve palsies, especially vagal paragangliomas, in the late clinical course of the disease.[32]

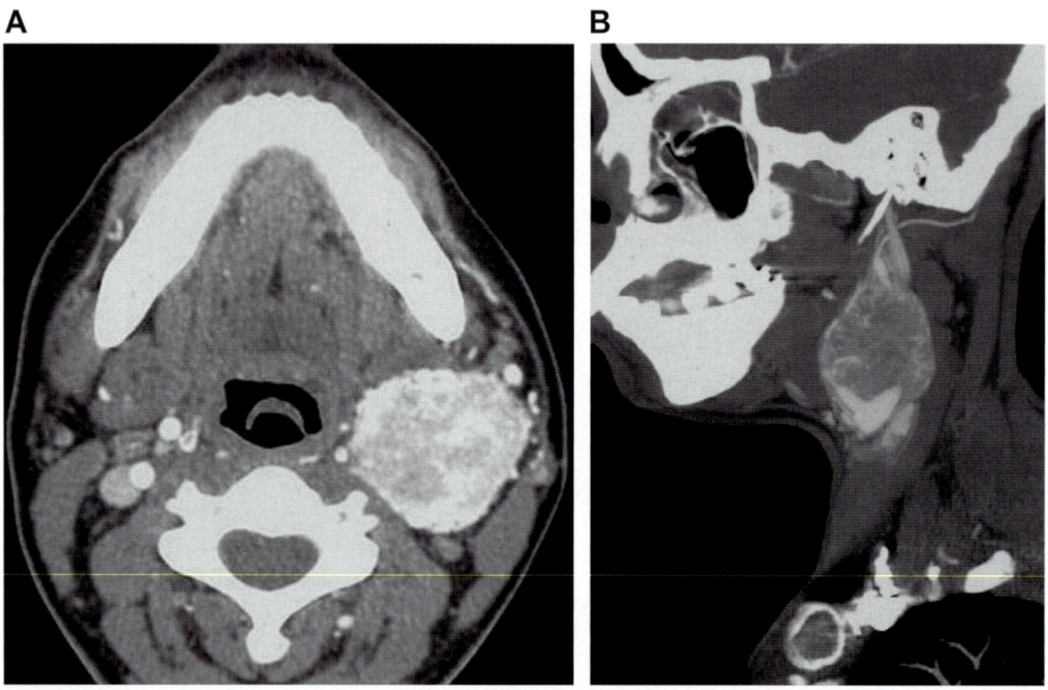

Fig. 16. Carotid body paraganglioma. Axial (*A*) and sagittal (*B*) images from a CT angiogram demonstrate a large left carotid body paraganglioma splaying the internal and external carotid arteries (*B*). (*Courtesy of* William P. Dillon, MD, San Francisco, CA.)

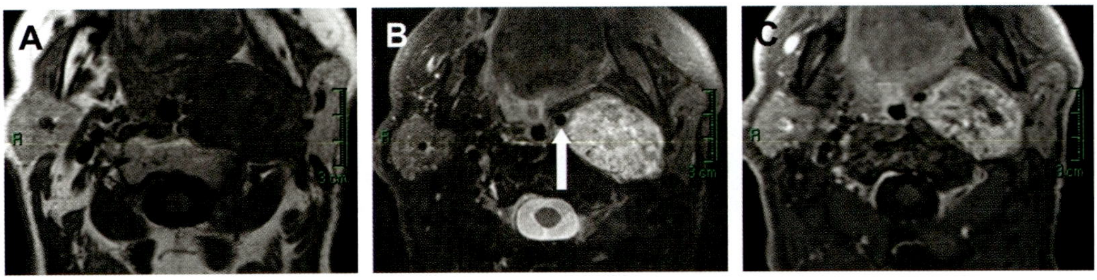

Fig. 17. Vagal schwannoma. (*A*) Axial T1-weighted MR imaging shows an isointense left carotid space mass. (*B*) Lesion is hyperintense on T2-weighted MR imaging and displaces the ICA anteriorly and medially (*arrow*). (*C*) Axial postcontrast T1-weighted MR imaging demonstrates heterogeneous enhancement. (*Courtesy of* C. Doug Phillips, MD, Charlottesville, VA.)

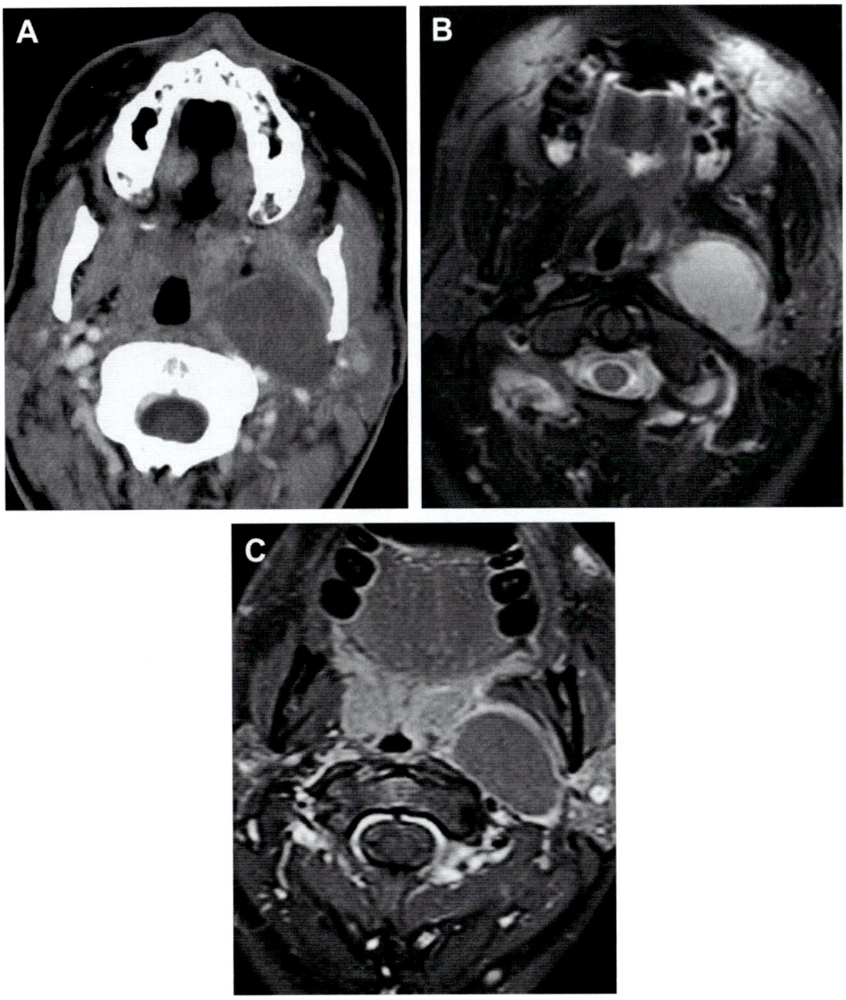

Fig. 18. Atypical second brachial cleft cyst in a 21-year-old woman with decreased cough and gag and left Horner's syndrome. (*A*) Postcontrast axial CT image of the neck at the level of the maxilla demonstrates a hypodense left parapharyngeal space lesion. Axial T2-weighted MR imaging reveals that the lesion is homogeneously hyperintense (*B*) and demonstrates no abnormal enhancement on the postcontrast T1-weighted image (*C*).

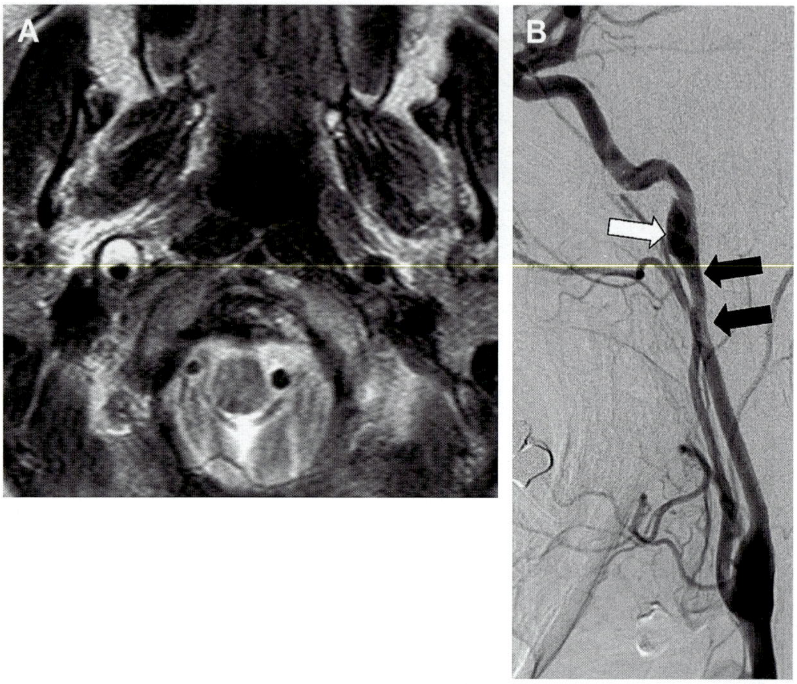

Fig. 19. ICA dissection in a patient who has right CN XII palsy after trauma. (*A*) Axial T2-weighted MR imaging shows crescentic high signal intensity in the lumen of the right ICA, narrowing the flow void. (*B*) Conventional angiography confirms the dissection (*black arrows*) and also visualizes a pseudoaneurysm superior to the level of the dissection (*white arrow*).

Schwannomas in the suprahyoid segment of the neck usually present as slow-growing masses.[57] When they arise in the carotid space, they displace the ICA anteriorly and medially (**Fig. 17**). Most of these tumors originate from the vagus nerve. Less commonly, they can originate from the glossopharyngeal nerve or the sympathetic chain.[58]

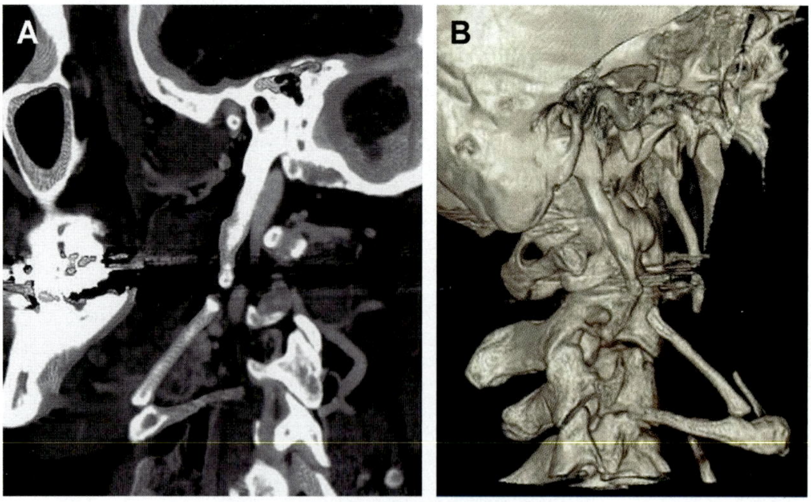

Fig. 20. Eagle's syndrome in a 45-year-old man with a history of tongue and posterior pharyngeal pain accentuated with tongue protrusion, in addition to occasional knife-like pain radiating to the right ear. Parasagittal right reformatted CT image (*A*) and right three-dimensional volume-rendered image (*B*) show complete ossification of the stylohyoid ligament. Identical ossification of the stylohyoid ligament was also found on the left side (not shown).

Second brachial cleft cysts are benign congenital lesions typically located anterolateral to the parapharyngeal space between the sternocleidomastoid muscle posteriorly and the submandibular gland anteriorly. They may rarely present atypically in the parapharyngeal space, however, causing impairment of multiple lower cranial nerves (**Fig. 18**).[59]

Malignant tumors, such as nasopharyngeal and oropharyngeal squamous cell carcinomas, can extend and compress the lower cranial nerves within the suprahyoid neck.[60] Additionally, other malignant tumors, such as lymphoma, have been reported as a cause of lower cranial nerve palsy.[61]

Dissection of the ICA, which is usually associated with hemicranial headache, Horner's syndrome, and cerebral ischemic symptoms, can also present with lower cranial nerve palsies.[62] Different theories have been proposed to explain the cranial nerve palsy associated with ICA dissection, including (1) aneurysmal dilatation of the ICA causing mechanical compression of the nerves within the carotid sheath and (2) impairment of blood supply to the cranial nerves. This second theory better explains the associated cranial nerve palsies in ICA dissections that occur without aneurysm formation.[62]

MR imaging, especially spin-echo T1-weighted precontrast sequences, is specific for identification of ICA dissection, demonstrating hematoma in the subintimal or subadventitial layers as a hyperintense crescent lesion (**Fig. 19**). It is superior to conventional angiography when there is no associated lumen abnormality or in cases resulting in nonspecific occlusion.[63] ICA dissections typically spare the proximal 2 cm involving the middle and distal segments. Most dissections end abruptly at the base of the skull, where the ICA enters the carotid canal.[64] Other vascular causes of lower cranial nerve palsies in the suprahyoid neck include ICA aneurysms[65,66] and iatrogenic insults in patients who have had an endarterectomy.[67]

Isolated glossopharyngeal neuralgia is rare, characterized by unilateral pain in the posterior oropharynx, ear lobe, and ipsilateral face.[3] It can be divided into a primary (idiopathic) type or a secondary type, in which a cause can be identified (trauma, inflammatory conditions, vascular deformities, aneurysms,[66] or tumors).[3] An interesting cause of secondary glossopharyngeal neuralgia results from compression of the nerve by an elongated styloid process, the so-called "Eagle's syndrome." It resembles primary glossopharyngeal neuralgia; however, in most cases, the pain is more constant and dull in character.[68] Evaluation of possible Eagle's syndrome is best performed by CT, demonstrating calcification or ossification of the stylohyoid ligament (**Fig. 20**).

Infectious diseases, including carotid space abscesses and deep neck infections, along the cranial nerve pathways can lead to cranial nerve involvement.[69] Penetrating neck trauma can also disrupt the nerve pathways.

Infrahyoid or Mediastinal Segment

The vagus nerve is the only one of the lower four cranial nerves that continues into the infrahyoid carotid space and mediastinum. Within the mediastinum, the left RLN can be affected in isolation because it loops under the aortic arch. Pathologic processes producing isolated paralysis of the

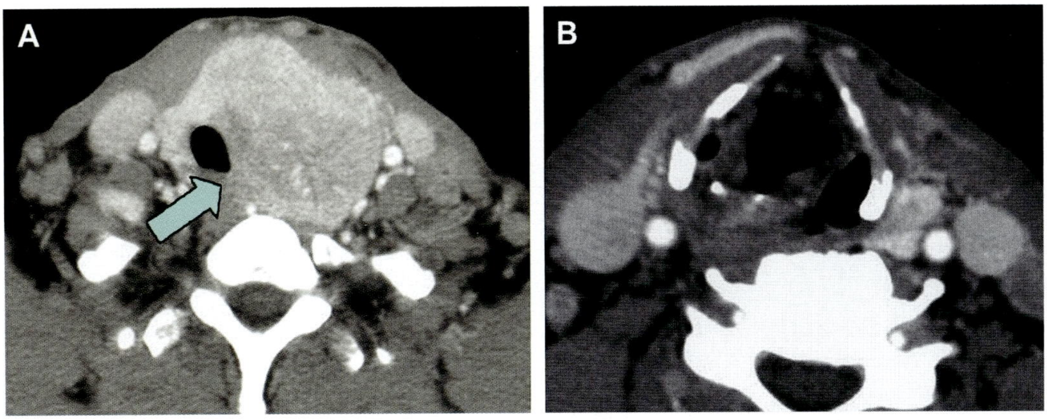

Fig. 21. Thyroid follicular neoplasm in a 67-year-old man with isolated left vocal cord paralysis. (*A*) Axial contrast-enhanced CT images of the neck at the thyroid level demonstrate heterogeneous enlargement with associated calcification of the left thyroid lobe and isthmus extending to involve the left tracheoesophageal groove (*arrow*). (*B*) More superiorly, an axial contrast-enhanced CT image shows left patulous piriform sinus and thickening and medialization of the aryepiglottic fold, compatible with left vocal cord paralysis. (*Courtesy of* Deborah L. Reede, MD, Brooklyn, NY.)

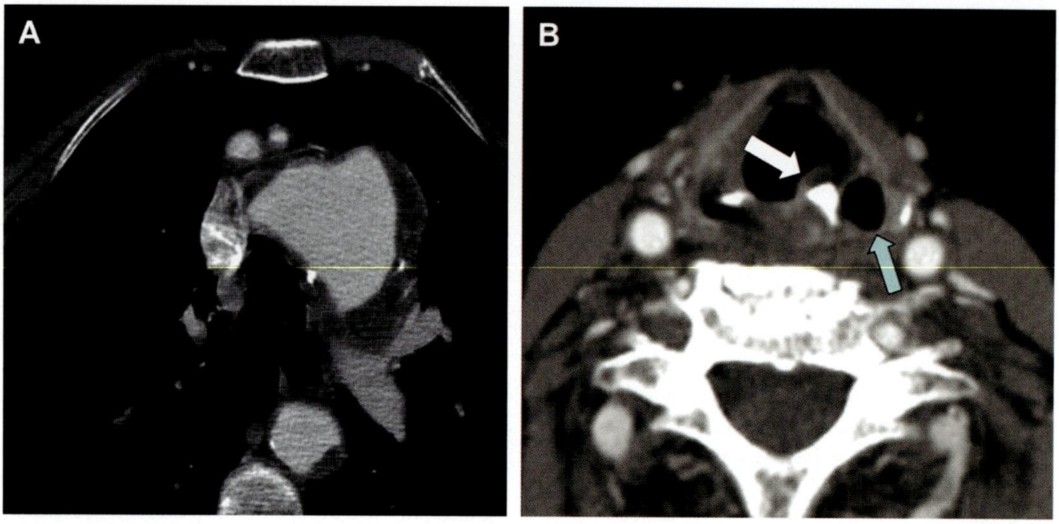

Fig. 22. Aortic arch aneurysm with thrombus in a 78-year-old man with new onset of hoarseness. (*A*) Contrast-enhanced axial CT at the level of the aortopulmonary window reveals dilatation of the aortic arch with associated thrombus. (*B*) Contrast-enhanced axial CT at the level of the larynx reveals ipsilateral enlargement of the piriform sinus (*gray arrow*) and rotation with anteromedial positioning of the arytenoid cartilage (*white arrow*), consistent with left recurrent laryngeal nerve (RLN) paralysis. (*Courtesy of* William P. Dillon, MD, San Francisco, CA.)

vagus nerve or its branches must be located in the infrahyoid or mediastinal segment. Patients present clinically with isolated vocal cord paralysis without involvement of proximal vagal function. Lesions in the infrahyoid segment can be considered as extrathyroid or intrathyroid. Aerodigestive tract squamous cell carcinoma is a common extrathyroidal etiology.[70] Intrathyroidal pathologic findings consist of benign and malignant thyroid tumors and parathyroidal carcinoma (**Fig. 21**).[71] In a review by Chiang and colleagues,[72] extracapsular spread of thyroid tumors was the most important risk factor for postoperative RLN palsy. RLN palsy is a known complication after thyroid surgery[72] and anterior cervical diskectomy or fusion.[73]

Mediastinal pathologic conditions may affect the left RLN in isolation, particularly pathologic findings in the region of the aortopulmonary window. The most common etiology is a bronchogenic neoplasm.[61] Other etiologies include lymphoma, bronchogenic cyst, aortic aneurysm (**Fig. 22**), and cardiomegaly.[6,74]

SUMMARY

The lower four cranial nerves can be affected by an acute or chronic process that has an impact on the way the patient presents clinically. Knowledge of nerve pathways and relations to surrounding structures is fundamental when evaluating patients who have lower cranial nerve symptoms. A systematic "segment-based" approach helps to narrow the differential diagnosis.

REFERENCES

1. Syms MJ, Singson MT, Burgess LP. Evaluation of lower cranial nerve deficits. Otolaryngol Clin North Am 1997;30(5):849–63.
2. Logermann JA. Mechanism of normal and abnormal swallowing. In: Cummings CW, Fredrickson JM, Harker LA, et al, editors. Otolaryngology—head and neck surgery. 2nd edition. St. Louis (MO): Mosby; 1993. p. 1704–12.
3. Claes J. Nervus glossopharyngeus (N. IX). Acta Otorhinolaryngol Belg 1986;40(1):207–14.
4. Castillo M, Mukherji SK. Magnetic resonance of cranial nerves IX, X, XI and XII. Top Magn Reson Imaging 1996;8(3):180–6.
5. Claes J, Jaco P. The nervus vagus. Acta Otorhinolaryngol Belg 1986;40(1):215–41.
6. Jacobs CJ, Harnsberger HR, Lufkin RB, et al. Vagal neuropathy: evaluation with CT and MR imaging. Radiology 1987;164(1):97–102.
7. Wilson-Pauwels P, Akesson E, Stewart PA, et al. Vagus nerve. In: Cranial nerves in health and disease. 2nd edition. London: BC Decker; 2002. p. 181–203.
8. De Cock M. Nervus accessorius (N. XI). Acta Otorhinolaryngol Belg 1986;40(1):243–57.
9. Yousry I, Moriggl B, Schmid UD, et al. Detailed anatomy of the intracranial segment of the hypoglossal nerve: neurovascular relationships and landmarks on magnetic resonance imaging sequences. J Neurosurg 2002;96(6):1113–22.

10. Tatu L, Moulin T, Bogousslavsky J, et al. Arterial territories of the human brain: brainstem and cerebellum. Neurology 1996;47(5):1125–35.
11. Brust JCM. Cerebral infarction. In: Rowland LP, editor. Merritt's textbook of neurology. 9th edition. Baltimore (MD): Williams & Wilkins; 1995. p. 253.
12. Khatri R, Leach J, Flaherty ML. False-negative diffusion-weighted imaging with lateral medullary infarction. Neurology 2006;67(10):E19.
13. Oppenheim C, Stanescu R, Dormont D, et al. False-negative diffusion-weighted MR findings in acute ischemic stroke. AJNR Am J Neuroradiol 2000;21(8):1434–40.
14. Barinagarrementeria F, Cantú C. Primary medullary hemorrhage. Report of four cases and review of the literature. Stroke 1994;25(8):1684–7 [comment in: Stroke 1995;26(4):706–7].
15. Zimmerman RS, Spetzler RF, Lee KS, et al. Cavernous malformations of the brain stem. J Neurosurg 1991;75(1):32–9.
16. Jha S, Das A, Gupta S, et al. Syringomyelia with syringobulbia presenting only with paralysis of 9th and 10th cranial nerves. Acta Neurol Scand 2002;105(4):341–3.
17. Kahana E, Leibowitz U, Alter M. Brainstem and cranial nerve involvement in multiple sclerosis. Acta Neurol Scand 1973;49(3):269–79.
18. Nakashima I, Fujihara K, Okita N, et al. Clinical and MRI study of brain stem and cerebellar involvement in Japanese patients with multiple sclerosis. J Neurol Neurosurg Psychiatry 1999;67(2):153–7 [comment in: J Neurol Neurosurg Psychiatry 1999;67(2):139].
19. Velázquez JM, Montero RG, Garrido JA, et al. [Lower cranial nerve involvement as the initial manifestation of Lyme borreliosis]. Afectación de nervios craneales bajos como manifestación inicial de la borreliosis de Lyme. Neurologia 1999;14(1):36–7 [in Spanish].
20. Smoker WR, Corbett JJ, Gentry LR, et al. High-resolution computed tomography of the basilar artery: 2. Vertebrobasilar dolichoectasia: clinical-pathologic correlation and review. AJNR Am J Neuroradiol 1986;7(1):61–72.
21. Panda S, Goyal V, Gupta V, et al. Vertebrobasilar dolichoectasia presenting as lower cranial nerve palsy. Neurol India 2004;52:279.
22. Chow M, Addas B, Sangalang V, et al. Cavernous malformation of the hypoglossal nerve: case report and review of the literature. Can J Neurol Sci 2002;29(2):191–4.
23. McKeon A, Murphy S, McNamara B, et al. Isolated hypoglossal nerve palsy due to compression by a dissecting vertebral artery. Eur Neurol 2005;53(3):162–4.
24. Garg RK. Tuberculosis of the central nervous system. Postgrad Med J 1999;75(881):133–40 [comment in: Postgrad Med J 1999;75(886):511].
25. Smith JK, Matheus MG, Castillo M. Imaging manifestations of neurosarcoidosis. AJR Am J Roentgenol 2004;182(2):289–95.
26. Christoforidis GA, Spickler EM, Recio MV, et al. MR of CNS sarcoidosis: correlation of imaging features to clinical symptoms and response to treatment. AJNR Am J Neuroradiol 1999;20(4):655–69.
27. Goyal M, Malik A, Mishra NK, et al. Idiopathic hypertrophic pachymeningitis: spectrum of the disease. Neuroradiology 1997;39(9):619–23.
28. Matano S, Shirasaki H, Terahata S, et al. Thickening of multiple cranial nerves in a patient with extranodal peripheral T-cell lymphoma. J Neuroimaging 2006;16(2):167–9.
29. Steinbok P. Clinical features of Chiari I malformations. Childs Nerv Syst 2004;20(5):329–31.
30. Ruff ME, Oakes WJ, Fisher SR, et al. Sleep apnea and vocal cord paralysis secondary to type I Chiari malformation. Pediatrics 1987;80(2):231–4.
31. Caldemeyer KS, Mathews VP, Azzarelli B, et al. The jugular foramen: a review of anatomy, masses, and imaging characteristics. Radiographics 1997;17(5):1123–39.
32. Rao AB, Koeller KK, Adair CF. From the archives of the AFIP. Paragangliomas of the head and neck: radiologic-pathologic correlation. Armed Forces Institute of Pathology. Radiographics 1999;19(6):1605–32.
33. Chakeres DW, LaMasters DL. Paragangliomas of the temporal bone: high-resolution CT studies. Radiology 1984;150(3):749–53.
34. Larson TC, Aulino JM, Laine FJ. Imaging of the glossopharyngeal, vagus, and accessory nerves. Semin Ultrasound CT MR 2002;23(3):238–55.
35. Gilmer-Hill HS, Kline DG. Neurogenic tumors of the cervical vagus nerve: report of four cases and review of the literature. Neurosurgery 2000;46(6):1498–503.
36. Laine FJ, Underhill T. Imaging of the lower cranial nerves. Magn Reson Imaging Clin N Am 2002;10(3):433–49.
37. Drevelegas A. Extra-axial brain tumors. Eur Radiol 2005;15(3):453–67.
38. Eldevik OP, Gabrielsen TO, Jacobsen EA. Imaging findings in schwannomas of the jugular foramen. AJNR Am J Neuroradiol 2000;21(6):1139–44.
39. Sekhar LN, Wright DC, Richardson R, et al. Petroclival and foramen magnum meningiomas: surgical approaches and pitfalls. J Neurooncol 1996;29(3):249–59.
40. Roberti F, Sekhar LN, Kalavakonda C, et al. Posterior fossa meningiomas: surgical experience in 161 cases. Surg Neurol 2001;56(1):8–20 [discussion: 20–1][comment in: Surg Neurol 2001;56(1):66].
41. Macdonald AJ, Salzman KL, Harnsberger HR, et al. Primary jugular foramen meningioma: imaging appearance and differentiating features. AJR Am J Roentgenol 2004;182(2):373–7.

42. Erdem E, Angtuaco EC, Van Hemert R, et al. Comprehensive review of intracranial chordoma. Radiographics 2003;23(4):995–1009.
43. Soo MY. Chordoma: review of clinicoradiological features and factors affecting survival. Australas Radiol 2001;45(4):427–34.
44. Laigle-Donadey F, Taillibert S, Martin-Duverneuil N, et al. Skull-base metastases. J Neurooncol 2005; 75(1):63–9.
45. Greenberg HS, Deck MD, Vikram B, et al. Metastasis to the base of the skull: clinical findings in 43 patients. Neurology 1981;31(5):530–7.
46. Chong VF, Khoo JB, Fan YF. Fibrous dysplasia involving the base of the skull. AJR Am J Roentgenol 2002;178(3):717–20.
47. Chang JT, Lin CY, Chen TM, et al. Nasopharyngeal carcinoma with cranial nerve palsy: the importance of MRI for radiotherapy. Int J Radiat Oncol Biol Phys 2005;63(5):1354–60.
48. Roh JL, Sung MW, Kim KH, et al. Nasopharyngeal carcinoma with skull base invasion: a necessity of staging subdivision. Am J Otolaryngol 2004;25(1): 26–32.
49. Lee AW, Foo W, Law SC, et al. Staging of nasopharyngeal carcinoma: from Ho's to the new UICC system. Int J Cancer 1999;84(2):179–87.
50. Ng SH, Chang TC, Ko SF, et al. Nasopharyngeal carcinoma: MRI and CT assessment. Neuroradiology 1997;39(10):741–6.
51. Chong VF, Mukherji SK, Ng SH, et al. Nasopharyngeal carcinoma: review of how imaging affects staging. J Comput Assist Tomogr 1999;23(6):984–93.
52. Slattery WH, Brackmann DE. Skull base osteomyelitis. Malignant external otitis. Otolaryngol Clin North Am 1996;29(5):795–806.
53. Rowlands RG, Lekakis GK, Hinton AE. Masked pseudomonal skull base osteomyelitis presenting with a bilateral Xth cranial nerve palsy. J Laryngol Otol 2002;116(7):556–8.
54. Legros B, Fournier P, Chiaroni P, et al. Basal fracture of the skull and lower (IX, X, XI, XII) cranial nerves palsy: four case reports including two fractures of the occipital condyle—a literature review. J Trauma 2000;48(2):342–8.
55. Urculo E, Arrazola M, Arrazola M, et al. Delayed glossopharyngeal and vagus nerve paralysis following occipital condyle fracture. Case report. J Neurosurg 1996;84(3):522–5.
56. Demisch S, Lindner A, Beck R, et al. The forgotten condyle: delayed hypoglossal nerve palsy caused by fracture of the occipital condyle. Clin Neurol Neurosurg 1998;100(1):44–5.
57. Leu YS, Chang KC. Extracranial head and neck schwannomas: a review of 8 years experience. Acta Otolaryngol 2002;122(4):435–7.
58. Som PM, Curtin HD. Parapharyngeal and masticator space lesions. In: Son PM, Curtin HD, editors. Head and neck imaging. 4th edition. St. Louis (MO): Mosby; 2003. p. 1965–6.
59. Shin JH, Lee HK, Kim SY, et al. Parapharyngeal second branchial cyst manifesting as cranial nerve palsies: MR findings. AJNR Am J Neuroradiol 2001;22(3):510–2.
60. Hardin CW, Harnsberger R, Osborn AG, et al. CT in the evaluation of normal and diseased oral cavity and oropharynx. Semin Ultrasound CT MR 1986;7:131–53.
61. Remley KB, Latchaw RE. Imaging of cranial nerves IX, X, and XI. Functional anatomy and pathology. Neuroimaging Clin N Am 1993;3(1):171–91.
62. Mokri B, Silbert PL, Schievink WI, et al. Cranial nerve palsy in spontaneous dissection of the extracranial internal carotid artery. Neurology 1996;46(2):356–9.
63. Schievink WI. Spontaneous dissection of the carotid and vertebral arteries. N Engl J Med 2001;344(12): 898–906 [comment in: N Engl J Med 2001;345(6): 467].
64. Provenzale JM. Dissection of the internal carotid and vertebral arteries: imaging features. AJR Am J Roentgenol 1995;165(5):1099–104.
65. Wilding LJ, Howlett DC, Anderson HJ, et al. Extracranial internal carotid artery aneurysm presenting as symptomatic hypoglossal and glossopharyngeal nerve paralysis. J Laryngol Otol 2004;118(2):150–2.
66. Lim YM, Lee SA, Kim DK, et al. Aneurysm of the extracranial internal carotid artery presenting as the syndrome of glossopharyngeal pain and syncope. J Neurol Neurosurg Psychiatry 2002;73(1):87–8.
67. Sweeney PJ, Wilbourn AJ. Spinal accessory (11th) nerve palsy following carotid endarterectomy. Neurology 1992;42:674–5.
68. Slavin KV. Eagle syndrome: entrapment of the glossopharyngeal nerve? Case report and review of the literature. J Neurosurg 2002;97(1):216–8.
69. Gunawardana SS, Earley AR, Pollard AJ, et al. Twelfth nerve palsy due to a retropharyngeal tuberculous abscess. Arch Dis Child 2004;89(6):579.
70. Harnsberger HR, Dillon WP. Major motor atrophic patterns in the face and neck: CT evaluation. Radiology 1985;155(3):665–70.
71. Remley K, Harnsberger R, Smoker WRK, et al. CT and MRI in the evaluation of glossopharyngeal, vagal, and spinal accessory neuropathy. Semin Ultrasound CT MR 1987;8(3):284–300.
72. Chiang FY, Wang LF, Huang YF, et al. Recurrent laryngeal nerve palsy after thyroidectomy with routine identification of the recurrent laryngeal nerve. Surgery 2005;137(3):342–7.
73. Baron EM, Soliman AM, Gaughan JP, et al. Dysphagia, hoarseness, and unilateral true vocal fold motion impairment following anterior cervical diskectomy and fusion. Ann Otol Rhinol Laryngol 2003;112(11):921–6.
74. Rice DC, Putnam JB. Recurrent bronchogenic cyst causing recurrent laryngeal nerve palsy. Eur J Cardiothorac Surg 2002;21(3):561–3.

Horner's Syndrome: Clinical and Radiographic Evaluation

Deborah L. Reede, MD[a,b,*], Ernst Garcon, MD[c], Wendy R.K. Smoker, MS, MD, FACR[d], Randy Kardon, MD, PhD[e]

KEYWORDS

- Horner's syndrome evaluation

Horner's syndrome (HS) occurs when there is interruption of the oculosympathetic pathway (OSP). This article reviews the anatomy of the OSP and clinical findings associated with lesions located at various positions along this pathway. The imaging findings of lesions associated with HS at various levels of the OSP, classified as preganglionic HS (first- and second-order neuron HS) or postganglionic HS (third-order neuron HS), are demonstrated.

ANATOMY OF THE OCULOSYMPATHETIC PATHWAY

The OSP supplies sympathetic innervation to the sweat glands (ipsilateral body and face), dilator muscles of the eye, and retractor muscles of the upper and lower eyelids. This pathway consists of three neurons and two relay centers (ciliospinal center of Budge-Waller and the superior cervical ganglion).

First-Order Neuron (FON)

The first-order neuron (FON) of the OSP is located in the posterior lateral aspect of the hypothalamus (**Fig. 1**). Postganglionic fibers (PGF) from this neuron descend in the reticular formation through the brainstem, cervical spinal cord, and proximal thoracic spinal cord and synapse in the second-order neurons (SON). The SON is located in the intermediolateral (IML) gray substance of the spinal cord at the level C8-T2 (Ciliospinal Center of Budge-Waller).[1–3]

Second-Order Neuron (SON)

The SON is located in the IML gray substance of the spinal cord between C8 and T2 (ciliospinal center of Budge-Waller) (see **Fig. 1**). The PGF exit in the ventral spinal roots (white rami communicantes) of C8, T1, and T2. These fibers pass through the inferior cervical or stellate ganglion (fusion of inferior cervical and first thoracic ganglia) and middle cervical ganglion without synapsing and eventually synapse in the superior cervical ganglion.

The inferior cervical and first thoracic ganglions are fused in 80% of the population. This results in the formation of a large ganglion called the stellate ganglion. This ganglion (inferior cervical or stellate) is located posterior to the vertebral artery between the transverse process of the C7 vertebra and the first rib. The middle cervical ganglion is at the level of the cricoid cartilage and has two or more

[a] State University of New York Health Science Center at Brooklyn, Brooklyn, NY, USA
[b] Department of Radiology, Long Island College Hospital, 339 Hicks Street, Brooklyn, NY 11201, USA
[c] Department of Radiology, University of Arkansas Medical Science, 4301 Markham Street, Little Rock, AR 72205, USA
[d] Department of Radiology, University of Iowa Hospitals and Clinics, 200 Hawkins Drive, 0453-G JCP, Iowa City, IA 52242, USA
[e] Department of Ophthalmology and Visual Sciences, University of Iowa Hospitals and Clinics and Veterans Administration, 200 Hawkins Drive, Iowa City, IA 52242, USA
* Corresponding author. Department of Radiology, Long Island College Hospital, 339 Hicks Street, Brooklyn, NY 11201.
E-mail address: dreede@chpnet.org (D.L. Reede).

Neuroimag Clin N Am 18 (2008) 369–385
doi:10.1016/j.nic.2007.11.003
1052-5149/08/$ – see front matter

neuroimaging.theclinics.com

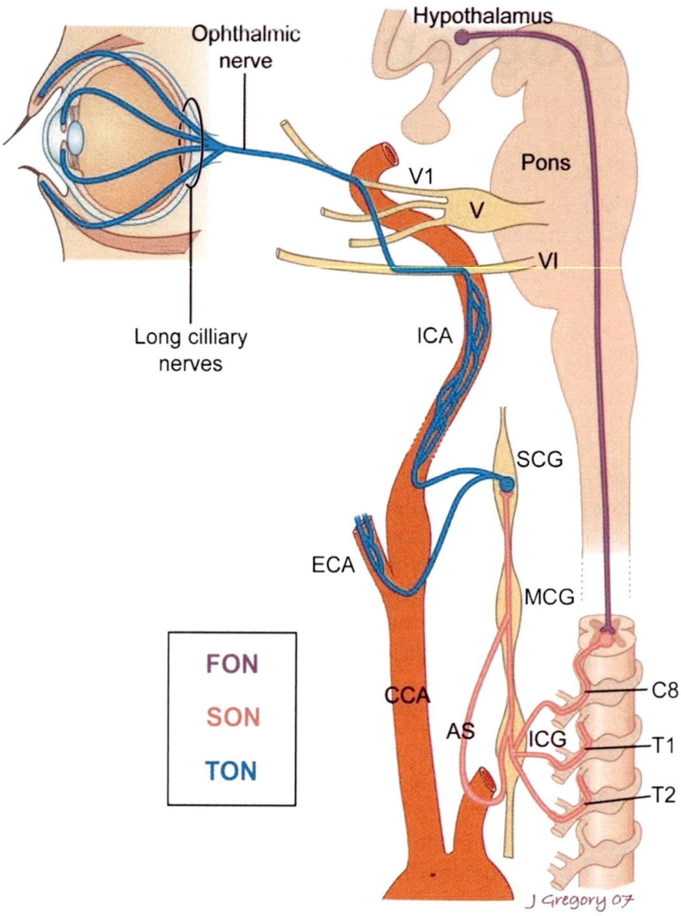

Fig. 1. Anatomy of the oculosympathetic pathway. AS, ansa subclavia; ECA, external carotid artery; ICA, internal carotid artery; ICG, inferior cervical ganglion; MCG, middle cervical ganglion; SCG, superior cervical ganglion; FON, first-order neuron; SON, second-order neuron; TON: third-order neuron.

connections to the inferior cervical or stellate ganglia.[4] This ganglion will be referred to as the inferior cervical ganglion in this article.

Third-Order Neuron (TON)

The superior cervical ganglion (TON) is located at the level of C2-C3, posterior to the carotid sheath and anterior to the longus colli muscle. There are numerous PGF with many anastomoses; however, only pertinent to a discussion of HS are the anterior fibers, which ascend and travel with the internal and external carotid arteries. The PGF of the TON travel in the adventitia of the internal carotid artery (carotid plexus) for a short distance and then attach to the cavernous sinus. Once in the cavernous sinus they attach to the abducens nerve (CN VI) and then onto the ophthalmic nerve (V1). The fibers then travel with the long ciliary nerve, a branch of the ophthalmic nerve (V1), through the superior orbital fissure (see **Fig. 1**). These fibers innervate the rectractor muscles of the upper and lower eyelids (Müller's muscles), dilator muscles of the pupil, lacrimal glands, and orbital vasomotor fibers. Fibers traveling with the external carotid artery follow the internal maxillary artery to the face and innervate the sweat glands of the face. Therefore, a lesion distal to the carotid bifurcation will not be associated with significant impairment of facial sweating. There are a few nerve fibers responsible for sweat to the forehead and lateral aspect of the nose that travel with the internal carotid artery (ICA). This explains the loss of sweat production in these areas with lesions distal to the carotid bifurcation.[1–3]

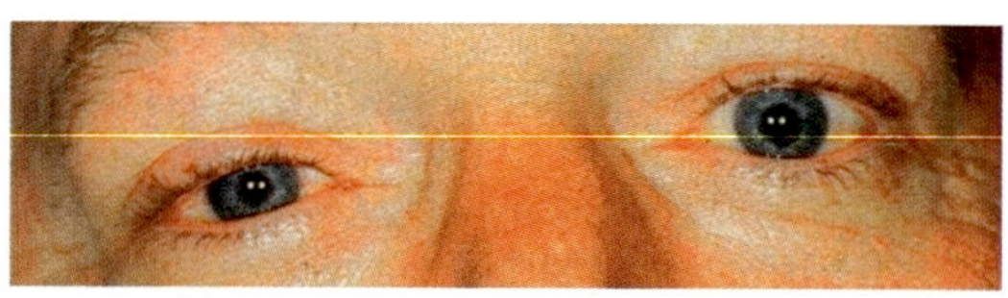

Fig. 2. Horner's eye findings. Classic clinical eye findings are demonstrated in this patient with a right Horner syndrome (ptosis of the upper eyelid, elevation of the lower eyelid, and miosis).

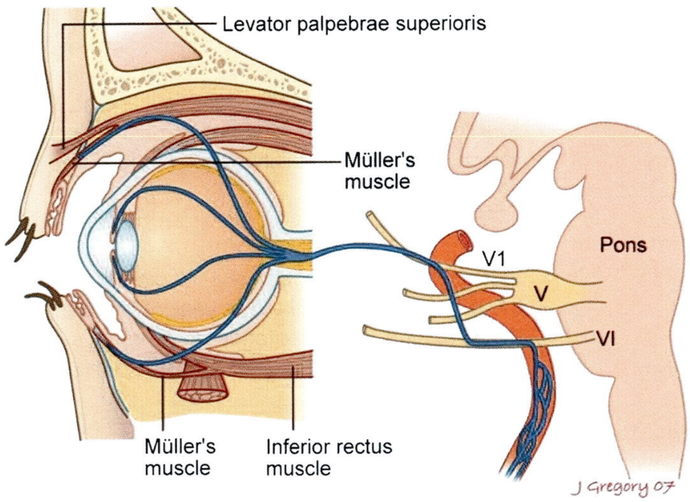

Fig. 3. Müller's muscles. The Müller's muscle in the upper eyelid arises from the undersurface of the levator palpebrae superioris muscle. Interruptions of the sympathetic innervation to this muscle cause ptosis of the upper eyelid. The Müller's muscle in the lower lid will elevate the lower eyelid slightly in HS ("upside-down ptosis").

HORNER'S SYNDROME CLINICAL FINDINGS

Johann Friedrich Horner first described the classic clinical triad of symptoms seen in HS, (ptosis, miosis, and anhidrosis) in 1869 (**Fig. 2**).[5]

Ptosis refers to a moderate drop of the upper eyelid. The levator palpebrae superioris muscle elevates the upper eyelid. This muscle is innervated by the oculomotor nerve (CN III). Müller's muscle in the upper eyelid is a thin sheet of smooth muscle arising from the undersurface of the levator palpebrae superioris muscle (**Fig. 3**). It also elevates the upper eyelid and controls the resting position of the upper eyelid (when the eye is open). It is innervated by the sympathetic nervous system, and therefore, interruptions of the sympathetic nerve supply result in ptosis.[2]

Miosis is a decrease in pupil size as a result of paralysis of the iris dilator muscles. This occurs when there is an interruption of the sympathetic innervation to the dilator muscle of the pupil (**Fig. 4**). The sphincter and dilator muscles of the pupil are innervated respectively by the sympathetic and parasympathetic systems. When the sympathetic system is interrupted, there are no forces to

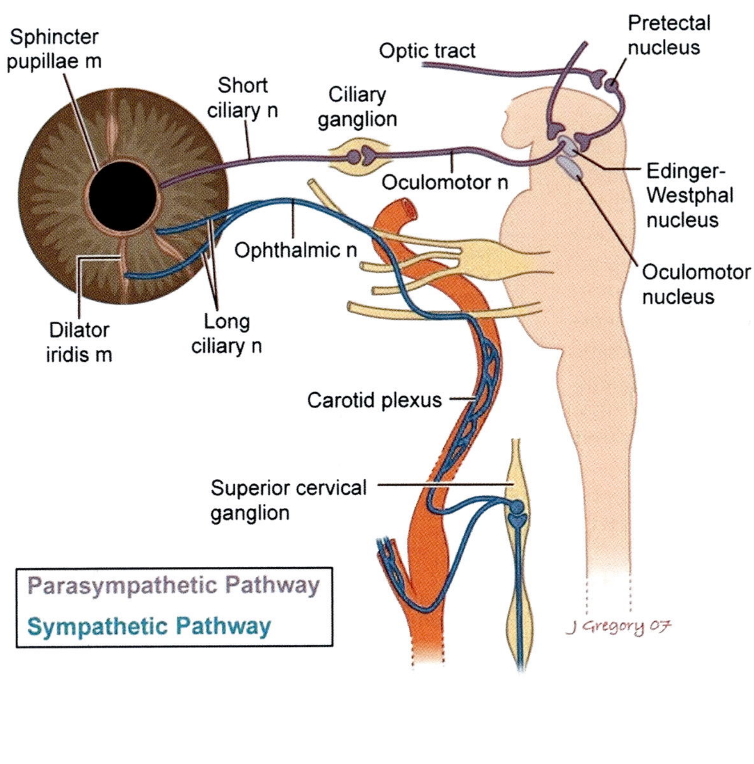

Fig. 4. Sympathetic and parasympathetic innervation of the iris. The sympathetic fibers innervate the dilator iridis muscles, which are responsible for dilating the iris. The sphincter pupillae muscle is innervated by the parasympathetic system. When the sympathetic innervation is interrupted, the parasympathetic system is unapposed and the pupil dilates.

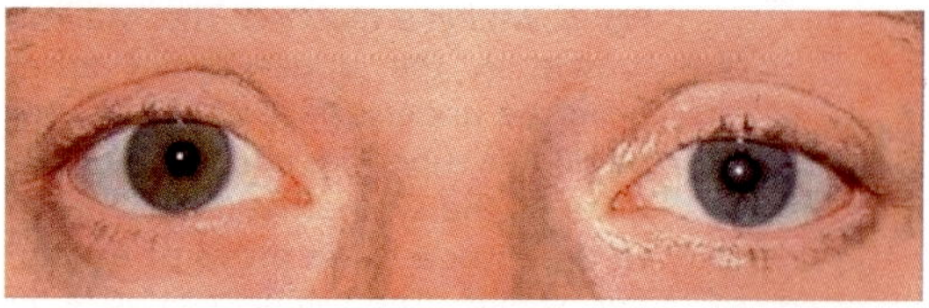

Fig. 5. Iris heterochromia. The light-colored right iris is secondary to abnormal pigment development because of interruption of the OSP in the first year of life. Miosis and ptosis (of both the upper and lower eyelids) are also present.

counteract the sphincter muscle, therefore the pupil will decrease in size.[2]

Anhidrosis occurs when there is interruption of sympathetic innervation to the sweat glands, resulting in a lack of sweat production. Unilateral absence of sweat to the forehead, face, or body is a good indication of HS. Different patterns in the distribution of anhidrosis are associated with FON, SON, and TON HS.[2] Anhidrosis is often not readily noticed by patients and it can be difficult to diagnose, thus it is not a routinely measurable sign.

Other Clinical Findings

Upside-down ptosis is best appreciated when the upper eyelid is in the resting position. Sympathetic fibers innervate retractor fibers in the lower eyelid (also called Müller's muscle), which arise from the fascial extension of the inferior rectus muscle (see **Fig. 3**). The lower lid will rise slightly in HS ("upside-down" ptosis). This, in conjunction with the upper eyelid changes, causes narrowing of the palpebral fissure and may give the false appearance of enophthalmos (see **Fig. 2**).[6]

Conjunctival hyperemia is a transient early sign of acute HS that is rarely present after the first few weeks. The conjunctiva is the mucous membrane that lines the eyelid and surface of the globe. Sympathetic denervation leads to vasodilatation of the capillaries in the conjunctiva (blood-shot eyes).[2,7]

Dilation lag refers to slower dilatation of the sympathetic denervated pupil in the dark when compared with the normal pupil. The sympathetic denervated pupil dilates slower than the normal pupil because the dilator muscles are innervated by the sympathetic nervous system.

Dilation lag is best observed when photographs of the eye are taken in the dark after 5 and 15 seconds.[2]

Iris heterochromia occurs when there is interruption of the OSP during the first year of life, resulting in a light-colored iris (**Fig. 5**). This finding is occasionally seen in HS, particularly in congenital lesions. In patients with brown eyes, the light-colored pupil is usually abnormal, however in patients with light-colored eyes the darker pupil is usually on the abnormal side. This finding, however, is not useful in the perinatal period because iris color is not established until several months of age.

The precise etiology for iris heterochromia in HS has not been established. It has been suggested that an intact OSP is required for pigmentation of the iris to develop in the first year of life, because the formation of pigmentation granules by stromal melanocytes is controlled by the sympathetic nervous system.[2,8]

Harlequin sign refers to the unilateral facial flushing seen in pediatric patients with congenital HS. The areas that do not flush correspond with anhidrotic areas. There is also a decrease in the skin temperature on the affected side. These findings are the result of impaired sympathetic vasodilatation.[9]

CLASSIFICATION

HS can be classified as preganglionic or postganglionic, based on the location of a lesion in the OSP with reference to the superior cervical ganglion (**Fig. 6**).

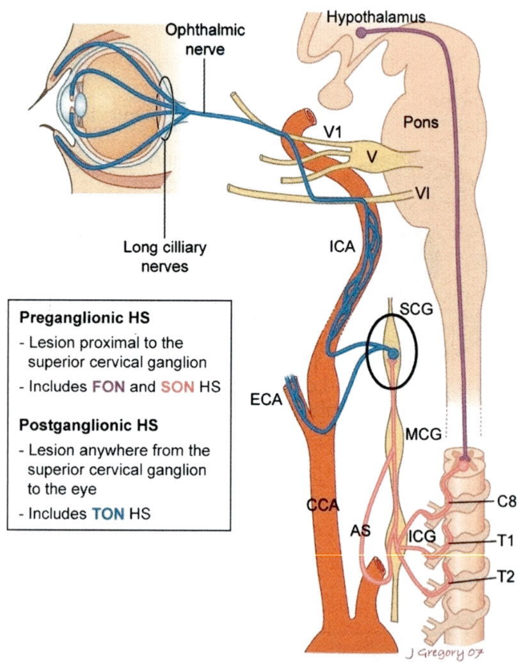

Fig. 6. Horner's classification. The superior cervical ganglion (SCG) divides the OSP into preganglionic and postganglionic segments.

The preganglionic segment is the segment of the OSP proximal to the superior cervical ganglion. It can be further subdivided into two subsegments:

1. The central, or FON, subsegment is located between the hypothalamus and IML before the FON PGF synapse in the ciliospinal center of Budge-Waller.
2. The peripheral, or SON, subsegment refers to the portion of the pathway from the SON before the PGF synapse with the superior cervical ganglion.

The postganglionic, or TON, segment is the portion of the pathway between the superior cervical ganglion and the eye.

To reiterate, the preganglionic segments include both the first- and second-order neurons; the third-order neuron is postganglionic.

CLINICAL EVALUATION

Anisocoria (unequal pupil size) may be a result of aging or sympathetic or parasympathetic dysfunction. Examination of the pupil in the dark will help determine the etiology (**Fig. 7**). The question to be answered is: "Is the pupil inequality greater in the dark or in the light?" If the inequality is greater in the light, this is consistent with a parasympathetic lesion. Examination of the eye in the dark will help differentiate physiologic anisocoria from sympathetic dysfunction. There is no dilation in patients with physiologic anisocoria. The sympathetic denervated pupil dilates slower than the normal pupil in the dark; therefore, the presence of dilation lag is consistent with interruption of the sympathetic pathway. This diagnosis should be confirmed by pharmacological testing. Patients with physiologic anisocoria do not have dilation lag.[2]

Pharmacological testing using cocaine and hydroxyamphetamine can be performed to confirm the diagnosis of HS and localize the lesion in the

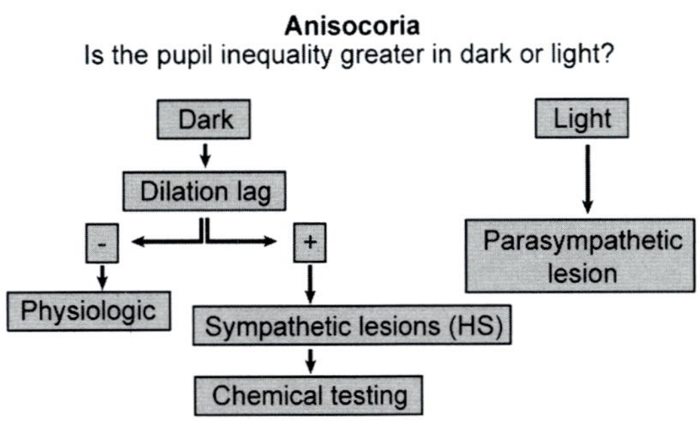

Fig. 7. Algorithm for the evaluation of anisocoria.

preganglionic or postganglionic segment of the OSP.

Initially, a 5% to 10% cocaine solution is placed in both eyes. This blocks the reuptake of norepinephrine in the synaptic junctions of the postganglionic fibers to the dilator muscles of the iris. If the sympathetic pathway is intact, norepinephrine is released from the nerve endings to the dilator muscles and the pupil dilates. Patients with HS have a poor response (minimal or no response) to cocaine. The affected pupils will dilate less than the normal pupil (**Fig. 8**). The upper eyelid will elevate slightly after the administration of cocaine. This should be followed by instillation of hydroxyamphetamine that will localize a lesion to the preganglionic or postganglionic segment of the OSP. Because cocaine inhibits the uptake of hydroxyamphetamine into the nerve terminals, there should be at least 3 days between the administration of cocaine and the localizing hydroxyamphetamine test to ensure maximum sensitivity to hydroxyamphetamine.[10] Hydroxyamphetamine releases norepinephrine from the presynaptic intraneural stores to the dilator muscles. The affected pupil in patients with preganglionic HS (FON and SON) will dilate. Pupil dilation is not seen in postganglionic HS (TON), because norepinephrine is depleted from the nerve endings (**Fig. 9**).[10]

PREGANGLIONIC LESIONS

First-Order Neuron Lesions

Location

Lesions that cause a FON HS are found anywhere from the hypothalamus to the level of the IML before the FON PGF synapse with the SON in the ciliospinal center of Budge-Waller (see **Fig. 1**).

Clinical findings

Miosis may be the only evidence of a FON HS. The anhidrosis distribution is ipsilateral to the entire half of the body (**Fig. 10**). Cerebellar, brain stem, or cervical spinal cord symptoms are usually present.[11]

Pharmacological testing

There is minimal or no pupil dilatation after the administration of cocaine. Dilation will increase after the administration of hydroxyamphetamine (see **Fig. 10**).

Imaging

The initial imaging study will depend on the clinical presentation. Patients with FON HS and brain or brain stem symptoms should be evaluated with MRI of the brain ± magnetic resonance angiography (MRA). If the patient has a FON HS without

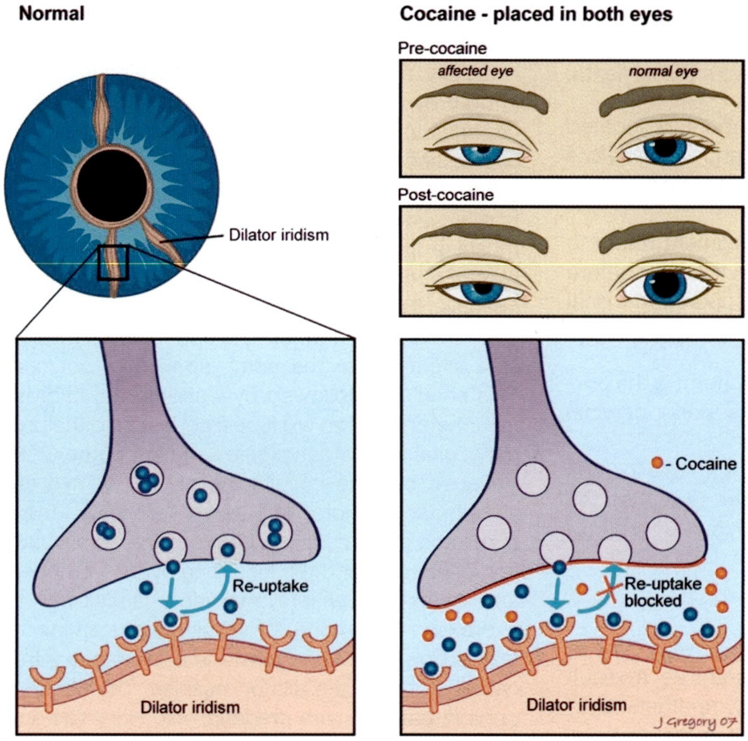

Fig. 8. Sympathetic nerve ending after cocaine administration. Under normal conditions there is continuous release of the norepinephrine (NE) from the presynaptic nerve terminals and reuptake of the NE into the sympathetic nerve terminals. Cocaine blocks the reuptake of NE, which leads to an accumulation of NE in the synaptic cleft. This leads to pupil dilatation. If the OSP is not intact the pupil will not dilate as much as the normal pupil. The eye findings in a patient with Horner's Syndrome pre and post cocaine administration are demonstrated above.

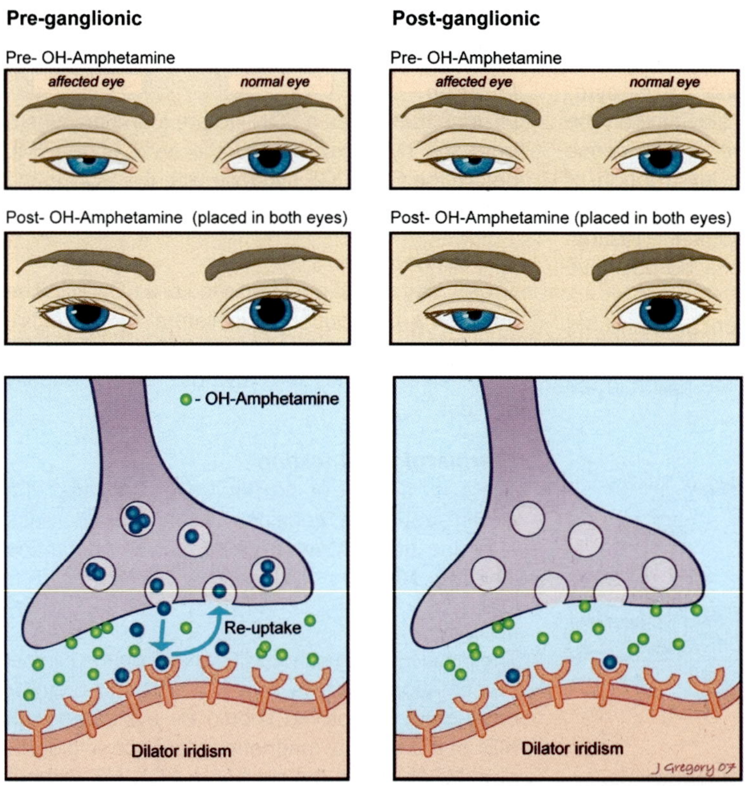

Fig. 9. Postganglionic nerve ending post-OH-amphetamine. OH-amphetamine promotes the release of norepinephrine from the postganglionic nerve terminals. The pupil will dilate in patients with preganglionic HS after the administration of OH-amphetamine. The pupil will not dilate in patients with postganglionic HS because norepinephrine is depleted from the nerve endings.

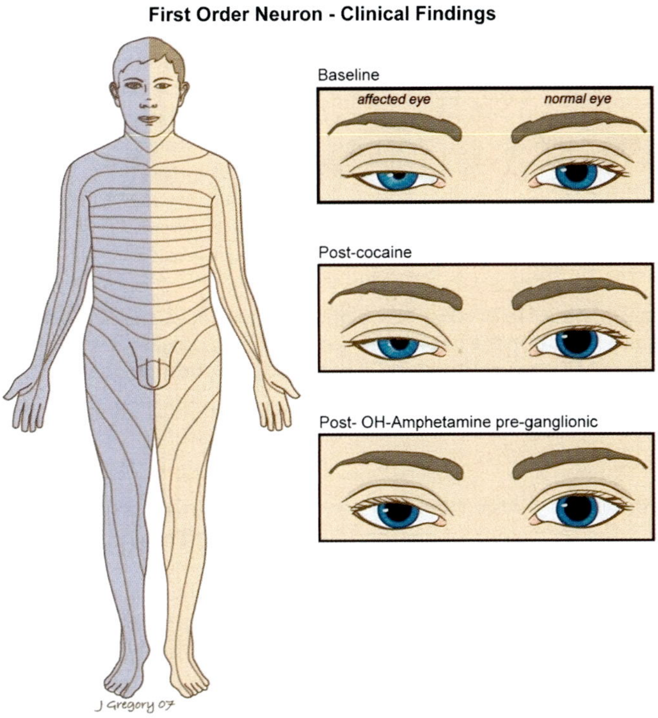

Fig. 10. First-order neuron clinical findings. The pupil size after the administration of cocaine shows a poor response but does increase in size after the administration of hydroxyamphetamine. Anhidrosis distribution in FON lesions is ipsilateral to the entire half of the body.

brain or brain stem symptoms, the first areas evaluated with an MRI should be the cervical and upper thoracic spine.[12]

FON HS Pathology

Hypothalamic lesions

The FON is located in the posterolateral aspect of the hypothalamus. Tumors, hemorrhage, or infarcts in this region may result in a FON HS (**Fig. 11**).[11]

Lateral medullary plate syndrome (Wallenberg syndrome)

Brain stem infarcts are the most common cause of FON HS. Occlusion of the posterior inferior cerebellar artery (PICA) or vertebral arteries can produce infarcts in the region of the lateral medullary plate (LMP). Infarcts in the LMP produce a number of neurologic deficits, including cranial nerve (CN) palsies and FON HS because of the neural structures found in this region (**Fig. 12**). The clinical triad of HS, ipsilateral ataxia, and

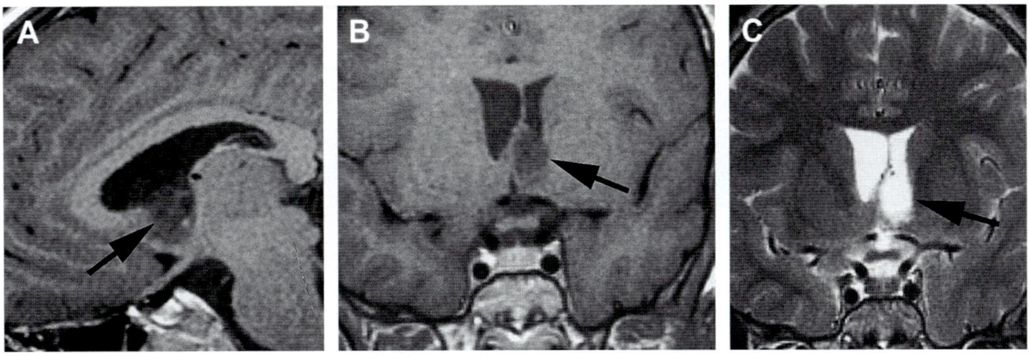

Fig. 11. Hypothalamic pilocytic astrocytoma. This 13-year-old male presented with headaches and left anisocoria. Pharmacological testing localized the lesion in the preganglionic segment. Sagittal (*A*) and coronal (*B*) T1-weighted image post-contrast and coronal (*C*) T2-weighted image shows a cystic nonenhancing mass (*arrows*) in the hypothalamus inferior to the foramen of Monro.

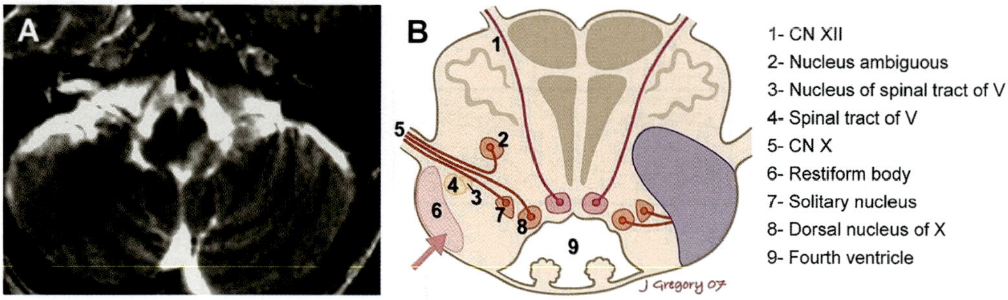

Fig. 12. Wallenberg syndrome (lateral medullary plate infarct). Axial T2-weighted image (*A*) at the level of the medulla demonstrates an area of increased signal intensity in the left lateral medullary plate consistent with an infarct. Diagram of the medulla (*B*) shows the location of the neural structures in this region. The postganglionic fibers of the FON are located in the restiform body (inferior cerebellar peduncle).

contralateral hypalgesia is seen in patients with LMP infarcts.[13]

Syringohydromyelia

This intramedullary cyst contains cerebrospinal fluid (CSF) and can cause compression of gray and white matter (**Fig. 13**). Syringohydromyelia is a slowly progressive disease that primarily involves the cervical spinal cord. Extension into the medulla and upper thoracic cord can occur. The typical symptoms include upper limb weakness and atrophy, as well as anesthesia to pinprick and temperature sensation. HS can be seen in conjunction with these findings or as an isolated finding in patients with this condition. HS in this condition can alternate from eye to eye.[14–16] Alternating HS can also be seen in cervical spinal cord injuries and Brown Sequard's syndrome.[17,18]

Multiple sclerosis

The presence of HS in a patient with a history of a demyelinating disease such as multiple sclerosis (MS) suggests the possibility of spinal cord involvement. MS plaques tend to occur in the dorsolateral aspect of the cord where the OSP travel through the cord (**Fig. 14**). Both gray and white matter can be involved.

Spinal cord neoplasms

Primary lesions of the spinal cord and intramedullary metastases that occur in the region where the

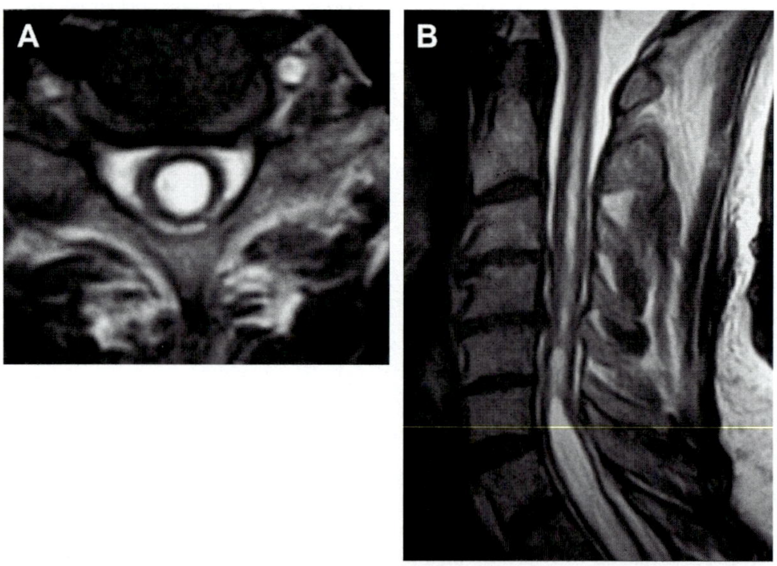

Fig. 13. Syringohydromyelia. Axial (*A*) and sagittal T2-weighted image (*B*) of the cervical cord show a cystic spinal cord lesion extending from C6 to T1. There is expansion of the involved central canal and spinal cord.

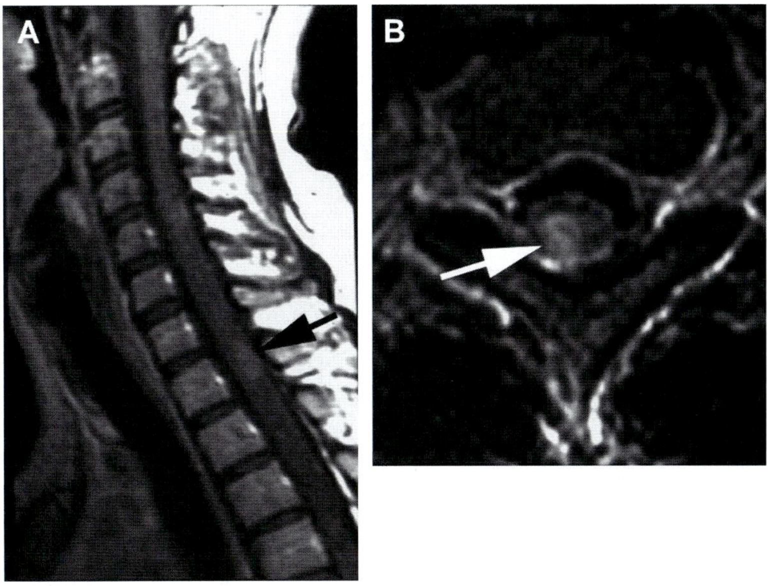

Fig. 14. Multiple sclerosis. Post-gadolinium sagittal T1-weighted image (*A*) of the cervical spine demonstrates a focus of abnormal enhancement in the posterolateral aspect of the cord. Post-gadolinium enhanced axial T1-weighted image (*B*) with fat suppression shows an area of enhancement in the right posterolateral aspect of the spinal cord.

OSP travels through the cord can produce FON HS (**Fig. 15**).

Other lesions that can produce FON HS include, trauma and inflammatory disease (poliomyelitis, transverse myelitis).[11,17,18]

Second-Order Neuron Lesions

Location

Lesions that produce this type of HS can involve the SON in the ciliospinal center of Budge- Waller or its PGF before they synapse with the superior

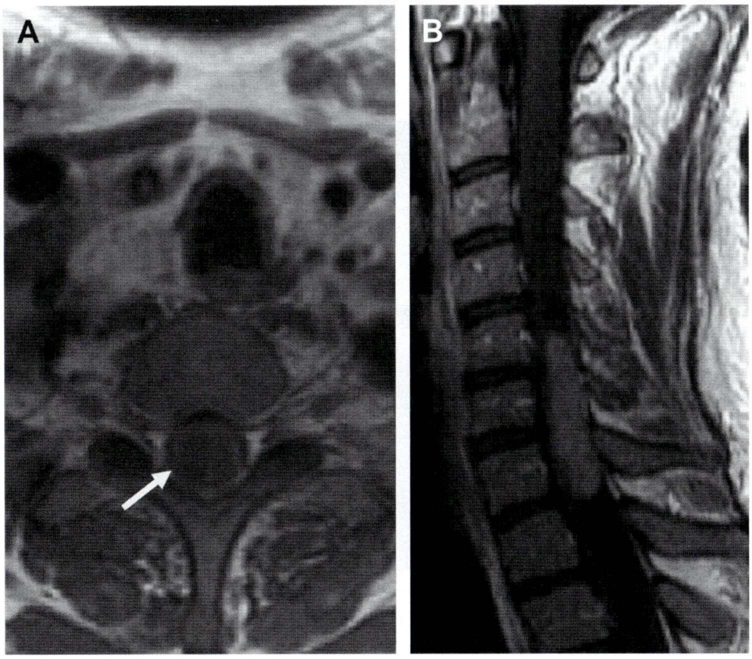

Fig. 15. Ependymoma of the cervical cord. This 38-year-old female presented with neck pain and a right preganglionic HS. Axial T1-weighted image (*A*) shows a mass on the right side of the cord (*arrow*) that enhances on the postcontrast sagittal T1-weighted image (*B*). The mass extends from C5 to the C7-T1 intervertebral disk space.

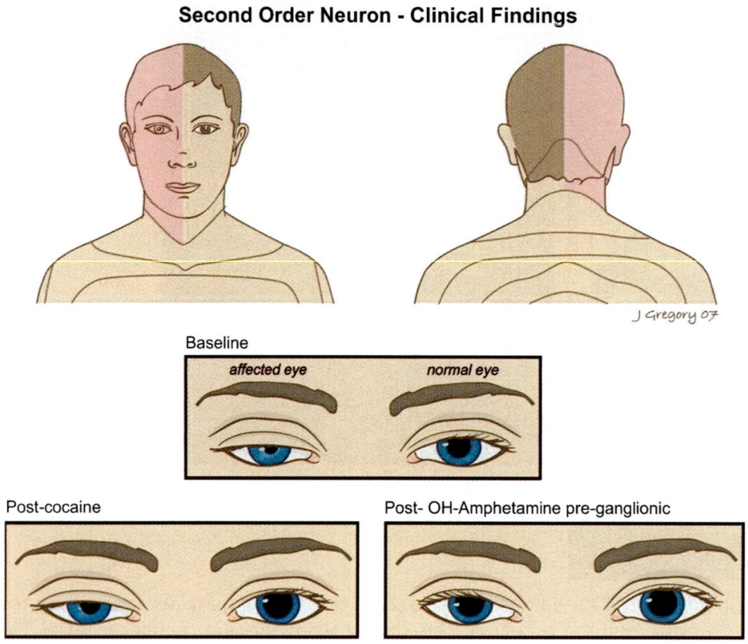

Fig. 16. Second-order neuron clinical findings. The pupil size after the administration of cocaine shows a poor response but does increase in size after the administration of hydroxyamphetamine. Anhidrosis distribution is ipsilateral to the face and neck in SON HS.

cervical ganglion (see **Fig. 1**). Most cases of preganglionic HS are secondary to lesions in this location.

Clinical findings

Patients with SON HS often have the full syndrome of ptosis, miosis, and anhidrosis. The anhidrosis distribution is ipsilateral to the face and neck (**Fig. 16**). A brachial plexopathy may also be present.

Pharmacological testing

There is minimal or no pupil dilatation after the administration of cocaine. Dilation increases after the administration of hydroxyamphetamine (see **Fig. 16**).

Imaging

Scans (CT or MR) of the neck should cover the area from the level of the superior cervical ganglion (angle of the mandible/C2-C3) to T2 (12). Lesions

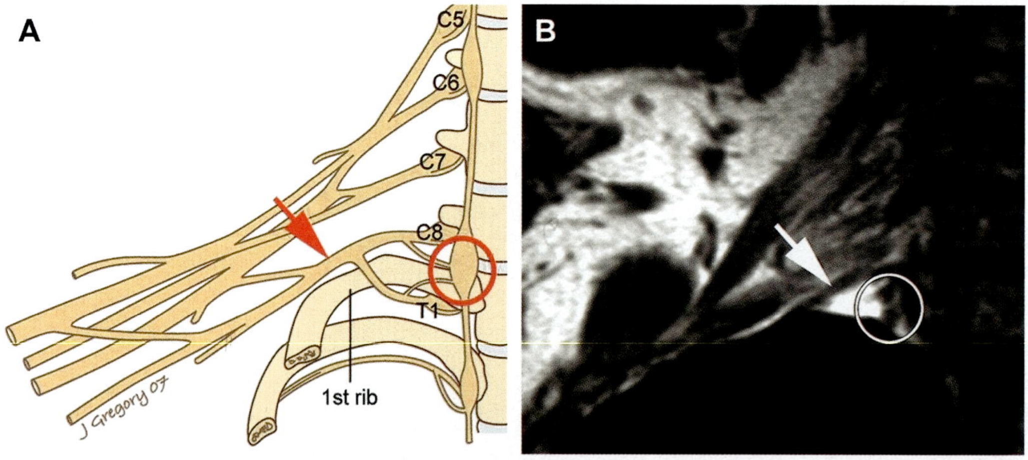

Fig. 17. Relationship of the brachial plexus and sympathetics. The illustration (*A*) shows the relationship of the inferior trunk of the brachial plexus (*arrow*), first rib, and inferior cervical ganglion (○). Coronal T1-weighted MR image (*B*) shows the C8 nerve root (*arrow*) superior to the ICG (○).

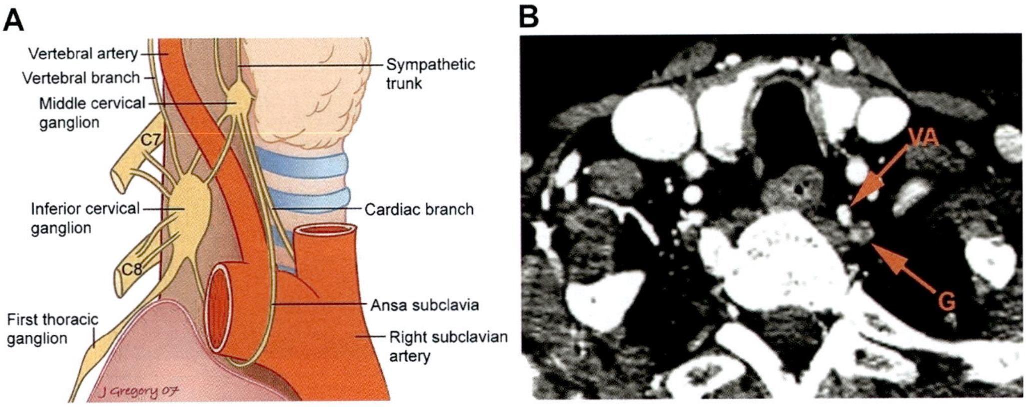

Fig. 18. Relationship of the inferior and middle cervical ganglion to the vertebral artery. There are numerous fibers connecting the MCG and ICG, which are located anterior and posterior to the vertebral artery (*A*) respectively. The normal ICG (G) can occasionally be identified posterior to the vertebral artery (VA) on cross-sectional imaging (*B*).

involving the SON and/or its PGF in the spine (C8-T2), nerve roots, or neck can produce a SON HS.

SON HS Pathology

Pancoast tumors

Pancoast tumors are bronchogenic carcinomas (squamous cell or adenocarcinoma) located in the lung apex (superior sulcus). These lesions can cause a brachial plexopathy when the inferior trunk of the brachial plexus and/or C8/T1 nerve roots are involved. A SON HS occurs when there is involvement of the inferior cervical or stellate ganglion (fused first thoracic and inferior cervical ganglion) or SON postganglionic fibers before they synapse with the superior cervical ganglion (SCG) (**Figs. 17–19**).[19,20]

Sympathetic schwannoma

These benign nerve sheath tumors account for 20% to 30% of tumors in the post-styloid portion of the parapharyngeal space (**Fig. 20**). These lesions usually arise from the vagus nerve or sympathetic chain. Lesions can also originate in the ganglion (see **Figs. 18 and 19**). Nerve sheath tumors arising from the sympathetic chain are uncommon. Horner's syndrome is rarely a part of the initial presentation but is often encountered after surgical intervention.[21–23]

Neuroblastic tumors

There are three tumors in this category: neuroblastoma, ganglioneuroblastoma, and ganglioneuroma. Neuroblastic tumors are the third most common neoplasm of early childhood and the most common tumor in the first year of life.[24] These tumors arise from neural crest blast cells in the adrenal medulla or the cervical sympathetic chain. Seventy-five percent to 90% of these lesions occur in the abdomen. Less than 5% of these lesions occur in the neck.[25–28] Histologically, the three types are different developmental stages of the same disease. Ganglioneuromas are the most differentiated and neuroblastomas the least differentiated with the most potential for metastasis. All three cell types can be seen in one lesion.[26] Those occurring in the cervical and thoracic region have a better prognosis than abdominal neuroblastic tumors.

Cervical neuroblastic tumors should be ruled out in children who present with HS and iris heterochromia, without a history of cervical trauma (**Fig. 21**).

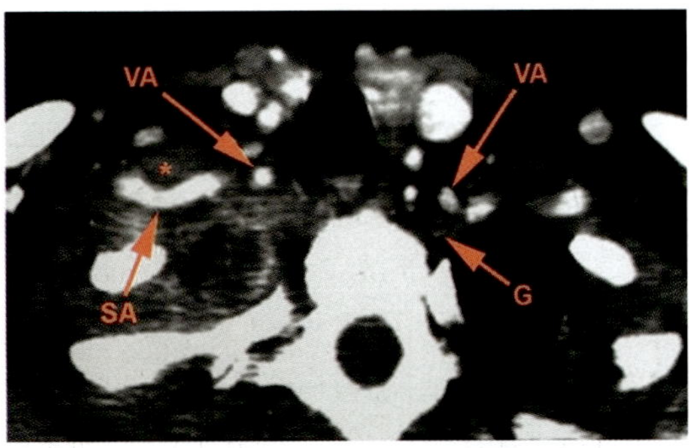

Fig. 19. Pancoast tumor. This 58-year-old male presented with weight loss, right brachial plexopathy, and SON HS. Contrast-enhanced CT at the level of the thoracic inlet shows a necrotic mass in the right lung apex. The mass abuts the posterior aspect of the right subclavian artery (SA) where the inferior trunk of the brachial plexus is located. The normal left ICG (G) is seen posterior to the vertebral artery (VA). The right ICG is encased by tumor.

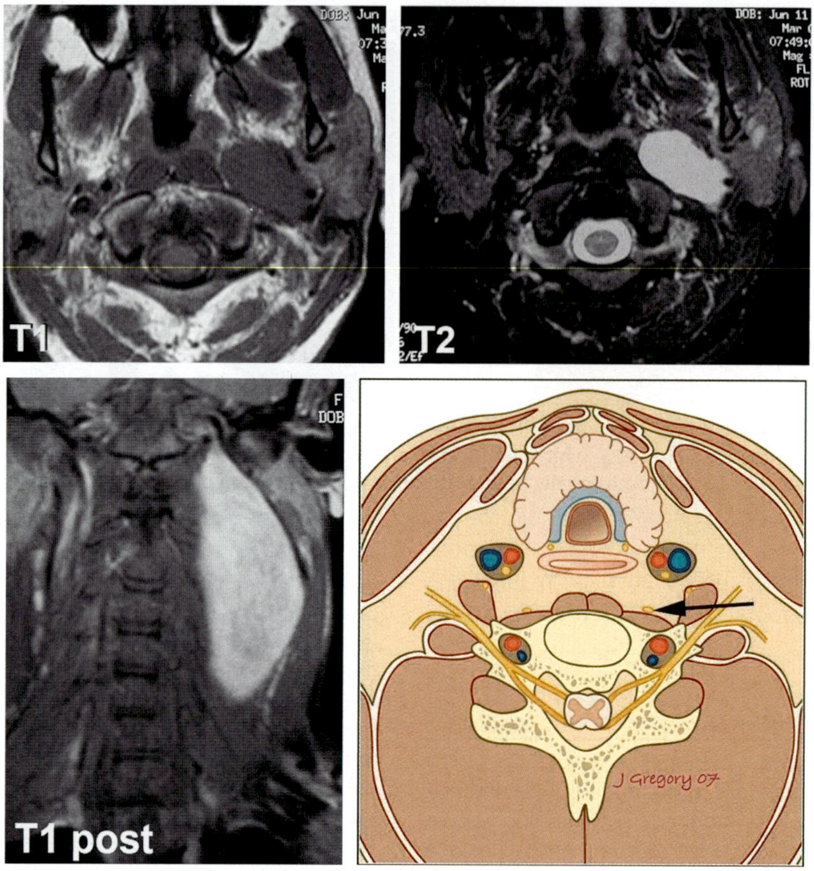

Fig. 20. Sympathetic chain schwannoma. Axial T1-weighted MR image shows a mass slightly hypointense to muscle in the left post-styloid parapharyngeal space causing anterior lateral displacement of carotid sheath structures. This mass increases in signal intensity on the T2 sequence and enhances heterogeneously after contrast administration. The normal anatomic relationship of the sympathetic chain (*arrow*) and the carotid sheath are shown in the illustration.

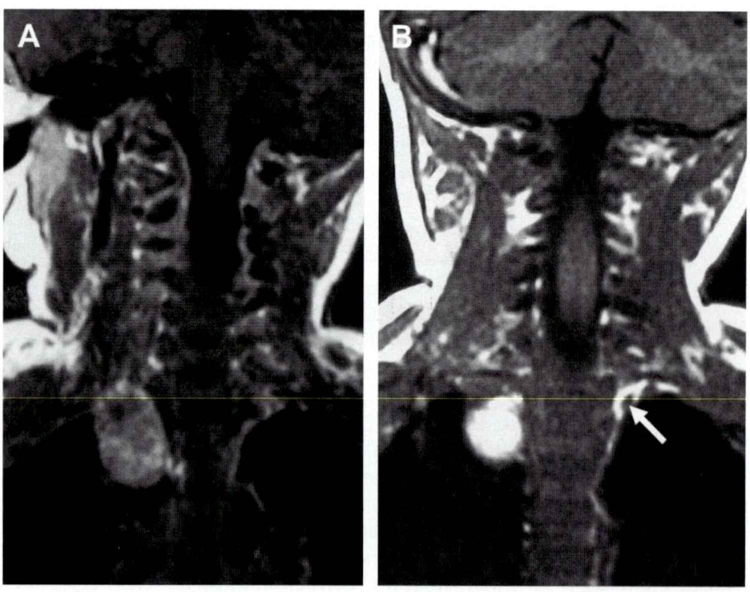

Fig. 21. Inferior cervical ganglion neuroblastoma. This 10-year-old boy presented with left iris heterochromia and SON HS. Axial T1-weighted image (*A*) shows a mass in the right lower neck that is causing an indentation on the right lung apex. Postgadolinium T1-weighted image (*B*) shows enhancement in the lesion. The normal left ICG is identified on the left (*arrow*).

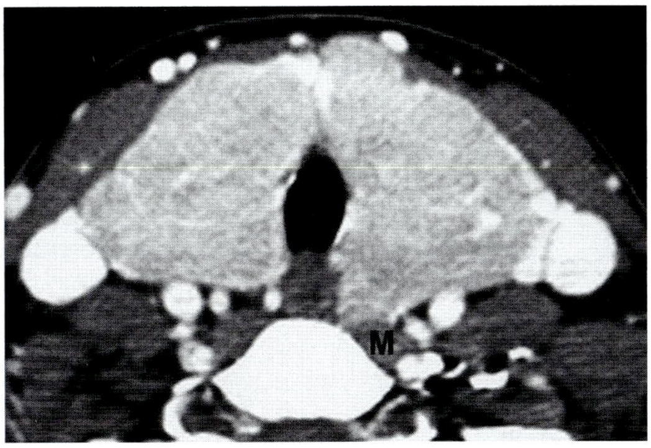

Fig. 22. Goiter. Contrast-enhanced CT of the neck shows an enlarged thyroid gland in this patient with SON HS. The posterior aspect of the left lobe abuts the prevertebral muscles (M). The cervical sympathetic chain is compressed between the enlarged thyroid and prevertebral muscles.

Goiter

Benign thyroid lesions rarely cause HS or nerve palsies. These findings are encountered more often in patients with thyroid malignancies. Occasionally, an enlarged thyroid gland may cause extrinsic compression on adjacent nerves and produce neurologic findings (**Fig. 22**).[28,29]

Other causes of SON HS include surgery or trauma to the upper thorax or neck, primary spinal nerve root tumors and lesions that destroy or compress the nerve roots (osteophytes, nerve root avulsions and tumors), first thoracic disk herniation, jugular venous.

Jugular venous ectasia, subclavian artery aneurysm, and neck masses causing compression of the cervical sympathetic chain.[30–34]

POSTGANGLIONIC LESIONS

Third-Order Neuron Lesions

Location

Lesions occurring anywhere from the superior cervical ganglion to the eye can produce a TON HS.

Clinical findings

The full syndrome of ptosis, miosis, and anhidrosis is usually present. Anhidrosis of the ipsilateral face and neck is seen with lesions involving the SCG. Lesions distal to the SCG have anhidrosis limited to the ipsilateral nose and forehead (**Fig. 23**). Proptosis, chemosis, or conjunctival hyperemia is often present in association with TON HS when an orbital lesion is the etiology.[11]

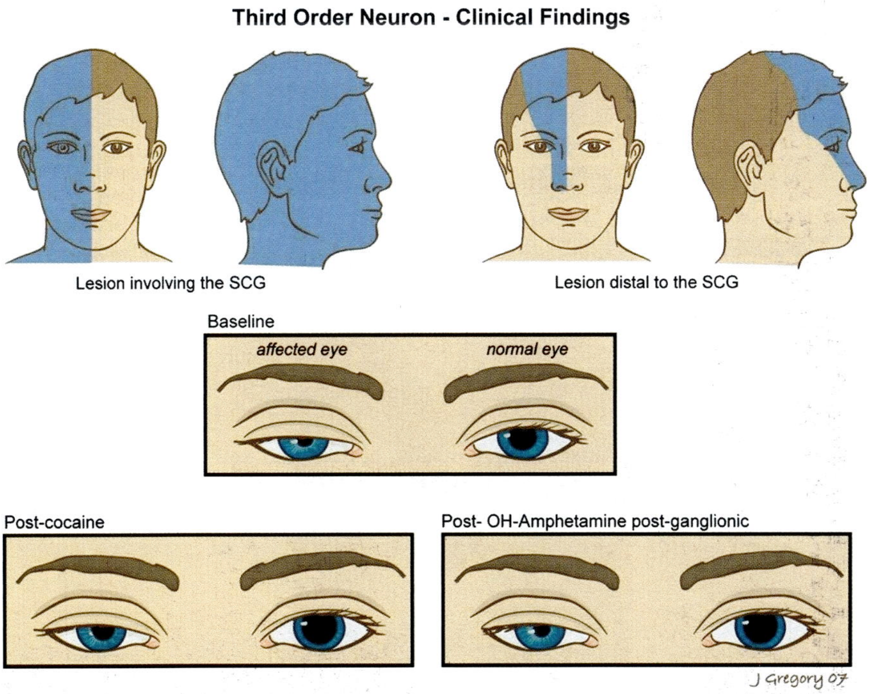

Fig. 23. Third-order neuron clinical findings. The pupil size after the administration of cocaine shows a poor response and does not increase in size after the administration of hydroxyamphetamine. The anhidrosis distribution is ipsilateral to the face and neck in lesion involving the superior cervical ganglion (SCG). If the lesion is distal to the SCG, anhidrosis is limited to the ipsilateral nose and forehead.

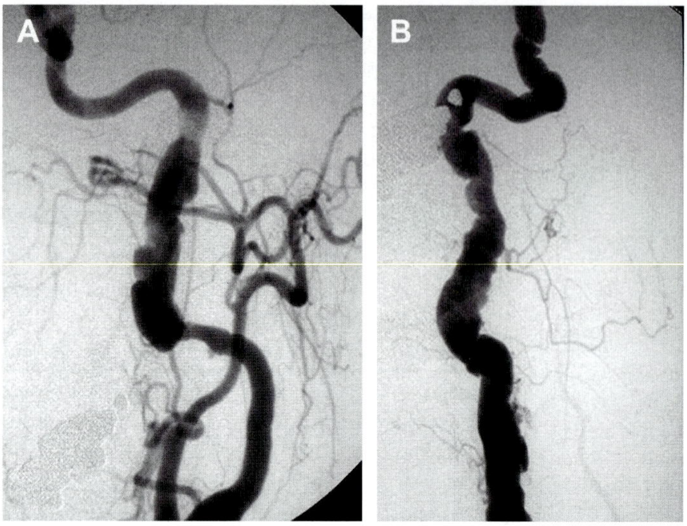

Fig. 24. Fibromuscular dysplasia (FMD). An anteroposterior view from an angiogram of the right internal carotid (*A*) and vertebral (*B*) arteries show areas of dilation and stenoses consistent with a "string of beads" appearance. This is consistent with a type 1 FMD. This patient presented with TON HS.

Pharmacological testing

The pupil does not dilate after the administration of cocaine and the degree of dilatation does not increase after hydroxyamphetamine (see **Fig. 23**).

Imaging

If there are no other clinical findings imaging is usually not performed because the cause of the HS is likely secondary to a benign condition. If a lesion cannot be localized clinically and imaging is requested, scan (CT or MR) should be obtained from the superior cervical ganglion inferiorly (angle of the mandible/C2-C3) through the orbit superiorly.[12] Coexisting clinical findings will dictate the area that should be scanned.

TON HS Pathology

Lesion that dilates or compresses the carotid artery can put pressure on the carotid plexus and cause a TON HS.

Fibromuscular dysplasia (FMD)

This vasculopathy of unknown etiology causes proliferative changes in the intima and media of

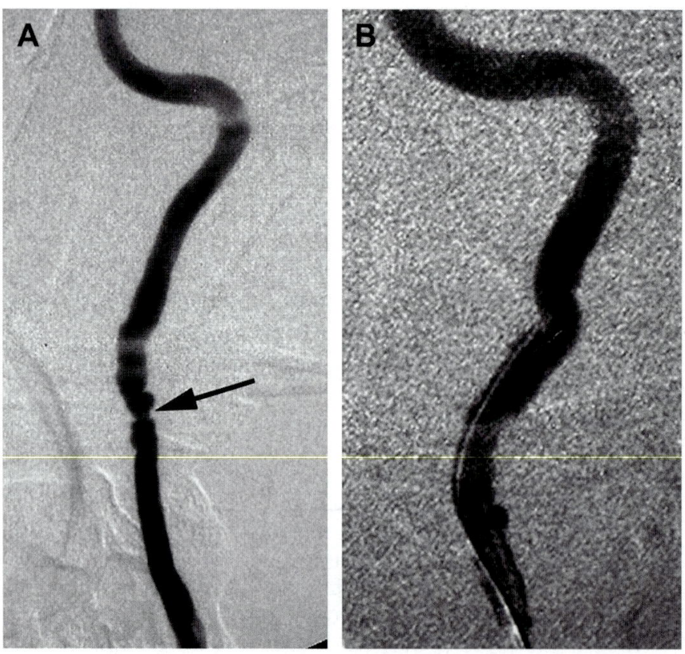

Fig. 25. Fibromuscular dysplasia pre- and postangioplasty. Selective internal carotid artery injection shows a segmental area of dilatation and narrowing consistent with FMD (*A*). There is a focal area of stenosis in the lesion (*arrow*). The patient was successfully treated with balloon angioplasty (*B*), but developed a TON HS postangioplasty.

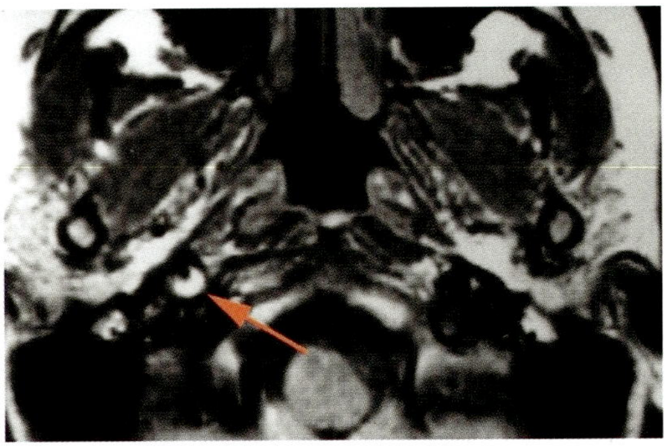

Fig. 26. Carotid dissection. Axial T1-weighted MR image shows an area of increased signal intensity (*arrow*) in the periphery of the right ICA that represents clot in the area of a dissection.

the cervical internal carotid artery. Typically it produces a "string of pearls" appearance on conventional angiography or MRA. The carotid bifurcation and proximal ICA are usually spared. The dilated portions of the carotid artery can cause compression of the cervical sympathetic plexus and produce a TON HS (**Fig. 24**). HS can also occur after therapeutic angioplasty as a complication (**Fig. 25**).

Carotid dissection

Internal carotid artery dissection should be suspected if a patient has a history of periorbital and/or facial pain, ipsilateral visual loss, ipsilateral hemicranial headache, and HS following trauma. The carotid plexus is compressed by the hematoma associated with the carotid dissection. HS is present in 40% to 50% of patients and may be transient. CT/computer tomography angiography or MR/MRA is the imaging modality of choice for the evaluation of these patients (**Fig. 26**).[35–39]

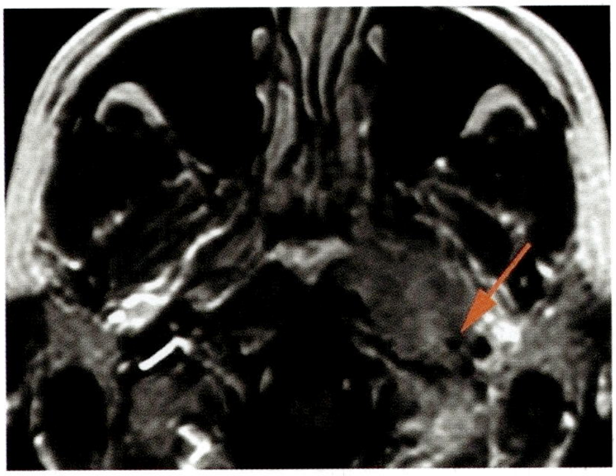

Fig. 27. Nasopharyngeal carcinoma. This 26-year-old female presented with left TON HS. Postgadolinium axial T1-weighted MR image shows a heterogeneously enhancing left nasopharyngeal mass encasing the left internal carotid artery (*arrow*). The peri-carotid tumor is compressing the sympathetic fibers, thus accounting for the TON HS.

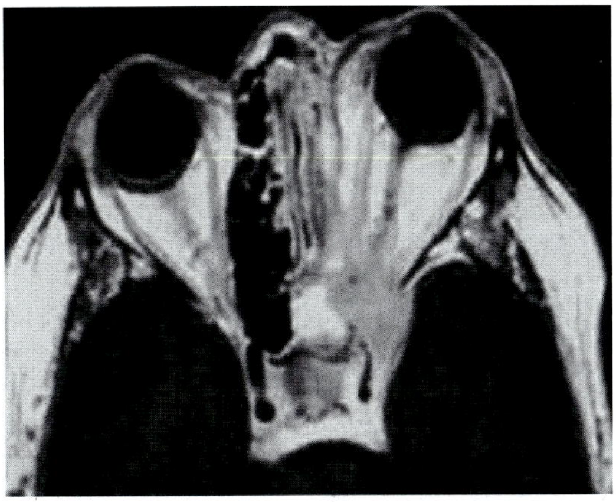

Fig. 28. Invasive aspergillosis. This 45-year-old immune-compromised male presented with left proptosis, chemosis, conjunctival hyperemia, and TON HS. Axial T1-weighted MR image shows a mass involving the left orbital apex and cavernous sinus.

Skull base, parasellar lesions, and orbital lesions

Palsies of CN III, IV, V1, V2, and VI, in association with a TON HS, may indicate the presence of a skull base or parasellar lesion (**Fig. 27**). Proptosis, chemosis, and conjunctival hyperemia are often present in patients with orbital lesions (**Fig. 28**).[9]

Other causes of TON HS include cluster or migraine headaches, trauma, infection, aneurysms of the petrous portion of the ICA, arteritis of the ICA, and agenesis of the internal carotid artery.[40–44]

SUMMARY

The clinical symptoms of HS may cause little if any functional impairment in most patients. However, since both benign and malignant processes are associated with HS, a thorough clinical evaluation is required. Once a lesion is localized clinically within the OSP by a combination of physical examination and pharmacological testing, the radiologic examination can be appropriately tailored.

ACKNOWLEDGMENTS

We thank Jill K. Gregory, MFA, CMI, Medical Illustrator.

REFERENCES

1. Amonoo-Kuofi HS. Horner's syndrome revisited: with an update of the central pathway. Clin Anat 1999;12: 345–61.
2. Thompson HS. The pupil. In: Hart WM Jr, editor. Adler's physiology of the eye. 9th edition. St. Louis (MO): Mosby-Year Book; 1992. p. 412–41.
3. Burde RM, Savino PJ, Trobe JD. Anisocoria and abnormal papillary light reactions. In: Kist KM, editor. Clinical decisions in neuro-ophthalmology. 2nd edition. St. Louis (MO): Mosby-Year Book; 1992. p. 321–46.
4. Snell RS, Lemp MA. The autonomic nervous system. In: Clinical anatomy of the eye. Boston: Blackwell Scientific Publications; 1989. p. 297–317.
5. Horner JF. On a form of ptosis. Klin Monatsbl Augenheilkd 1869;7:193–8.
6. Lepore FE. Enophthalmos and Horner's syndrome. Arch Neurol 1983;40:460.
7. Smith G, Dyches TJ, Burden RM. Topographic analysis of Horner's syndrome. Otolaryngol Head Neck Surg 1986;94:451–7.
8. Weinstein JM, Lweifel TJ, Thompson HS. Congenital Horner's syndrome. Arch Ophthalmol 1980;98: 1074–8.
9. Morrison DA, Bibby K, Woodruff G. The "harlequin" sign and congenital Horner's syndrome. J Neurol Neurosurg Psychiatry 1997;62(6):626–8.
10. Wilhelm H, Welhelm B, Kriegbaum C. Interaction of the indirectly acting topical sympathomimetics cocaine and pholegrine. Ger J Ophthalmol 1996;5: 168–70.
11. Nagy AN, Hayman LA, Diaz-Marchan PJ, et al. Horner's syndrome due to first-order neuron lesions of the oculosympathetic pathway. AJR Am J Roentgenol 1997;169:581–4.
12. Digre KB, Smoker WRK, Johnston P, et al. Selective MR imaging approach for evaluation of patients with Horner's syndrome. AJNR Am J Neuroradiol 1992; 13:223–7.
13. Sacco RL, Freddo L, Bello JA, et al. Wallenberg's lateral medullary syndrome: clinical-magnetic resonance imaging correlations. Arch Neurol 1993;50:609–14.
14. Pomeranz H. Isolated Horner syndrome and syrinx of the cervical spinal cord. Am J Ophthalmol 2002; 133:702–4.
15. Ellis CJK. Editorial commentary: isolated Horner's syndrome and syringomyelia. J Neurol Neurosurg Psychiatry 2000;69:3–4.
16. Kerrison JB, Biousse V, Newman NJ. Isolated Horner's syndrome and syringomyelia. J Neurol Neurosurg Psychiatry 2000;69:131–2.
17. Ottomo M, Heimburger RF. Alternating Horner syndrome and hyperhidrosis due to dural adhesions following cervical spinal cord injury. J Neurosurg 1980; 53:97–100.
18. Shen CC, Wang YC, Yang DY, et al. Brown-Sequard syndrome associated with Horner's syndrome in cervical epidural hematoma. Spine 1995;20:244–7.
19. Detterbeck FC. Pancoast (superior sulcus) tumors. Ann Thorac Surg 1997;63:1810–8.
20. Attar S, Krasna MJ, Sonett JR, et al. Superior sulcus (pancoast) tumor: experience with 105 patients. Ann Thorac Surg 1998;66:193–8.
21. Rosner M, Fisher W, Mulligan L. Cervical sympathetic schwannoma: case report. Neurosurgery 2001;49:1452–4.
22. Hood RJ, Jensen ME, Reibel JF, et al. Schwannoma of the cervical sympathetic chain. Ann Otol Rhinol Laryngol 2000;109:48–51.
23. Clements DM, Hedges AR, Tudor GR. Horner's syndrome following excision of a vagal paraganglioma. Int J Clin Pract 2002;56:626–7.
24. Lopez IB, Schwartz A. Neuroblastoma. Pediatr Clin North Am 1985;32:755–78.
25. Shimada H, Ambros I, Dehner L, et al. Terminology and morphologic criteria of neuroblastic tumors. Cancer 1999;86:349–63.
26. Aljassim AHH. Cervical ganglioneuroblastoma. J Laryngol Otol 1987;101:296–301.
27. Moukheiber AK, Nicollas R, Roman S, et al. Primary pediatric neuroblastic tumors of the neck. Int J Pediatr Otorhinolaryngol 2001;60:155–61.
28. Levin R, Newman SA, Login IS. Bilateral Horner's syndrome secondary to multinodular goiter. Ann Intern Med 1986;105:550–1.
29. Cengiz K, Aykin A, Demirci A, et al. Intrathoracic goiter with hyperthyroidism, tracheal compression, superior vena cava syndrome and Horner's syndrome. Chest 1990;97:1005–6.
30. Kumar R, Buckley TF. First disc protrusion. Spine 1986;11:499–501.
31. Inci S, Bertan V, Kansu T, et al. Horner's syndrome due to jugular venous ectasia. Childs Nerv Syst 1995;11:533–5.
32. Delabrousse E, Kastler B, Bernard Y, et al. MR diagnosis of a congenital abnormality of the thoracic aorta with an aneurysm of the right subclavian artery presenting as a Horner's syndrome in an adult. Eur Radiol 2000;10:650–2.
33. Ekatodramis G, Macaire P, Borgeat A. Prolonged Horner syndrome due to neck hematoma after continuous interscalene block. Anesthesiology 2001;95: 801–3.
34. Bell RL, Atweh N, Ivy ME, et al. Traumatic and iatrogenic Horner syndrome: case reports and review of the literature. J Trauma 2001;51:400–4.
35. Auer D, Karnath HO, Nagele T, et al. Case report: noninvasive investigation of pericarotid syndrome: role of MR angiography in the diagnosis of internal carotid dissection. Headache 1995;35:163–8.
36. Guy N, Deffond D, Gabrillargues J, et al. Spontaneous internal carotid artery dissection with lower

cranial nerve palsy. Can J Neurol Sci 2001;28: 265–9.
37. Chan CC, Paine M, O'Day J. Carotid dissection: a common cause of Horner's syndrome. Clin Experiment Ophthalmol 2001;29:411–5.
38. Leira EC, Bendixen BH, Kardon RH, et al. Brief, transient Horner's syndrome can be the hallmark of a carotid artery dissection. Neurology 1998;50: 289–90.
39. Brown J, Danielson R, Donahue SP, et al. Horner's syndrome in subadventitial carotid artery dissection and the role of magnetic resonance angiography. Am J Ophthalmol 1995;119:811–3.
40. Khurana RK. Bilateral Horner's syndrome in cluster type headaches. Headache 1993;33:449–51.
41. Coley SC, Clifton A, Britton J. Giant aneurysm of the petrous internal carotid artery: diagnosis and treatment. J Laryngol Otol 1998;112:196–8.
42. Zander DR, Just N, Schipper HM. Aneurysm of the intrapetrous internal carotid artery presenting as isolated Horner's syndrome: case report. Can Assoc Radiol J 1998;49:46–8.
43. Ryan FH, Kline LB, Gomez C. Congenital Horner's syndrome resulting from agenesis of the internal carotid artery. Ophthalmology 2000;107: 185–8.
44. Dinc H, Alioglu Z, Erdöl H, et al. Agenesis of the internal carotid artery associated with aortic anomaly in a patient with congenital Horner's syndrome. AJNR Am J Neuroradiol 2002;23:929–31.

Denervation Atrophy of Motor Cranial Nerves

Wendy R.K. Smoker, MS, MD, FACR[a,*], Deborah L. Reede, MD[b,c]

KEYWORDS

• Cranial nerves • Denervation • Atrophy

Muscles undergoing denervation demonstrate a predictable sequence of imaging findings, best appreciated in those muscles innervated by the mandibular and hypoglossal nerves. Denervation changes in smaller muscles are usually only appreciated in the late chronic stage of denervation. It is incumbent on the radiologist to be aware of these changes so as not to interpret these muscles as harboring a tumor or being involved by an inflammatory process. This article reviews the stages of denervation and provides an explanation for the changes identified on MR imaging. The muscles innervated by each motor cranial nerve are reviewed and emphasis is placed on those muscles that can routinely be identified on cross-sectional imaging, physical examination findings that result from insults to each of the motor cranial nerves are presented, and various stages of denervation atrophy for the muscles innervated by each of these nerves are illustrated.

STAGES OF DENERVATION

Well-known magnetic resonance (MR) signal abnormalities in denervated skeletal muscle are described in the literature for peripheral and cranial nerves.[1–5] Long-standing chronic denervation atrophy, and its associated extensive fatty infiltration, is usually readily apparent on CT studies,[6] but MR imaging permits identification of changes that occur earlier in the denervation process.[7] Russo and colleagues[7] and others have categorized the MR appearance of denervated muscle roughly, according to the chronicity of the process, into acute, subacute, early chronic, and late chronic patterns. These patterns are most evident when larger muscles are affected. It has also been suggested that different nerves may demonstrate differences in the progression of denervation.[8] Kato and colleagues[8] noted that changes in signal intensity and in contrast enhancement of muscles supplied by the hypoglossal nerve appeared earlier than in muscles supplied by V3 and that the volume of the denervated tongue musculature decreased earlier than the volume of the muscles of mastication. This would further complicate attempts to "stage" denervation.

Russo and colleagues[7] described muscles undergoing acute denervation (patients who have "acute" symptoms) as demonstrating increased muscle volume, pathologic T2 prolongation, and abnormal enhancement, but there was no evidence of fatty replacement. Those muscles thought to be in the subacute stages of denervation also showed pathologic T2 prolongation and abnormal enhancement but did not demonstrate increased muscle volume and did evidence some slight fatty infiltration.[7] Early chronic atrophic changes were those of mild fatty infiltration and no increased T2 signal intensity or pathologic enhancement, with relative preservation of muscle volume, whereas changes of long-standing denervation atrophy involved marked fatty infiltration and loss of muscle volume (**Table 1**).[7]

The exact duration of denervation needed to produce these various stages is not clear. Some clinical reports define the beginning of denervation as the onset of symptoms,[8] but the reliability of such timing is inherently limited, given the fact

[a] Department of Radiology, University of Iowa Hospitals and Clinics, 200 Hawkins Drive, 0453-G JCP, Iowa City, IA 52242, USA
[b] State University of New York Health Science Center at Brooklyn, Brooklyn, NY, USA
[c] Department of Radiology, Long Island College Hospital, 339 Hicks Street, Brooklyn, NY 11201, USA
* Corresponding author.
E-mail address: wendy-smoker@uiowa.edu (W.R.K. Smoker).

Neuroimag Clin N Am 18 (2008) 387–411
doi:10.1016/j.nic.2007.12.011
1052-5149/08/$ – see front matter

Table 1
Stages of motor denervation

	Acute	Subacute	Early Chronic	Late Chronic
Muscle volume	↑	–	–	↓
T2 prolongation	+	+	–	–
Fatty infiltration	–	+	+	++
Abnormal enhancement	+	+	–	–

Abbreviations: ↑, increased; ↓, decreased; +, present; ++, strongly present.

that the temporal relation between the onset of symptoms and the denervation process is, most likely, highly variable. The one patient described by Russo and colleagues[7] who demonstrated subacute changes at 8 months underwent a follow-up MR imaging examination that revealed late chronic changes at 20 months. In their study, all patients demonstrating long-standing chronic denervation changes had a known pathologic process of at least 20 months' duration.[7] Davis and colleagues[1] reported changes of subacute denervation in the muscles of mastication in a patient 6 months after brain stem hemorrhage. In their study of denervated peripheral skeletal muscle, Fleckenstein and colleagues[3] arbitrarily defined acute denervation as less than 1 month's duration, subacute denervation as between 1 and 12 months, and chronic denervation as greater than 1 year. In their discussion, however, Dill-Macky and colleagues[9] consider the acute phase as "within one month of denervation" and the subacute phase as between 1 and 3 months. It becomes apparent that the literature is inconsistent with regard to the exact timing of the changes associated with denervation atrophy.

BASIS FOR CHANGES ON MR IMAGING

T2 Prolongation

Multiple investigators have reported T2 prolongation during acute and subacute stages of denervation involving the muscles of mastication and muscles of the tongue.[1,5,7,8] It has been suggested that the explanation for T2 prolongation noted in muscles undergoing denervation relates to the size of the extracellular fluid space (extracellular water), which has a much longer T2 prolongation than intracellular water.[10] In their experimental study on rats, Kikuchi and colleagues[11] demonstrated that subsequent normalization of T2 signal intensity correlated with normalization of extracellular volume changes. Polak and colleagues[12] observed skeletal muscle T2 prolongation in an animal model 2 weeks after ligation of the sciatic nerve. Although there was no change in the overall water content, they noted a relative increase in extracellular water with a concomitant decrease in intracellular water.[12] Small differences in water compartmentation may result in substantial signal intensity changes on T2-weighted imaging. Fleckenstein and colleagues[3] suggested that it might be useful to consider the observed T2 prolongation to be "edema-like" rather than a reflection of true edema, given that true edema implies an absolute increase in tissue water content. This would not explain the associated increased muscle volume in reported cases of acute denervation atrophy, however, suggesting that there may well be a component of true edema. May and colleagues[13] prefer to use the term *muscle edema* to describe the increased muscle signal intensity on T2-weighted images identified in a variety of pathologic conditions, including polymyositis, dermatomyositis, mild injuries, radiation therapy, rhabdomyolysis, and sickle cell crisis in addition to subacute denervation. Wessig and colleagues[14] suggested that increased blood volume is the most important factor altering MR relaxation times. In their study on rats, they found marked capillary enlargement before any other histologic abnormality and noted that changes of the mean capillary area exactly paralleled the increase, maximum, and subsequent decrease in T2 relaxation times.[14] Hayashi and colleagues[15] also concluded that changes in T2 relaxation times were caused by an enlarged blood volume, reporting a linear correlation between T2 relaxation times and increased blood volume measured by ^{19}F nuclear magnetic resonance (NMR) spectroscopy. More recently, however, Bendszus and colleagues[16] have offered evidence that contradicts the increase in blood flow as an explanation for the T2 prolongation. They demonstrated T2 prolongation in rat muscles as early as 24 hours after sciatic nerve transaction and believe it is the redistribution of fluid from the intracellular to the extracellular space that is responsible for the MR signal changes.[16]

West and colleagues[4] found signal intensity on short-tau-inversion-recovery (STIR) imaging, especially sensitive to T1 and T2 prolongation associated with acute or subacute denervation, to be increased as early as 4 days after the onset of clinical denervation, which is significantly earlier than changes detected on electromyography (EMG). Overall, the STIR sequence is considered to be more sensitive than the spin-echo T2-weighted sequence because of its fat suppression characteristics and ability to enhance differences between water and tissue content.[10,12] In their article evaluating STIR imaging in 90 patients with clinical evidence of peripheral nerve injury or radiculopathy, McDonald and colleagues[17] reported that STIR imaging had a relative sensitivity of 84% and specificity of 100% for detecting denervation but was less sensitive than needle EMG. They suggested that there may be a shorter time frame of abnormality for STIR MR imaging compared with EMG in detecting denervation or that there is a threshold of muscle edema induced by denervation that is required to increase signal intensity sufficiently so that it can be identified on STIR images.[17]

Contrast Enhancement

Normal skeletal muscle is known to enhance slightly after gadolinium contrast administration.[18] In particular, the extraocular muscles, highly specialized with a unique degree of differentiation, normally demonstrate more prominent enhancement than other skeletal muscles, probably because of the fact that they possess more prominent extravascular and extracellular spaces and richer vascularity.[19] Contrast material is usually present in the extracellular, intravascular, and interstitial spaces. Therefore, a muscle undergoing atrophy, with its expanded extracellular space, would demonstrate greater relative enhancement than normal muscle.[20] Additionally, studies have demonstrated that denervated muscle has relatively increased vascularity per volume of muscle compared with normal muscle.[21,22] Denervated muscles maintain the total number of capillaries supplying the muscles, but the number of capillaries per unit area increases such that it has been suggested that this luxury perfusion also contributes to contrast enhancement, although the luxury perfusion may be somewhat diminished by capillary necrosis.[21–24]

PROBLEM AND THE CHALLENGE

It should come as no surprise that, given the MR imaging appearance of muscles undergoing acute or subacute denervation, there have been instances in which these muscles have been erroneously mistaken as harboring a tumor or infection. The authors are personally aware of at least three patients who underwent biopsies of such muscles. (Many more instances have probably occurred but never been reported.) Had the radiologist been aware of the MR imaging appearance of the sequential stages associated with denervation atrophy, these procedures may well not have taken place. It thus becomes important to remember these stages, especially when evaluating imaging abnormalities of the larger muscle bundles, such as those supplied by the mandibular division of the trigeminal nerve (muscles of mastication) and the hypoglossal nerve (tongue musculature), so as not to consider these muscles as being involved by other pathologic conditions.[1,7,8]

These various stages of motor denervation have not been described on MR imaging for many of the smaller muscles supplied by motor cranial nerves, most likely because of their small volumes. The primary finding of denervation in smaller muscles on CT and MR imaging is decreased muscle volume, typically without visualization of fatty replacement. Interestingly, however, despite the large size of the muscles innervated by the spinal accessory nerve (trapezius and sternocleidomastoid), the various stages of motor denervation have not been reported in these muscles and researchers have not been able to identify changes of acute or subacute denervation or fatty replacement within these muscles on cross-sectional imaging studies.

When a muscle of the head and neck exhibits changes of denervation, one must first determine if this is an isolated finding or whether all muscles supplied by the same nerve are affected. Obviously, to do this, one must know what muscles are supplied by each of the motor cranial nerves and be able to identify them on cross-sectional imaging. In some instances, patterns of denervation involving muscles supplied by more than one cranial nerve may be identified (especially IX, X, XI, $\pm$ XII). The second task involves an assessment of the entire course of the implicated nerve(s), from the brain stem to the abnormal muscle(s), in an attempt to identify the causative lesion. This should be performed with MR imaging, because CT has limited usefulness for assessment of cranial nerves. Imaging of the cranial nerve should be performed in at least two planes, T1- and T2-weighted sequences should be acquired, and fat-suppressed postcontrast T1-weighted images should be obtained.

In the remainder of this article, the muscles innervated by the motor cranial nerves are briefly reviewed and the findings on clinical examination resulting from damage to each of these nerves are presented. For most nerves, emphasis is directed toward single nerve denervation and not extensive pathologic findings involving multiple cranial nerves (ie, cavernous sinus lesions involving cranial nerves III, IV, V, and VI). The anatomy of each motor cranial nerve has been presented elsewhere in this issue and is thus not duplicated here.

OCULOMOTOR NERVE—CRANIAL NERVE III

After the oculomotor nerve exits the skull, it enters the orbit by way of the superior orbital fissure, passes through the annulus of Zinn, and is classically described as dividing into superior and inferior divisions. The superior division innervates the superior rectus and levator palpebrae superioris muscles, whereas the inferior division innervates the inferior and medial rectus, inferior oblique muscles, and the pupil (**Fig. 1**).[25,26] These muscles can be identified on CT and MR imaging, usually individually, although the levator palpebrae superioris and superior rectus muscles are often visualized as a single muscle bundle. It is recognized that some reports exist in the literature that challenge this traditionally held description of oculomotor nerve divisional anatomy. Some investigator have reported patients who have superior division oculomotor nerve palsy caused by disease in the midbrain and subarachnoid space,[27–29] leading to proposals that functional segregation of oculomotor nerve fibers occurs before the anatomic bifurcation of the oculomotor nerve. Other uncommon causes of superior division oculomotor nerve paresis that have been reported include diabetes,[30,31] sphenoid sinusitis,[32] and ophthalmoplegic migraines.[33] Cases of oculomotor nerve inferior division[29] and isolated extraocular muscle palsies[34] have also been reported.

A third nerve palsy results in the following (**Fig. 2**)[35,36]:

I. Exotropia: outward deviation of the eye in primary gaze
II. Inability to adduct, depress, and elevate the eye (eye deviates outward and downward), resulting in diplopia
III. Ptosis (from paresis of the levator muscle): drooping of the eyelid such that it covers the globe with an inability to raise the eyelid voluntarily
IV. The pupil may be larger and partially reactive or unreactive. Imaging typically demonstrates a diminutive caliber of the affected muscles (late chronic stage) without changes in signal or enhancement, although, on occasion, earlier stages of denervation may be identified. Rare reports of bilateral oculomotor palsies, paresis, or denervation from a variety of causes also exist (**Fig. 3**).[37–39]

TROCHLEAR NERVE—CRANIAL NERVE IV

After traversing the superior orbital fissure, the trochlear nerve courses to supply a single muscle, the superior oblique muscle (**Fig. 4**).[25] Dysfunction of the unilateral trochlear nerve and resulting superior oblique palsy result in subtle neurologic deficit compared with other cranial nerves: (1) decrease in torsion and depression, (2) vertical diplopia in downward gaze or in primary position (patients often present with difficulty in descending stairs because of an inability to look down), and (3) head tilt representing compensatory adjustment that can mask the symptoms (**Fig. 5**).[35,36,40] Rare reports of bilateral trochlear nerve dysfunction place the pathologic change at the level of the superior medullary velum.[41] Researchers have only

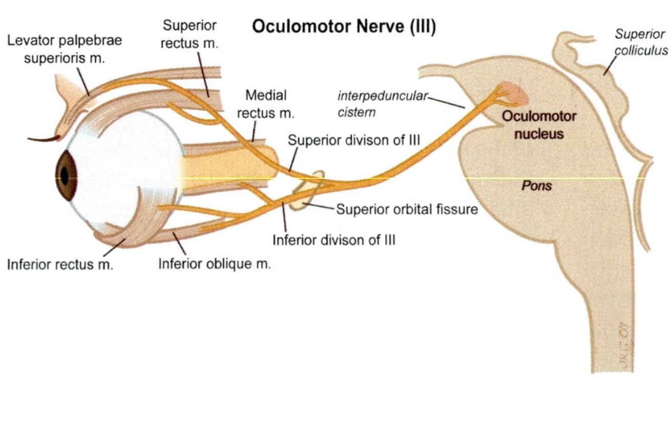

Fig. 1. Diagram of muscles innervated by divisions of the oculomotor nerve.

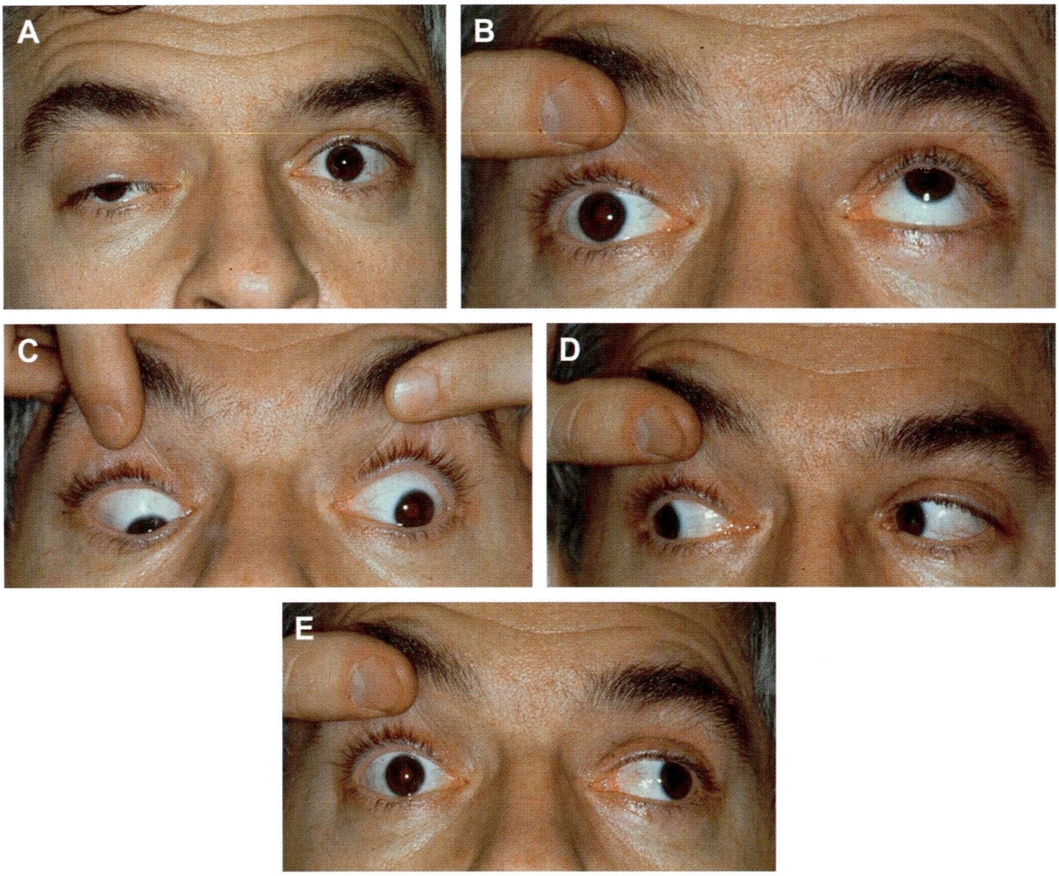

Fig. 2. Clinical examination: right third nerve paresis in a 33-year-old man with a pituitary adenoma. Photographs in primary gaze (*A*), upward gaze (*B*), downward gaze (*C*), right lateral gaze (*D*), and left lateral gaze (*E*). Note right ptosis in primary gaze (*A*), paralysis of upward gaze (*B*), and paralysis of left lateral gaze attributable to an inability to adduct (*E*).

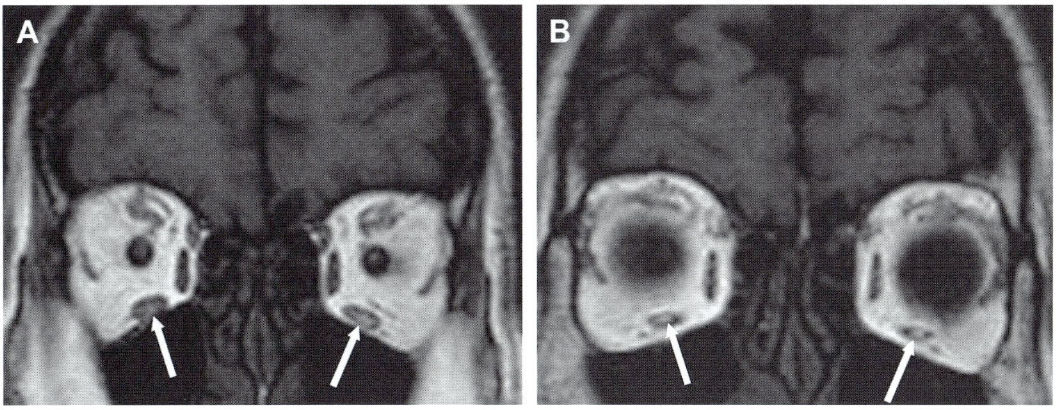

Fig. 3. Bilateral oculomotor nerve denervation atrophy in a 43-year-old man (presumed viral). (*A*, *B*) T1-weighted coronal MR imaging. Muscles innervated by the third nerve are diminutive bilaterally, and fatty changes are identified in the inferior rectus muscles bilaterally (*arrows*).

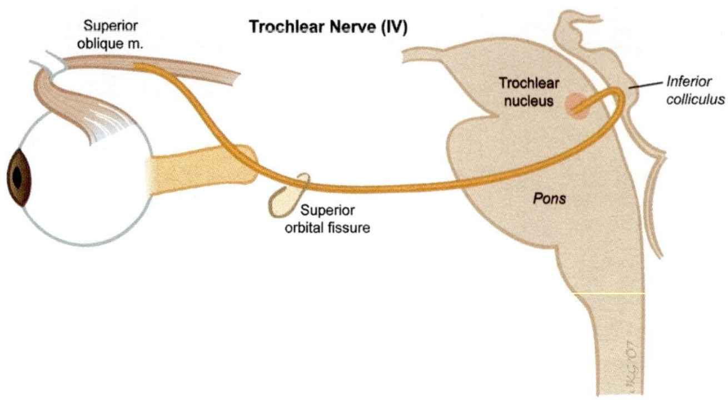

Fig. 4. Diagram of the trochlear nerve and superior oblique muscle.

encountered changes of late chronic atrophy (significant atrophy without signal changes), identified as a small superior oblique muscle, which is most easily appreciated on coronal imaging (**Fig. 6**).

MANDIBULAR NERVE MOTOR COMPONENT—CRANIAL NERVE V_3

The mandibular nerve exits the skull by way of the foramen ovale to enter the high masticator space, first giving rise to small nerves that innervate the tensor tympani and tensor veli palatini muscles before dividing into its two major branches: the larger masticator and smaller mylohyoid nerves. The masticator nerve supplies motor innervation to the muscles of mastication (medial and lateral pterygoid, temporalis, and masseter muscles). The mylohyoid nerve provides innervation to the mylohyoid and anterior bellies of the digastric muscles (**Fig. 7**).

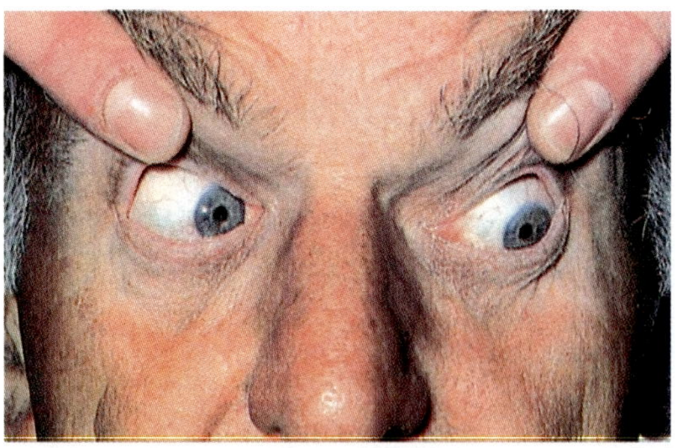

Fig. 5. Clinical examination: right fourth nerve palsy in a 65-year-old man with a 6-month history of vertical image separation. Note reduced downward and inward gaze of the right eye. (*From* Perkin D, Rose FC, Blackwood W, et al. Atlas of clinical neurology. London: Gower Medical Publishing; 1986; with permission.)

Loss of V3-innervated muscle volume produces a "hollow concavity" of the cheek (masseter muscle atrophy) or the temporal fossa (temporalis muscle atrophy) (**Fig. 8**A, B). It also produces weakness of the muscles of mastication, such that the jaw deviates toward the affected side as a result of the unopposed action of the contralateral muscles (see **Fig. 8**C).[26] Denervation of the tensor veli palatini muscle results in a diminutive torus tubarius, eustachian tube dysfunction, and accumulation of mastoid fluid, whereas denervation of the tensor tympani muscle may result in loss of acoustic dampening.[7] Because of the large size of the masticatory muscles, all phases of denervation are able to be appreciated, depending on the proximity of imaging to the onset of symptoms (**Figs. 9–11**). Researchers have yet to visualize anything but the late chronic phase of denervation in those muscles supplied by the mylohyoid nerve, presumably because of their diminutive size (**Fig. 12**).

ABDUCENS NERVE—CRANIAL NERVE VI

After traversing the superior orbital fissure and coursing through the annulus of Zinn, the abducens nerve goes on to supply a single extraocular muscle, the lateral rectus muscle (**Fig. 13**).[25] Denervation atrophy and unilateral paresis of the abducens nerve results in (1) esotropia-unopposed medial rectus function, causing the eye to turn inward, and (2) horizontal diplopia, an inability to direct the eye laterally (abduction) (**Fig. 14**).[35,40] Imaging demonstrates a small lateral rectus muscle (**Fig. 15**). To date, fatty infiltration of the lateral rectus muscle associated with late chronic denervation has not been identified.

FACIAL NERVE—CRANIAL NERVE VII

After exiting the petrous bone at the stylomastoid foramen, the facial nerve immediately enters the

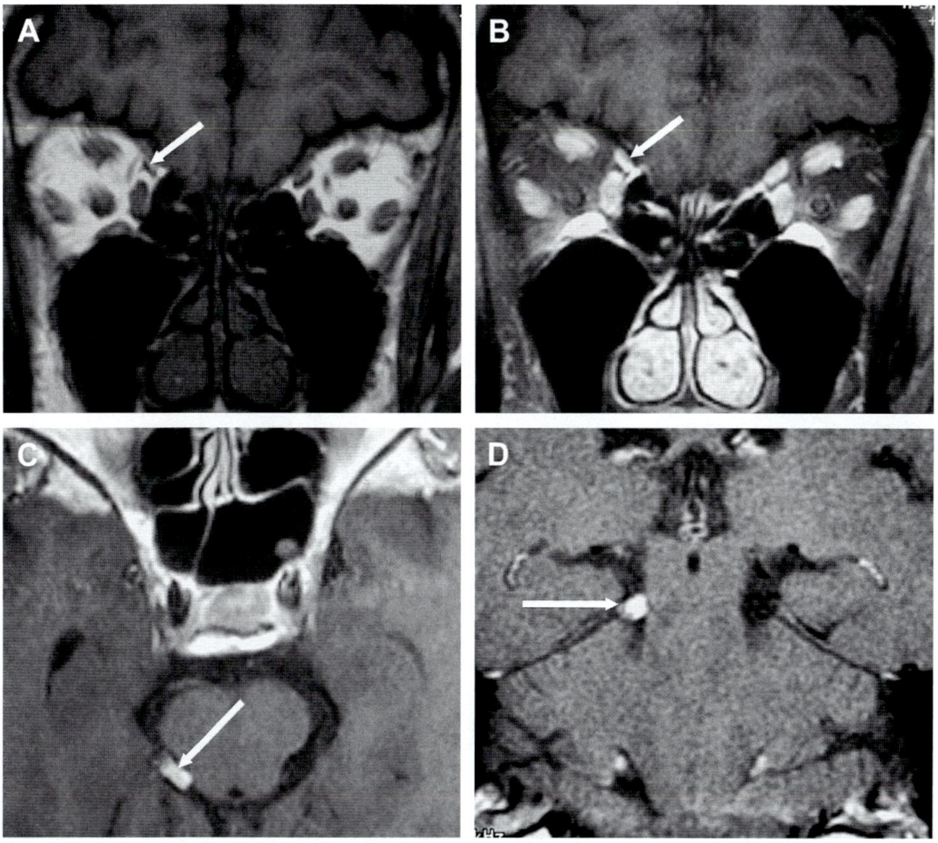

Fig. 6. Right superior oblique palsy in a 58 year-old women with a (presumed) trochlear nerve schwannoma. Coronal precontrast (*A*) and fat-suppressed postcontrast (*B*) T1-weighted MR imaging demonstrates marked atrophy of the right superior oblique muscle (*arrows*). Axial (*C*) and coronal (*D*) postcontrast T1-weighted MR imaging through the brain stem reveals the right fourth nerve schwannoma (*arrows*).

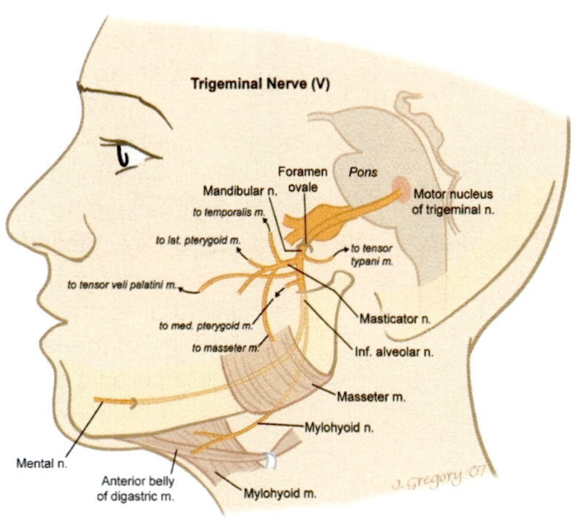

Fig. 7. Diagram of the muscles innervated by branches of the mandibular nerve (V_3).

parotid gland and divides into its five terminal branches for motor innervation to the muscles of facial expression, posterior belly of the digastric muscle, buccinator, stylohyoid, occipitalis, and platysma muscles (the small branch to the stapedius muscle emerges separately from the nerve before its terminal branching) (**Fig. 16**). Loss of motor VII function typically leads to loss of facial expression with flattening of the nasolabial fold and drooping of the lip with an inability to smile symmetrically (orbicularis oris) (**Fig. 17**).[26] In cases of peripheral insult, there is additional involvement of the forehead, with an inability to close the eye because of involvement of the orbicularis oculi (**Fig. 18**). To date, researchers have only appreciated late chronic VII denervation changes with muscle volume loss in the buccinator, posterior belly of the digastric muscle,

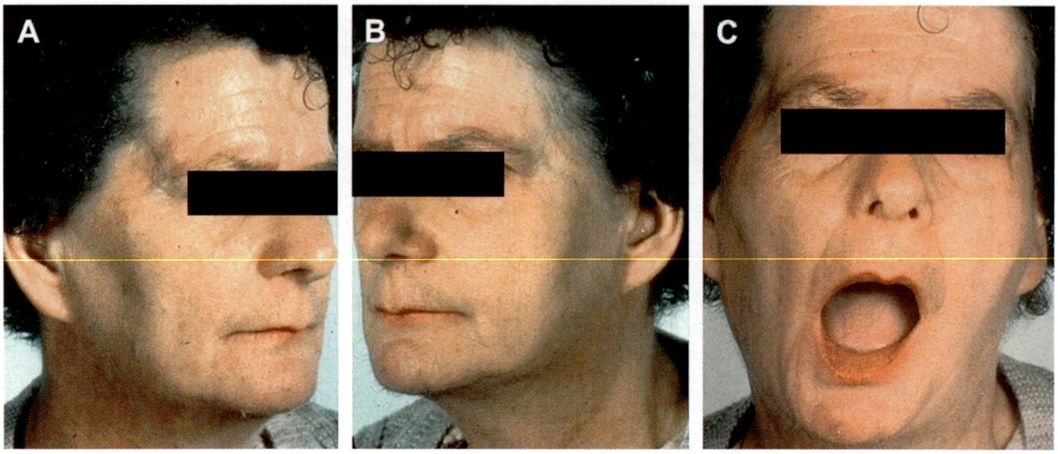

Fig. 8. Clinical examination: left V_3 paresis. Photographs are seen in closed-mouth right oblique (*A*), closed-mouth left oblique (*B*), and open-mouth (*C*) positions. Note the hollow concavity of the right cheek (masseter muscle atrophy) and temporal fossa (temporalis muscle atrophy) in (*A*) compared with the normal left side in (*B*). (*C*) On opening the mouth, the jaw deviates toward the right, the side of pathologic findings, because of unopposed action of the right pterygoid muscles. (*From* Perkin D, Rose FC, Blackwood W, et al. Atlas of clinical neurology. London: Gower Medical Publishing; 1986; with permission.)

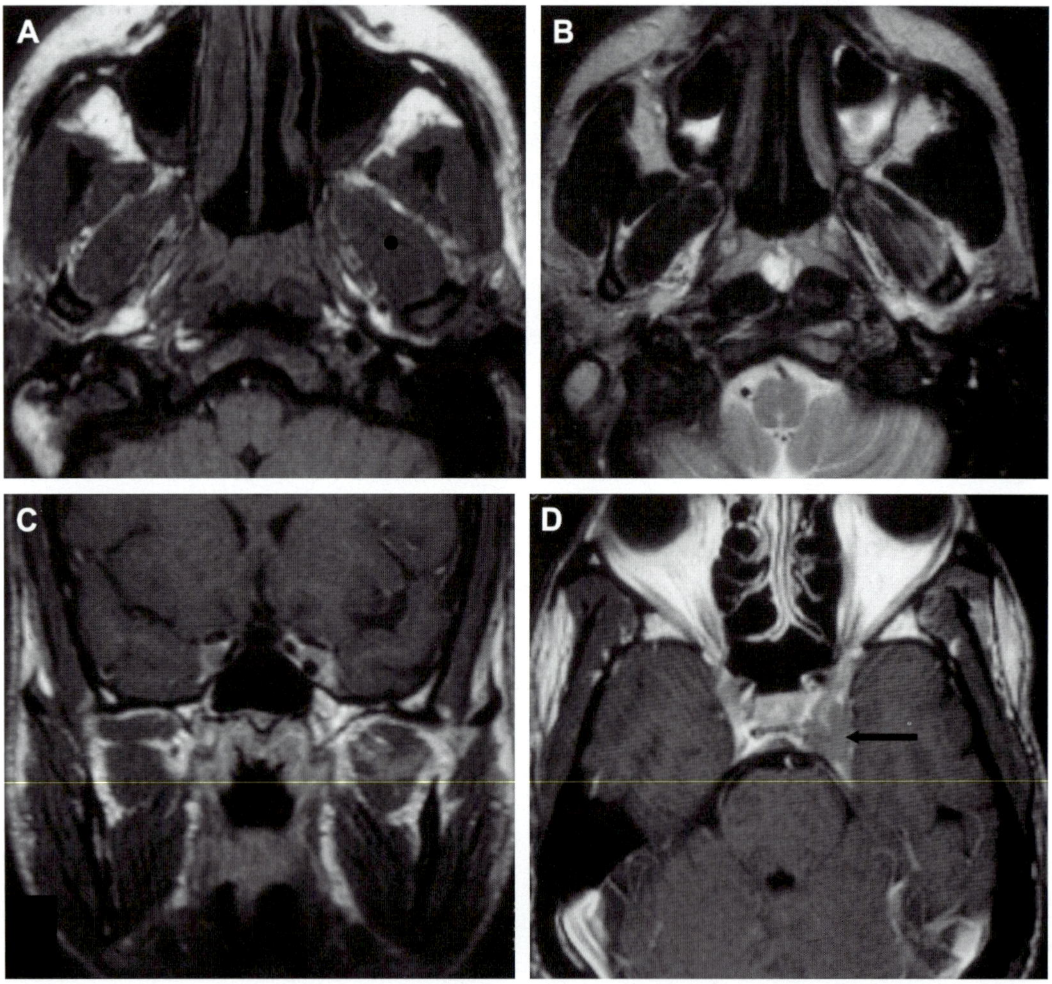

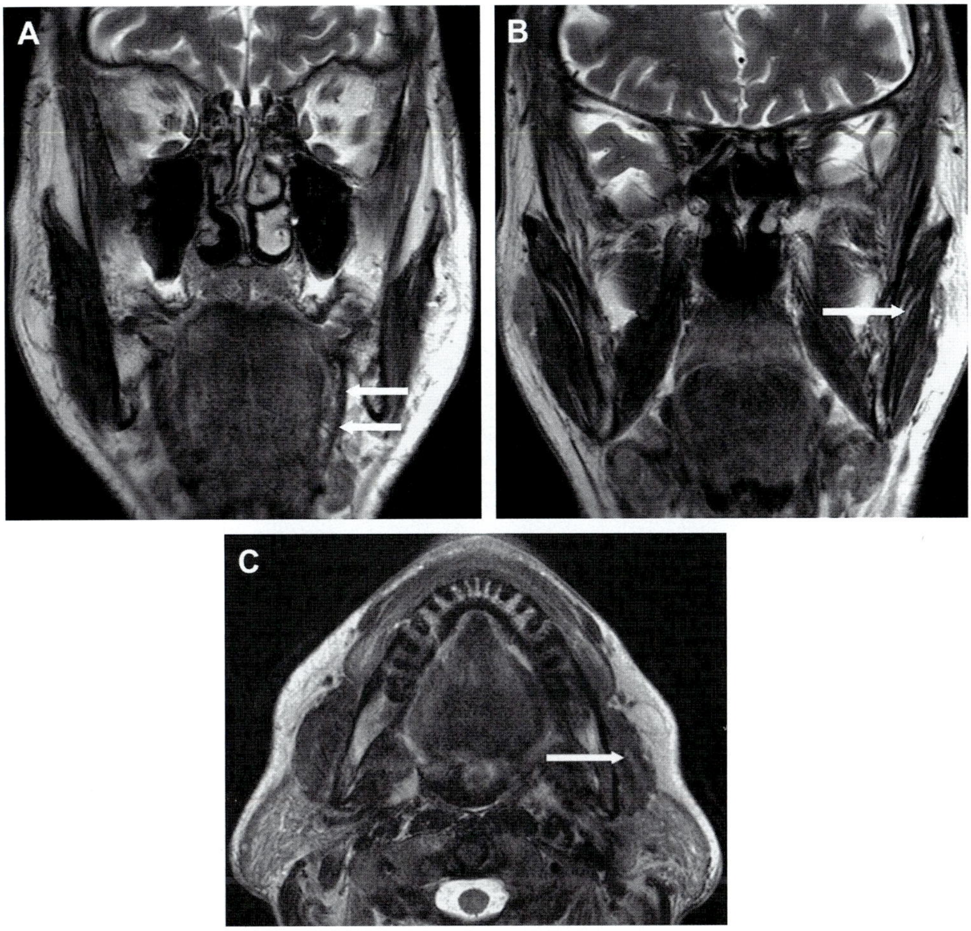

Fig. 10. Subacute left V_3 denervation atrophy in a 52-year-old man status post-trigeminal rhizotomy. Coronal (*A, B*) and axial (*C*) T2-weighted MR imaging. There is decreased volume in muscles innervated by the left V_3 nerve, which is subtle in some but especially notable in the left mylohyoid (*double arrow*) and masseter (*single arrow*) muscles. Significant fatty infiltration is not present.

Fig. 9. Acute left lateral pterygoid muscle denervation atrophy in a 64-year-old man with metastatic lymphoma to the left cavernous sinus. (*A*) Axial T1-weighted MR imaging reveals enlargement of the left lateral pterygoid muscle (*dot*). (*B*) Axial T2-weighted MR imaging demonstrates pathologic T2 prolongation in the enlarged muscle. (*C*) Coronal postcontrast T1-weighted MR imaging shows pathologic enhancement within the muscle. (*D*) Axial postcontrast T1-weighted imaging reveals the causative cavernous sinus lymphoma metastasis (*arrow*).

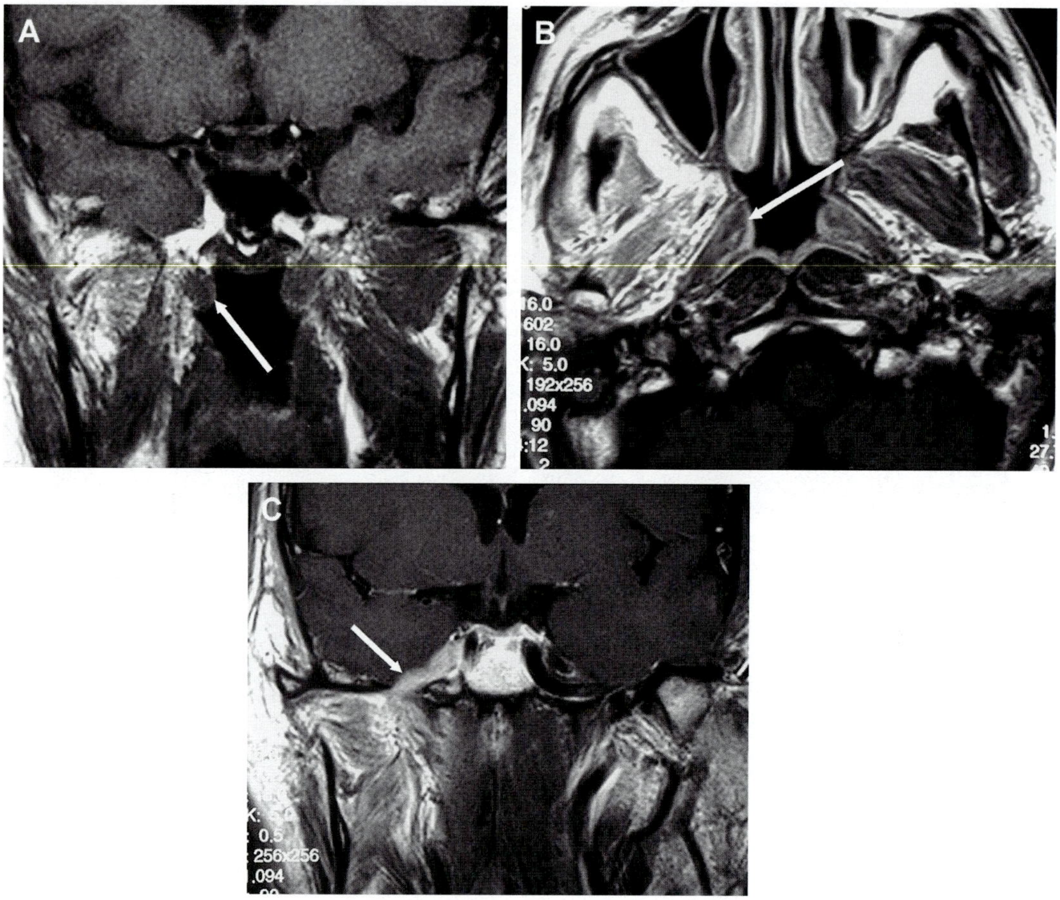

Fig. 11. Late chronic right V_3 denervation atrophy in a 45-year-old man with a V_3 schwannoma. Coronal T1-weighted (*A*) and axial (*B*) and coronal (*C*) postcontrast T1-weighted MR imaging. (*A, B*) Note the diminutive size of the right torus tubarius (*arrow*) because of atrophy of the tensor veli palatini muscle. (*C*) Causative lesion (*arrow*) is shown.

platysma, and various muscles of facial expression (**Figs. 19–21**).

GLOSSOPHARYNGEAL NERVE—CRANIAL NERVE IX

After its exit from the skull by way of the pars nervosa of the jugular foramen, cranial nerve IX enters the high nasopharyngeal carotid space within the carotid sheath. It gives rise to a single motor branch providing innervation to the stylopharyngeus muscle.[42,43] The glossopharyngeal nerve also contributes fibers to the pharyngeal plexus that, along with the vagus nerve, provide motor innervation to the palatoglossus and palatopharyngeus muscles, superior and middle pharyngeal constrictor muscles, and levator veli palatini muscle (**Fig. 22**).[42,43] It should be noted that some consider the palatoglossus muscle as receiving sole innervation from the glossopharyngeal nerve rather than from the pharyngeal plexus.[43] Compression of cranial nerve IX may produce glossopharyngeal neuralgia, with the primary clinical manifestations related to various sensory branches (eg, otalgia, tachycardia, bradycardia, hypotension, loss of taste to the posterior one third of the tongue) rather than to its motor branch.[44] The main symptom produced by dysfunction of the stylopharyngeus muscle is dysphagia, a symptom also produced by pathologic conditions of the vagus nerve and by a large number of diverse causes. Dysphagia is thus unreliable as a sole clinical indicator of

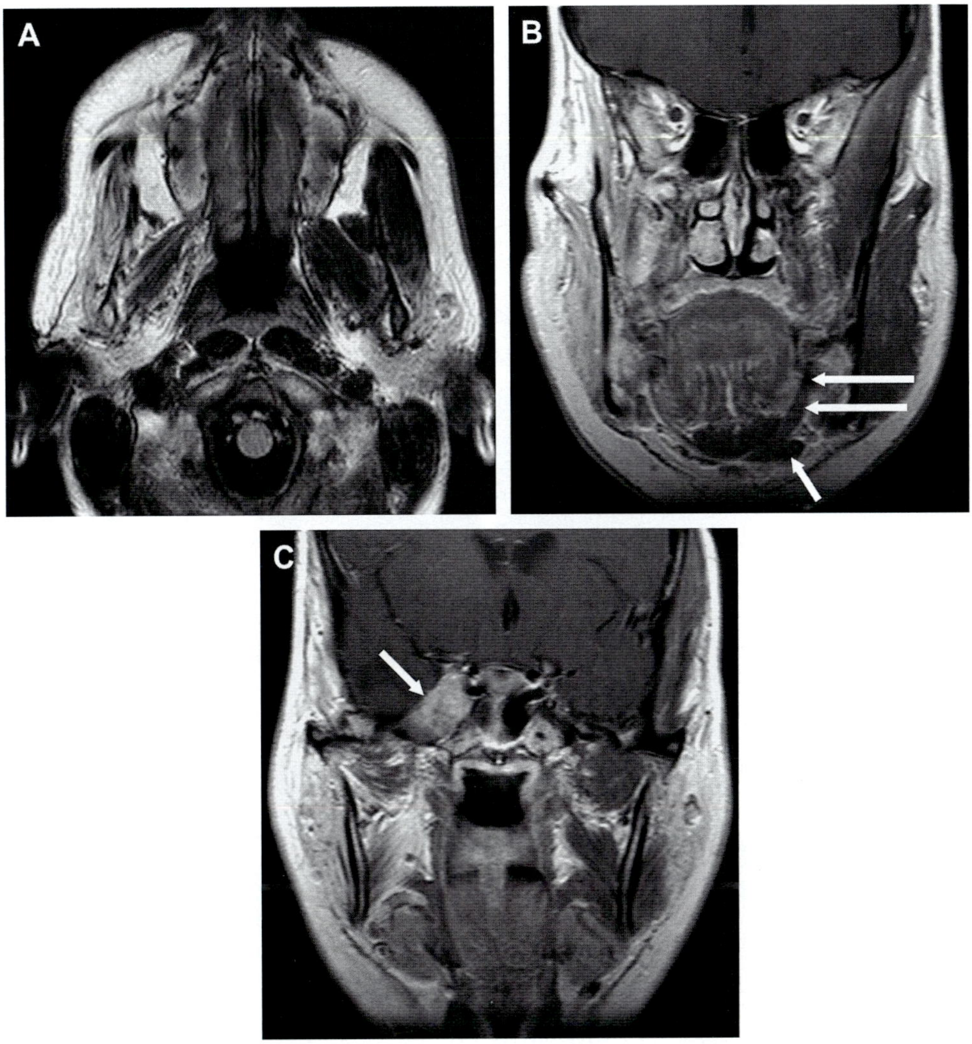

Fig. 12. Late chronic right V_3 denervation atrophy in a 51-year-old man with a Meckel's cave meningioma. (*A*) Axial T1-weighted MR imaging demonstrates severe atrophy and complete fatty replacement of all the muscles innervated by right the V_3 nerve. (*B, C*) Coronal postcontrast T1-weighted MR imaging. Especially note the complete atrophy of the right mylohyoid muscle and anterior belly of the digastric muscle, the normal left mylohyoid muscle (*long arrows*), and the anterior belly of the digastric muscle (*short arrow*). (*C*) Causative meningioma (*arrow*) is shown.

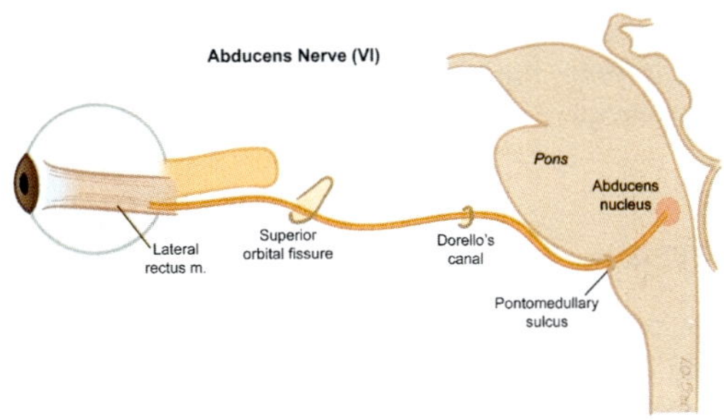

Fig. 13. Diagram of the abducens nerve and the lateral rectus muscle.

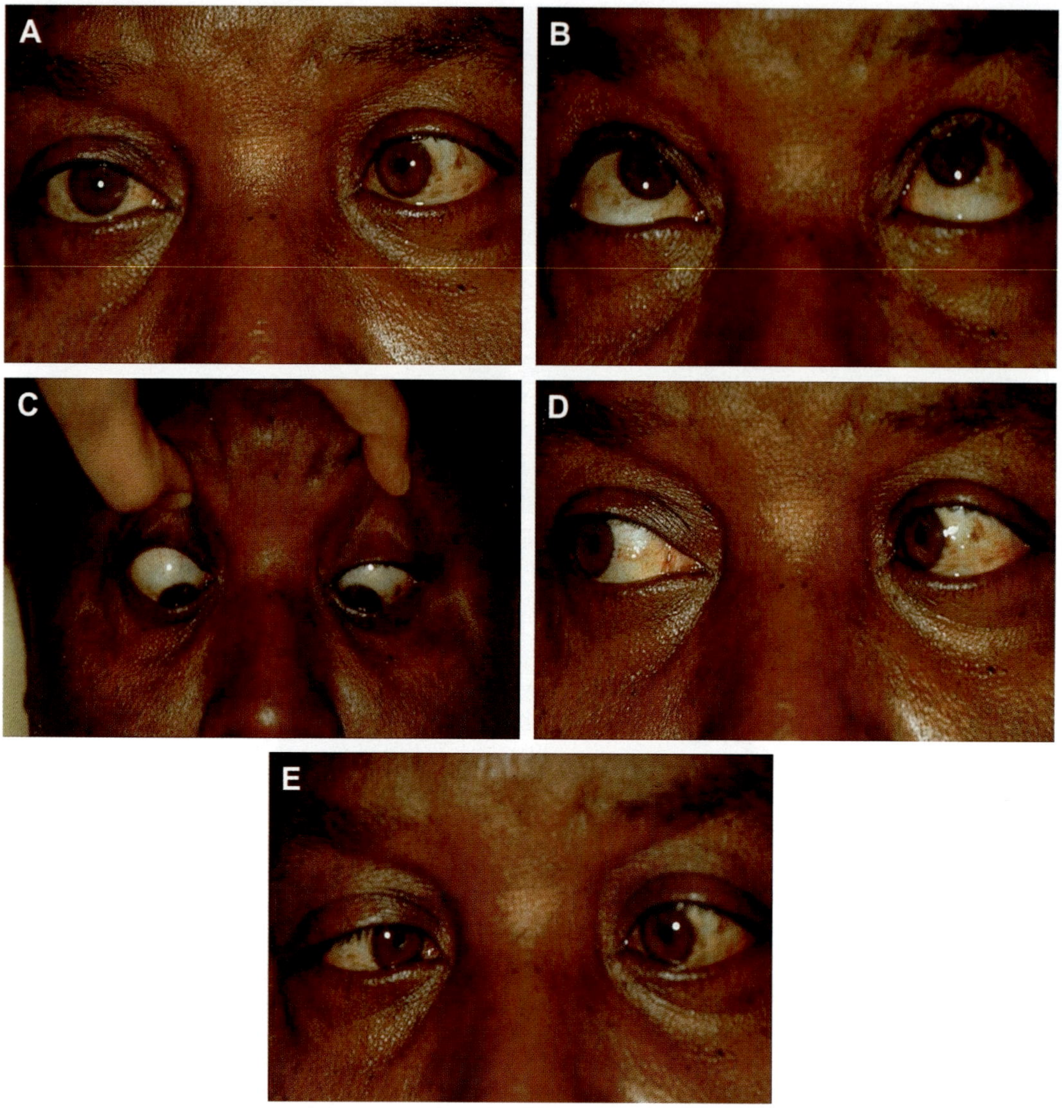

Fig. 14. Clinical examination: left cranial nerve VI palsy in a 59 year-old man with a cavernous sinus meningioma. Clinical photographs in primary gaze (*A*), upward gaze (*B*), downward gaze (*C*), right lateral gaze (*D*), and left lateral gaze (*E*). Note that the left eye wanders medially in primary gaze (*A*) and demonstrates paralysis on left lateral gaze because of an inability to abduct (*E*).

glossopharyngeal nerve pathologic change. The stylopharyngeus muscle cannot be isolated for clinical testing. To date, researchers have not been able to identify denervation atrophic changes of the stylopharyngeus muscle.

VAGUS NERVE—CRANIAL NERVE X

The vagus nerve is a complex cranial nerve that has been covered in its entirety elsewhere in this issue. After exiting the skull through the pars vascularis of the jugular foramen, cranial nerve X enters the nasopharyngeal carotid space and, from the nodose (inferior) ganglion, gives rise to two motor branches: the pharyngeal plexus and superior laryngeal nerve.[42,43] The pharyngeal plexus provides primary innervation to the superior and middle pharyngeal constrictor muscles, muscles of the soft palate (palatoglossus [ie, anterior tonsillar pillar] and palatopharyngeus [ie, posterior tonsillar pillar]), and levator veli palatini muscle. The superior laryngeal nerve provides motor supply to cricothyroid and inferior pharyngeal constrictor muscles by way of its external branch.

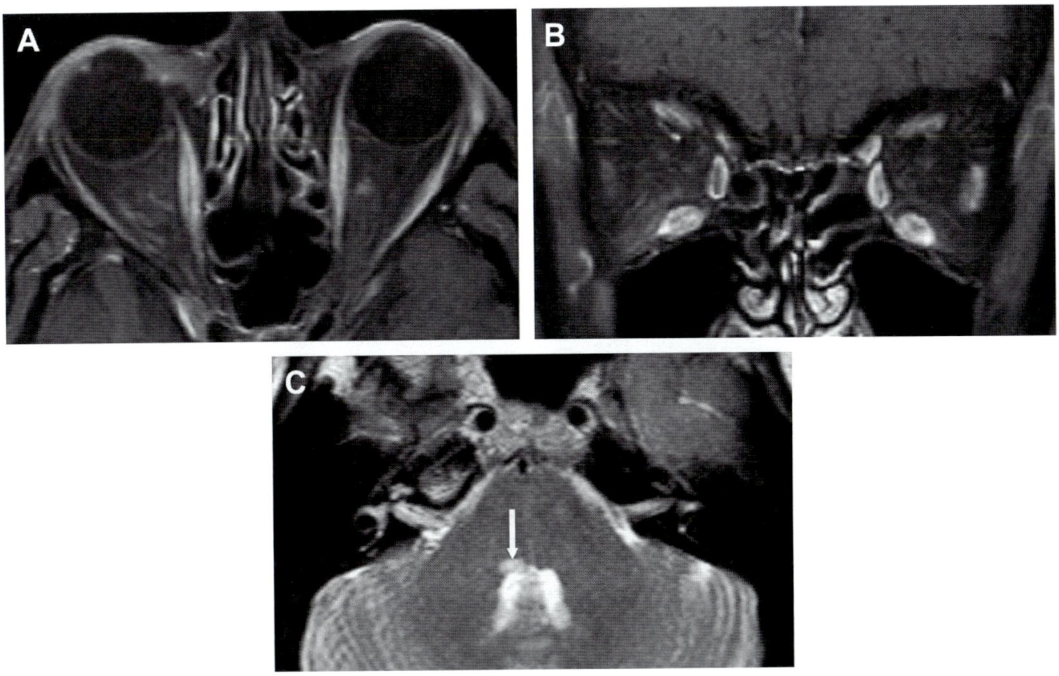

Fig. 15. Right cranial nerve VI denervation atrophy in a 27-year-old woman with multiple sclerosis. Axial (*A*) and coronal (*B*) fat-suppressed postcontrast T1-weighted MR imaging demonstrates decreased size of the right lateral rectus muscle compared with the left. (*C*) Axial T2-weighted MR imaging reveals a multiple sclerosis plaque in the right sixth nerve nucleus at the level of the facial colliculus (*arrow*).

More inferiorly, the recurrent laryngeal nerves originate at different levels on the two sides and primarily innervate the endolaryngeal muscles, with the exception of the cricothyroid muscle (**Fig. 23**).

On clinical examination, patients who have paresis of cranial nerve X proximal to the origin of

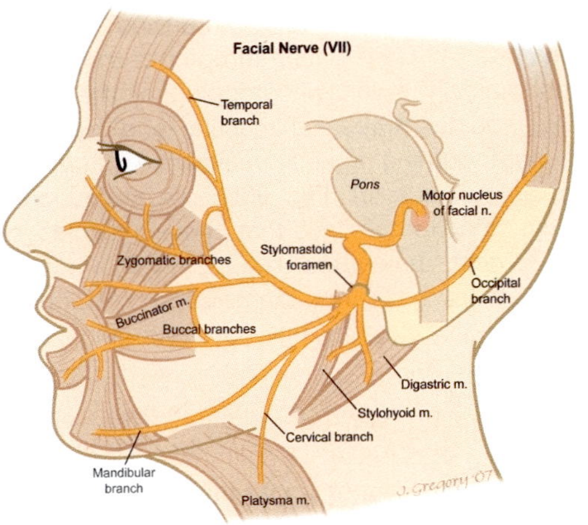

Fig. 16. Diagram of muscles innervated by the facial nerve.

the pharyngeal plexus demonstrate paralysis of the soft palate with drooping of the affected side of the palate at rest, deviation of the uvula away from the side of pathologic change on phonation, and ipsilateral complete vocal cord paralysis (**Fig. 24**).[26] Insults to the distal vagus nerve or recurrent laryngeal nerve are not associated with soft palate paralysis.

On cross-sectional imaging, denervation atrophy affecting the proximal vagus nerve typically manifests as decreased volume of the pharyngeal constrictor muscles with "ballooning-out" of the ipsilateral oropharyngeal or hypopharyngeal airway (**Fig. 25**A).[45] Because of the presence of the pharyngobasilar fascia at the level of the nasopharynx, pharyngeal airway distortion does not occur at this level. Researchers have not been able to recognize a decrease in muscle fibers of the palate, presumably because of their diminutive size. Only occasionally can changes of acute denervation be identified in the fibers of the superior pharyngeal constrictor muscle (**Fig. 25**B). More inferiorly, imaging findings consist of those described in association with vocal cord paralysis: paramedian position of the vocal cord, anteromedial positioning of the arytenoid cartilage,

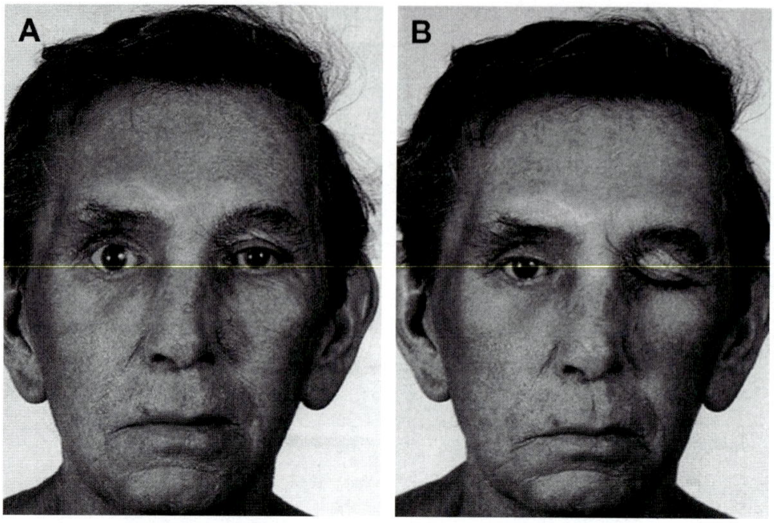

Fig. 17. Clinical examination: lower motor neuron right facial nerve paralysis. Photographs with eyes open (*A*) and eyes closed (*B*). Note involvement of all facial muscles with drooping of the mouth, flattening of the nasolabial fold, and inability to close the eye. (*From* Perkin D, Rose FC, Blackwood W, et al. Atlas of clinical neurology. London: Gower Medical Publishing; 1986; with permission.)

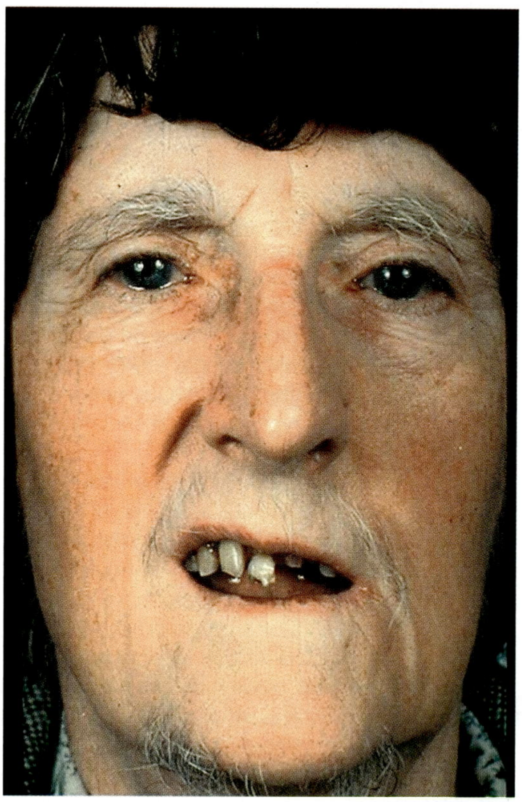

Fig. 18. Clinical examination: upper motor neuron left facial nerve paralysis. Clinical photograph shows a similar appearance to the lower face as that seen in the patient presented in Fig. 17; however, note sparing of the upper facial muscles. (*From* Perkin D, Rose FC, Blackwood W, et al. Atlas of clinical neurology. London: Gower Medical Publishing; 1986; with permission.)

ipsilateral laryngeal ventricle dilatation, denervation atrophy of the thyroarytenoid muscle, ipsilateral medial positioning and thickening of the aryepiglottic fold, ipsilateral dilatation of the pyriform sinus, ipsilateral subglottic fullness, and ipsilateral vallecular dilatation.[45,46] An additional indicator of recurrent laryngeal nerve paralysis is denervation atrophy of the posterior cricoarytenoid muscle (**Figs. 26–28**).[47]

SPINAL ACCESSORY NERVE—CRANIAL NERVE XI

The spinal accessory nerve exits the skull base through the pars vascularis of the jugular foramen and provides only motor innervation to the large sternocleidomastoid and trapezius muscles (**Fig. 29**).[42,43] Denervation atrophy of these muscles clinically results in drooping of the ipsilateral shoulder (trapezius muscle) and weakness on head turning against resistance (sternocleidomastoid muscle) (**Fig. 30**).[26] As stated previously, despite the fact that these muscles are the largest innervated by the cranial nerves, the authors have not identified any stages of denervation except the late chronic stage (**Fig. 31**).

HYPOGLOSSAL NERVE—CRANIAL NERVE XII

After exiting the skull by way of the hypoglossal canal, the hypoglossal nerve courses through the

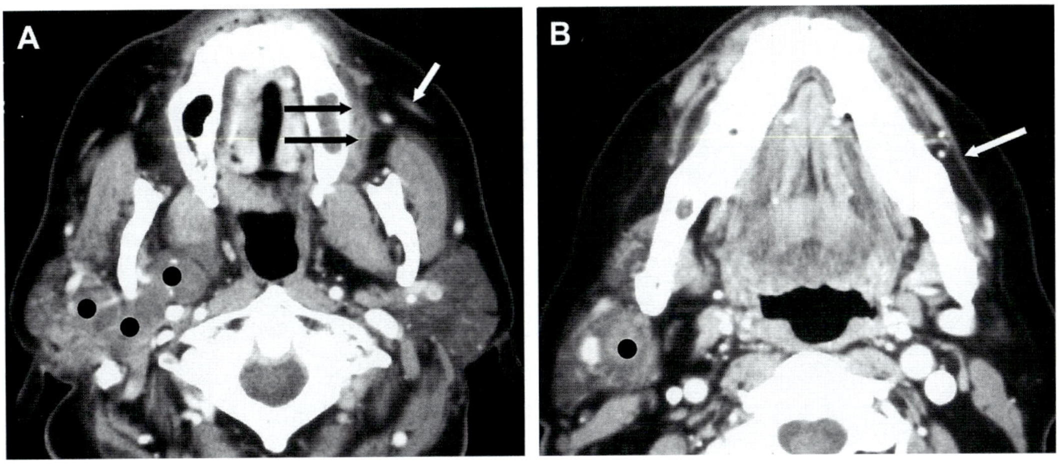

Fig. 19. Right seventh nerve denervation atrophy in a 47-year-old man with a facial nerve plexiform neurofibroma (neurofibromatosis II). (*A*, *B*) Axial postcontrast CT images. (*A*) There is atrophy of the fibers of the right buccinator and zygomaticus muscles. The normal buccinator (*black arrows*) and zygomaticus (*white arrow*) muscles are labeled on the left. (*B*) Note severe atrophy of the right platysma muscle in comparison to the normal left platysma muscle (*arrow*). Dots indicate the plexiform neurofibroma in both images.

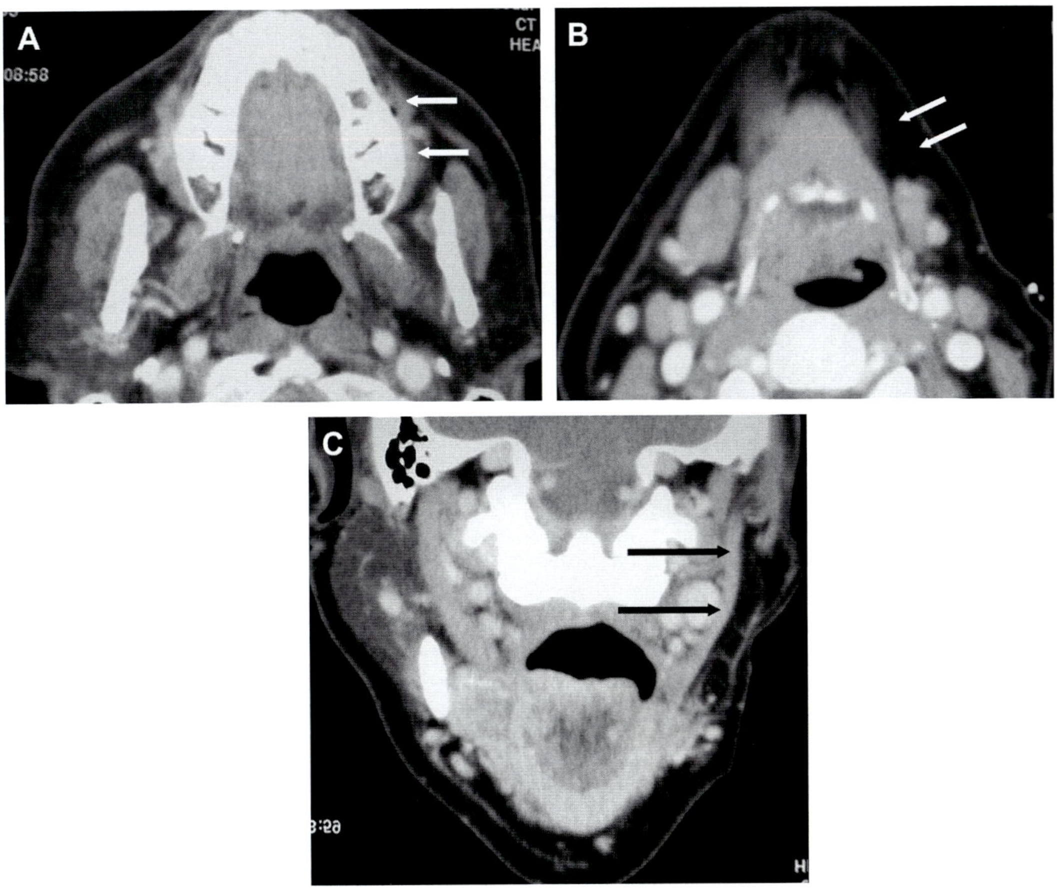

Fig. 20. Left seventh nerve denervation atrophy in a 47-year-old woman who noted left facial weakness status after a right parotid pleomorphic adenoma resection. Axial (*A*, *B*) and coronal (*C*) postcontrast CT images. (*A*) Note slightly decreased size of the right buccinator muscle (*arrows*). (*B*) There is marked loss of the right platysma fibers (*arrows*). (*C*) There is atrophy of the left posterior digastric muscle (*arrows*).

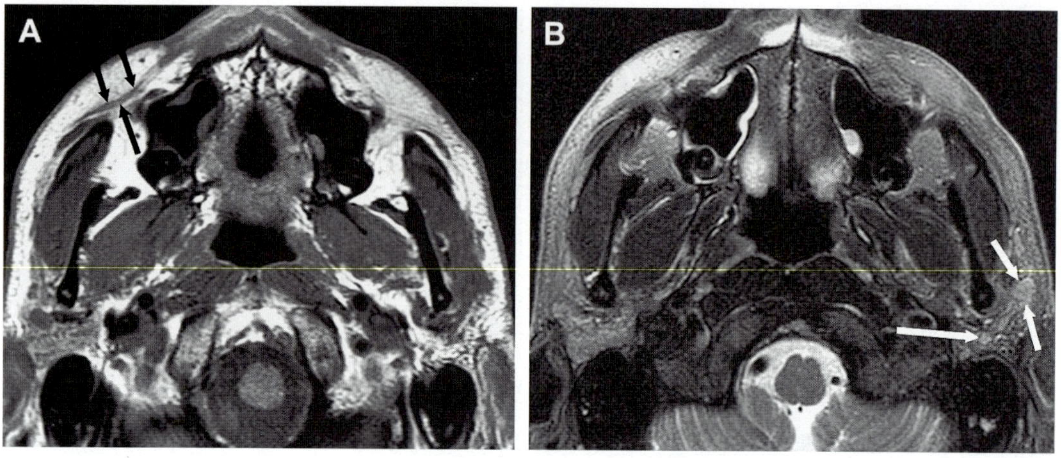

Fig. 21. Partial left peripheral seventh nerve palsy in a 57-year-old man with high-grade carcinoma of the left parotid gland, not otherwise specified. (*A*) Axial T1-weighted MR imaging demonstrates atrophy of the left quadratus labii superioris muscle, with the normal muscle indicated on the right (*arrows*). There was no volume loss of other muscles innervated by the facial nerve. (*B*) Axial fat-suppressed T2-weighted MR imaging shows the small tumor (*small arrows*) and the pathologically proved perineural extension along the mastoid segment of the seventh nerve (*long arrow*). (*Courtesy of* Christine M. Glastonbury, MD, San Francisco, CA.)

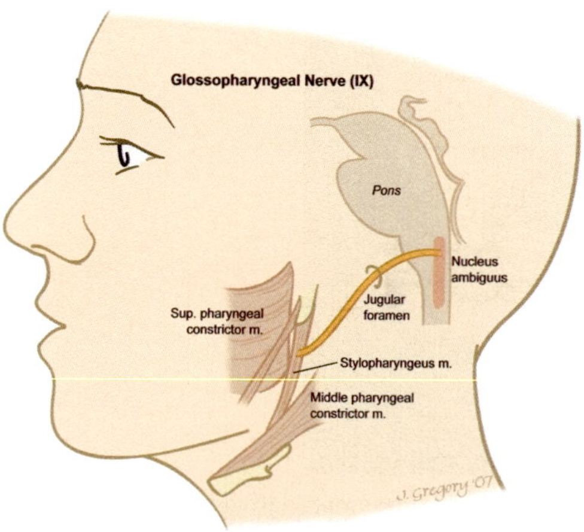

Fig. 22. Diagram of muscles innervated by branches of the glossopharyngeal nerve.

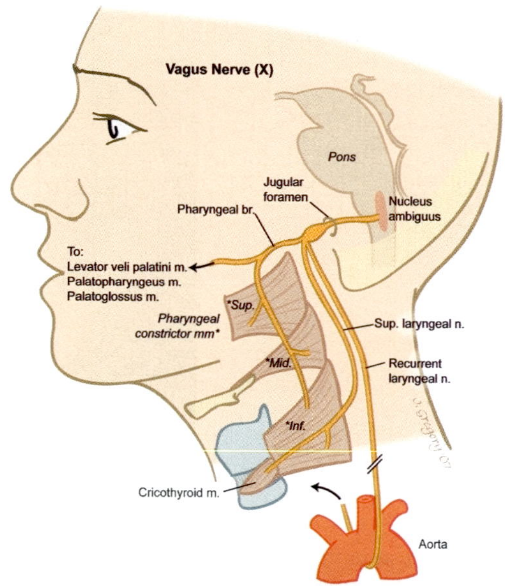

Fig. 23. Diagram of muscles innervated by branches of the vagus nerve.

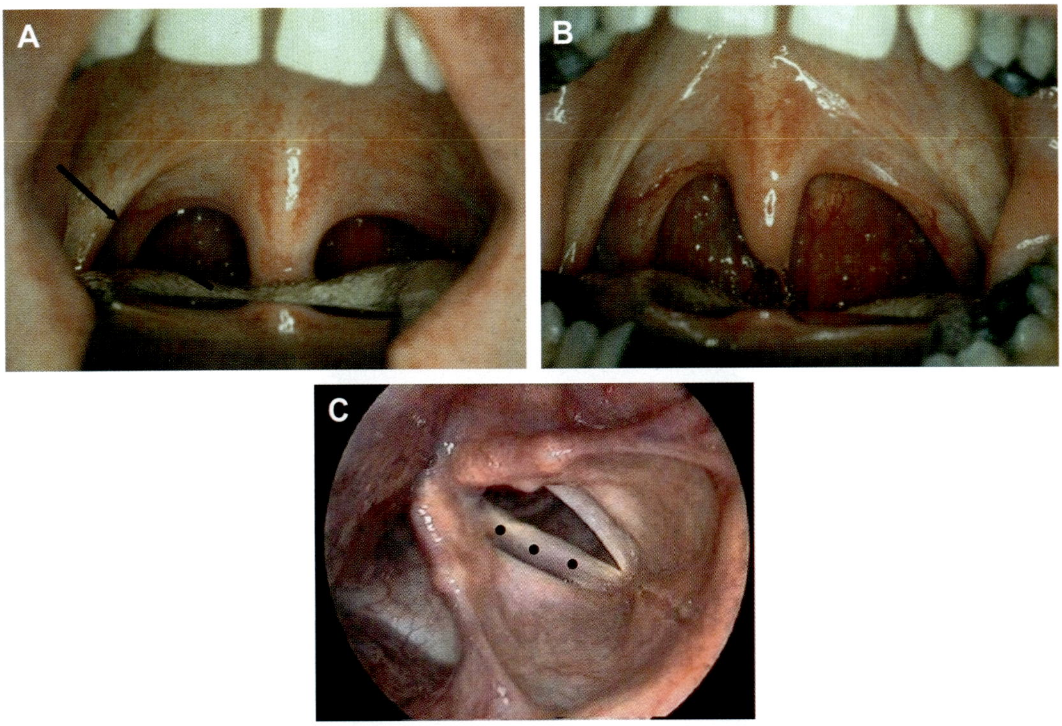

Fig. 24. Clinical examination: (*A*, *B*) left vagus nerve paralysis. (*A*) With the palate at rest, note drooping of the left aspect of the palate with decreased prominence of the muscle ridges (tonsillar pillars) produced by the anterior palatoglossus and posterior palatopharyngeus muscles compared with the normal right muscles (*arrows*). (*B*) On "ah" phonation, there is deviation of the uvula to the right. (*C*) Endoscopy of the larynx shows medialization and thickening of the left vocal cord (*dots*). (*A*, *B*: *From* Perkin D, Rose FC, Blackwood W, et al. Atlas of clinical neurology. London: Gower Medical Publishing; 1986; with permission.)

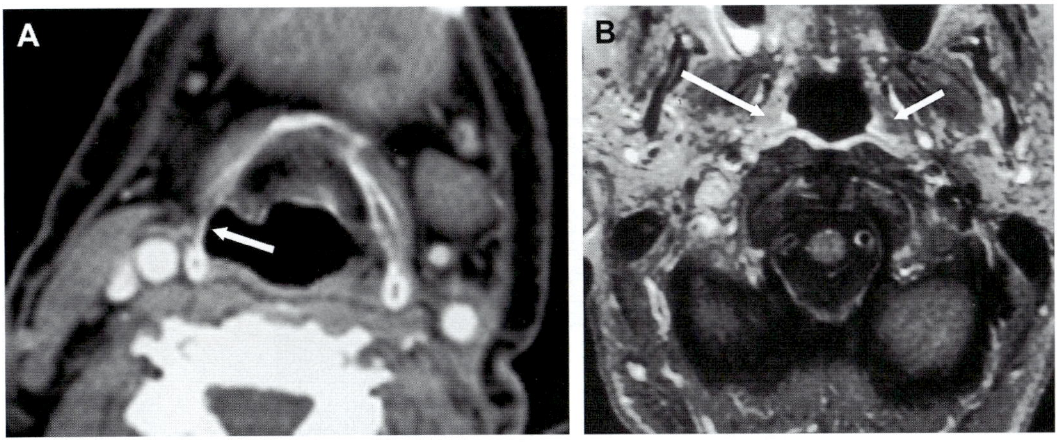

Fig. 25. Findings in proximal vagal dysfunction (different patients). (*A*) Axial CT scan shows loss of pharyngeal constrictor muscle fibers on the right, with subsequent ballooning of the airway (*arrow*) from long-standing chronic denervation and a jugular paraganglioma. (*B*) Axial postcontrast T1-weighted MR imaging demonstrates a normal-sized left superior pharyngeal constrictor muscle (*short arrow*) compared with abnormally enhancing normal-sized muscle fibers on the right (*long arrow*) attributable to acute denervation caused by a jugular paraganglioma.

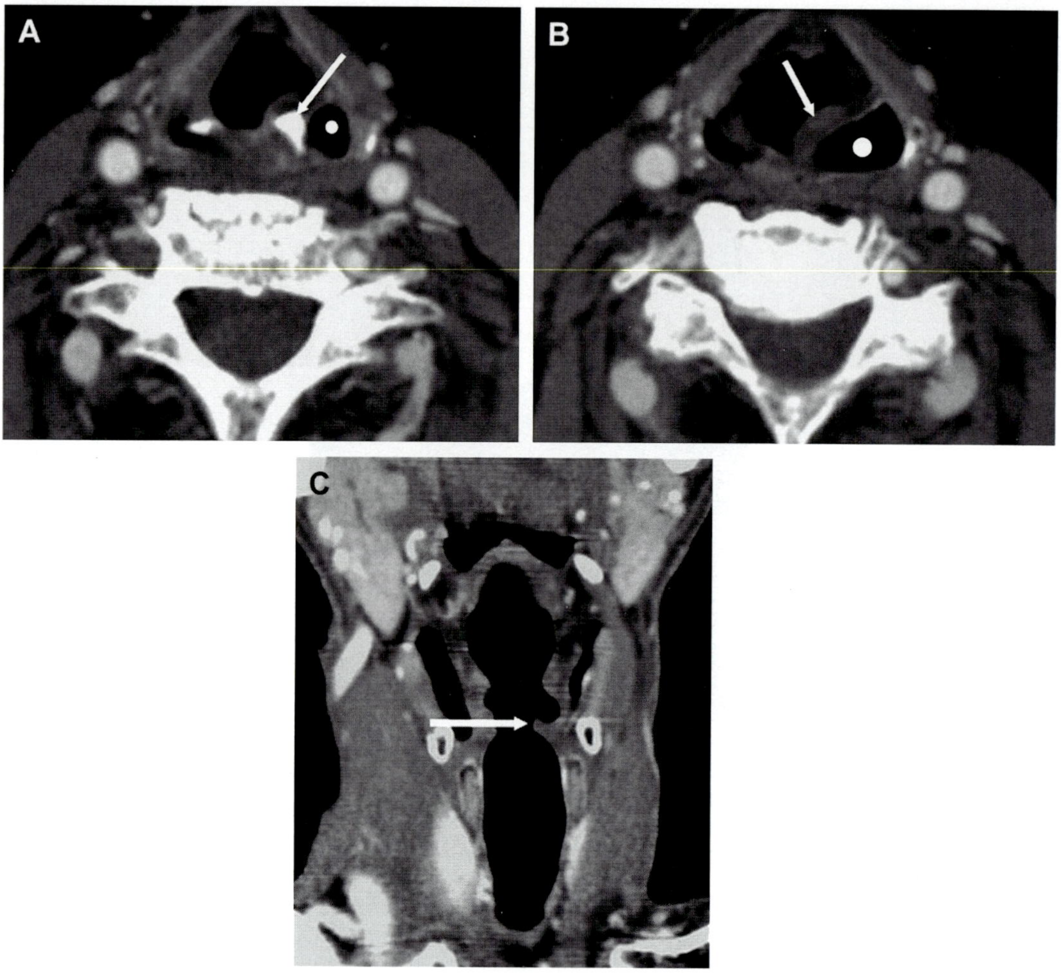

Fig. 26. Left distal vagal nerve paralysis in a patient with acute hoarseness (normal proximal function) from an aortic arch aneurysm. Axial CT scans with contrast through the larynx. (*A*) Note rotation and anteromedial positioning of the left arytenoid cartilage (*arrow*). (*B*) There is thickening and medial positioning of the left aryepiglottic fold (*arrow*). Dilatation of the pyriform sinus is also noted (*dot*). (*C*) Coronal CT reformatted image demonstrates characteristic "pointing" of the thinned left vocal cord (*arrow*). (*Courtesy of* William P. Dillon, MD, San Francisco, CA.)

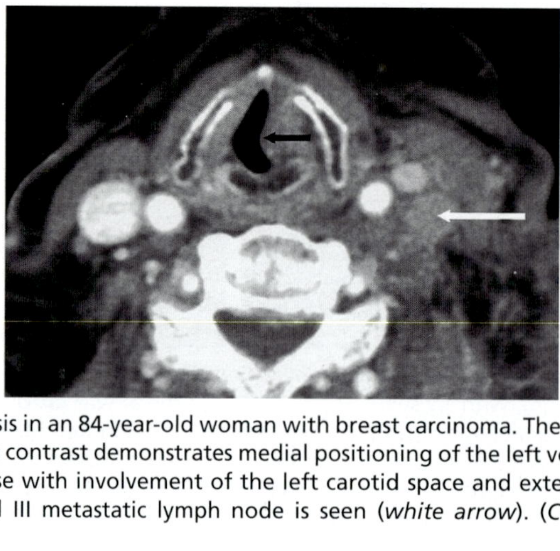

Fig. 27. Left vocal cord paralysis in an 84-year-old woman with breast carcinoma. The cough and gag reflexes were normal. An axial CT scan with contrast demonstrates medial positioning of the left vocal cord (*black arrow*). There is extensive metastatic disease with involvement of the left carotid space and extension to the left tracheoesophageal groove. A left level III metastatic lymph node is seen (*white arrow*). (*Courtesy of* William P. Dillon, MD, San Francisco, CA.)

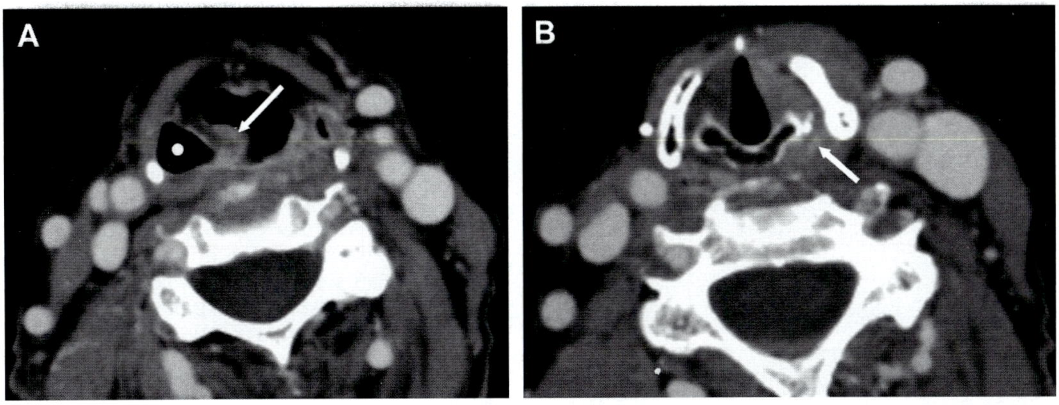

Fig. 28. Right distal vagal nerve paralysis in a 57-year-old woman, status postthyroidectomy, with complaints of "voice problems." (*A*, *B*) Axial CT images with contrast through the lower neck. (*A*) Note thickening and medial positioning of the right aryepiglottic fold (*arrow*) and patulous pyriform sinus (*dot*). (*B*) There is atrophy of the right posterior cricoarytenoid muscle fibers, with the normal posterior cricoarytenoid muscle located on the left (*arrow*).

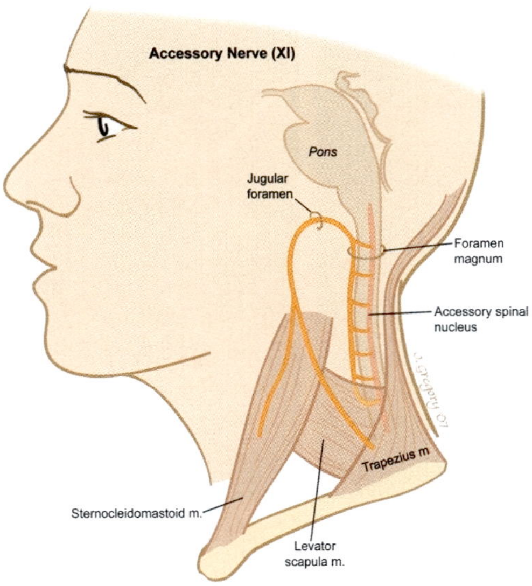

Fig. 29. Diagram of muscles innervated by the spinal accessory nerve.

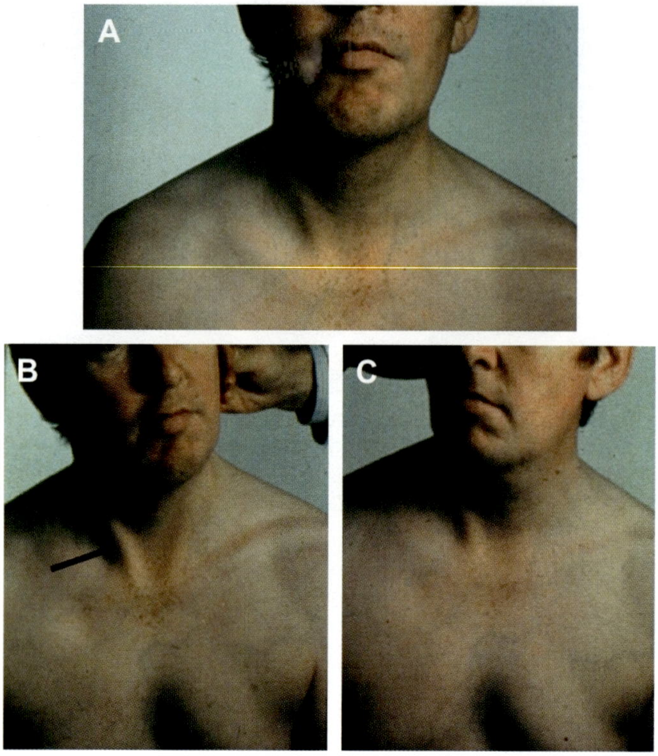

Fig. 30. Clinical examination: left spinal accessory nerve palsy. (*A*) Patient is in a neutral position, at rest. Notice flattening and drooping of the left shoulder (trapezius muscle atrophy). (*B*) Head is turned to the left against resistance. There is noticeable contraction of the right sternocleidomastoid muscle (*arrow*). (*C*) Head is turned to the right against resistance. There is no visible left sternocleidomastoid muscle contraction. (*From* Perkin D, Rose FC, Blackwood W, et al. Atlas of clinical neurology. London: Gower Medical Publishing; 1986; with permission.)

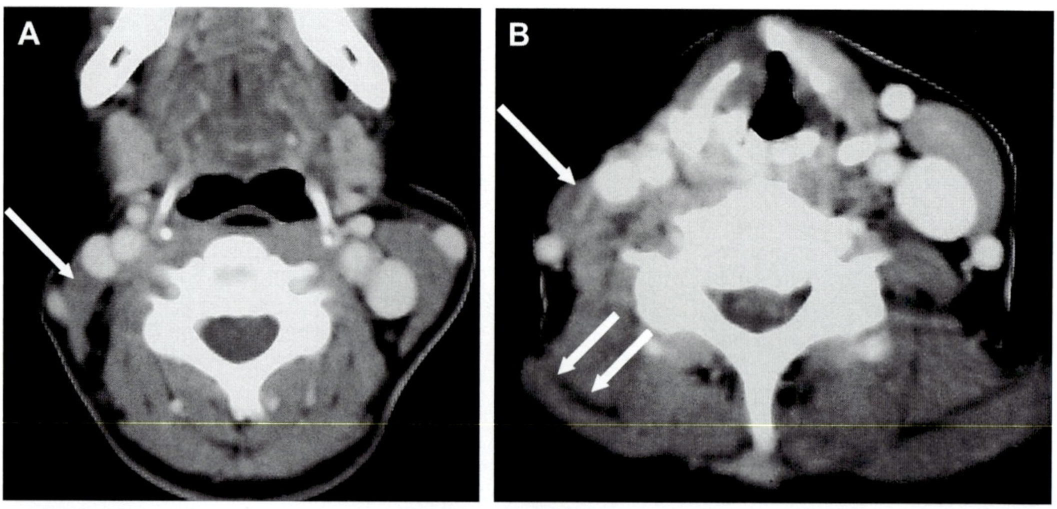

Fig. 31. Isolated left spinal accessory nerve palsy in a 41-year-old woman, presumed postviral. (*A, B*) Axial CT images with contrast. Note denervation atrophy of the right sternocleidomastoid (*single arrows*) and trapezius (*double arrows*) muscles. Note normal tongue musculature and normal oropharyngeal airway contour (10th and 12th nerves intact).

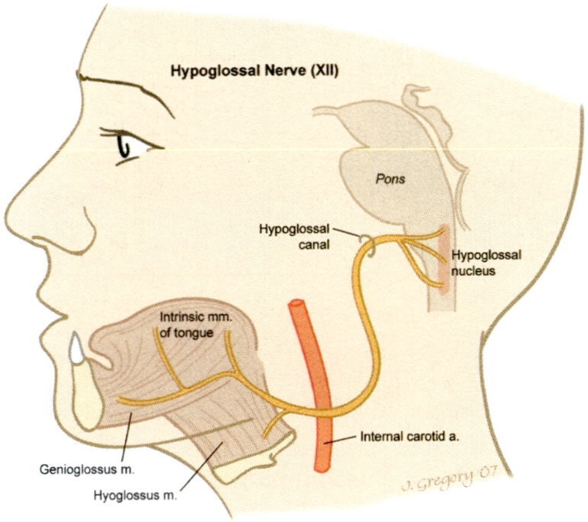

Fig. 32. Diagram of muscles innervated by the hypoglossal nerve.

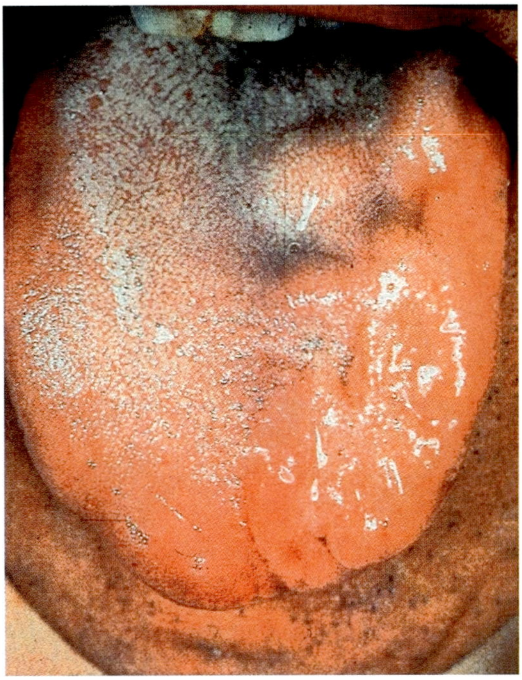

Fig. 33. Clinical examination: left hypoglossal nerve denervation atrophy. Note decreased volume of the left hemitongue and a smooth surface, devoid of normal papillae. (*From* Perkin D, Rose FC, Blackwood W, et al. Atlas of clinical neurology. London: Gower Medical Publishing; 1986; with permission.)

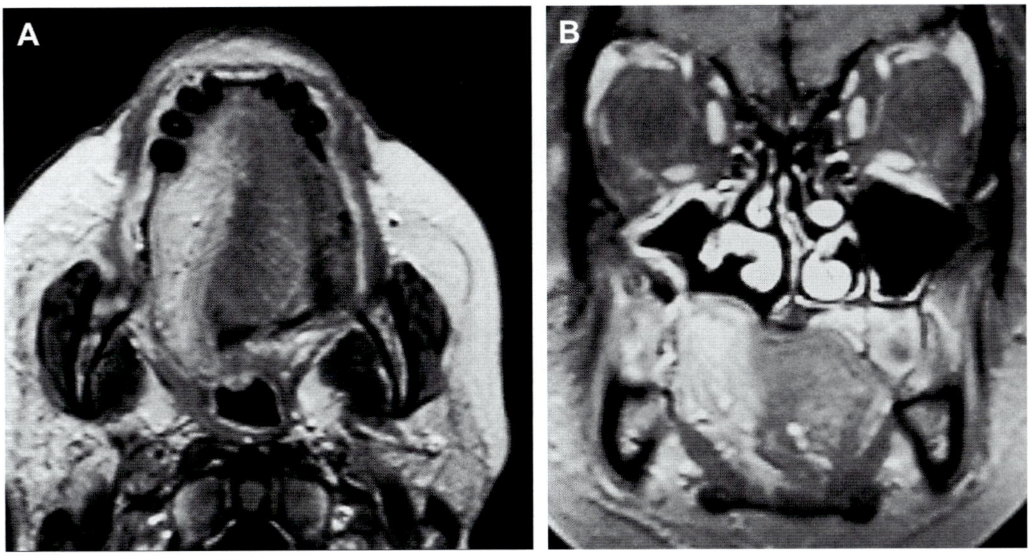

Fig. 34. MR imaging of late chronic right hypoglossal denervation atrophy in a 40-year-old woman status post-right maxillectomy and hard palate resection for squamous cell carcinoma. Axial (*A*) and coronal (*B*) postcontrast T1-weighted MR imaging demonstrates complete fatty replacement and volume loss of the right hemitongue, which is significantly prolapsed back into the oropharynx. Postoperative changes are appreciated in (*B*).

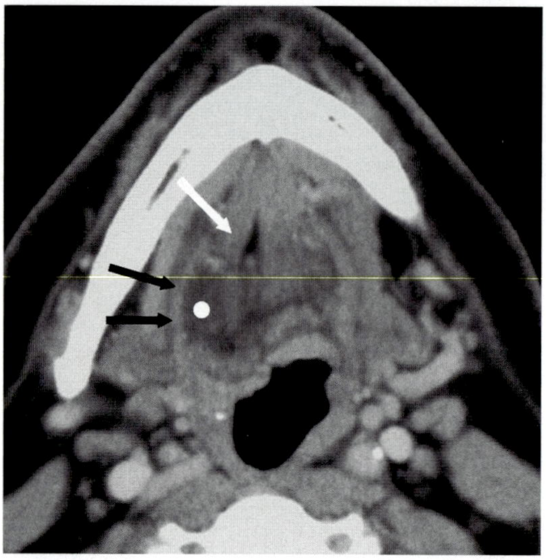

Fig. 35. CT of late chronic right hypoglossal nerve denervation atrophy in a 48-year-old diabetic man with right skull base osteomyelitis. An axial CT image with contrast clearly demonstrates fatty atrophy of the intrinsic tongue muscles (*dot*) and a marked decrease in size of the extrinsic hyoglossus (*black arrows*) and genioglossus (*white arrow*) muscles. Note deviation of the midline fatty septum to the right.

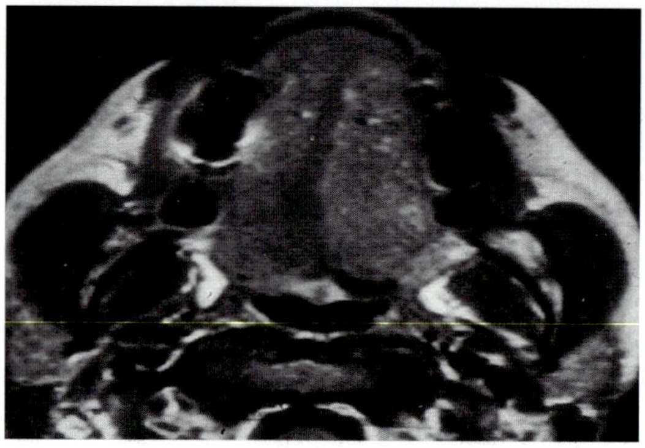

Fig. 36. Acute and subacute left hypoglossal denervation atrophy in a 9-year-old boy 2 weeks status post-tonsillectomy. Axial T1-weighted MR imaging. Note enlargement of the left hemitongue and some evidence of early fatty infiltration.

high nasopharyngeal carotid space with the other lower cranial nerves. The nerve courses inferiorly to supply the extrinsic and intrinsic muscles of the tongue (**Fig. 32**). Patients who have denervation atrophy of muscles innervated by the hypoglossal nerve demonstrate loss of hemitongue volume, loss of the normal papillae (smooth appearance), and deviation of the tongue toward the side of pathologic change on protrusion (imbalanced action of genioglossus muscles) (**Fig. 33**).[26] The various stages of denervation on MR imaging and CT have been reported in the literature.[6,7,48–51] Most common, of course, are marked fatty infiltration and prolapse of the tongue posteriorly into the oropharynx, which are changes associated with long-standing chronic atrophy (**Fig. 34**). As for the mandibular nerve, earlier stages of denervation are also able to be identified for the hypoglossal nerve, probably because tongue muscle denervation is able to be noted clinically at an earlier stage than denervation associated with most other cranial nerves (**Figs. 35 and 36**).

COMBINED CRANIAL NERVE PALSIES

The pathologic cases illustrated have emphasized the findings of denervation atrophy associated with isolated cranial nerve insults. Not infrequently, however, multiple cranial nerves are affected by a single lesion. This is especially the case of lesions that affect the lower four cranial nerves. One such case, produced by a jugular paraganglioma, is illustrated in **Fig. 37**.

SUMMARY

Muscles undergoing denervation demonstrate a variety of imaging appearances in the various stages. It is incumbent on the radiologist to be aware of these changes so as not to interpret these muscles as harboring a tumor or being involved by an inflammatory process. Knowledge of cranial nerve anatomy and the muscles they innervate enables identification of denervation patterns that could implicate more than one nerve and directs the search for the causative lesion.

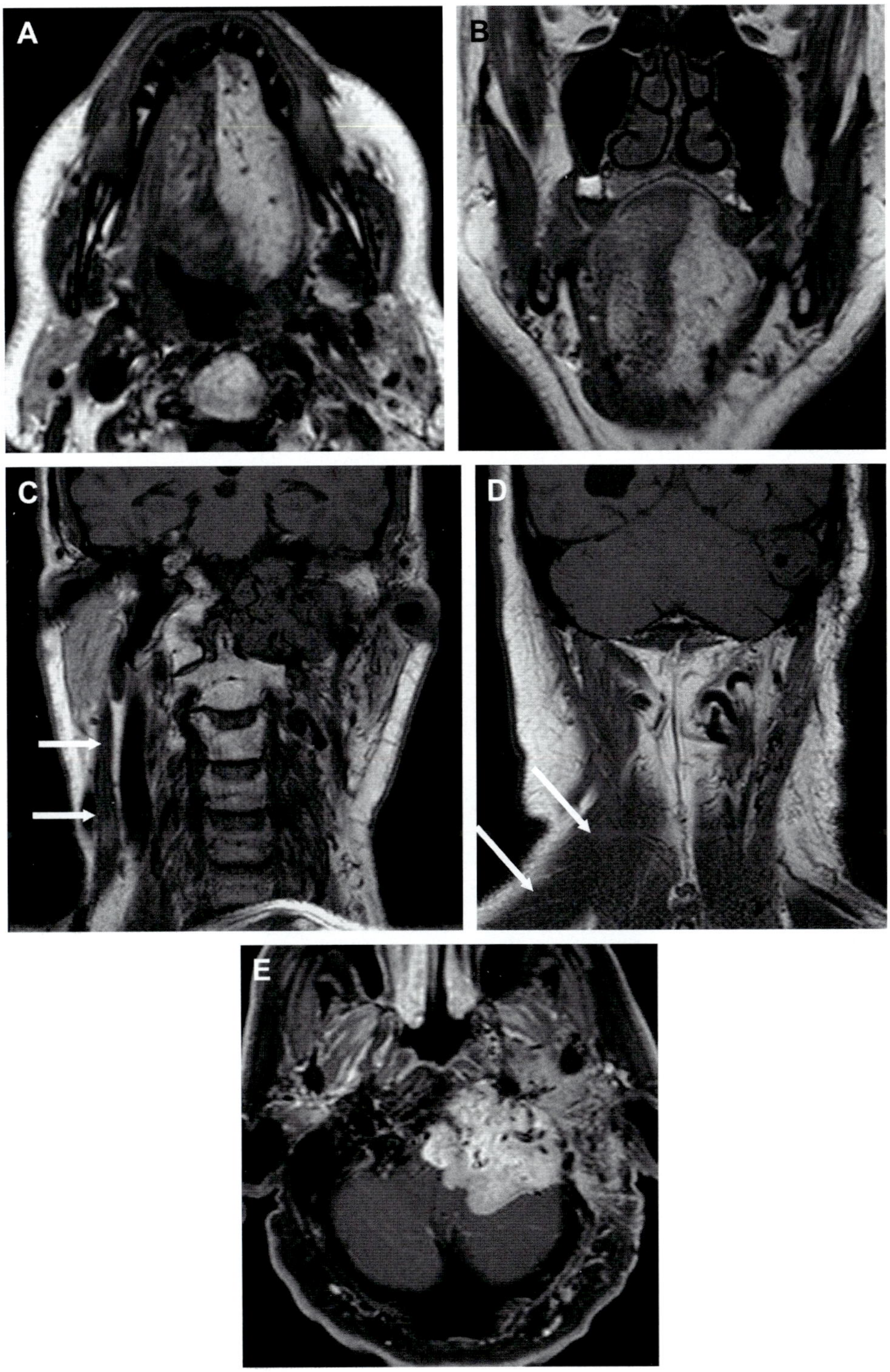

Fig. 37. Combined ninth through 12th nerve denervation atrophy in a 54-year-old woman with a jugular paraganglioma. Axial (*A*) and coronal (*B*) T1-weighted MR imaging demonstrates fatty replacement of the left hemitongue with only mild volume loss. (*C*) Coronal T1-weighted MR imaging through the level of the posterior skull base demonstrates a large mass with numerous flow voids replacing the left jugular tubercle, left occipital condyle, and left lateral mass of C1. Note complete atrophy of the left sternocleidomastoid muscle fibers and the normal right sternocleidomastoid muscle (*arrows*). (*D*) Coronal T1-weighted MR imaging through the posterior aspect of the neck reveals atrophy of the left trapezius muscle and the normal right trapezius muscle (*arrows*). (*E*) Axial fat-suppressed postcontrast T1-weighted MR imaging demonstrates the large destructive jugular paraganglioma with numerous flow voids (patient had symptoms of decreased cough and gag reflexes as well).

REFERENCES

1. Davis SB, Mathews VP, Williams DW. Masticator muscle enhancement in subacute denervation atrophy. AJNR Am J Neuroradiol 1995;16:1292–4.
2. Hutchins LG, Harnsberger HR, Cardin CW, et al. The radiologic assessment of trigeminal neuropathy. AJNR Am J Neuroradiol 1989;10:1275–82.
3. Fleckenstein JL, Watamull D, Conner KE, et al. Denervated human skeletal muscle: MR imaging evaluation. Radiology 1993;187:213–8.
4. West GA, Haynor DR, Goodkin R, et al. Magnetic resonance imaging signal changes in denervated muscles after peripheral nerve injury. Neurosurgery 1994;35:1077–85.
5. Shellhas KP. MR imaging of muscles of mastication. AJR Am J Roentgenol 1989;153:847–55.
6. Harnsberger HR, Dillon WP. Major motor atrophic patterns in the face and neck: CT evaluation. Radiology 1985;155:165–70.
7. Russo CP, Smoker WRK, Weissman JL. MR appearance of trigeminal and hypoglossal motor denervation. AJNR Am J Neuroradiol 1997;18: 1375–83.
8. Kato K, Tomura N, Takahashi S, et al. Motor denervation on tumors of the head and neck: changes in MR appearance. Magn Reson Med Sci 2002;1: 157–64.
9. Dill-Macky M, Song S, Silbert PL. Magnetic resonance imaging features of subacute brachial neuritis. Australas Radiol 2000;44:98–100.
10. Polak JF, Jolesz FA, Adams DF. NMR of skeletal muscle differences in relaxation parameters related to extracellular/intracellular fluid spaces. Invest Radiol 1988;23:107–12.
11. Kikuchi Y, Nakamura T, Takayama S, et al. MR imaging in the diagnosis of denervated and reinnervated skeletal muscles: experimental study in rats. Radiology 2003;229:861–7.
12. Polak JF, Jolesz FA, Adams DF. Magnetic resonance imaging of skeletal muscle prolongation of T1 and T2 subsequent to denervation. Invest Radiol 1988; 23:365–9.
13. May DA, Disler DG, Jones EA, et al. Abnormal signal intensity in skeletal muscle at MR imaging: patterns, pearls, and pitfalls. Radiographics 2000;20: S295–315.
14. Wessig C, Koltzenburg M, Reiners K, et al. Muscle magnetic resonance imaging of denervation and reinnervation: correlation with electrophysiology and histology. Exp Neurol 2004;185:254–61.
15. Hayashi Y, Ikata T, Takai H, et al. Effect of peripheral nerve injury on nuclear magnetic resonance relaxation times of rat skeletal muscle. Invest Radiol 1997;32:135–9.
16. Bendszus M, Koltzenburg M, Wessig C, et al. Sequential MR imaging of denervated muscle: experimental study. AJNR Am J Neuroradiol 2002; 23:1427–31.
17. McDonald CM, Carter GT, Fritz RC, et al. Magnetic resonance imaging of denervated muscle: comparison to electromyography. Muscle Nerve 2000;23: 1431–4.
18. Elster AD, Jackels SC, Allen NS, et al. Europium-DTPA: a gadolinium analogue traceable by fluorescence microscopy. AJNR Am J Neuroradiol 1989; 10:1137–44.
19. Kaissar G, Kim JH, Bravo S, et al. Histologic basis for increased extraocular muscle enhancement in gadolinium-enhanced MR imaging. Radiology 1991;179:541–2.
20. Uetani M, Hayaski K, Matsunaga N, et al. Denervated skeletal muscle: MR imaging work in progress. Radiology 1993;189:511–5.
21. Hudlicka O. Blood flow and oxygen consumption in muscles after section of ventral roots. Circ Res 1967; 20:570–7.
22. Bondy SC, Purdy JL, Carroll JE, et al. The rate of nutrient supply to normal and denervated slow and fast muscle, and its relation to muscle blood flow. Exp Neurol 1976;51:678–83.
23. Carpenter S, Karpati G. Necrosis of capillaries in denervation atrophy of human skeletal muscle. Muscle Nerve 1982;5:250–4.
24. Hassler O. The angioarchitecture of normal and denervated skeletal muscle. Neurology 1970;20:1161–4.
25. Laine FJ, Smoker WRK. Cranial nerves III, IV, and VI. Neuroimaging Clin N Am 1993;3:85–103.
26. Perkin D, Rose FC, Blackwood W, et al. Cranial nerve, neuro-ophthalmological and neuro-otological syndromes. In: Perkin D, Rose FC, Blackwood W , et al. editors. Atlas of clinical neurology. Philadelphia: JB Lippincott Co.; 1986. p. 12.1–12.22.
27. Guy J, Savino PJ, Schatz NJ, et al. Superior division paresis of the oculomotor nerve. Ophthalmology 1985;92:777–84.
28. Guy JR, Day AL. Intracranial aneurysms with superior division paresis of the oculomotor nerve. Ophthalmology 1989;96:1071–6.
29. Ksiazek SM, Repka MX, Maguire A, et al. Divisional oculomotor nerve paresis caused by intrinsic brainstem disease. Ann Neurol 1989;26:714–8.
30. Bregman DK, Harbour R. Diabetic superior division oculomotor nerve palsy. Arch Ophthalmol 1988; 106:1169–70.
31. Masucci EF, Kurtzke JF. Diabetic superior branch palsy of the oculomotor nerve. Ann Neurol 1980;7:493–6.
32. Stefanis L, Przedborski S. Isolated palsy of the superior branch of the oculomotor nerve due to chronic erosive sphenoid sinusitis. J Clin Neuroophthalmol 1993;13:229–31.
33. Katz B, Rimmer S. Ophthalmoplegic migraine with superior ramus oculomotor paresis. J Clin Neuroophthalmol 1989;9:181–3.

34. Castro O, Johnson LN, Mamourian AD. Isolated inferior oblique paresis from brain-stem infarction: perspective on oculomotor fascicular organization in the ventral midbrain tegmentum. Arch Neurol 1990;47:235–7.
35. Barr ML. Cranial nerves. In: The human nervous system. 3rd edition. New York: Harper & Row; 1979. p. 101–19.
36. Walsh TJ. Diplopia. In: Walsh TJ, editor. Neuro-ophthalmology: clinical signs and symptoms. 2nd edition. Philadelphia: Lea & Febiger; 1985. p. 89–126.
37. Good WV, Barkovich AJ, Nickel BL, et al. Bilateral congenital oculomotor nerve palsy in a child with brain anomalies. Am J Ophthalmol 1991;111:555–8.
38. Getenet JC, Vighetto A, Nighoghossian N, et al. Isolated bilateral third nerve palsy caused by a mesencephalic hematoma. Neurology 1994;44:281–2.
39. Okamoto K, Ito J, Tokiguchi S, et al. Atrophy of bilateral extraocular muscles. J Neuroophthalmol 1996;16:286–8.
40. Chusid JG. The cranial nerves. In: Correlative neuroanatomy and functional neurology. 17th edition. Los Altos (CA): Lange Medical Publishers; 1979. p. 84–110.
41. Guy JR, Friedman WF, Mickle JR. Bilateral trochlear nerve paresis in hydrocephalus. J Clin Neuroophthalmol 1989;9:105–11.
42. Grey H. Anatomy, descriptive and surgical. 15th edition. Pickering T, Howden R, editors. New York: Bounty Books; 1977.
43. Sobotta J. Atlas of human anatomy. 14th edition. Putz R, Pabst R, editors. Munchen (Germany): Elsevier Urban & Fischer; 2006. p. 8–11.
44. Remley KB, Latchaw RE. Imaging of cranial nerves IX, X, and XI. Neuroimaging Clin N Am 1993;3:171–91.
45. Chin SC, Edelstein S, Chen CY, et al. Using CT to localize side and level of vocal cord paralysis. AJR Am J Roentgenol 2003;180:165–70.
46. Jacobs CJM, Harnsberger HR, Lufkin RB, et al. Vagal neuropathy: evaluation with CT and MR imaging. Radiology 1987;164:97–102.
47. Romo LV, Curtin HD. Atrophy of the posterior cricoarytenoid muscle as an indicator of recurrent laryngeal nerve palsy. AJNR Am J Neuroradiol 1999;20:467–71.
48. Smoker WRK, Harnsberger HR, Osborn AG. The hypoglossal nerve. Semin Ultrasound CT MR 1987;8:301–12.
49. Smoker WRK. The hypoglossal nerve. Neuroimaging Clin N Am 1993;3:193–206.
50. Naidich TP, Pudlowski RM, Leeds NE, et al. Hypoglossal palsy: computed tomography demonstration of denervation hemiatrophy of the tongue associated with glomus jugulare tumor. J Comput Assist Tomogr 1978;2:630–2.
51. Murakami R, Baba Y, Nishimura R, et al. MR of denervated tongue: temporal changes after radical neck dissection. AJNR Am J Neuroradiol 1998;19:515–8.

Perineural Tumor Spread

Roberto Maroldi, MD*, Davide Farina, MD, Andrea Borghesi, MD,
Anna Marconi, MD, Enza Gatti, MD

KEYWORDS

- Cranial nerve neoplasms
- Head and neck neoplasms • Trigeminal nerve
- Neoplasm invasiveness • MR • CT
- Radiography

Perineural spread (PNS) refers to the extent of tumor cells or other nonneoplastic lesions along the tissues of the nerve sheath. In head and neck malignancies, perineural spread has been described in surgical and imaging literature for decades.

Although PNS was previously associated with worsening prognosis, increasing evidence shows that cure is possible.[1,2] In patients who have PNS from squamous cell carcinoma of the skin, a cure rate of approximately 80% can be achieved when both symptoms and imaging findings (for PNS) are absent.[1]

In addition, in symptomatic patients the lesions limited to peripheral nerves or with minimal/moderate PNS tumor burden have a better local control rate, although a similar survival rate, compared with patients who have central or macroscopic disease.[3,4]

This pattern of neoplastic spread can be clinically unsuspected while it conveys the tumor cells beyond the surgical and radiation fields of treatment. Therefore, if PNS is undetected or its extent is underestimated by imaging techniques, treatment will probably not control the disease.

Two additional points help radiologists understand the clinical significance of PNS assessment. First, in most head and neck neoplasms, the primary lesion and its gross extent have already been detected and estimated at clinical examination. Second, treatment of the neck is mainly dictated by the site and size of the primary tumor. Therefore, the evaluation of possible PNS through imaging may influence treatment planning more than identifying the primary tumor or assessing nodal disease.[5]

INCIDENCE, EPIDEMIOLOGY, AND MOST FREQUENT MALIGNANT TUMORS SHOWING PERINEURAL SPREAD

Overall, the incidence of PNS ranges from 2.5% to 5%.[6] Although it may occur with any head and neck malignancy, PNS is more frequently associated with carcinoma arising from minor or major salivary glands (more often adenoid cystic carcinoma [ACC]), mucosal or cutaneous squamous cell carcinoma (SCC), basal cell carcinoma (BCC), melanoma, lymphoma, and sarcoma.

PNS along a major (named) nerve has been observed in up to 28% of ACC arising from major or minor salivary and nonsalivary glands.[7] Immunohistochemical studies have shown a high expression of neural cell adhesion molecules in ACC. These molecules could facilitate the mechanism of PNS.[8,9]

Also the desmoplastic melanoma has a striking propensity to invade nerves. This ability has been related to a high expression of the p75 neurotrophin receptor (highly expressed also in a small series of ACC). During development, the interaction of nerve growth factor with the p75 receptor located on Schwann cells promotes the migration of Schwann cell to the nerve.[10,11]

Although the adjacent nerves are invaded in up to 30% of desmoplastic melanoma, spread along cranial nerves is expected in no more than 1% to 2%.[12,13]

Among tumors of the skin, SCC spreads more frequently along cranial nerves (5%–14%) than BCC, though in recurrent BCC the incidence of PNS significantly increases.[14]

Even in the absence of neurologic abnormalities, accurate imaging is recommended to assess or

Department of Radiology, University of Brescia, Radiologia 2 – Spedali Civili, I-25123 Brescia, Italy
* Corresponding author.
E-mail address: maroldi@med.unibs.it (R. Maroldi).

Neuroimag Clin N Am 18 (2008) 413–429
doi:10.1016/j.nic.2008.01.001

rule out PNS along nerves whose distribution corresponds to the innervation of glands, mucosa, and skin areas of the face.

Therefore, radiologists must be aware of the relevant cranial nerve anatomy and examine not only the nerves close to the primary tumor site but also the whole neural pathways that can be accessed through PNS. Equally critical is the knowledge of the radiologic appearance of perineural tumor extension and of the best imaging strategies to detect PNS.

NEURAL PATHWAYS RELEVANT FOR PERINEURAL SPREAD

In most cases the peripheral branches of the second (V2) or third division (V3) of the trigeminal nerve and the descending branch of the facial nerve serve as conduits for perineural tumor spread into the skull base.

Preexisting neural pathways, such as the vidian nerve, greater superficial petrosal nerve (GSPN), and auriculotemporal nerve (ATN), account for neoplastic dissemination from trigeminal branches to those of the facial nerve (and vice versa).[15–17] Less frequently, the ophthalmic nerve (V1) or hypoglossal nerve are involved.[18,19] PNS along other nerve routes has been reported in few patients.[20,21] Perineural tumor spread is usually antegrade (toward the central nervous system), but retrograde spread may also occur.

Trigeminal Nerve

The trigeminal nerve is the largest of the cranial nerves, with a diameter of approximately 2.5 mm when measured a few millimeters from the entry point into the pons.[22] The nerve exits the ventral surface of the pons and traverses the prepontine cistern. Once it reaches the petrous apex, the nerve runs through a defect of the dura and enters Meckel's cave, which is located lateral to the cavernous sinus. Meckel's cave is a trigeminal cistern filled with cerebrospinal fluid (CSF) and enclosed by two dural layers: the external layer, derived from the internal layer of cranial periosteum, and the internal layer, the true meningeal dura mater.

The sensory rootlets of the trigeminal nerve reach the concave gasserian ganglion, placed on the floor of Meckel's cave. The ganglion has a semilunar shape. The concave surface (posteromedial) is outlined by the CSF. From the (opposite) convex surface, which blends with the dura of the floor of Meckel's cave, originate the three branches of the trigeminal nerve. The ophthalmic nerve (V1) and the maxillary nerve (V2) are purely sensory, whereas the mandibular nerve (V3) has both sensory and motor functions.

The ophthalmic nerve divides into three branches (lacrimal, frontal, and nasociliary nerves) immediately before entering the superior orbital fissure. These nerves supply branches to the lacrimal gland and conjunctiva; to the skin of the eyelids, eyebrow, forehead, and nose; to the cornea, ciliary body, and iris; and to the mucosa of the nasal cavity.

Although PNS along V1 can occur with malignancies arising from the mucosa investing the nasoethmoid complex or from intraorbital neoplasms, it is generally caused by cutaneous malignant neoplasms (SCC or BCC, melanoma). In this setting, the two terminal branches of the frontal nerve are the most likely to be invaded: the supraorbital nerve (largest branch, runs between the orbital vault and the levator palpebrae superioris, leaves the orbit through the supraorbital foramen) and the supratrochlear nerve (runs medially to the pulley for the superior oblique muscle).[23]

Numbness or pain in the forehead or upper eyelid skin and conjunctiva are associated with involvement of the two terminal branches of the frontal nerve.[24,25]

The maxillary nerve shows a particular bayonet course (**Fig. 1**). The nerve runs straightly along the foramen rotundum, and then turns laterally into the upper pterygopalatine fossa (PPF) and inferior orbital fissure before bending anteriorly into the orbit, through the infraorbital groove, where it gives rise to the zygomatic and the infraorbital nerves. The zygomatic nerve passes along the lateral orbital wall, exits the orbit laterally, and pierces the temporal fascia to supply the skin over the lateral/upper cheek and the temple.

The infraorbital nerve can be regarded as the terminal branch of V2. It reaches the infraorbital canal and leaves the orbit through the infraorbital foramen, giving off three terminal branches: the palpebral, labial, and nasal nerves. These nerves innervate the skin of the lower eyelid, lower cheek, upper lip and gingiva, and skin of the lateral side of the external nose.

The infraorbital nerve also provides the middle and anterosuperior alveolar nerves. The posterosuperior alveolar nerve branches separately from the main trunk of V2 at the PPF.

Within the PPF, two ganglionic branches spring from the maxillary nerve and connect V2 with the pterygopalatine ganglion. Parasympathetic, sympathetic, and sensory fibers enter the ganglion, although only the parasympathetic fibers synapse in the ganglion.

These preganglionic parasympathetic fibers originate from the brainstem (superior salivary nucleus), pass with the nervus intermedius of the

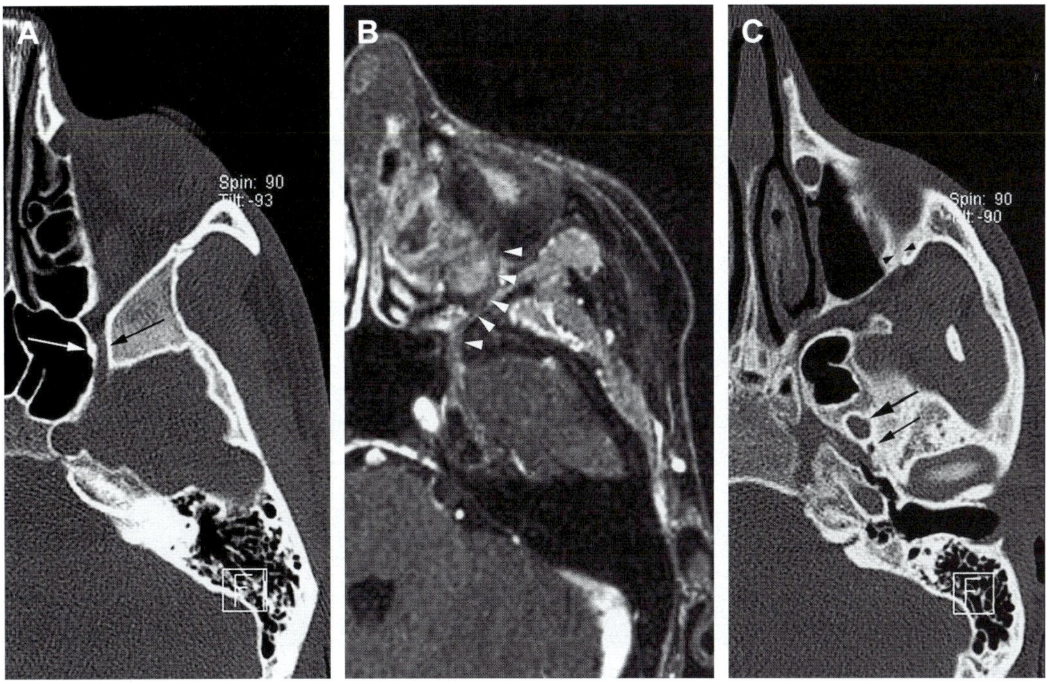

Fig. 1. Axial CT image with bone window setting at the level of the round (*A*) and oval (*C*) foramen and 1-mm thick axial contrast-enhanced three-dimensional gradient-echo T1 volumetric interpolated brain examination image (*B*). The maxillary nerve runs straight through the foramen rotundum (*arrows in A*) to reach the upper portion of the pterygopalatine fossa and inferior orbital fissure. The nerve describes a bayonet-like path (*white arrowheads*) that bends anteriorly to reach the infraorbital canal (*black arrowheads*) in which the infraorbital nerve, its terminal branch, is located. Foramen ovale (*large arrow in C*) and foramen spinosum (*small arrow in C*).

facial nerve, and leave the facial canal of the temporal bone as the GSPN. The nerve runs on the anterior surface of the petrous apex. At the foramen lacerum the GSPN is joined by the deep petrosal nerve, carrying postganglionic sympathetic fibers from the sympathetic plexus on the internal carotid artery. They form the pterygoid (vidian) nerve, which passes through the pterygoid canal and ends in the pterygopalatine ganglion.

Because of this connection with the ganglion, the branches of the maxillary nerve arising from the pterygopalatine ganglion contain not only sensory fibers but also autonomic fibers, which are distributed to glands and blood vessels. Among these branches are the superior nasal and nasopalatine nerves, pharyngeal nerve, and greater and lesser palatine nerves.

The superior nasal and nasopalatine nerves leave the pterygopalatine fossa through the sphenopalatine foramen. They supply the mucosa of the lateral nasal fossa, the nasal septum, and the oral mucosa around the incisive canal of the hard palate. The pharyngeal (pterygopalatine) nerve passes through the pterygovaginal canal to supply the nasopharyngeal mucosa.

The greater and lesser palatine nerves run downward from the ganglion, through the greater palatine canal, and on the palate diverge, exiting at the greater and lesser palatine foramen, respectively (**Fig. 2**). The greater palatine nerve innervates the posteroinferior lateral nasal wall mucosa and the hard palate mucosa (except around the incisive papilla). The lesser palatine nerve supplies the soft palate mucosa.

PNS along the peripheral branches of V2 is most frequently associated with neoplasms arising from the mucosa investing the oral cavity or oropharynx, particularly the hard and soft palate, and sinonasal tract. It can be observed in cutaneous malignancies arising from the facial skin innervated by V2 branches.

In several patients, PNS along V2 may be asymptomatic. Symptoms suggesting the involvement of peripheral branches of V2 or a more central extent include facial paresthesia or anesthesia in the V2 territory, atypical trigeminal neuropathy with facial pain, or concurrent impairment of other cranial nerves.[26–29]

The mandibular nerve is the largest division of the trigeminal nerve. It leaves the skull base

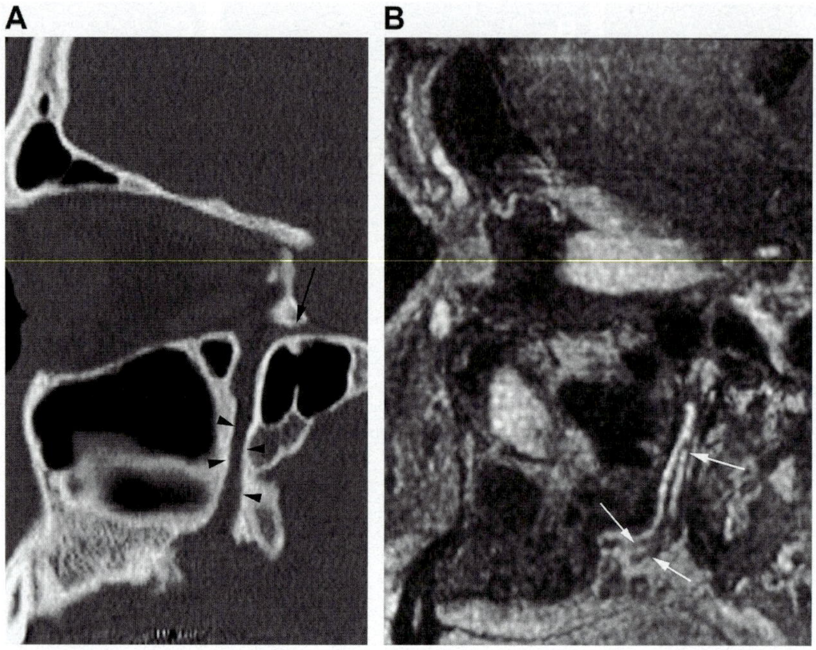

Fig. 2. CT image reconstructed in the sagittal plane with bone window setting (*A*) and 0.5-mm–thick contrast-enhanced three-dimensional gradient-echo T1 volumetric interpolated brain examination images reconstructed in the sagittal plane (*B*). The pterygopalatine fossa acts as a crossroad for the maxillary nerve, through the round foramen (*black arrow*), and for the palatine nerves. Although CT allows excellent delineation of the bony canal of the greater palatine nerve (*black arrowheads*), high-resolution MR imaging may directly display the nerves, surrounded by a venous plexus (*white arrows*).

through the oval foramen and courses between the medial pterygoid muscle and its fascia (medially) and the lateral pterygoid muscle (laterally). A few millimeters below the foramen ovale, V3 divides into a small anterior trunk (mainly motor) and a large posterior trunk, mainly sensory (**Fig. 3**A–C).

The anterior division distributes the masseteric nerve, deep temporal nerves, nerve to the lateral pterygoid muscle (all are motor branches), and buccinator (buccal) nerve, which supplies sensory fibers for the mucosa and skin of the cheek. PNS along these branches may cause atrophy of corresponding masticator muscles. Involvement of these branches usually occurs with neoplasms arising from the masticator space, nasopharynx, or oropharynx, or through retrograde spread along the inferior alveolar nerve.[30]

The posterior trunk of V3 divides into three nerves: the ATN, lingual nerve, and inferior alveolar nerve.

The ATN is mainly sensory but carries autonomic fibers for the parotid gland, derived from small branches connecting to the otic ganglion. The postganglionic parasympathetic fibers from the VII and IX nerves are carried to the otic ganglion by the lesser superficial petrosal nerve.[31] The ATN is the first branch of the posterior division of V3. The nerve then splits into two roots that encircle the middle meningeal artery (**Fig. 3**D–F) and then merge again to continue as a short trunk, which runs close to the medial aspect of the temporomandibular joint.[17] The ATN then pierces the parotid fascia and enters the retromandibular parotid gland, where it lies immediately above the bifurcation of the external carotid artery into the superficial temporal and internal maxillary arteries. Just posterior to the masseter muscle, two rami connect the ATN to the facial nerve. These connections provide sensory fibers for the zygomatic, buccal, and mandibular divisions of the facial nerve to the skin. Other branches of the ATN supply the temporomandibular joint and the skin of the anterosuperior portion of the auricle, the external acoustic meatus, and the temporal region.

Symptoms related to PNS along the ATN include periauricular pain and otalgia. The occurrence of facial weakness (suggesting VII nerve palsy), temporomandibular joint dysfunction, or pain, and V3 palsy indicate extensive tumor spread. Neoplasms arising from skin or parotid gland may follow the ATN neural pathway, sometimes with simultaneous spread along the facial nerve.[17]

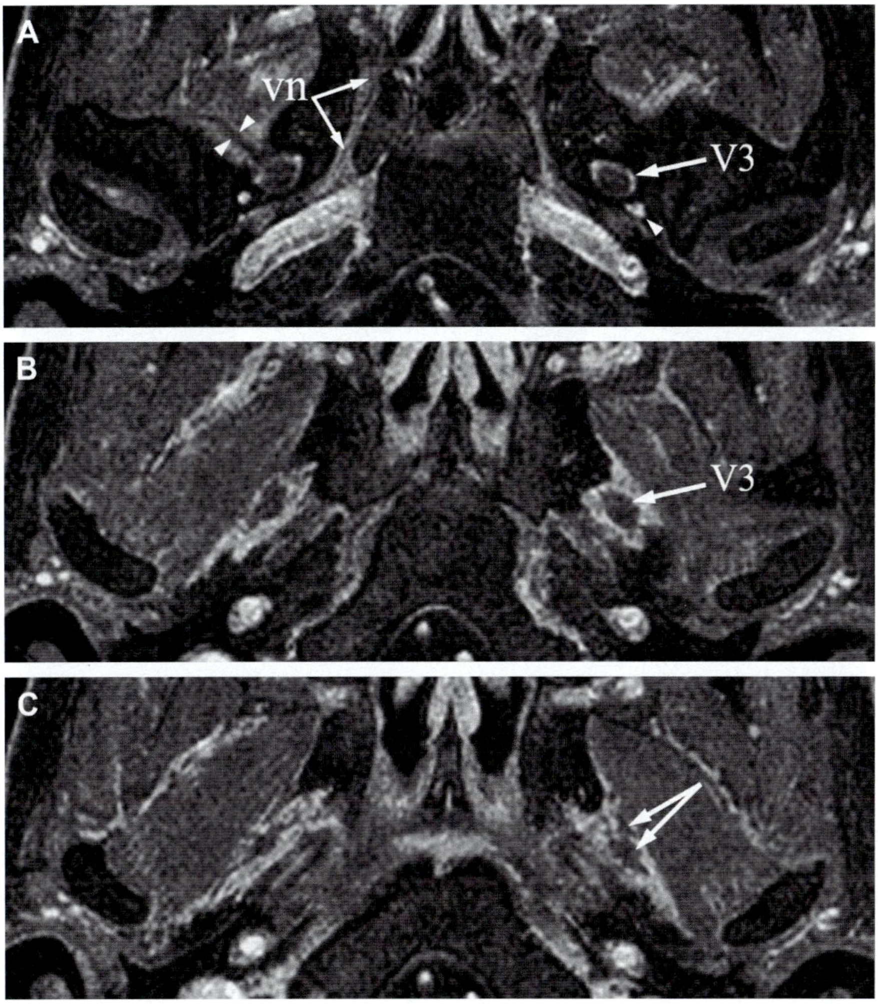

Fig. 3. Axial (*A–C, E–F*) and parasagittal (*D*) reconstructed 0.5-mm–thick contrast-enhanced three-dimensional GE T1 VIBE images. The mandibular nerves (V3) are imaged at the oval foramen (*A*). At the lower aspect of the foramen, the middle deep temporal branch leaves the right V3 (*facing arrowheads*). The vidian nerve (vn) runs along the pterygoid canal, surrounded by venous structures. The middle meningeal artery is seen posterior and lateral to the foramen ovale (*single arrowhead*). Both at the oval foramen and immediately below, V3 appears as a hypointense oval structure completely surrounded by venous signal (*B*). Few millimeters below, the nerve divides into the anterior and posterior trunks (*white arrows in C*). The parasagittal multiplanar reconstruction (*D*) shows the anterior (*white arrowhead*) and posterior (*black arrowhead*) trunks of V3. Part of the auriculotemporal nerve is seen (*black arrows*). On the axial images (*E, F*), the auriculotemporal nerve (*black arrowheads*) surrounds the middle meningeal artery (*straight black arrows*) and then bends laterally to run in the retromandibular parotid gland (*white arrows*). IAN, inferior alveolar nerve; XII, hypoglossal nerve.

Although the lingual nerve is a sensory nerve, it also contains parasympathetic fibers because of its fusion with the chorda tympani branch of the facial nerve. The nerve runs beneath the lateral pterygoid muscle and then bends forward and downward in the space between the medial pterygoid muscle and the ramus of the mandible to reach the lingual alveolar ridge of the mandible. The nerve then courses along the floor of the mouth lateral to the hyoglossus muscle, twists twice around the submandibular gland duct, and enters the tongue behind the sublingual gland. The lingual nerve supplies the mucosa of the anterior two thirds of the tongue, the floor of the mouth, the lingual gingiva of the mandibular teeth, and the buccal mucosa. The chorda tympani provides parasympathetic fibers for the submandibular ganglion (which distributes postganglionic fibers to the sublingual and submandibular glands) and sensory fibers associated with taste for the

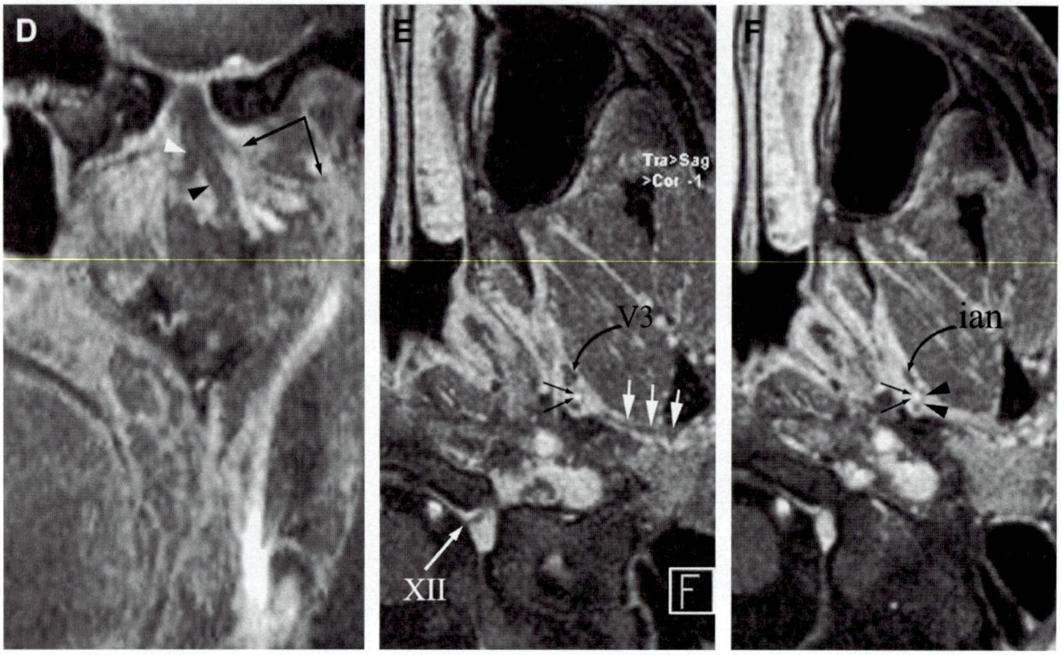

Fig. 3. (*continued*)

anterior two thirds of the tongue. Dysgeusia, sensory impairment, and pain may be associated with lingual nerve invasion.

The inferior alveolar nerve is the third branch of the posterior trunk of V3. In addition to sensory fibers, it carries motor fibers for the mylohyoid muscle and the anterior belly of the digastric muscle (the mylohyoid nerve). The inferior alveolar nerve descends along the medial surface and inferior border of the lateral pterygoid muscle and then enters the mandibular foramen together with the inferior alveolar artery. The main distribution of the nerve is to the mandibular teeth. A cutaneous branch supplying the skin of the chin and inferior lip is the mental nerve. It exits the mandible through the mental foramen.

Involvement of the mental nerve can cause dysesthesia or numbness from the chin to the lower lip extending to the midline, often associated with anesthesia of the mucosal surface of the cheek, anterior gums, or lips. However, with alveolar nerve invasion up to the mandibular foramen, symptoms also are noted in the teeth and gums of the posterior ipsilateral mandible.[32] Masticator space extent may cause denervation of the mylohyoid muscle and anterior belly of the digastric muscle.

The otic ganglion lies immediately below the foramen ovale on the medial surface of V3. It primarily supplies the parotid gland. Parasympathetic fibers (from the inferior salivary nucleus) reach the ganglion through the glossopharyngeal nerve, tympanic plexus in the middle ear, and lesser superficial petrosal nerve, which passes through the foramen ovale. Its sympathetic root consists of a filament from the plexus surrounding the middle meningeal artery. The sensory root is the ATN.

Facial Nerve

The facial nerve emerges from the groove between the medulla and pons. It has a large motor root and a smaller sensory root (nervus intermedius). The nerve crosses the cerebellopontine angle cistern with the vestibulocochlear nerve and runs through the internal auditory canal to reach the fundus. It then enters the facial canal, which it follows to the end at the stylomastoid foramen. On emerging from the stylomastoid foramen, the facial nerve courses downward, lateral to the styloid process and medial to the digastric muscle, to enter the parotid gland. At this level, the nerve divides into the temporofacial and cervicofacial branches, which show a variable intraglandular pattern of branching. From this parotid plexus usually emerge five branches for facial and cranial muscles (buccinator, orbicularis oculi, muscles of the upper and lower lips). The two segments of the facial nerve that are most likely to be involved in PNS are the descending portion of the intratemporal course of the nerve (the mastoid part) and the GSPN.

Neoplasms arising from or invading the parotid gland account for most PNS along the mastoid segment of the facial nerve.[33] Primary tumors include adenoid cystic carcinoma, adenocarcinoma, mucoepidermoid carcinoma, and SCC. Among neoplasms secondarily invading the gland are cutaneous carcinoma and melanoma.

Further retrograde spread up to the geniculate ganglion and, less frequently, through the labyrinthine or intracanalicular segments is possible. Different degrees of facial palsy may accompany PNS.

The GSPN was described in the section discussing trigeminal nerve anatomy as a neural connection between the facial nerve and V2. Parasympathetic fibers travel by way of the GSPN and then the vidian nerve to reach the pterygopalatine ganglion and distribute to the mucosa through V2 peripheral branches. This path serves as a duplicate conduit for retrograde PNS by tumors that reach the pterygopalatine ganglion, the usual pathway being the maxillary nerve and Meckel's cave. As a result, a hard palate adenoid cystic carcinoma spreading through the greater palatine nerve and reaching the pterygopalatine ganglion may subsequently follow either the V2 or the parasympathetic path (or both), ultimately extending into the temporal bone.[16]

Hypoglossal Nerve

The hypoglossal nerve is a motor nerve supplying the musculature of the tongue. It originates from the medulla oblongata as 10 to 12 nerve roots that are fusing into 1 or 2 trunks piercing the dura mater and entering the hypoglossal canal of the occipital bone. The nerve emerges deep to the carotid sheath and runs downward close to the vagus nerve between the internal jugular vein and the internal carotid artery. It loops around the occipital artery, continues forward passing below the submandibular gland, lateral to the hyoglossus muscle, to be distributed to the muscles of the tongue.

Although PNS from tongue neoplasms has been described,[34] the nerve is more frequently involved by nasopharyngeal carcinoma accessing the retrostyloid compartment of the parapharyngeal space.[19]

NORMAL ASPECT OF CRANIAL NERVES THROUGH CISTERNS, FORAMINA, AND FISSURES, AND OUTSIDE THE SKULL BASE

On cross-sectional imaging, the detectability of normal cranial nerves and their major branches depends on their size and the difference in signal intensity between nerve and surrounding structures. Generally, nerve segments traveling through cisterns are more easily shown by T2-weighted MR sequences, which enhance the difference in signal intensity between CSF and nerves. High-resolution three-dimensional T2-weighted fast

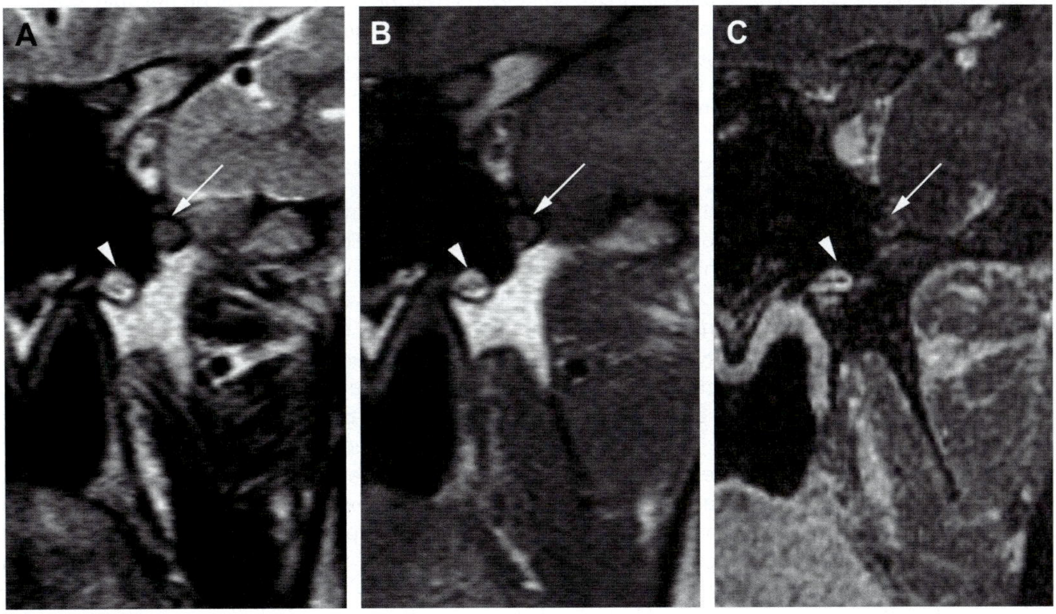

Fig. 4. Coronal spin-echo (SE) T2 (*A*), SE T1 (*B*), and contrast-enhanced three-dimensional gradient-echo T1 VIBE (*C*) images. The maxillar nerve (*arrows*) appears as a dot like structure which is surrounded, on the VIBE image by a thin incomplete venous ring. Hyperintensity is seen around the vidian nerve (*arrowheads*) on both unenhanced and contrast-enhanced images, caused by the presence of both fat tissue and a venous plexus.

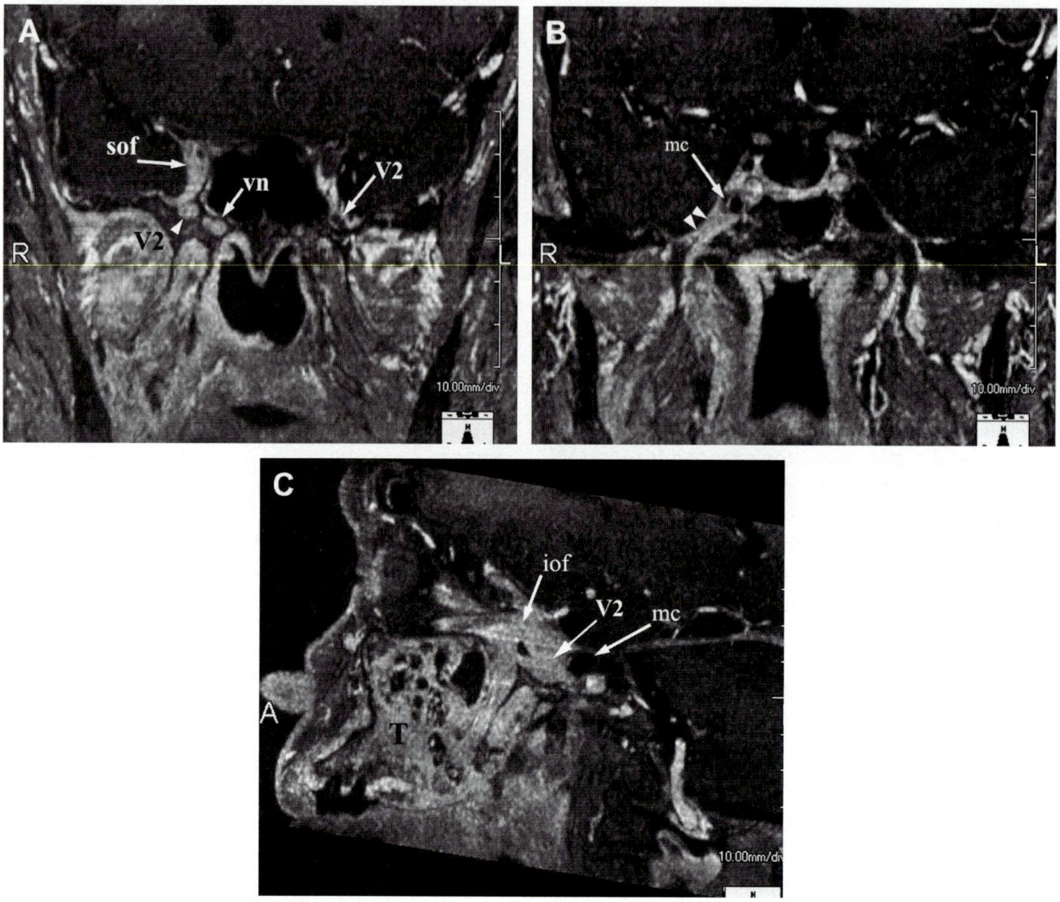

Fig. 5. Coronal (*A, B*) and sagittal (*C*) reconstructed 1-mm–thick contrast-enhanced three-dimensional GE T1 VIBE images. Adenoid cystic carcinoma of the right maxillary sinus (T). The tumor spreads through the pterygopalatine fossa and extends into the vidian canal (vn) and round foramen (*V2 + white arrowhead*) reaching Meckel's cave (mc) posteriorly. Note the normal appearance of the contralateral maxillary nerve as it runs through the round foramen (V2) surrounded by a venous plexus. Although the tumor is close to the oval foramen (*white arrowheads in B*), no signs of PNS along the mandibular nerve are seen. Both the superior (sof) and inferior (iof) orbital fissures are invaded by the neoplasm.

spin-echo (SE) sequences (FSE or FASE) or the three-dimensional gradient-echo (GE) T2-weighted Fourier transformation constructive interference in steady state (3DFT-CISS) sequence provide high-contrast resolution and submillimetric spatial detail. Therefore, these techniques allow one to image the dense rootlet network of the trigeminal nerve within Meckel's cave before it enters the gasserian ganglion[35] or to clearly separate the facial nerve from the acoustic and vestibular nerves in the internal acoustic canal. Contrast-enhanced 3DFT-CISS has also been suggested for a detailed depiction of the gasserian ganglion and Meckel's cave.

Instead of CSF, some venous plexuses and veins surrounding the nerves allow some nerve segments crossing the skull-base foramina and canals to be seen on MR imaging. Examples include the maxillary (**Fig. 4**) and mandibular nerves (see **Fig. 3**A–C), which are surrounded by perineural venous plexuses[36,37] and the hypoglossal nerve, which courses through its canal accompanied by the anterior condylar vein.[38,39] On contrast-enhanced SE or GE T1-weighted images, these nerves appear as hypointense round or linear sharp structures surrounded by enhancing veins. Using submillimetric postcontrast sequences, such as the volumetric interpolated brain examination (VIBE) sequence, can depict that the hypointense signal of the maxillary nerve fills 50% of the diameter of the round foramen while the mandibular nerve fills 75% of the diameter of the oval foramen. The hypoglossal nerve, which is three to five times smaller, occupies only 20% of the hypoglossal canal diameter.

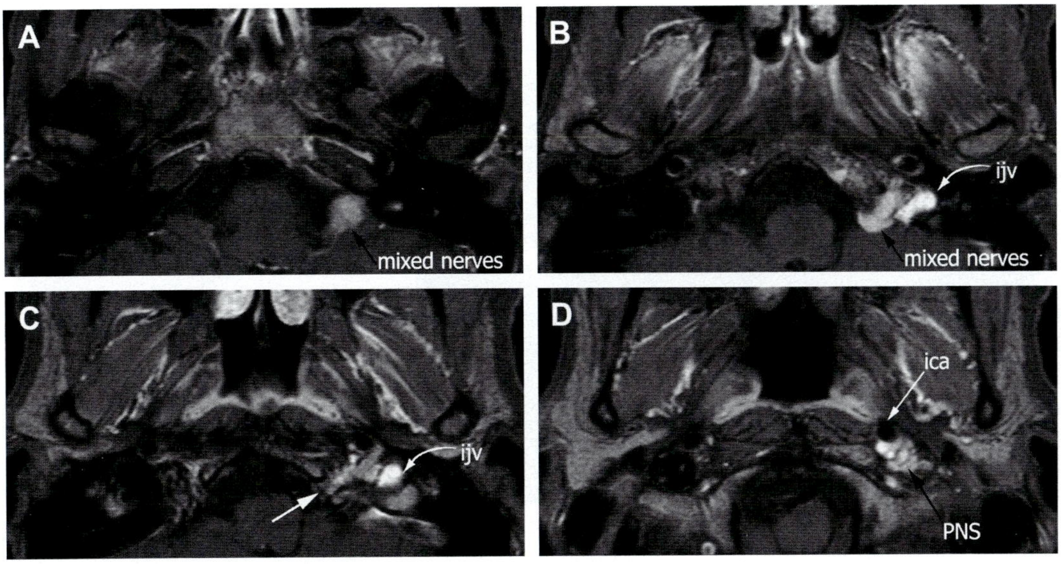

Fig. 6. Axial contrast-enhanced fat-suppressed T1-weighted SE images. Adenoid cystic carcinoma of the base of the tongue. Tumor tissue is seen in the lateral part of the prepontine cistern following the cisternal segments of the mixed nerves (*black arrow in A and B*) and into the hypoglossal canal (*white arrow in C*). PNS in the carotid space, posterior to the partially compressed internal jugular vein (ijv), leads the tumor toward these lower cranial nerves (*D*). ICA, internal carotid artery.

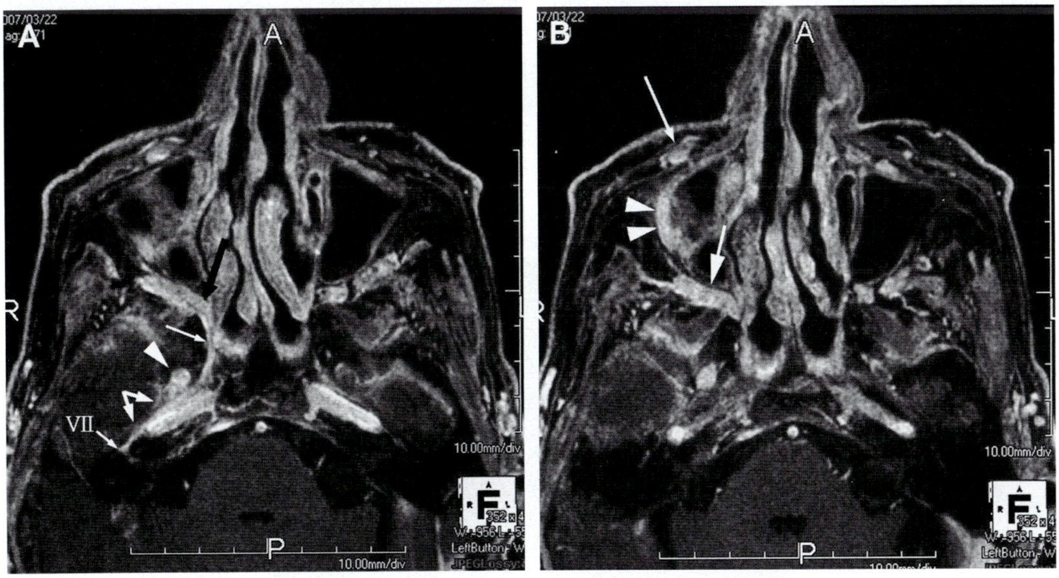

Fig. 7. Axial reconstructed 1-mm–thick contrast-enhanced three-dimensional GE T1 VIBE images. Adenoid cystic carcinoma of the hard palate. The tumor reaches the pterygopalatine fossa (*black arrow in A*) and continues along the infraorbital nerve (*arrowheads in B*), the maxillary nerve within the pterygopalatine fossa (*large arrow in B*), and the vidian nerve (*small arrow in A*). Linear enhancement along the anterior surface of the petrous bone (*double arrow*) and at the level of the geniculate ganglion (*VII + arrow*) indicates perineural spread along the greater superficial petrosal nerve. Thickening and enhancement of the mandibular nerve in the oval foramen (*arrowhead in A*). Tumor tissue is also seen in the subcutaneous fat tissue, anterior to the right maxillary sinus (*long arrow in B*), at the peripheral end of the infraorbital nerve.

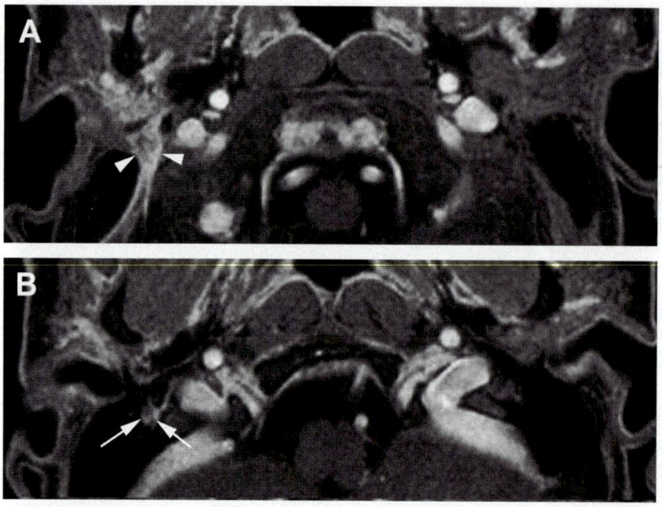

Fig. 8. Axial reconstructed 1-mm–thick contrast-enhanced three-dimensional GE T1 VIBE images. Adenoid cystic carcinoma of the right parotid gland. (*A*) Tumor tissue reaches the stylomastoid foramen (*arrowheads*). (*B*) Enhancement is seen along the mastoid tract of facial nerve indicating PNS (*arrows*).

On high-resolution fat-saturation VIBE, the two trigeminal branches are normally surrounded by a 1-mm thick enhanced layer of perineural venous coating (see **Fig. 3**D–F), which separates the nerve from the inner bony surface of the foramina. Therefore, when sectioned perpendicular to their main course, the intraforaminal segments of V2 and V3 show a "target" appearance. The inner

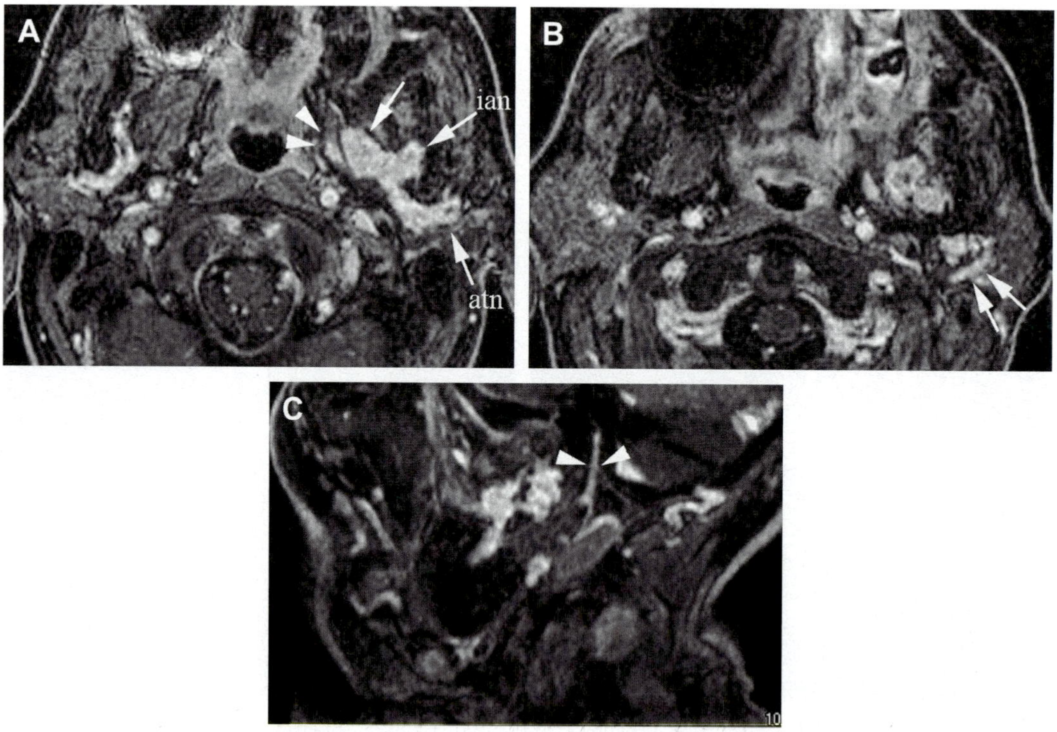

Fig. 9. Axial (*A, B*) and sagittal oblique (*C*) reconstructed 0.5-mm–thick contrast-enhanced three-dimensional GE T1 VIBE images. Adenoid cystic carcinoma of the floor of the mouth. Neoplastic tissue is seen in the masticator space (*white arrow*), deep to the medially displaced medial pterygoid muscle (*white arrowhead in A*), and is probably caused by PNS along the lingual nerve. Two additional paths of tumor spread can be observed: anterolateral, probably following the inferior alveolar nerve (ian), and posterolateral, along the auricolotemporal nerve (atn). PNS is also detected along the intraparotid (*white arrows in B*) and mastoid segment (*white arrowheads in C*) of the facial nerve, probably following the anatomic connections between the facial and mandibular nerves.

hypointense dot (corresponding to the nerve) is usually larger than the perineural vascular plexus coating. The opposite is observed for the XIIth nerve in the hypoglossal canal where the venous layer appears larger (2–3 mm) than the central hypointense nerve.

When imaged along their main axis, the transverse plane for the XIIth nerve, the nerves show a sort of "tram-track-like" pattern, where the sharp hypointense nerve and enhancing venous plexus run parallel.

Enhancement along the facial canal can also be seen in normal nerves, mostly at the geniculate ganglion level. It probably corresponds to the circumneural facial arteriovenous plexus. In contrast to the maxillary, mandibular, and hypoglossal nerves, the thin facial nerve cannot be discriminated from the venous plexus within its narrow canal.[40]

Immediately outside the skull base foramina, the high signal of fat tissue on T1-weighted sequences helps identify the cranial nerve branches, such as the mandibular nerve below the oval foramen,

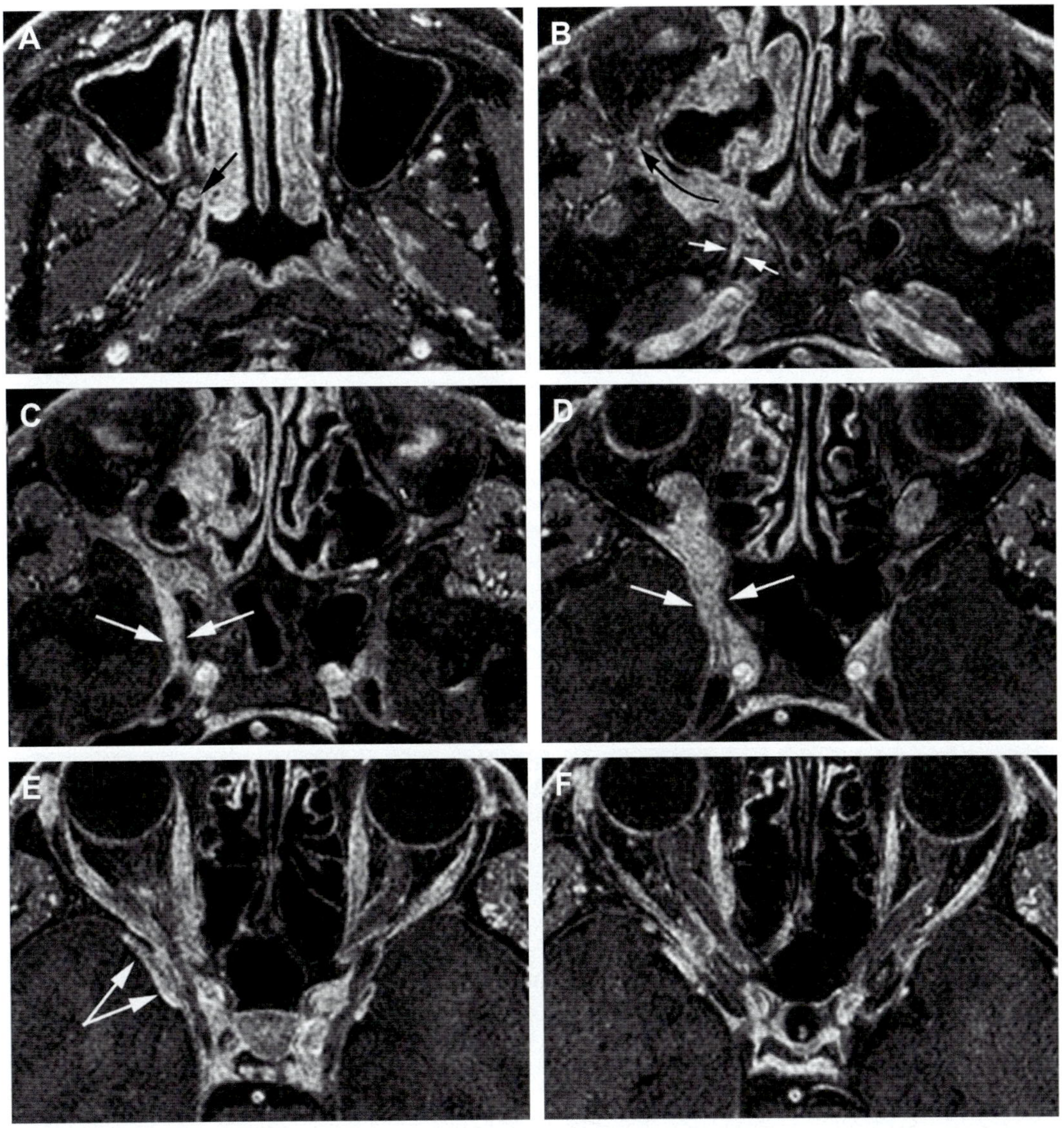

Fig. 10. Axial reconstructed 1-mm–thick contrast-enhanced three-dimensional GE T1 VIBE images. Adenoid cystic carcinoma of the hard palate. Perineural tumor spread along the greater palatine nerve (*black arrow in A*) is reaching the pterygopalatine fossa. The neoplasm then continues both antegradely along the infraorbital nerve (*curved arrow in B*) and retrogradely along the vidian (*white arrows in B*) and maxillary nerve (*white arrows in C*). In addition, antegrade tumor spread is seen at the level of the superior orbital fissure, possibly following the course of the ophthalmic nerve (*white arrows in D*). Thickening and enhancement of the dura close to the lateral orbital wall is detected (*white arrows in E*).

the maxillar nerve coursing through the fat-filled PPF, or the vidian nerve within the pterygoid canal.

Fat also allows detection of the inferior alveolar nerve entering the mandibular foramen, whereas the remaining course of the nerve through the whole canal can be imaged only on postcontrast sequences, where it appears surrounded by vascular structures.

Outside and immediately below the skull base, the enhancing (and large) pterygoid venous plexus provides sufficient contrast resolution to show, through high-resolution VIBE images, the anterior and posterior trunks of the mandibular and, in some patients, most of the ATN and inferior alveolar nerve course.[41]

IMAGING FINDINGS OF PERINEURAL SPREAD

The single nerve fibers, axons and their covering derived from Schwann cells, are separated by loose vascular connective tissue and extracellular fluid (endoneurium). Several nerve fibers and endoneurium are bundled into fascicles, each one surrounded by a dense connective sheath (perineurium). The perineurium and the tight junctions between the endothelial cells of the endoneurial capillaries isolate the extracellular endoneurial fluid from the general extracellular space.[42] Large nerves contain several bundles of fascicles, the trigeminal nerve being composed of 45 to 55 bundles.[35] These bundles are enveloped by a dense connective layer (epineurium), which is the outermost sheath of the nerve.

At the skull base, the epineurium is continuous with the dura mater. At the peripheral end of the nerve branches, the thickness of the epineurium progressively decreases, ultimately blending into the perineurium.

Perineural invasion is the term used to indicate infiltration of nerve compartments or nerve sheaths at the primary tumor site, which is undetectable with imaging techniques.

Further extent of tumor cells along the nerve, to reach distant locations, is a form of direct neoplastic spread defined as *perineural spread*. The areas of nerve invasion can be microscopically continuous with the main tumor mass; however, the invasion may also appear macroscopically discontinuous (skip lesions).[43]

Although the term *perineural spread* should be limited to tumor spreading along the perineurium that envelopes the nerve bundles, the term actually encompasses neoplasms invading all compartments and their neural sheaths or neoplasms involving single compartments, such as the space between the epineurium and the nerve bundles, or single sheaths, mainly the perineurium.[5]

As the tumor grows, segmental nerve damage usually occurs, inducing increased permeability of the endoneurial capillaries and eventually causing destruction of the perineurium.[44–46] The rupture of the blood–nerve barrier allows leakage and accumulation of iodinated or paramagnetic contrast agents, accounting for segmental nerve enhancement on MR imaging (**Fig. 5**).

MR imaging has been shown to be more sensitive than CT for detecting segmental nerve enhancement.[13,47,48]

Several MR imaging techniques have been proposed, most based on fat-suppression imaging (**Fig. 6**).[16,47,49] Fat suppression has the advantage of increasing the conspicuity of the enhancing

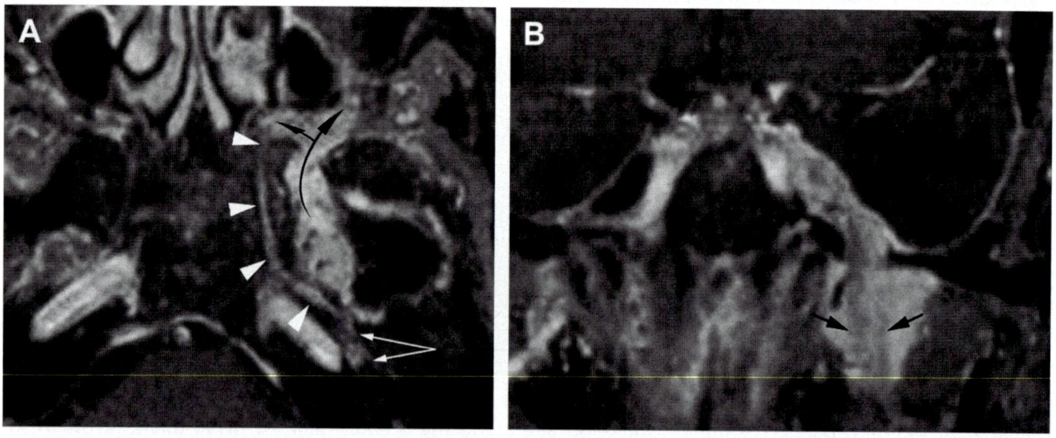

Fig. 11. Axial (*A*) and coronal (*B*) reconstructed 1-mm–thick contrast-enhanced three-dimensional GE T1 VIBE images. Dumbbell-shaped middle cranial fossa meningioma with extracranial extension along the maxillary nerve reaching the pterygopalatine fossa (*curved arrows*), and along the mandibular nerve into the masticator space (*black arrows*). The enhancing vidian nerve (*arrowheads*) is seen bending posterolateral towards the anterolateral surface of the petrous apex, along the course of the greater superficial petrosal nerve (*white arrows*).

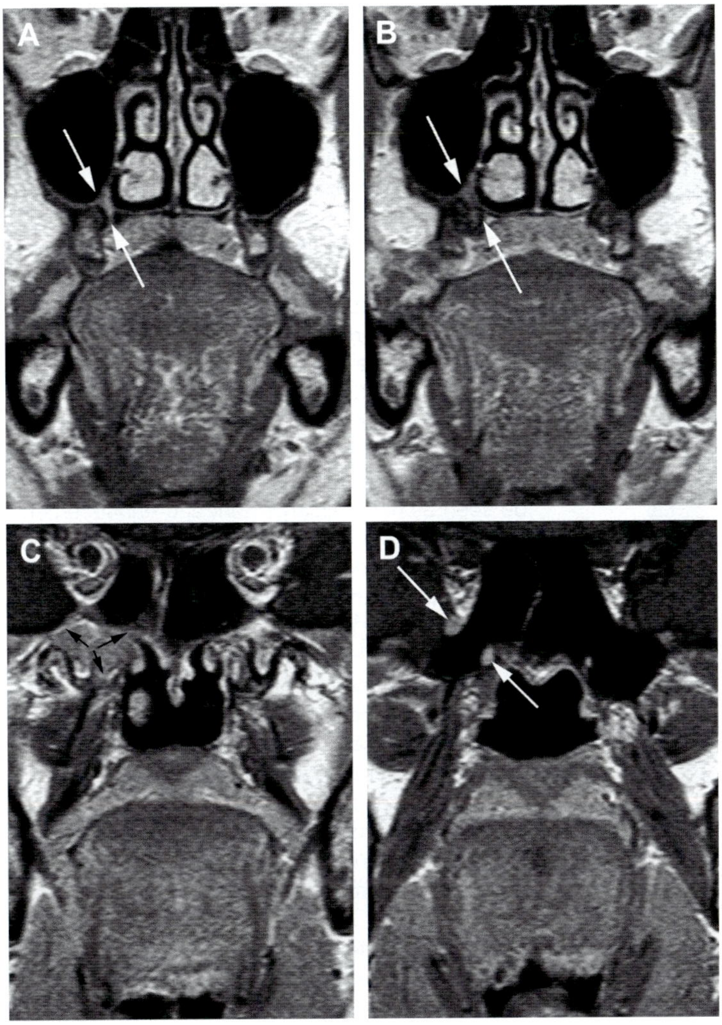

Fig. 12. Coronal contrast-enhanced SE T1 images. Adenoid cystic carcinoma of the hard palate. The tumor invades the greater palatine foramen (*arrows in A and B*) and resurfaces in the pterygopalatine fossa (*arrows in C*), replacing the fat adjacent to the sphenopalatine artery. Retrograde spread along both the vidian and maxillary nerve are also seen (*arrows in D*).

abnormal nerve through diminishing or nulling the signal of fat, which surrounds the extraforaminal nerve course and the foramina. Nevertheless, if a frequency-selective fat-suppression technique is used, susceptibility artifacts may obscure the skull-base foramina, particularly in the area of the sphenoid sinus.[5]

The use of high-spatial resolution SE T1, pre- and postcontrast administration, has been reported to overcome this limitation. Appropriate windowing should allow detection of abnormal nerve enhancement, without artifacts related to susceptibility.[5]

We prefer to use isotropic high-spatial resolution postcontrast fat-saturation VIBE with a voxel size ranging from 0.5 to 0.7 mm. These images allow a detailed evaluation of the skull-base foramina without artifacts (**Fig. 7**). The spatial resolution of the images allow the normal nerve and surrounding vascular plexus to be clearly imaged.[41,50]

Segmental nerve enhancement, however, is not unique to PNS. It can be present in several non-neoplastic lesions that cause blood–nerve barrier disruption, such as inflammation, ischemia, infarct, trauma, demyelination, and axonal degeneration.[43] These conditions may account for false-positive MR imaging findings.

Moreover, for nerves such as the V2, V3, XII, and inferior alveolar nerves, which cross foramina and canals, the "target" or "tram-track-like" enhancement patterns are normally present and should not be interpreted as an abnormal finding.[36] Conversely, if these enhancement patterns are shown in the labyrinthine or mastoid segments of the facial nerve (**Fig. 8**), rupture of the blood–nerve barrier should be suspected.[40]

Abnormal enhancement of the central nerve on the "target" or "tram-track-like" image without nerve enlargement correlates with PNS.[3,51] Further growth of tumor cells along the nerve causes

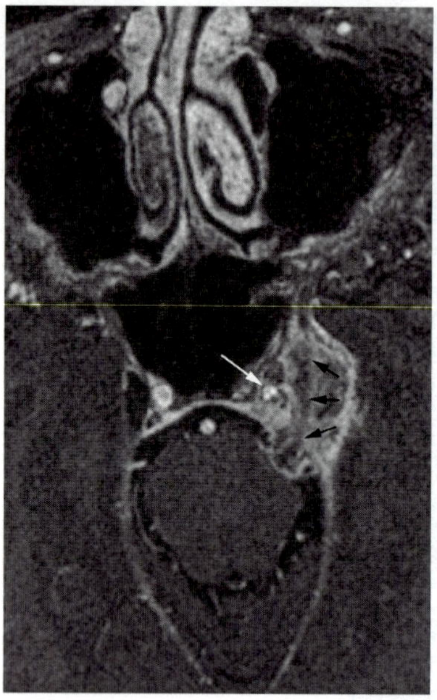

Fig. 13. Axial reconstructed 1-mm–thick contrast-enhanced three-dimensional GE T1 VIBE image. Squamous cell carcinoma of the oropharynx invading both the parapharyngeal and masticator space. Meckel's cave is completed occupied by tumoral tissue growing along the maxillary nerve (*black arrows*) and retrogradely spreading along the cisternal segment of the trigeminal nerve. Note the encasement of the internal carotid artery (*white arrow*).

increased nerve diameter with or without abnormal nerve enhancement on MR imaging (**Figs. 9 and 10**).

Detection of an enlarged nerve before the occurrence of remodeling or erosion of the foramina is possible on CT, if the nerve is mainly surrounded by fat. The infraorbital nerve is an example of a nerve segment that is completely surrounded by fat tissue, and whose abnormal enlargement can therefore be detected on axial or coronal CT.[52,53]

As nerve segments enlarge, remodeling, widening, and eventually erosion of fissures, foramina, and canals occurs, causing them to be more easily detected on CT (**Fig. 11**).[53–56]

However, the enlarged nerve may recover its normal diameter when it passes through a bony canal instead of remodeling or eroding it, causing skip areas on the tract (**Fig. 12**). Once it exits the foramen or canal, PNS regains a macroscopic size. This resurfacing phenomenon is a mechanism of perineural extension that deserves particular attention on CT and MR imaging. It can be observed with hard or soft palate tumors that resurface into the PPF. On CT, obliteration of the fat tissue within the PPF is a key sign.[53] Coronal or sagittal high-spatial resolution MR imaging not only shows the abnormal mass within the PPF but also can directly track the abnormal nerve enhancement in the greater or lesser palatine foramina and canals. When this mechanism of PNS involves the maxillar nerve at the round foramen, the tumor resurfaces in the gasserian ganglion or Meckel's cave.

Retrograde (central) spread along the peripheral branches of the trigeminal nerve eventually leads the tumor to Meckel's cave, the gasserian ganglion, and less frequently to the cisternal segment of the fifth nerve (**Fig. 13**).

On CT or MR imaging, replacement of the fluid signal in Meckel's cave by a solid and enhancing lesion indicates invasion of the trigeminal cistern. Further spread along the cisternal segment can be seen as nerve enlargement and enhancement. On CT and MR imaging, cavernous sinus invasion can be seen as an enlargement of the cavernous sinus with lateral bulging and increased convexity.[18,47,54,55,57] However, on CT, the enhancing tumor tissue tends to be hardly separable from the venous-filled cavernous sinus.

When high-resolution postcontrast GE sequences are used, distinguishing the signal from tumor and venous structures becomes easier, not only because of the smaller voxels but also because of improvement in contrast resolution.[50] The 0.5-mm isotropic VIBE sequence is started approximately 2 minutes after intravenous contrast administration. At that moment, the maximal contrast resolution acquired during the central k-space will correspond with the wash-out phase in most epithelial tumors. This strategy increases the chance that the tumor will show a lower signal intensity than the cavernous sinus. In addition, the intracavernous wall of the carotid artery can be nicely shown because of the high signal intensity of blood bordering the internal (carotid lumen) and external surfaces of the wall (enhancing cavernous sinus), which therefore appears as a hypointense ring on the axial plane.

If PNS causes damage to a motor branch of a cranial nerve, the corresponding innervated musculature undergoes flaccid paresis, paralysis, and atrophy. The effects of denervation on muscles can be detected with CT and MR imaging. CT can detect only late changes related to the reduced volume (atrophy, fatty replacement) of the affected musculature, occurring at least 12 to 20 months after nerve damage (**Fig. 14**).

MR imaging is more sensitive than CT. In case of mandibular nerve damage, increased hyperintensity on T2 and abnormal muscle enhancement are common findings in the acute (within 1 month) and subacute phases (up to 12–20 months). In the

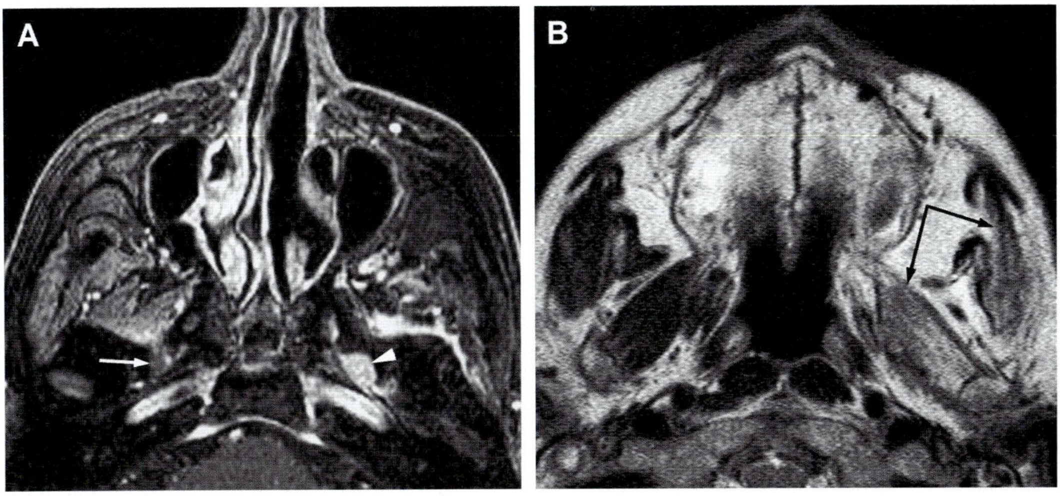

Fig. 14. Axial reconstructed 1-mm–thick contrast-enhanced three-dimensional GE T1 VIBE image (*A*) and axial SE T2 image (*B*). Adenoid cystic carcinoma of the floor of the mouth. Perineural tumor spread along the mandibular nerve through the left oval foramen (*arrowhead*) is indicated by thickening and asymmetric enhancement of the nerve. Compare with the normal contralateral nerve (*white arrow*). Fatty degeneration of the muscles of mastication, caused by denervation, can be seen as high signal intensity on T2-weighted images (*black arrows in B*).

acute phase, increased volume of the affected muscles is also observed. As the denervation progresses to the subacute phase, the muscle volume decreases. The muscles become more intense on T1 when fat begins to replace the muscular fibers.

The early chronic phase is characterized by further fatty changes of the affected muscles without volume loss, T2 hyperintensity, or abnormal enhancement. Volume loss with muscular atrophy and extensive fatty replacement are late changes.[58–60]

Similar findings are observed in hypoglossal denervation, although without clear distinction between the early and late chronic phases. On CT and MR imaging, late changes can be recognized as atrophy of the ipsilateral tongue, which also falls posteriorly in the supine position.[19] Motor denervation of the facial nerve causes a hyperintense signal on T2 and enhancement of the small muscles of facial expression after contrast administration.[58]

REFERENCES

1. Mendenhall WM, Amdur RJ, Williams LS, et al. Carcinoma of the skin of the head and neck with perineural invasion. Head Neck 2002;24(1):78–83.
2. Zupi A, Mangone GM, Piombino P, et al. Perineural invasion of the lower alveolar nerve by oral cancer: a follow-up study of 12 cases. J Craniomaxillofac Surg 1998;26(5):318–21.
3. Williams LS, Mancuso AA, Mendenhall WM. Perineural spread of cutaneous squamous and basal cell carcinoma: CT and MR detection and its impact on patient management and prognosis. Int J Radiat Oncol Biol Phys 2001;49(4):1061–9.
4. Galloway TJ, Morris CG, Mancuso AA, et al. Impact of radiographic findings on prognosis for skin carcinoma with clinical perineural invasion. Cancer 2005; 103(6):1254–7.
5. Curtin HD. Detection of perineural spread: fat suppression versus no fat suppression. AJNR Am J Neuroradiol 2004;25(1):1–3.
6. Fowler BZ, Crocker IR, Johnstone PA. Perineural spread of cutaneous malignancy to the brain: a review of the literature and five patients treated with stereotactic radiotherapy. Cancer 2005;103(10): 2143–53.
7. Garden AS, Weber RS, Morrison WH, et al. The influence of positive margins and nerve invasion in adenoid cystic carcinoma of the head and neck treated with surgery and radiation. Int J Radiat Oncol Biol Phys 1995;32(3):619–26.
8. Hutcheson JA, Vural E, Korourian S, et al. Neural cell adhesion molecule expression in adenoid cystic carcinoma of the head and neck. Laryngoscope 2000; 110(6):946–8.
9. Gandour-Edwards R, Kapadia SB, Barnes L, et al. Neural cell adhesion molecule in adenoid cystic carcinoma invading the skull base. Otolaryngol Head Neck Surg 1997;117(5):453–8.
10. Iwamoto S, Odland PB, Piepkorn M, et al. Evidence that the p75 neurotrophin receptor mediates

perineural spread of desmoplastic melanoma. J Am Acad Dermatol 1996;35(5 Pt 1):725–31.
11. Miknyoczki SJ, Klein-Szanto AJ, Ruggeri BA. Neurotrophin-Trk receptor interactions in neoplasia: a possible role in interstitial and perineural invasion in ductal pancreatic cancer. Crit Rev Oncog 1996; 7(1–2):89–100.
12. Kalina P, Bevilacqua P. Perineural extension of facial melanoma. Neuroradiology 2005;47(5):372–4.
13. Chang PC, Fischbein NJ, McCalmont TH, et al. Perineural spread of malignant melanoma of the head and neck: clinical and imaging features. AJNR Am J Neuroradiol 2004;25(1):5–11.
14. Lo JS, Snow SN, Reizner GT, et al. Metastatic basal cell carcinoma: report of twelve cases with a review of the literature. J Am Acad Dermatol 1991;24(5 Pt 1):715–9.
15. Blandino A, Gaeta M, Minutoli F, et al. CT and MR findings in neoplastic perineural spread along the vidian nerve. Eur Radiol 2000;10(3):521–6.
16. Ginsberg LE, De Monte F, Gillenwater AM. Greater superficial petrosal nerve: anatomy and MR findings in perineural tumor spread. AJNR Am J Neuroradiol 1996;17(2):389–93.
17. Schmalfuss IM, Tart RP, Mukherji S, et al. Perineural tumor spread along the auriculotemporal nerve. AJNR Am J Neuroradiol 2002;23(2):303–11.
18. Majoie CB, Hulsmans FJ, Verbeeten B Jr, et al. Perineural tumor extension along the trigeminal nerve: magnetic resonance imaging findings. Eur J Radiol 1997;24(3):191–205.
19. Chong VF, Fan YF. Hypoglossal nerve palsy in nasopharyngeal carcinoma. Eur Radiol 1998;8(6): 939–45.
20. Streams BN, Eaton JS, Zelac DE. Perineural spread of squamous cell carcinoma involving the spinal accessory nerve in an immunocompromised organ transplant recipient. Dermatol Surg 2005;31(5): 599–601.
21. Ginsberg LE, Eicher SA. Great auricular nerve: anatomy and imaging in a case of perineural tumor spread. AJNR Am J Neuroradiol 2000;21(3): 568–71.
22. Erbay SH, Bhadelia RA, O'Callaghan M, et al. Nerve atrophy in severe trigeminal neuralgia: noninvasive confirmation at MR imaging–initial experience. Radiology 2006;238(2):689–92.
23. Ginsberg LE. MR imaging of perineural tumor spread. Magn Reson Imaging Clin N Am 2002; 10(3):511–25.
24. Lau CH, Taylor S. The eye in malignant disease. Hosp Med 2003;64(3):177–9.
25. McNab AA, Francis IC, Benger R, et al. Perineural spread of cutaneous squamous cell carcinoma via the orbit. Clinical features and outcome in 21 cases. Ophthalmology 1997;104(9):1457–62.
26. Boerman RH, Maassen EM, Joosten J, et al. Trigeminal neuropathy secondary to perineural invasion of head and neck carcinomas. Neurology 1999;53(1): 213–6.
27. Bridgman JB, Snape L. Facial sensory loss—a need for suspicion. N Z Dent J 1998;94(416):65–8.
28. Slavin ML, Abramson AL. Squamous cell carcinoma of the pterygopalatine fossa (retroantral space). J Clin Neuroophthalmol 1986;6(4):254–7.
29. Dolan EJ, Schwartz ML, Lewis AJ, et al. Adenoid cystic carcinoma: an unusual neurosurgical entity. Can J Neurol Sci 1985;12(1):65–8.
30. Ariji Y, Fuwa N, Tachibana H, et al. Denervation atrophy of the masticatory muscles in a patient with nasopharyngeal cancer: MR examinations before and after radiotherapy. Dentomaxillofac Radiol 2002; 31(3):204–8.
31. Gray H, Williams PL, Bannister LH. Gray's anatomy: the anatomical basis of medicine and surgery. 38th edition. New York: Churchill Livingstone; 1995.
32. Harris CP, Baringer JR. The numb chin in metastatic cancer. West J Med 1991;155(5):528–31.
33. Selesnick SH, Burt BM. Regional spread of non-neurogenic tumors to the skull base via the facial nerve. Otol Neurotol 2003;24(2):326–33.
34. Silvester KC, Barnes S. Adenoid cystic carcinoma of the tongue presenting as a hypoglossal nerve palsy. Br J Oral Maxillofac Surg 1990;28(2):122–4.
35. Ziyal IM, Sekhar LN, Ozgen T, et al. The trigeminal nerve and ganglion: an anatomical, histological, and radiological study addressing the transtrigeminal approach. Surg Neurol 2004;61(6):564–73 [discussion: 73–4].
36. Williams LS, Schmalfuss IM, Sistrom CL, et al. MR imaging of the trigeminal ganglion, nerve, and the perineural vascular plexus: normal appearance and variants with correlation to cadaver specimens. AJNR Am J Neuroradiol 2003;24(7):1317–23.
37. Yousry I, Moriggl B, Schmid UD, et al. Trigeminal ganglion and its divisions: detailed anatomic MR imaging with contrast-enhanced 3D constructive interference in the steady state sequences. AJNR Am J Neuroradiol 2005;26(5):1128–35.
38. Caruso RD, Rosenbaum AE, Chang JK, et al. Craniocervical junction venous anatomy on enhanced MR images: the suboccipital cavernous sinus. AJNR Am J Neuroradiol 1999;20(6):1127–31.
39. Voyvodic F, Whyte A, Slavotinek J. The hypoglossal canal: normal MR enhancement pattern. AJNR Am J Neuroradiol 1995;16(8):1707–10.
40. Martin-Duverneuil N, Sola-Martinez MT, Miaux Y, et al. Contrast enhancement of the facial nerve on MRI: normal or pathological? Neuroradiology 1997; 39(3):207–12.
41. Maroldi R, Nicolai P. Imaging in treatment planning for sinonasal diseases. Berlin: Springer; 2005. New York.
42. Maravilla KR, Bowen BC. Imaging of the peripheral nervous system: evaluation of peripheral neuropathy

and plexopathy. AJNR Am J Neuroradiol 1998;19(6):1011–23.

43. Nemzek WR, Hecht S, Gandour-Edwards R, et al. Perineural spread of head and neck tumors: how accurate is MR imaging? AJNR Am J Neuroradiol 1998;19(4):701–6.
44. Carter RL, Foster CS, Dinsdale EA, et al. Perineural spread by squamous carcinomas of the head and neck: a morphological study using antiaxonal and antimyelin monoclonal antibodies. J Clin Pathol 1983;36(3):269–75.
45. Kobayashi S, Yoshizawa H, Hachiya Y, et al. Vasogenic edema induced by compression injury to the spinal nerve root. Distribution of intravenously injected protein tracers and gadolinium-enhanced magnetic resonance imaging. Spine 1993;18(11):1410–24.
46. Sartoretti-Schefer S, Wichmann W, Valavanis A. Idiopathic, herpetic, and HIV-associated facial nerve palsies: abnormal MR enhancement patterns. AJNR Am J Neuroradiol 1994;15(3):479–85.
47. Caldemeyer KS, Mathews VP, Righi PD, et al. Imaging features and clinical significance of perineural spread or extension of head and neck tumors. Radiographics 1998;18(1):97–110 [quiz: 47].
48. Ginsberg LE, DeMonte F. Imaging of perineural tumor spread from palatal carcinoma. AJNR Am J Neuroradiol 1998;19(8):1417–22.
49. Barakos JA, Dillon WP, Chew WM. Orbit, skull base, and pharynx: contrast-enhanced fat suppression MR imaging. Radiology 1991;179(1):191–8.
50. Maroldi R, Ambrosi C, Farina D. Metastatic disease of the brain: extra-axial metastases (skull, dura, leptomeningeal) and tumour spread. Eur Radiol 2005;15(3):617–26.
51. Williams LS. Advanced concepts in the imaging of perineural spread of tumor to the trigeminal nerve. Top Magn Reson Imaging 1999;10(6):376–83.
52. Blandino A, Gaeta M, Volta S, et al. Perineural metastatic spread along the infraorbital nerve in malignant neoplasms of the skin. Findings with computerized tomography and magnetic resonance in 2 cases. Radiol Med (Torino) 1995;90(1–2):129–31.
53. Curtin HD, Williams R, Johnson J. CT of perineural tumor extension: pterygopalatine fossa. AJR Am J Roentgenol 1985;144(1):163–9.
54. Parker GD, Harnsberger HR. Clinical-radiologic issues in perineural tumor spread of malignant diseases of the extracranial head and neck. Radiographics 1991;11(3):383–99.
55. Woodruff WW Jr, Yeates AE, McLendon RE. Perineural tumor extension to the cavernous sinus from superficial facial carcinoma: CT manifestations. Radiology 1986;161(2):395–9.
56. Pandolfo I, Gaeta M, Blandino A, et al. Perineural spread of nasopharyngeal carcinoma: radiological and CT demonstration. Eur J Radiol 1988;8(4):231–5.
57. Laine FJ, Braun IF, Jensen ME, et al. Perineural tumor extension through the foramen ovale: evaluation with MR imaging. Radiology 1990;174(1):65–71.
58. Fischbein NJ, Kaplan MJ, Jackler RK, et al. MR imaging in two cases of subacute denervation change in the muscles of facial expression. AJNR Am J Neuroradiol 2001;22(5):880–4.
59. Russo CP, Smoker WR, Weissman JL. MR appearance of trigeminal and hypoglossal motor denervation. AJNR Am J Neuroradiol 1997;18(7):1375–83.
60. Davis SB, Mathews VP, Williams DW 3rd. Masticator muscle enhancement in subacute denervation atrophy. AJNR Am J Neuroradiol 1995;16(6):1292–4.

Arterial Vascularization of the Cranial Nerves

Augustin Ozanne, MD*, Vitor Pereira, MD, Timo Krings, MD, PhD, Frédérique Toulgoat, MD, Pierre Lasjaunias, MD, PhD

KEYWORDS

• Cranial nerves • Arteries • Angiography • Imaging
• Anatomy • Skull base

Most cranial nerves are peripheral nerves. They originate from one or multiple brain stem nuclei and course through the skull base to innervate the orbit and derivatives from the six branchial arches mostly within the head and neck region. Understanding of the arterial vascularization of the cranial nerves is derived from anatomic,[1] microsurgical,[2,3] and angiographical[4,5] studies. Under normal conditions, the caliber of these arteries, is small, ie, between 100 and 300 microns. Thus they can be visualized during digital subtraction angiography (DSA) only with superselective injections. Although noninvasive imaging methods have improved considerably and are able to demonstrate the course of the cranial nerves,[6–11] they remain insufficient to detect their arterial vascularization.

Few pathologies may lead to specific involvement of the vascularization of the cranial nerves. Diabetes or viral infections may be the cause of vasculitis of these small vessels and subsequent nerve ischemia and deficit. This is described for example in Bell's palsy where the viral involvement is responsible for a breakdown of the blood-nerve barrier resulting in gadolinium enhancement on MRI.[12]

Some pathologic processes induce enlargement of dural arteries and subsequently of arteries to the cranial nerves without compromising their supply: these encompass highly vascularized and/or dural tumors (paragangliomas, juvenile angiofibromas, meningiomas) or dural arteriovenous shunts. The endovascular treatment of these pathologies requires a careful understanding of the regional anatomy and their vascular source as well as possible dangerous anastomoses between the cranial nerve supply and the central nervous system to avoid complications.

The phylogeny and neuroembryology remain essential to understand anatomic variations that may be encountered.[5,13] At the spinal level every metameric artery is supplying its corresponding nerve root, from its origin at the spinal cord to the foramen. The metameric distribution, although less obvious, will help to understand the vascularization of the cranial nerves at the cervicocephalic level.

The aim of this chapter is to discuss the arterial supply of the cranial nerves from their exit out of the brain stem to their exit from the cranial cavity. The dural vascular network and its anastomoses between external carotid, internal carotid, and vertebral artery through the respective foramina of the skull base are also considered. Outside the cranial cavity, the arterial nerve root supply is derived from other branches of the external carotid artery and will not be further detailed. Being outpouchings of the brain rather than true cranial nerves, the first and second nerves are not considered as peripheral nerves and for didactic and practical reasons are not considered in this text. Briefly, the first cranial nerve is supplied by the olfactory artery and ethmoidal branches of the ophthalmic artery. The optic nerve is supplied by the proximal ophthalmic artery as a remnant of the ventral and dorsal ophthalmic arteries.

For better comprehension of embryology and anatomic correlations, in the following description, the cranial nerves were grouped as belonging to different embryonic systems. For each group, the embryologic and phylogenic part is described

Bicêtre Hospital, Department of Neuroradiology, National Center for Malformative Neurovascular Diseases, 78 rue du General Leclerc, 94275 Le Kremlin Bicêtre, France
* Corresponding author.
E-mail address: augustin.ozanne@bct.aphp.fr (A. Ozanne).

Neuroimag Clin N Am 18 (2008) 431–439
doi:10.1016/j.nic.2007.12.010
1052-5149/08/$ – see front matter

after brief overviews of the cranial nerve anatomy and their respective arterial descriptive anatomies are given.

GROUP OF EXTRAOCULAR NERVES AND OPHTHALMIC ROOT OF THE TRIGEMINAL NERVE: III, IV, VI, AND V1

Cranial Nerves: Descriptive Anatomy

The cranial nerves of this group emerge from the brain stem at different points, course into the subarachnoid cisterns of the skull base and posterior fossa, to enter subsequently into the cavernous sinus (**Figs. 1 and 2**). The third nerve is exiting the brain from the medial sulcus at the medial surface of the cerebral peduncle and courses through the interpeduncular fossa between the anterosuperior cerebellar artery and the posterior cerebral artery. It passes over the basal attachment of the tentorium to the posterior part of the roof of the cavernous sinus (oculomotor triangle).[2,14,15] After penetrating the roof of the sinus, the oculomotor nerve courses inside its lateral wall passing forward through the superior orbital fissure to innervate intraorbital structures.

The fourth nerve originates from a controlateral nuclei and is the only one to emerge from the dorsal surface of the brain stem. It turns around the cerebral peduncle and courses anteriorly, within the cerebellomesencephalic, quadrigeminal, and ambient cisterns, parallel to the anterosuperior cerebellar and posterior cerebral artery and basal vein until it enters the cavernous sinus, just lateral to the oculomotor nerve. The trochlear nerve runs inside the inner layer of the lateral wall of the cavernous sinus, below the third nerve to leave this region via the superior orbital fissure.[2,16]

The sixth nerve arises from the lower portion of the pons and courses along the cerebellopontine angle's cistern to reach Dorello's canal or petroclival venous confluence[17] at the apex of the petrous bone. Inside the cavernous sinus, the nerve runs in its lower part, on the lateral surface of the internal carotid artery (ICA) and below the

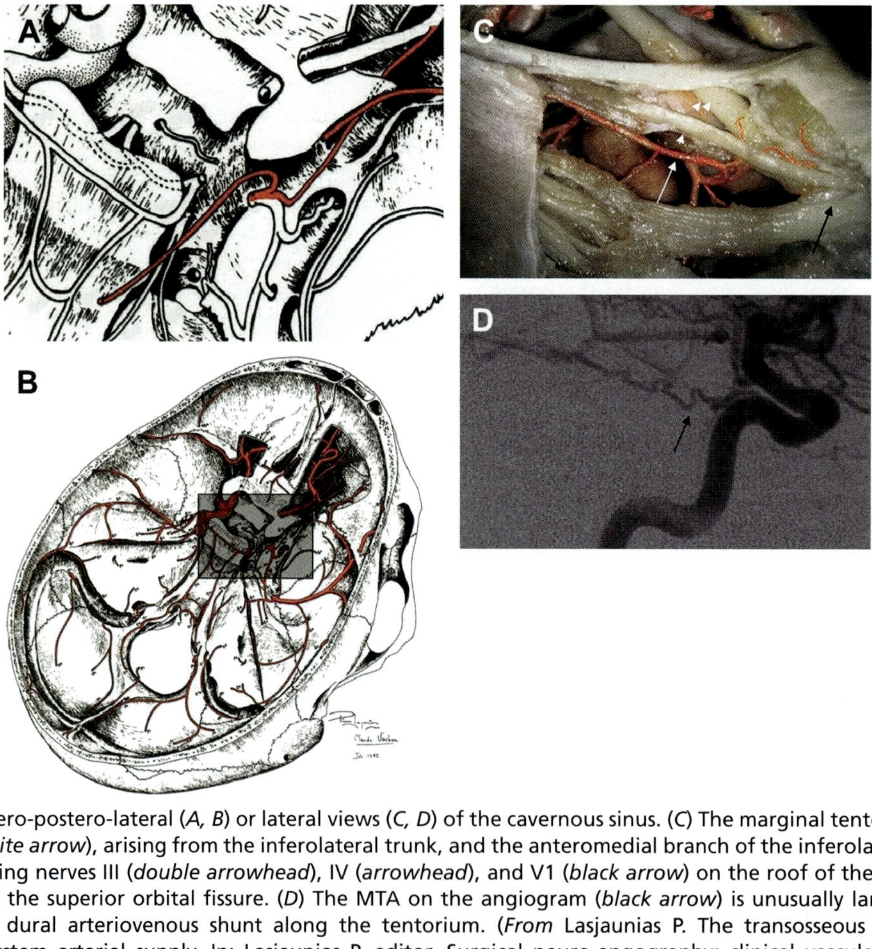

Fig. 1. Supero-postero-lateral (*A, B*) or lateral views (*C, D*) of the cavernous sinus. (*C*) The marginal tentorial artery (MTA) (*white arrow*), arising from the inferolateral trunk, and the anteromedial branch of the inferolateral trunk are supplying nerves III (*double arrowhead*), IV (*arrowhead*), and V1 (*black arrow*) on the roof of the cavernous sinus or in the superior orbital fissure. (*D*) The MTA on the angiogram (*black arrow*) is unusually large, as it is feeding a dural arteriovenous shunt along the tentorium. (*From* Lasjaunias P. The transosseous peripheral nervous system arterial supply. In: Lasjaunias P, editor. Surgical neuro-angography: clinical vascular anatomy and variations. Heidelberg: Springer; 2001. p. 467–75; with permission.)

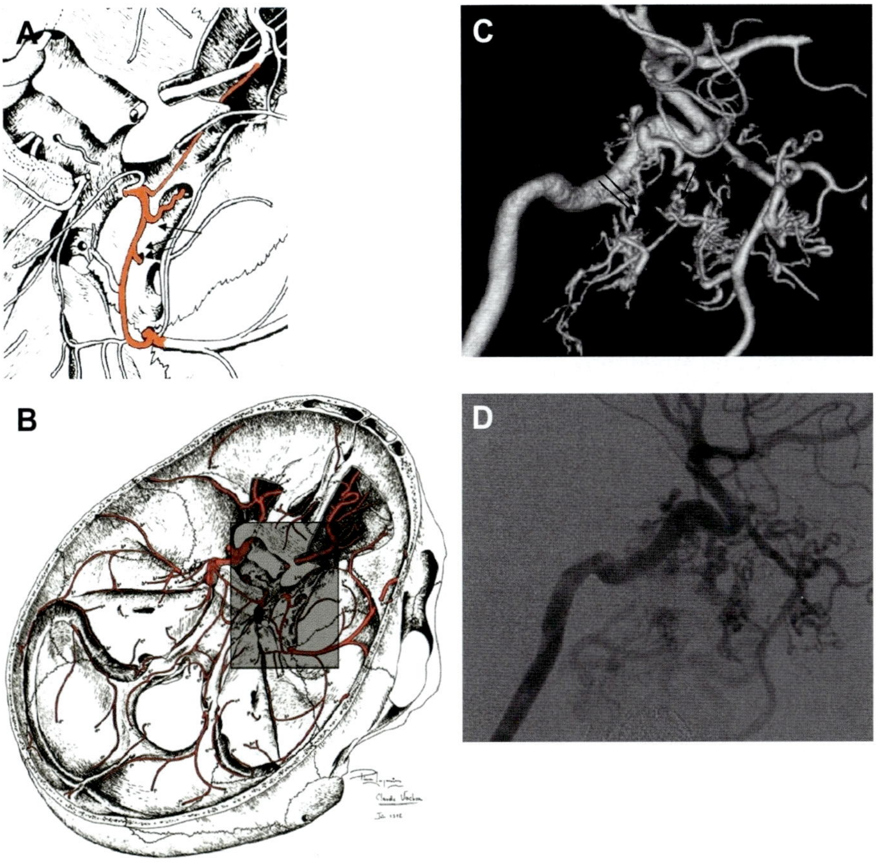

Fig. 2. Arteries of the foramen rotundum and foramen ovale supplying V2 and V3. Supero lateral (*A, B*) and lateral view of angiogram, on 3D (*C*) and conventional lateral view (*D*), of the right cavernous sinus show branches of the inferolateral trunk arising from the cavernous internal carotid: the artery of the foramen rotundum (*arrow*) and the artery of foramen ovale (*double arrow*) supply the V2 and V3 roots respectively. Note on *A* that the artery of the ovale foramen is coursing through the accessory Vesalius foramen and not the ovale foramen (*double arrow*), artery of the foramen rotundum (*black arrow*). The DSA was performed in a case of arteriovenous malformation of the mandible, whose external carotid had been previously ligated before beeing referred. (*From* Lasjaunias P. The transosseous peripheral nervous system arterial supply. In: Lasjaunias P, editor. Surgical neuro-angography: clinical vascular anatomy and variations. Heidelberg: Springer; 2001. p. 467–75; with permission.)

inferolateral trunk until it enters the superior orbital fissure in its medial aspect.[2,18]

Arterial Descriptive Anatomy

Contribution from the vertebrobasilar system to the proximal cisternal course of the cranial nerves

In their cisternal course, after they emerge from the brain stem, nerves III, IV, and VI receive arterial supply from branches of the vertebrobasilar system. The third nerve may receive arterial supply in the vicinity of the posterior perforating substance from the basilar artery or from the posterior cerebral artery; subsequently this arterial supply may also concern parts of the thalamus. There are either two lateral arteries or one common trunk. The fourth nerve is supplied by branches from the anterosuperior cerebellar artery or from circumferential arteries of the P1 segment of the posterior cerebral artery.

Contribution from dural and transosseous arteries

The dural arteries contribute to the supply of the cranial nerves in their dural and transosseous course. Nerves III and IV nerves are supplied by the marginal artery of the tentorium cerebelli on the roof of the cavernous sinus. The marginal artery of the tentorium is an arcade between orbital vessels and branches of the carotid siphon. Many anatomic variations may be observed in this region.[19] The artery may arise from the middle meningeal artery, the ophthalmic or lacrimal artery, the inferolateral trunk, or the posterior group of collaterals of the internal carotid artery.

The sixth nerve is supplied by a clival network along its course anterior to the pons. Medial and lateral clival arteries are caudally fed by the hypoglossal and jugular branch of the neuromeningeal trunk of the ascending pharyngeal artery. Cranially, the medial and lateral clival arteries arising from branches of the ascending segment of the carotid siphon supply this nerve.

The anteromedial branch of the inferolateral trunk is supplying nerves III, IV, VI, and V1 in the cavernous sinus and the superior orbital fissure.

Arterial Embryology and Phylogeny

This group of cranial nerves (III, IV, VI, and V1) is under the control of the dorsal ophthalmic artery, whose vestige is the inferolateral trunk of the carotid siphon. The metameric structures they are linked to are the prebranchial somites. The medial clival artery and the posteroinferior hypophyseal trunk belong to the remnant of the primitive maxillary artery. The lateral clival artery is the remnant of the trigeminal artery.

GROUP OF TRIGEMINAL GANGLION AND TRIGEMINAL NERVES V2, V3, AND VM, AND FACIAL NERVE VII AND VESTIBULOCOCHLEAR NERVE VIII

Trigeminal Ganglion and Trigeminal Nerves V2, V3, and Vm

Cranial nerve descriptive anatomy

The fifth nerve emerges from the lateral surface of the pons (see **Fig. 2**; **Fig. 3**). Both the sensory roots and the motor portion cross the subarachnoid space below the superior petrosal sinus to reach the upper edge of the petrous bone at the level of Meckel's cave and the trigeminal ganglion (gasserian ganglion). The motor and sensory roots are regrouped and diverged into the three major roots, ophthalmic (V1), maxillary (V2) and mandibular nerves (V3), to reach their foramina as indicated in (**Table 1**).[2,20]

Arterial descriptive anatomy

Contribution from the vertebrobasilar system to the proximal cisternal course of the cranial nerves The trigeminal nerve in its proximal cisternal course, after emerging from the pons, is supplied by the vestigial artery of the trigeminal artery that arises from the basilar artery.

Contribution from dural and transosseous arteries The trigeminal ganglion in Meckel's cave is supplied by the lateral artery of the trigeminal ganglion that arises from the vertical portion of the intracavernous ICA, and by cavernous branches from the middle meningeal artery. V2 is supplied by the artery of the foramen rotundum, which is fed by the inferolateral trunk that arises from the cavernous horizontal segment of the internal carotid artery. The artery of the foramen rotundum courses through the foramen rotundum and anastomoses with the distal maxillary artery. V3 and Vm have a common course through the oval foramen: they are supplied by the accessory meningeal artery, which represents an anastomosis between the posterior branch of the inferolateral trunk of the carotid siphon and the proximal maxillary artery. There is a hemodynamic balance between the accessory meningeal artery and the posterior branch of the inferolateral trunk. The variation in size of the accessory meningeal artery is significant and depends on its soft tissue supply. Depending on the depth of the course of the maxillar artery, the accessory meningeal artery may originate from a common trunk with the middle meningeal artery

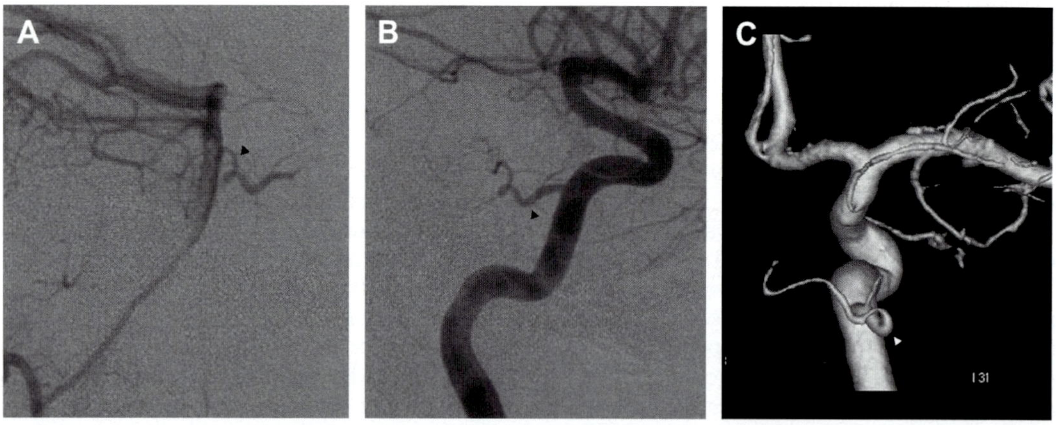

Fig. 3. Persistant trigeminal artery (*arrowheads*). This case illustrates the persistance of the embryonic trigeminal artery, from the basilar artery (*A*) and the petrosal carotid artery, lateral (*B*) and posterior (*C*) view. Remnant or persisting embryonic artery, it supplies the trigeminal nerve at its cisternal course.

Table 1
Arterial contribution to the vascularization of the cranial nerves and skull base foramina

Cranial Nerves	Intracranial Feeders: Intracisternal Vertebrobasilar Origin	Intracranial Feeders: Epidural Internal Carotid Artery (ICA) Origin	Skull Base Foramen	External Carotid Arteries Feeders
III	PCA	MAT Anteromedial branch of the ILT	Superior orbital fissure	Ophthalmic, or lacrimal, or MMA tentorial branches
IV	ASCA	MAT Anteromedial branch of the ILT	Superior orbital fissure	Ophthalmic, or lacrimal, or MMA tentorial branches
V_1	Remnant of the trigeminal artery	MAT Anteromedial branch of the ILT	Superior orbital fissure	Ophthalmic, or lacrimal, or MMA tentorial branches
V_2	Remnant of the trigeminal artery	Medial branch of the ILT to the artery of the foramen rotundum	Foramen rotundum	Artery of the foramen rotundum (distal maxillar artery)
V_3 and V_m	Remnant of the trigeminal artery	Posterior branch of the ILT, to the accessory meningeal artery	Foramen ovale	Accessory meningeal artery (proximal maxillar artery)
VI		Clival arteries from ICA MAT and anteromedial branch of the ILT	Superior orbital fissure	Clival arteries from neuromeningeal trunk of APA
VII	Auditory artery, branch of the AICA		Facial Canal Facial Canal Stylomastoid foramen	Petrous branch of MMA Stylomastoid artery from posterior auricular artery or Occipital artery
VIII	Auditory artery, branch of the AICA			
IX	Vertebral artery		Jugular Foramen (Pars nervosa)	Neuromeningeal trunk of APA (jugular branch)
X	Vertebral artery		Jugular Foramen (Pars nervosa)	Neuromeningeal trunk of APA (jugular branch)
XI	Vertebral artery		Jugular Foramen (Pars nervosa)	Neuromeningeal trunk of APA (jugular branch)
XII	Vertebral artery		Hypoglossal canal	Neuromeningeal trunk of APA (hypoglossal branch)

Abbreviations: AICA, anterior internal carotid artery; APA, ascending pharyngeal artery; ASCA, anterosuperior cerebellar artery; ICA, internal carotid artery; ILT, inferolateral trunk; MAT, marginal artery of the tentorium; MMA, middle meningeal artery; PCA, posterior cerebral artery.

(in case of a superficial course of the maxillar artery) or directly from the maxillar artery (in case of a deep course). V3 and Vm are also supplied by cavernous branches from the middle meningeal artery.

Vestibulocochlear Nerve and Facial Nerve

Cranial nerve descriptive anatomy

The seventh nerve includes sensory and motor fibers and emerges from the pontomedullary junction caudal to the origin of the trigeminal nerve (**Fig. 4**). It enters the pontocerebellar cistern and courses anteriorly above the eighth nerve before entering the internal auditory canal until it reaches the facial nerve canal and soon after the geniculate ganglion. It gives off intrapetrous branches before exiting the canal at the stylomastoid foramen.

Owing to its anatomic and functional division, the eighth nerve or vestibulocochlear complex leaves the brain stem at the lateral part of pontomedullary junction, anterior to the flocculus of the cerebellum, to enter the cerebellopontine cistern and, thereafter, the internal acoustic canal together with the labyrinthine branch of the anteroinferior cerebellar artery (AICA).[14,21]

Arterial descriptive anatomy

Contribution from the vertebrobasilar system to the proximal cisternal course of the cranial nerves In their

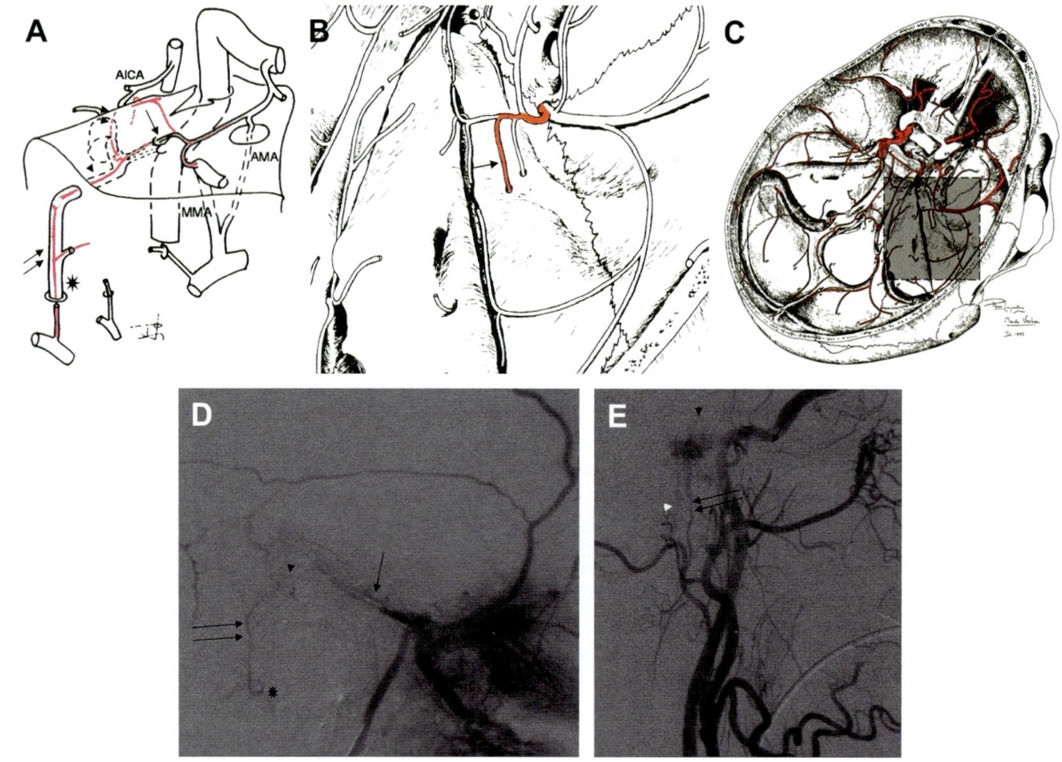

Fig. 4. Facial arch supplying the second and third segments of the facial nerve. (*A*) Postero-lateral view of the petrous bone, with nervous and vascular structures. Facial arch: at the level of the spinous foramen the arterial petrous branch arises from the middle meningeal artery (MMA) to course along the great petrosal nerve, the geniculate ganglion, then the tympanic segment, to anastomose to the stylomastoid artery along the third vertical segment of the facial nerve. Note the internal auditory artery (*double arrowhead*) arising from the anteroinferior cerebellar artery (AICA). (*B, C*) Supero-postero-lateral view of the petrous bone shows the petrous branch arising from the middle meningeal artery after its emergence from the spinous foramen, and coursing along the great petrosal nerve (*black arrow*). Note laterally the superior tympanic artery along the small petrosal nerve and the relationship with the petrous branch of the accessory meningeal artery. (*D*) Right lateral view angiogram in a patient treated for juvenile angiofibroma. The selective injection of the middle meningeal artery is opacifying the facial arch: the petrous branch (*arrow*), is coursing along the second tympanic (*arrowhead*) then the third stylomastoid (*double arrow*) segments of the facial nerve, to anastomose with the stylomastoid artery. Note the stylomastoid foramen (*asterisks*). (*E*) Right lateral view in a patient embolized for a tympanic paraganglioma: two stylomastoid arteries are arising from occipital artery (*double arrow*) and from posterior auricular artery (*white arrowhead*). (*From* Lasjaunias P. The transosseous peripheral nervous system arterial supply. In: Lasjaunias P, editor. Surgical neuro-angography: clinical vascular anatomy and variations. Heidelberg: Springer; 2001. p. 467–75; with permission.)

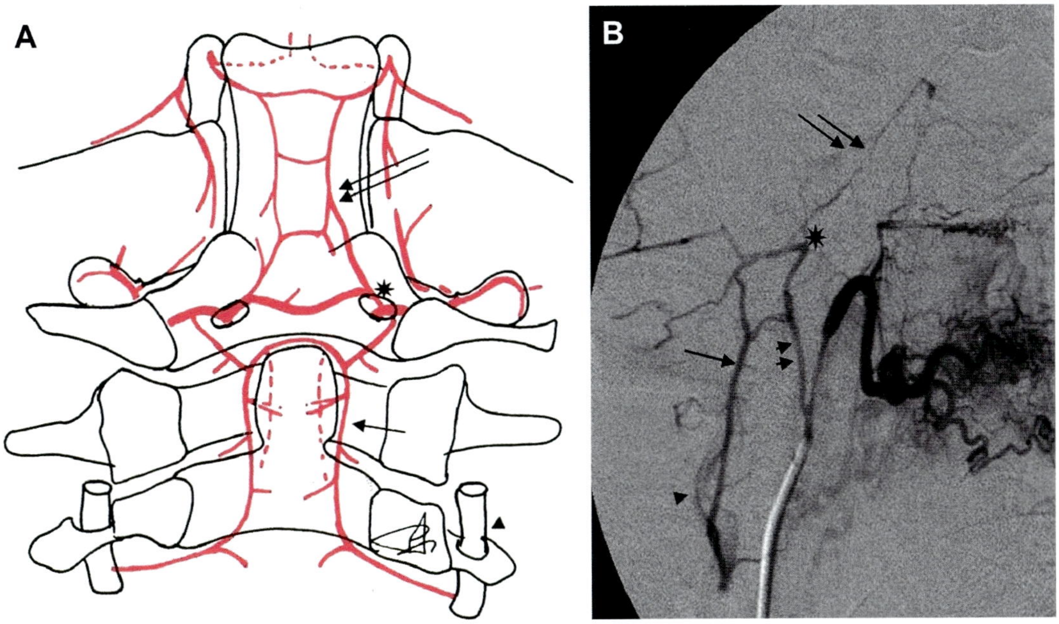

Fig. 5. Clival epidural arterial network anastomosed to the odontoid arch. (*A*) This shows the anastomosis between medial clival arteries (*double arrow*) and the hypoglossal branch (through the hypoglossal canal: supply of the XII) (*asterisk*) of the ascending pharyngeal artery; between lateral clival arteries and jugular branch of the ascending pharyngeal artery (through the pars nervosa of the jugular foramen: supply of the IX, X, XI). The clival network supplies nerve VI in its cisternal course. It is anastomosed with the odontoid arch (*arrow*) caudally and with the internal carotid cranially. (*B*) Selective injection of the ascending pharyngeal artery in a case of Cerebrofacial Arteriovenous Metameric Syndrome type II, lateral view, opacifies the epidural clival network (*double arrow*) through the neuromeningeal trunk (*double arrowhead*) and the hypoglossal artery through the hypoglossal canal (*asterisk*). Note the anastomosis with the odontoid arch (*arrow*) and opacification of the vertebral artery (*arrowhead*) at the third cervical space. (*From* Lasjaunias P. The transosseous peripheral nervous system arterial supply. In: Lasjaunias P, editor. Surgical neuro-angography: clinical vascular anatomy and variations. Heidelberg: Springer; 2001. p. 467–75; with permission.)

cisternal course from the brain stem to the medial part of the internal acoustic meatus, the facial and the vestibulocochlear nerves are supplied by branches issued from the vertebrobasilar system. These branches arise from the internal auditory artery originating from the cerebellolabyrintine branch of the AICA. The internal auditory artery is also supplying the first labyrinthic segment of the facial nerve, until the geniculate ganglion.

Contribution from dural and transosseous arteries

The second (tympanic) and third (mastoid) segments of the facial nerve are supplied by an arterial arcade that includes the petrosal branch from the middle meningeal artery (MMA) to the stylomastoid branch of the posterior auricular artery, called the facial arch. The petrosal branch arises from the middle meningeal artery after its emergence into the cranial cavity through the foramen spinosum. It courses retrogradely along with the superficial petrosal nerve to join the geniculate ganglion. The arcade toward the stylomastoid artery follows the intrapetrous facial nerve in the facial canal, horizontally, at the tympanic portion and then vertically, at the mastoid portion. The balance point between the two different sources and subsequently the functional role of the afferent arteries may vary: in 10% the stylomastoid artery supplies the facial arch to the geniculate ganglion; in 15% the stylomastoid artery is absent.[22] Thus, the petrous branch of the MMA is the prominent supply in the vast majority of cases. Small arterial supplies to the tympanic cavity may anastomose with the facial arch, such as the infratympanic artery (branch of the ascending pharyngeal artery), the anterior tympanic artery (branch of the maxillary artery), and the caroticotympanic artery (branch of the ICA). Classically, there is no anastomosis between the internal auditory artery and the petrous branch of the middle meningeal artery.[22]

Arterial embryology and phylogeny

This group (V2, V3, Vm, VII, and VIII) is related to the stapedial artery and its remnants. They are linked to the first branchial arch, ie, the trigeminal neural crest, and the second branchial arch, ie, the acousticofacial neural crest. The trigeminal artery is an embryonic artery between the ascending

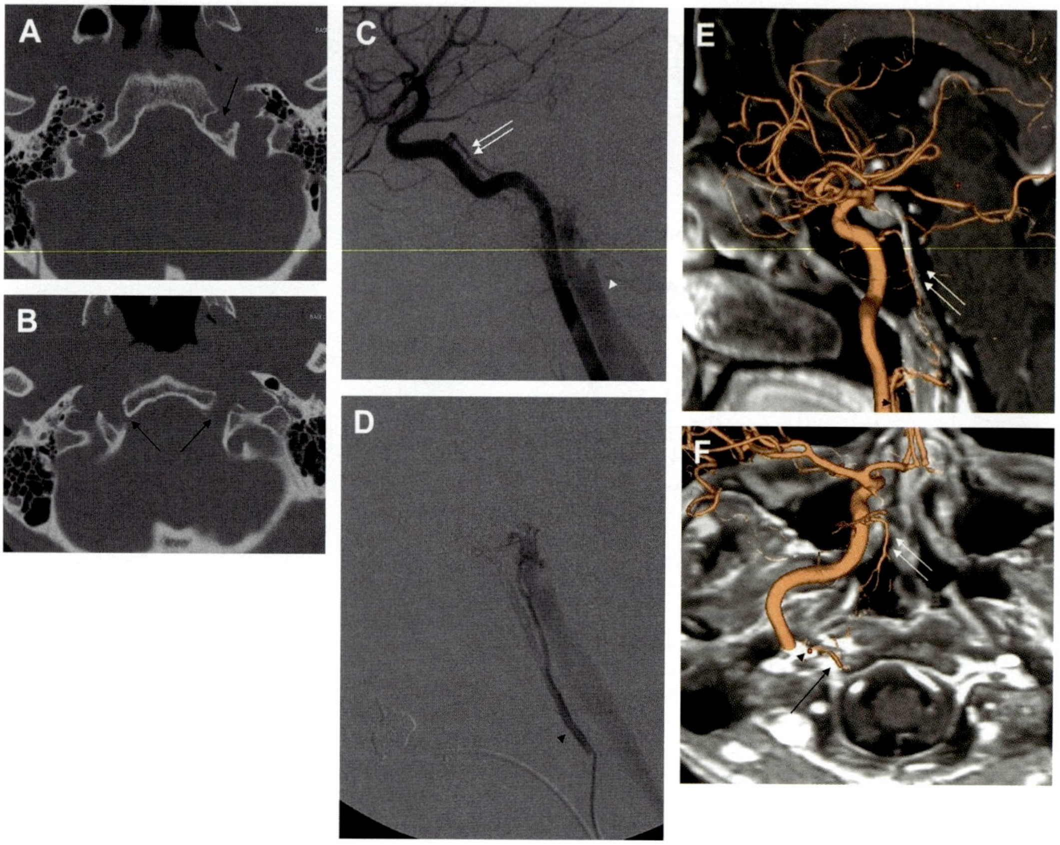

Fig. 6. Hypoglossal and internal carotid contribution to the clival network. Axial CT (*A, B*), lateral view conventional angiograms (*C, D*), and sagittal and axial MR images fused with 3D-angiogram, postero-lateral (*E*) and supero-posterior view (*F*) respectivily. Case of osteodural arteriovenous shunt revealed by pulsatile bruit. (*A, B, F*) Enlarged hypoglossal canal (*arrows*). (*C–F*) The neuromeningeal trunk of the ascending pharyngeal artery (*black arrowhead*) and medial branch of clival artery arising from the internal carotid artery (*double white arrowhead*) are supplying the arteriovenous shunt, draining into the jugular vein (*white arrowhead*).

petrous segment of the internal carotid (at the junction of the carotid segments C4-C5) and the basilar artery (between the anterosuperior cerebellar artery and the superior cerebellar artery).

THE GROUP OF THE GLOSSOPHARYNGEAL NERVE IX AND VAGAL NERVES X

Descriptive Anatomy

The glossopharyngeal and vagal nerves emerge as rootlets from the posterolateral portion of the medulla oblongata. Nerve IX rests on the jugular tubercule of the occipital bone just above nerve X and enters the lateral cerebellomedullary cistern until the jugular foramen. In this cisternal course, the rootlets are crossed by the first loop of the postero-inferior cerebellar artery (PICA).[3,23]

Arterial Descriptive Anatomy

The intradural course of these nerves is supplied by the ipsilateral vertebral artery, the basilar artery, and by the artery for the lateral part of the medulla. In their intraforaminal course, the supply is coming from the jugular branch of the neuromeningeal trunk of the ascending pharyngeal artery. This jugular branch also anastomoses with the lateral clival artery in the inferior petrosal sinus.

Embryology and Phylogeny

This group belongs to the pharyngeal system and their arterial supply is under the control of the jugular branch of the neuromeningeal trunk of the ascending pharyngeal artery.

THE GROUP OF THE SPINAL BRANCH OF THE ACCESSORY XI AND HYPOGLOSSAL XII NERVES

Descriptive Anatomy Including Arterial Description

The spinal accessory nerve rootlets emerge, widely separate, from the posterior edge of the postolivary sulcus below nerves IX and X, whereas the rootlets of the hypoglossal nerve come out more anteriorly, from the preolivary sulcus (**Figs. 5 and 6**). Nerve XI runs inferolateraly to the jugular foramen where it enters frequently together with the vagal nerve. This intradural course is supplied by the ipsilateral vertebral artery with collaterals from the lateral spinal and PICA branches. Inside the jugular foramen, nerve XI is supplied by the same jugular branch of the neuromeningeal trunk as nerves IX and X. The hypoglossal rootlets course anterolateral through the subarachnoid space behind the vertebral artery to arrive in the hypoglossal canal. This cisternal portion is vascularized by branches of vertebral, anterior spinal, and PICA arteries. At the level of the hypoglossal canal, it is supplied by the hypoglossal branch of the neuromeningeal trunk of the ascending pharyngeal artery (see **Fig. 4**).

Embryology and Phylogeny

This group belongs to an accessory-hypoglossal group, under the control of the posterior branch of the neuromeningeal trunk of the ascending pharyngeal artery (musculospinal and hypoglossal branches).

REFERENCES

1. Libersa C. Contribution to the study of arterial vascularisation of the cranial nerves [thesis]. France: Université de Lille; 1951. p. 104.
2. Rhoton AL Jr. The cavernous sinus, the cavernous venous plexus, and the carotid collar. Neurosurgery 2002;51:S375–410.
3. Rhoton AL Jr. The anterior and middle cranial base. Neurosurgery 2002;51:S273–302.
4. Lapresle J, Lasjaunias P. Cranial nerve ischaemic arterial syndromes. A review. Brain 1986;109(1): 207–16.
5. Lasjaunias P. The transosseous peripheral nervous system arterial supply. In: Lasjaunias P, editor. Surgical neuro-angography: clinical vascular anatomy and variations. Heidelberg (Germany): Springer; 2001. p. 467–75.
6. Casselman JW, Kuhweide R, Deimling M, et al. Constructive interference in steady state-3DFT MR imaging of the inner ear and cerebellopontine angle. AJNR Am J Neuroradiol 1993;14:47–57.
7. Doyon D. The cranial nerves. Icon Learning System; 2004.
8. Leblanc A. Système nerveux encéphalo-périphérique vascularisation, anatomie, imagerie. Berlin: Springer; 2001.
9. Yousry I, Camelio S, Schmid UD, et al. Visualization of cranial nerves I-XII: value of 3D CISS and T2-weighted FSE sequences. Eur Radiol 2000;10: 1061–7.
10. Castillo M. Imaging of the upper cranial nerves I, III-VIII, and the cavernous sinuses. Neuroimaging Clin N Am 2004;14:579–93.
11. Yagi A, Sato N, Taketomi A, et al. Normal cranial nerves in the cavernous sinuses: contrast-enhanced three-dimensional constructive interference in the steady state MR imaging. AJNR Am J Neuroradiol 2005;26:946–50.
12. Girard N, Raybaud C, Poncet M. 3D-FT MRI of the facial nerve. Neuroradiology 1994;36:462–8.
13. Padget D. The development of the cranial arteries in the human embryo. Contrib Embryol 1948;212.
14. Krisht A, Barnett DW, Barrow DL, et al. The blood supply of the intracavernous cranial nerves: an anatomic study. Neurosurgery 1994;34:275–9 [discussion: 279].
15. Uz A. Variations in the origin of the thalamoperforating arteries. J Clin Neurosci 2007;14:134–7.
16. Tubbs RS, Oakes WJ. Relationships of the cisternal segment of the trochlear nerve. J Neurosurg 1998; 89:1015–9.
17. Destrieux C, Velut S, Kakou MK, et al. A new concept in Dorello's canal microanatomy: the petroclival venous confluence. J Neurosurg 1997;87: 67–72.
18. Lu J, Zhu XL. Cranial arachnoid membranes: some aspects of microsurgical anatomy. Clin Anat 2007; 20:502–11.
19. Lasjaunias P. The artery of the free margin of the tentorium cerebelli. In: Lasjaunias P, editor. Surgical neuroangiography, clinical vascular anatomy and variations. Berlin: Springer; 2001.
20. Marinkovic S, Gibo H, Vucevic R, et al. Anatomy of the cavernous sinus region. J Clin Neurosci 2001; 8(Suppl 1):78–81.
21. Scolozzi P, Dorfl J, Tribolet N. Microsurgical anatomy of the subtentorial supracerebellar and infracerebellar approach to the trigeminal and facial nerves. J Clin Neurosci 1999;6:400–7.
22. Blunt MJ. The blood supply of the facial nerve. J Anat 1954;88:520–6.
23. Ozveren MF, Ture U, Ozek MM, et al. Anatomic landmarks of the glossopharyngeal nerve: a microsurgical anatomic study. Neurosurgery 2003;52:1400–10 [discussion: 1410].

Index

Note: Page numbers of article titles are in **boldface** type.

Neuroimag Clin N Am 18 (2008) 441–444
doi:10.1016/S1052-5149(08)00040-3
1052-5149/08/$ – see front matter

S

T

V

W